Smoking Cessation: Theory, Interventions and Prevention

SMOKING CESSATION: THEORY, INTERVENTIONS AND PREVENTION

JEROME E. LANDOW

EDITOR

Nova Science Publishers, Inc.
New York

LIBRARY OF CONGRESS CATALOGING-IN-PUBLICATION DATA

ISBN: 978-1-60021-591-9

Available Upon Request

Published by Nova Science Publishers, Inc. ✦ New York

CONTENTS

PREFACE

Smoking is the most common risk factor for the development of lung cancer, which is the leading cause of cancer death. It is also associated with many other types of cancer, including cancers of the esophagus, larynx, kidney, pancreas, and cervix. Smoking also increases the risk of other health problems, such as chronic lung disease and heart disease. Smoking during pregnancy can have adverse effects on the unborn child, such as premature delivery and low birth weight. The health benefits of smoking cessation (quitting) are immediate and substantial.

Almost immediately, a person's circulation begins to improve and the level of carbon monoxide in the blood begins to decline. (Carbon monoxide, a colorless, odorless gas found in cigarette smoke, reduces the blood's ability to carry oxygen.) A person's pulse rate and blood pressure, which may be abnormally high while smoking, begin to return to normal. Within a few days of quitting, a person's sense of taste and smell return, and breathing becomes increasingly easier.

People who quit smoking live longer than those who continue to smoke. After 10 to 15 years, a previous tobacco user's risk of premature death approaches that of a person who has never smoked. Quitting smoking reduces the risk for developing cancer, and this benefit increases the longer a person remains "smoke free."

Quitting smoking may cause short-term after-effects, especially for those who have smoked a large number of cigarettes for a long period of time. People who quit smoking are likely to feel anxious, irritable, hungry, more tired, and have difficulty sleeping. They may also have difficulty concentrating. Many tobacco users gain weight when they quit, but usually less than 10 pounds. These changes do subside. This new book presents new and important research in this bewildering field.

Chapter 1 - Despite a vast body of research on smoking, quit rates for people with a concurrent mental illness remain extremely low. Research has established that these groups smoke more heavily, for more years and in greater proportions than the general population - up to 90% for people with psychotic illnesses compared with approximately 25% for general populations in many countries. This problem is particularly so in psychiatric institutions and community hostels where people with mental illness reside in great numbers. Using the ethnographic method of qualitative inquiry, combined with grounded theory analysis of indepth semi-structured interviews with people with mental illness and the staff who interact with them, this research aimed to study the culture of smoking as it is experienced by these populations in their day-to-day lives. Entrenched historical and current systemic barriers to quitting were observed, emanating from the mental health system in general. In many respects, the hospital was identified as a 'total institution' that appeared to shape and guide the beliefs and attitudes about mental illness held by staff and patients. In this setting, cigarettes were identified as the currency by which economic, social and political exchange took place between the various players. An enculturation process was described by all participants. Once entered into escape from the smoking behaviour and reinforcement by the cultural milieu appeared to be extremely difficult for patients and staff. Likewise, the community hostels were described, by participants, as a mirror image of the psychiatric extended care wards with the same level of institutionalised formal and informal rules, routines and behaviours in respect of smoking and its reinforcement.

Chapter 2 - Cigarette smoking imperils roughly 6000 additional individuals in this country each day (that many youngsters light up for the first time daily); over 400,000 die annually as a result of having made the decision to smoke tobacco. The more we know about the factors influencing the decision to smoke, and the more we amass evidence in support of the decision to refrain, our power to effect positive change will be enhanced.

Given the imperfect efficacy of smoking cessation programs, prevention needs to be a top priority. Since many young people begin to smoke as a means of enhancing their social image, it may be helpful for them to learn more about the actual magnitude of negative stereotyping of smokers. Perhaps if they are better informed about the social hazards of smoking, they will be more likely to make the decision to refrain. Failing that, at least this information should make them less likely to smoke in public. This in itself should be beneficial, because reductions in public smoking should reduce pro-smoking norms.

A research project consisting of several studies conducted over a five year period was developed to increase campus awareness of the risks associated with campus smoking. In order to shift student norms, a large number of undergraduates, including several student leaders, participated actively in the research process. The studies assessed the reasons students smoke, the reasons many refrain, the social costs associated with public smoking, the impact of environmental manipulations on smoking behavior, and the effects of participation in campus smoking cessation programs. Several of the studies explored how students and teachers in high schools, colleges, law and medical schools view adolescents who smoke cigarettes. The results revealed pervasive, harsh negative stereotypes of smokers. Campus discussion of these findings increased students' awareness of the potential social, academic, and career repercussions of choosing to smoke.

Collectively, these studies were accompanied by an 8% reduction in the percentage of students reporting regular use of cigarettes (from 34% in 1999 to 26% in 2004). Since student involvement in this research project seems to have helped to interrupt a rising trajectory in undergraduate smoking on campus, this chapter will review the results of the studies comprising this project and explore various strategies for engaging students in smoking prevention and cessation programs.

Chapter 3 - Smoking among college students is widespread and represents a significant public health issue. Smoking cessation programs utilizing state-of-the-art theoretical concepts and computer technologies hold considerable promise for this category of young adults. Our research team has conducted a study aimed at designing, evaluating, and testing the impact of a theory-guided intervention utilizing a computer-assisted, counselor-delivered approach. This chapter provides background information on smoking among college students. It also describes our computer-based expert system used for data collection and addressing personal health risks and readiness to change smoking behavior, and the main outcomes from our study. A group-randomized, controlled trial was used to assess the intervention in a sample of 426 students (58.5% females; mean age, 22.8 ± 4.7 years) from 15 pair-matched community colleges located in the Houston, Texas area. The experimental intervention was delivered by a trained counselor who used the computerized expert system, motivational intervention approach, and personalized health feedback. At the 10-month follow-up assessment, the salivary cotinine-validated smoking cessation rates were 16.6% in the experimental condition and 10.1% in the standard care condition (p=0.068). Although the statistical significance between the study conditions was not reached, our results indicate that our computer-assisted intervention holds considerable promise in reducing smoking among community college students. Difficulties and solutions in terms of recruitment and retention of our young study participants are discussed. Feasible and effective tobacco control interventions targeting college students, along with adoption of smoke-free campus policies are warranted.

Chapter 4 - Since the first Surgeon General's report on smoking and health was published in 1964, there have been more than 12 million premature deaths attributable to smoking in the United States (American Cancer Society [ACS], 2006). In the United States, tobacco use is responsible for nearly one in five deaths, an estimated 438,000 premature deaths each year between 1997-2001 (ACS, 2006). In addition, it is estimated that another 8.6 million persons suffer from smoking-caused chronic conditions, including chronic bronchitis, emphysema, and cardiovascular disease. Moreover, smoking accounts for 30% of all cancer deaths and 87% of lung cancer deaths (ACS, 2006).

In 2003, the number of smokers in the world was estimated at about 1.3 billion people. This figure is expected to increase to at least 1.7 billion by 2025, with the doubling in the number of female smokers making the greatest contribution to the increase (ACS, 2006). In 2000, there were about 4.8 million smoking-related premature deaths worldwide, nearly evenly divided between developed and developing nations. Based on current patterns, smoking-attributable diseases will kill about 650 million of the world's 1.3 billion smokers alive today (ACS, 2003).

The Healthy People 2010 objectives regarding adult tobacco use in the United States (U.S. Department of Health and Human Services [U.S. DHHS], 2000) are to reduce the prevalence of cigarette smoking to 12%, cigar smoking to 1.2%, use of smokeless tobacco to 0.4%, and to increase cessation attempts among adults to 75.0%. A Centers for Disease Control (CDC) report indicated lagging progress on all four objectives (Mariolis, Rock, Asman, et al., 2006). In 2005, approximately 20.9% of U.S. adults were current cigarette smokers, the same percentage as in 2004, suggesting that the 8-year decline in smoking prevalence among adults in the United States might be stalling, mirroring a similar lack of decline in smoking among adolescents since 2002 (Mochizuki-Kobayashi, Fishburn, Baptiste, et al., 2006). In addition, in 2005, an estimated 2.2% of U.S. adults were current cigar smokers, 2.3% used smokeless tobacco, and 42.5% of current cigarette smokers had stopped smoking for at least 1 day in the preceding 12 months because they were trying to quit. (Mariolis, et al., 2006).

These figures demand the attention of the medical and public health communities, and physicians, in particular, have a unique and important role to play in the anti-smoking arena. In the United States, they literally see about 70% of smokers each year (Burns, 1994), and some, such as pregnant women and parents of newborn babies, on numerous occasions. Obstetricians are uniquely positioned to encourage expectant mothers to quit smoking, and pediatricians may utilize well baby visits to counsel parents about the harmful effects of environmental tobacco smoke (ETS), to encourage mothers who quit smoking during their pregnancy to remain abstinent, and to help parents who smoke to quit. On other occasions, pediatricians may play a role in the prevention of smoking onset in children and adolescents and help young people who smoke to quit (cf. Stein, Haddock, O'Byrne, et al., 2000).

Other primary care physicians, as well as specialists, may take advantage of their position in society to influence the health behavior of patients of all ages, not only by encouraging cessation of all tobacco use, but by offering effective assistance. As health care providers, physicians have a solemn obligation to help patients avoid illness and promote good health as well as treating the infirmed. With respect to tobacco prevention and control, physicians have played a leadership role in identifying the harm caused by tobacco products, formulating policy and legislation to protect the public, and the management of tobacco addiction in office, clinic, and hospital settings. However, more must and can be done.

The purpose of the present chapter is to provide an overview of what can be accomplished by practicing physicians who address tobacco in clinical settings. The chapter is less of a critical review and critique of the existing literature on the efficacy and effectiveness of physician intervention (cf. Lancaster and Stead, 2004) and more of a commentary on how contemporary physicians' may use their growing armamentarium and state-of-the-art interventions to help patients quit smoking. In so doing, the author presents a historical perspective to highlight the foundations on which contemporary approaches to physician office-based intervention on tobacco stand.

Chapter 5 - Even though a large body of research elucidating the negative health impact of cigarette smoking has become more widely known by the public in recent years, smoking remains as the single most preventable cause of morbidity and mortality in the U. S. In fact, according to the most recently available prevalence estimates, 20.9% of the American population over 18 years of age were smokers in 2005, which is unchanged from 2004 estimates (Schiller, Martinez, and Barnes, 2006, June). Continuing high levels of smoking among adults emphasize the need for additional research in areas that can inform our understanding and knowledge of smoking cessation behavior. Both the Theory of Reasoned Action (Fishbein and Ajzen, 1975) and the Theory of Planned Behavior (Ajzen, 1985) have been applied to modeling smoking behavior. Although the importance of elicitation or grounding research to subsequent model testing has been emphasized by Ajzen and Fishbein (1980) and others (e.g., Montaño, Kasprzyk, and Taplin, 1997), a search of the literature revealed that very few studies provided details of beliefs used to assess attitudes and social norms or how these beliefs were chosen for the measures developed. This study addressed that gap by conducting elicitation research with adult smokers recruited from an urban Midwestern university (n = 30) and from the community in which the university is located (n = 38). The purpose of the research reported in this chapter was to identify salient behavioral outcomes, social referents, and control beliefs for smoking cessation among adult men and women smokers. Content analysis was conducted on the responses to the elicitation questionnaire in order to determine salient modal beliefs related to quitting smoking. A discussion of the findings and implications is provided.

Chapter 6 - Although the smoking rate is declining in the general population, smoking remains highly prevalent among substance abusers. Very little is known about optimal treatments for the reduction of cigarette use in persons dually-dependent on nicotine and other substances, and investigators frequently exclude alcohol and drug abusers from anti-smoking research projects. Researchers are beginning to study the effectiveness of anti-smoking interventions, previously tested only in the general population, in people with other chemical dependencies. Issues impacting effectiveness of standard anti-smoking interventions in people with non-nicotine chemical dependencies include: timing of smoking cessation attempts relative to other substance use and relative to treatment for non-nicotine addictions, interrelated patterns of cigarette smoking with other substance use, and unique barriers to quitting or reasons for continued smoking among substance abusers. Novel anti-smoking strategies, which may be particularly effective for this dually-dependent population, are under development. Data indicate that substance-abusing populations, responsive to the systematic application of behavioral contingencies to reduce drug use, also benefit from behavioral strategies to reduce cigarette smoking.

Chapter 7 - It is believed by some scientists and lay-people that drug craving causes drug addiction, and indeed the assumption that craving is responsible for compulsive drug use is the cornerstone of many scientific and popular conceptualizations of addictive behaviour (Tiffany and Carter, 1998; Tiffany, 1990, 1992, 1997). The concept of "drug craving" has been prominent in the drug addiction literature since the 1950s. The World Health Organization held an Expert Committee meeting in 1954, in an attempt to define and clarify the concept of craving. This committee suggested that the term craving be excluded from scientific use because it has several everyday connotations which could lead to confusion (Jellinek et al., 1955). Despite this recommendation, and the continued expression of concern about the utility of the term craving in scientific explanations of addiction (e.g., Hughes, 1987; Wise, 1988) the use of the term in the scientific literature continued, and so did the debates concerning its definition. In 1992 a WHO/UNDCP committee defined drug craving as "the desire to experience the effect(s) of a previously experienced psychoactive substance" (UNDCP and WHO, 1992). Despite the intuitive appeal of this definition, it does not easily lend itself to the empirical investigation of the phenomenon of craving without further clarification of the scientific term "craving" as opposed to the popular generic understanding of the word. Further, many investigators employ the term "craving" without defining it precisely. Thus, there can be no guarantee of heterogeneity of the construct of craving across investigators, a fact that limits its utility (Kozlowski and Wilkinson, 1987; Merikle, 1999). This chapter reviews scientific conceptualizations of craving, specifically withdrawal and appetitive based concepts that have dominated the literature and the more recent conception of "incentive salience". It then considers the usefulness of these definitions in relation to cigarette addiction, and evaluate the assumption that craving is a key causal feature of addiction and investigate the claim that "a truly comprehensive theory of addictive disorders can ill afford to overlook this salient feature of addictive behaviour" (Tiffany 1990). Although the use of the term craving can be thought of as ambiguous for empirical research, the concept remains clinically useful. DSM-IV lists urges and cravings as part of the symptoms characteristic of some drug dependencies (American Psychiatric Association, 1994). The diagnostic usefulness of urges and cravings indicate that the behavioural manifestations of these constructs are important features of addictive disorders (Baker, Sherman and Morse 1987). Thus, the chapter concludes with a consideration of the relationship between conceptualizations of craving and relapse and an assessment the applicability of research into craving to smoking cessation strategies.

Chapter 8 - Approximately 1/3 of the adult population in industrial countries and 70% in several Asian countries are daily smokers. Tobacco is the greatest preventable cause of death worldwide. Smoking is an important risk factor for developing cardiovascular disorders, and smoking causes about 90% of COPD

The literature on smoking and smoking cessation in patients with cardiovascular diseases and COPD was reviewed, and original investigations were presented.

Smoking cessation is associated with an approximately 50% risk reduction for death five years after myocardial infarction or unstable angina. With longer follow up periods the benefit of smoking cessation increases even further. In COPD, smoking cessation is the only action that improves the long-term prognosis. In patients with cardiovascular diseases and COPD, smoking cessation programs with behavioral support over several months combined with nicotine replacements significantly increases quit rates. Such programs can probably be delivered by personnel without special education in smoking cessation using simple intervention principles. A long follow up period is probably the most important element in the programs. In patients with coronary heart disease smoking cessation interventions are extremely cost effective compared to all other treatment modalities. In COPD, cost effectiveness analyses have not been performed, but a smoking cessation program has shown improved survival compared to usual care.

In patients with cardiovascular diseases and COPD smoking cessation interventions with several months of follow up combined with nicotine replacements are effective and easily applicable in clinical practice. Wider implementation of such programs would be a cost effective way of saving lives.

Chapter 9 - In the last decade we have become increasingly aware of the detrimental effects of smoking on surgical outcome. During more than half a century scientists have identified the relationship between smoking and different types of complications relating to surgery and anesthesia, but only recently effective preoperative smoking intervention have been researched.

This chapter sets out to identify the effects of smoking on surgical outcomes, intra- as well as postoperatively. The effects of smoking relates to duration and amount of tobacco smoking as well of the type and setting of surgery. The patophysiological background for the changes in organ function induced by tobacco smoking will be explained.

In the recent years several authors have explored the effect of preoperative smoking intervention on the risk of postoperative complications as well as on patient smoking habits in the short and long term. The chapter includes a review of these trials. In addiction the effectiveness and appropriateness of different types of preoperative smoking intervention methods will be discussed.

Finally the chapter discusses national and international approaches to facilitate the implementation of effective preoperative smoking intervention programs.

Chapter 10 - Cigarette smoking has been linked to eating and weight-related issues in numerous basic and clinical studies. Typically, smoking and weight issues, such as weight concern, dietary restraint, and clinically significant eating disorders like Bulimia Nervosa have been positively correlated with smoking among women. Existing literature suggests that women smokers are less likely to quit smoking, are less successful in initial cessation attempts, and relapse at higher rates than male smokers (Grunberg, Winders, and Wewers, 1991). Female smokers are also more likely to report smoking cigarettes to manage negative mood and to control weight—factors that have been identified as influencing women's smoking patterns and success in quitting (Solomon and Flynn, 1993). Women are more concerned about postcessation weight gain, tend to get more weight-control benefits from smoking, and suffer more postcessation weight gain than men (Perkins, Mitchell, and Epstein, 1995; Pirke and Laessle, 1993). Women are also more likely to experience increased appetite as a nicotine withdrawal symptom than are men (e.g., Perkins et al., 1995). This chapter contains information about the relationship between smoking and weight/eating-related issues, ranging from basic laboratory studies with animals and humans, to clinical applications and smoking cessation treatment.

Chapter 11 - The aim of the authors study was to bring to light the motivational differences between the successful quitters and the smokers who just contemplate on quitting. They analyzed self-reported motivations of ex-smokers' smoking cessation and the reasoning of current smokers who consider quitting.

The study is based on the Hungarostudy Health Panel (HHP) which is the second wave of the Hungarostudy 2002, a national representative health survey of the adult Hungarian population. The Hungarostudy Health Panel was completed in 2006. In the follow-up study data of 3701 persons were analyzed. Cessation motivations were examined on the basis of various self-reported health status indicators, education, self-rated economic situation, and sources of social support. To the original questionnaire some new blocks were added; comparing to base-line, smoking habits have been deeper investigated with further inquiries.

About half of the respondents are never smokers, 21 percent have quitted and 28 percent reported thoughts about giving up smoking. More than half of the current smokers contemplate on smoking cessation. Among the people with a smoking history, ex-smokers and contemplating current smokers alike (38-40 %), disease prevention was mentioned as the single most important reason of cessation. Financial reasons were mostly mentioned by current smokers; ex-smokers were more likely to explain their decision with deteriorating health, especially with the occurrence of certain diseases. Cardio-vascular morbidity played the most important role in smoking cessation. Cancers, respiratory disease and diabetes also increased significantly the odds of quitting. High blood pressure stimulated quitting considerations but not cessation. Social pressure was an underlying reason of quitting among women and among older persons. Among current smokers, the cohabitants and the better-off tended to entertain thoughts of quitting.

Our study confirmed the great importance of the experience of cardiovascular diseases in the smoking cessation: although people emphasize preventive purposes of their cessation efforts, existing circulatory and heart problems play the major role both in actual cessation and in quitting considerations. The odds of having serious thoughts about quitting are almost three times higher among smokers who developed cardiovascular disease; ex-smokers also attribute their quitting to treated circulatory illnesses.

Chapter 12 - Past research has emphasized the impact of smoking to physical health; however, the impact to mental and social health has been less explored. The purpose of this prospective study is to estimate the risks of smoking and cessation to successful aging for the elderly in Taiwan.

The data came from face-to-face interviews in Taiwan that used an elderly population-based probability sample provided by the Population and Health Research Center, Bureau of Health Promotion. Data were followed from baseline 1993 and to 1999, and only the survivor samples (n=2,525) were selected for analysis. Smoking status was separated into 'never smoked,' 'quit,' 'light smoker' and 'heavy smoker' categories. Successful aging indicators included activities of daily living, cognitive function, depressive symptoms, and social support. Hierarchical logistic regression models were used for analysis of the 6-year prediction of failing in successful aging, by controlling for demographics, co-morbidities, and successful aging state at baseline.

The sample was made up of 53.6% elderly nonsmokers, 21.4% ex-smokers, 10.0% light smokers and 15.0% heavy smokers at the baseline year. Heavy smokers had a higher risk of depressive symptoms. Influences of smoking status to other successful aging loss were not significant though. Ex-smokers had higher physical disability and cognitive impairment, and heavy smokers had lower social support.

Elderly are more likely to be aware of the smoking risks to physical health which can help them quit smoking. They are, however, less likely to appreciate the risks of smoking to mental health. Smoking cessation projects should consider the holistic health problems of the elderly and develop strategies to eliminate the smoking risk to successful aging.

Chapter 13 - Feedback is an important mechanism to bring about behavioural change. Printed and computer-generated information, either generic or targeted, has been used extensively to improve smoking cessation. Biochemical feedback provides personalised information, which gives a source of comparison for the individual among their cohort and gives an assessment of risk, establishes the current status and provides a platform for a change opinion of the smoker. Carbon monoxide monitoring, although primarily used to verify smoking habit, it can provide feedback, which can encourage smokers to quit. However, lack of specificity and sensitivity of this test limits its suitability. Cotinine testing, the preferred method to verify and monitor smoking habit, is primarily laboratory based, which has problems of delay and data accessibility.

To provide a simple point-of-care test for cotinine and other nicotine metabolites, which retain the sensitivity and specificity of laboratory testing, yet provides an immediate result. To demonstrate that feedback from the test can improve smoking cessation advice.

A urine test was developed and used in an antenatal care setting. Immediate feedback about smoking levels increased awareness of tobacco intake on foetal development. A saliva test was also developed and used in general dental practice to interact with patients to improve understanding why smoking causes oral disease.

During the antenatal study in the case group there was a significant reduction in test-verified smoking (p<0.001), with 16% quitting and 33% significantly reducing their cigarette usage. There was a significant reduction in urinary nicotine metabolite concentration (NMC) by the end of pregnancy compared to the control group. In the dental study a similar pattern emerged, with 23% of the case group quitting compared to 7% in the control group.

Biochemical feedback from a rapid, point-of-care test for smoking can significantly improve smoking cessation interventions and bring about behavioural change.

Chapter 14 - Tobacco is the major independent risk factor for the development of oral cancer and potentially malignant lesions. It is also involved in the pathogenesis of periodontal disease. The members of the dental team can play an effective role in tobacco preventing and cessation as they provide preventive and therapeutic services to a basically healthy population on a regular basis.

In this paper, the authors present specific strategies to guide oral health professionals (i.e. dentist and dental hygienist) providing smoking cessation interventions.

The "Five A's" strategic approach represents a brief and effective protocol for smoking cessation that members of dental team can use with all patients in their office practice. This protocol involves asking each patient about tobacco use, advising users to quit, assessing their willingness to make a quit attempt, assisting them with the quitting process and arranging follow-up to prevent relapse. Intensive interventions, more effective than brief ones, can be further adopted with any smokers willing to make a quit attempt. Patients not ready to quit may be motivated to make a quit attempt by employing the "Five R's" approach. Dental professionals can encourage their patients to identify reasons why quitting is personally relevant and the oral health risks of tobacco use; dental professionals can also rewards that patients can experience from quitting and help the patients to identify roadblocks to quitting. All patients attempting to quit should also be encouraged to use the pharmacotherapy agents.

The "Stages of Change" model may be helpful to assist the clinician in assessing readiness to make a quit attempt. Tobacco users are categorised as belonging at any one time to one of five stages: Pre-contemplation (not thinking about stopping); Contemplation stopping; Preparing to stop; Action-making a quit attempt; Maintaining abstinence or relapsing. The intention is to help tobacco users move through the stages by using different interventions at different stages.

Growing evidence supports the efficacy of smoking cessation counselling by oral health professionals. Dentists and dental hygienists, therefore, should be trained on smoking cessation counselling and dental offices should incorporate this service into routine patient care. While the approach to smoking intervention provides a useful framework from which to begin, special considerations need to be given when treating various categories of tobacco users such as smokeless tobacco users, adolescents and women.

In: Smoking Cessation: Theory, Interventions and Prevention   ISBN: 978-1-60021-591-9
Editor: Jerome E. Landow   © 2008 Nova Science Publishers, Inc.

Chapter 1

"A DAY IN THE LIFE OF...": THE CULTURE OF CIGARETTE SMOKING FOR PSYCHIATRIC POPULATIONS

Sharon Lawn

Flinders Human Behavior and Health Research Unit,
Flinders University, Adelaide, South Austrailia

ABSTRACT

Despite a vast body of research on smoking, quit rates for people with a concurrent mental illness remain extremely low. Research has established that these groups smoke more heavily, for more years and in greater proportions than the general population - up to 90% for people with psychotic illnesses compared with approximately 25% for general populations in many countries. This problem is particularly so in psychiatric institutions and community hostels where people with mental illness reside in great numbers. Using the ethnographic method of qualitative inquiry, combined with grounded theory analysis of indepth semi-structured interviews with people with mental illness and the staff who interact with them, this research aimed to study the culture of smoking as it is experienced by these populations in their day-to-day lives. Entrenched historical and current systemic barriers to quitting were observed, emanating from the mental health system in general. In many respects, the hospital was identified as a 'total institution' that appeared to shape and guide the beliefs and attitudes about mental illness held by staff and patients. In this setting, cigarettes were identified as the currency by which economic, social and political exchange took place between the various players. An enculturation process was described by all participants. Once entered into escape from the smoking behaviour and reinforcement by the cultural milieu appeared to be extremely difficult for patients and staff. Likewise, the community hostels were described, by participants, as a mirror image of the psychiatric extended care wards with the same level of institutionalised formal and informal rules, routines and behaviours in respect of smoking and its reinforcement.

Note

The terms 'patient', 'client', or 'consumer' are often used in the literature to refer to people who are experiencing a mental illness and are receiving care and treatment for it. Throughout this chapter, people with mental illness will be referred to as 'patients', as much of the content of the text relates to hospital environments. People living in supported accommodation in the community will be referred to as 'residents'.

SMOKING AND MENTAL ILLNESS

Smoking rates for people with a concurrent mental illness continue to be extremely high and quit rates continue to be extremely low (Addington, el-Guebaly, Duchak and Hodgins, 1997; Glynn and Sussman, 1990; Goff, Henderson and Amico, 1992; Hughes, Hatzukami, Mitchell and Dahlgren, 1986; Watt and Hocking, 1996; Ziedonis and George, 1997). People with a mental illness are more likely to smoke, smoke for more years, smoke more heavily and use higher tar cigarettes (Kumari and Postma, 2005; Jochelson and Majrowski, 2006; McNeill, 2001; Tidey, Rohsenow, Kaplan and Swift, 2005). There is a growing literature emphasising the possibility of links between nicotine withdrawal and mental illness relapse that help to explain this phenomenon (Glassman, 1993; Glynn and Sussman, 1990; Greeman and McClellan, 1991; Hall, Munoz, Reus, Sees, Duncan, Humfleet and Harris, 1996; Stage, Glassman and Covey, 1996). Lasser, Boyd, Woolhandler, Himmelstein, McCormick and Bor (2000), in their survey of 4411 participants from the US National Co-Morbidity Survey, found that people were twice as likely to smoke in the presence co-morbid mental illness. They also found that approximately 45% of all cigarettes smoked in the United States are smoked by people with mental illness. This supports the concern of many that people with mental illness are disproportionately represented in the smoking population. Additionally, through the collection of tobacco excise by governments which then fund health services, they are contributing substantially to the cost of their own care (Lawn, 2001a).

Current smoking cessation interventions made available by mainstream anti-smoking campaigns do not appear to be adequately addressing the health needs of people with mental illness. The reasons for this remain unclear. The high incidence of smoking amongst all people with a mental illness is a concerning public health problem. In a fifteen-year follow-up of 179 patients with schizophrenia in the community, Brown, Birtwhistle, Roe and Thompson (1999) found that 22% had died, 11% from cardiovascular and respiratory diseases; this being twice the expected rate for the general population. Similarly, others have found an increased rate of heart and lung disease for people with mental illness who smoke (Himelhoch, Lehman, Kreyenbuhl, Daumit, Brown and Dixon, 2004; Kisely, Smith, Lawrence and Maaten, 2005; Mortenson and Juel, 1993). A major Australian survey of approximately 165,500 adults with mental illness (known as the Busselton Study), identified smokers with mental illness as being among those with the greatest risk of premature death from all major physical health problems as a consequence of their smoking and other risk behaviours such as alcohol and other substance abuse, obesity, poor diet and lack of exercise (Coghlan, Lawrence, Holman and Jablensky, 2001). The presence of fewer health promoting behaviours, low levels of exercise as a consequence of disabling symptoms and weight gain from psychiatric medications, and poorer nutrition for people with mental illness has also been proposed to help explain their greater risk of premature death (Hennekens, Hennekens, Hollar and Casey, 2005; Holmberg and Kane, 1999; Davidson, Judd, Jolley, Thompson and Hyland, 2001).

Co-Morbid Nicotine Dependence and Mental Illness

A review of the existing research on smoking and mental illness has found significant co-morbidity (Carosella, Ossip-Klein, and Owens, 1999; George and Krystal, 2000; Herran, de Santiago, Sandoya, Fernandez, Diez-Manrique, and Vazquez-Barquero, 2000; McNeill, 2001; Miller, Hemenway and Rimm, 2000; Poirier, Canceil, Bayle, Millet, Bourdel, Moatti, Olie, and Attar-Levy, 2002). The relationship between depressive states and smoking has been found to be established early in the person's life, with the presence of depression or depressive mood in childhood or adolescence significantly increasing the risk of smoking initiation at that time. Depression was found to precede smoking initiation in a number of studies although the direction of causality remains unclear (Breslau and Johnson, 2000; Escobedo, Kirch and Anda, 1996; Escobedo, Reddy and Giovini, 1998; Kandel and Davies, 1986; Stefanis and Kokkevi, 1986). Likewise, smoking has been causally linked to the onset of depression (Brown, Levinsohn, Seeley and Wagner, 1996; Johnson, Cohen, Dohrenwend, Link and Brook, 1999; Wu and Anthony, 1999). Others have proposed that smoking and depression share common genetic factors (Kendler, Neale, MacLean, Heath, Eaves and Kessler, 1993), and similar childhood and social risk factors (Fergusson, Lynskey and Horwood, 1996). A recent US study using two samples of 8704 and 6947 adolescents concluded that prior smoking is a powerful determinant of depression. They advocated the use of anti-depressants in non-depressed young smokers to assist them to quit (Goodman and Capitmas, 2000).

Between 74% and 92% of people with schizophrenia smoke, compared to 25% for the general population (Hughes, et al., 1986; Glynn and Sussman, 1990; Goff, et al., 1992; de Leon, Dadvand, Canusa and White, 1995; Watt and Hocking, 1996;). Smoking rates for people with schizophrenia are also higher than for people with other psychiatric illnesses (Ziedonis and George, 1997). Between 35% and 54% of people with BPAD are thought to be smokers (Goff, et al., 1992; de Leon, et al., 1995; Gonzalez-Pinto, Gutierrez, Ezcurra, Aizuru, Mosquera, Lopez and de Leon, 1998). McEvoy and Brown (1999) found that more than 80% of people with schizophrenia were established smokers by the time of their first episode of psychosis, suggesting that this high prevalence is directly related to the illness itself and the person's attempts to self-medicate their symptoms, and not to features of its treatment. Others have suggested that smoking may play a causal role in the onset of schizophrenia (Kelly and McCreadie, 1999). People with mental illness who smoke also require higher doses of neuroleptic medications, generally have more hospitalisations and earlier onset of their illness and have higher Brief Psychiatric Rating Scale scores (Goff, et al., 1992; Haywood, kravitz, Grossman, cananaugh, Davis and Lewis, 1995; Sandyk and Kay, 1991; Sonne, Brady and Morton, 1994; Ziedonis, Kosten, Glazer and Frances, 1994). They also have increased risk of suicide (Soyka, Albus, Kathmann, finelli, Hofstetter, Holzbach, Immler and Sand, 1993).

In their review of BPAD and substance use disorder, Strakowski and DelBello (2000) found that substance abuse by this group is state dependent, that is, more of the substance is used when the person with BPAD is manic. Others have identified cases of acute mania following abrupt nicotine withdrawal (Benezzi, 1989). People with BPAD and depression have been found to have significant problems with spatial and holistic tasks (Robertson and Taylor, 1985) and problems with attention, memory and visio-spatial function (Bulbena and Berrios, 1993). Van Gorp et al. (1998) found significant long-term cognitive impairment in people with long-standing BPAD, especially where they had a history of alcohol abuse. The implications of these findings for the person's ability to fulfil the cognitive planning and processing necessary to quit smoking are apparent.

The rate of co-morbid Borderline Personality Disorder and substance abuse has been found to be high, ranging from 55% upwards (Dulitt, fyer, Haas, Sullivan and Frances, 1990; Hatzitaskos, Soldatos, Kokkevi and Stefanis, 1999; Nace, 1990; Trull, Sher, Minks-Brown, Durbin and Burr, 2000). Substance abuse and a history of child sexual or physical abuse are common in people with this diagnosis (American Psychiatric Association, 2000). In a major review of seventeen studies on Borderline Personality Disorder and substance abuse conducted between 1987 and 1997, Trull et al. (2000) proposed several reasons for co-morbidity between the two conditions. The two are thought to share common risk factors for initiation, for example, childhood trauma (see also Brown and Anderson, 1991; Parrott, 2000; Sabo, 1997). Once co-morbidity develops, each disorder serves to maintain the other; that is, they have reciprocal effects in which the existence of one fosters greater chronicity of the other. Impulsivity and inhibition are characteristic of people with both conditions. Both are a means of affect regulation in the presence of affect instability, especially smoking to cope with negative affective states and tension (see also Hatzitaskos, et al., 1999).

Several theories have been proposed for the high incidence of smoking for people with mental illness generally. A brief review of the main theories follows:

Smoking to Self-Medicate Mental Illness

Smoking has been reputed to have anti-depressant effects in people with depression, with smoking cessation attempts being causally implicated in the relapse of these people's depression (Anda, Williamson, Escobedo, mast, Giovino and Remington, 1990; Breslau and Johnson, 2000; Carmody, 1989; Carton, Jouvent and Widlocher, 1994; Covey, Glassman and Stetner, 1990, 1997; Glassman, 1993; Hughes, et al., 1986; Kendler, et al., 1993; Kinnunen, Doherty, Militello and Garvey, 1996; Shiffman, Hickcox, Paty and Gnys, 1996; Tsoh, Humfleet, Munoz, Reus, Hartz and Hall, 2000; Worthington, Fava, Agustin, Alpert, Nierenberg, Pava and Rosenbaum, 1995). Khantzian (1985) had earlier found that self-medication by using drugs, was common among depressed persons. A French study by Carton et al., (1994) found that depressed smokers were more likely to smoke in negative emotional situations, were more likely to use smoking for its sedative and stimulant effect and were more likely to use cigarettes to regulate emotions. They also noted the sensation-seeking role of smoking for depressed smokers seeking to counteract anhedonia. Despite this research activity, the experiences of the depressed people themselves have received little attention. Research has largely focusing on pharmacological explanations of the associations between the two phenomena, arguing that self-medication is essentially nicotine withdrawal relief (Brown, 2004; Jarvis, 2004) or more complex interactions between nicotine dependence and psychiatric symptoms (Aguilar, Gurpegui, diaz and de Leon, 2005).

Nicotine's role in regulating a dysfunctional dopamine system, by augmenting dopamine release, has been proposed as the mechanism involved in smoking dependence for people with mental illness (Glassman, 1993). More generally, mesolimbic dopaminergic pathway activity in the brain has been found to be especially important in mediating reward in nicotine dependence (Koob, 1992; Pontieri, Tanda, Orzi, and DiChiara, 1996). Others have suggested that smoking is used to self-medicate the negative symptoms of schizophrenia, with nicotine acting on the dopamine system of the brain to help regulate it and overcome problems with motivation, commitment and affective flattening (Glassman, 1993; Lohr and Flynn, 1992; Sandyk and Kay, 1991; Ziedonis and George, 1997). The sedative/stimulant effect of nicotine is relevant here. Nicotine is an agonist/antagonist drug, acting as a stimulant at low dose and a sedative at high dose. With the amount that people with schizophrenia smoke it is most likely to be sedative rather than stimulating in its effect. The positive symptoms of schizophrenia (conceptual disorganisation, delusions and hallucinations) are also reported to be influenced by nicotine action, increasing symptomatology (Ziedonis, et al., 1994). However the chemistry of this interaction is less clear (Forchuk, Norman, Malla, Voz and Martin, 1997). The positive influence of nicotine on the release of dopamine in the brain, and therefore the role in reward and hedonistic pathways has been proposed for depressed smokers (Carton, et al., 1994; Glassman, 1993). Others have challenged the self-medication hypothesis for mental illness and drug use, suggesting that a model incorporating stress, personality traits and coping is more appropriate (Blanchard, Brown, Horan and Sherwood, 2000).

Smoking to Overcome Cognitive Deficits

It has also been suggested that smoking is used to overcome deficits in attention, concentration, memory and cognition related to schizophrenia (Adler, Hoffer, Wiser and Freedman, 1993; Addington and Duchak, 1997; Taiminen, et al., 1998). Nicotine has been shown to improve sensory gating so that smoking alleviates processing difficulties regarding sensory information in people suffering from schizophrenia. Auditory sensory gating deficits are found in more than 75% of people with schizophrenia. Adler et al. (1993) found that the auditory evoked response for people with schizophrenia is different to the general population and that these deficits are temporarily normalised by nicotine use for people with schizophrenia. In this way, nicotine stimulates the nicotinic receptors in the brain to normalise gating deficits, albeit with transient effects. If so, such deficits would make the quitting process more difficult to master, given the complex processes thought to be necessary to institute and maintain change (Bellack and DiClemente, 1999).

Mental Illness and Nicotine Withdrawal

Physical withdrawal from nicotine has been shown to worsen psychiatric symptoms in smokers and to increase the potential for illness relapse (Glynn and Sussman, 1990; Greeman and McClellan, 1991; Glassman, 1992, 1993). The pharmacological interactions of nicotine with psychiatric medications and its influence on dopaminergic activity in the brain has been mentioned. The psychological aspects of learning habit replacement and the need to find new ways to relieve anxiety and boredom may also be associated with problems of withdrawal. The symptoms associated with that withdrawal, such as increased agitation, restlessness, and insomnia are also common forerunners to illness relapse and may raise the person's fears even further. A complex web of learned responses, based on physical symptoms of withdrawal and subjective responses, may therefore guide the person's decision to keep smoking, rather than attempt to quit.

Nicotine, Cigarette Smoke and Neuroleptic Medication Interactions

The relationship between smoking and psychiatric medications is a complex one, with higher doses of medication often required when the person is a smoker due to the the action of cigarette smoke in increasing liver enzyme activity and therefore lowering the level of medication in the blood (Schein, 1995; Wilhelm, Arnold, Niven and Richmond, 2004). Smoking has also been shown to mitigate the side effects of neuroleptic medications that are widely used by psychiatric populations, to treat their mental illness. One such side effect, neuroleptic induced parkinsonism, has been increasingly found to be less common in smokers (Decina, Caracci, Sandyk, Berman, Mukherjee and Scapicchio, 1990; Goff, et al., 1992; Ziedonis and George, 1997). However, tardive dyskinesia and akathisia are more prevalent among smokers with schizophrenia due to their need to take higher doses of neuroleptic medication (Glassman, 1993; Hughes, et al., 1996; Yassa, Korpassy and Ally, 1987; Ziedonis and George, 1997). Recent biological in-vivo research with non-psychiatric populations has confirmed that smoking and the development of dependence are associated with increased dopamine activity in the basal ganglia of the brain and that smokers have special sensitivity to presynaptic dopaminergic activation by nicotine (Salokangas, et al, 2000). This is significant because dopamine activity is central to understanding the course and progress to mental illness. Nicotine and alcohol dependence are thought to be caused by a simliar dopamine-related mechanism (Tiihonen, et al., 1998). A further biological study has found connections between low dopaminergic neurotransmission and detached personality, being one of the first studies to test for biological explanations for psychological traits. They further speculate that a combination of genetic factors and environmental influences on brain development during childhood and adolescence are responsible and there may be links between motivation and reward processes also for this presentation (Laakso, et al., 2000). The role of nicotine in improving cognitive function has also been proposed, although it is unclear whether nicotine has direct positive effects on cognitive function in smokers or whether it plays a role in reversing cognitive deficits (Adler, et al., 1993; Taiminen, et al., 1998). Smoking has also been proposed to have a protective effect against dementia, but this has not been confirmed according to a report reviewing the evidence (Brayne, 2000).

OTHER INFLUENCES ON SMOKING IN PSYCHIATRIC SETTINGS

Several researchers have attempted to refocus their attention on the theory of dependence, realising that biological, psychological, and social variables account for only minor proportion of the variance in addictive behaviours while most of the variance remains unexplained (Miller, 1990). The self-medication theory of dependence, that proposes that people smoke to cope with adverse external pressures and internal negative states, assumes that if the adverse conditions are treated or changed the drug dependence will no longer fulfil this need and will vanish (Gold and Miller, 1994). For people with a mental illness, little exploration of what these people are medicating in their social world and where they gain their sense of self and meaning has occurred beyond looking at the physical symptoms of illness. Examining the nature of institutions and systems where people with mental illness receive treatment would seem important.

The Role of Institutions

Rhodes (1991), in her study of two United States acute psychiatric units, highlights the inherent contradictions that exist within mental health settings, where staff provide care and therapy but also act as agents of social control. Foucault (1977) describes psychiatric patients as the object of knowledge and the subject of discipline. He argues that staff are therefore placed in a paradoxical position. Foucault (1977) describes the historical context for power relationships and social control functions of mental health settings, focusing on the emergent asylums as sites of discipline and surveillance and the transfer of these values to current mental health treatment. Goffman (1961a, 1961b, 1961c) gives a detailed description of how power was displayed and used in the asylums of the past. Parallels to the present day psychiatric hospital are evident. On entering the total institution, the person was said to begin, "a series of abasements, degradations, humiliations and profanations of self" (Goffman, 1961c, p.23). This involved role dispossession and a lack of work that led to a demoralisation of the individual over time. In these settings, tobacco was used as a source of reward, with clients receiving a tobacco ration as part of a privilege system (Shlomowitz, 1990).

Interactions with institutions and other organised systems are based on power relationships established as part of the cultural beliefs and values of those in the setting. Cultural power means, "control over the means of value creation, interpretation and maintenance," (Jessop, 1972, p.58) and involves control over economic, political and social power. Within institutions and organisations, both culture and power relationships exert a significant influence on the behaviours of their members. It has been unclear what role smoking plays in this for those in psychiatric settings. The findings of our research (Lawn, 2001) suggest that these power relationships are often suspended when staff and patients "have a ciggy together" often to defuse increasing agitation, after a confrontation or as "a getting to know you exercise". Cigarette smoking is one "normal" thing that patients do and may be symbolically important in maintaining at least a symbolic contact with people who are well, to feel "normal".

Community hostels are another form of institution where many people with mental illness reside. The role of smoking in hostels has not been studied. Suto and Frank's (1994) qualitative study of ten people in a board and care hostel in California, found that hostels steeped in institutional routines had a significant influence on how people oriented to time and future; that they were very much oriented to the present or to a few hours into the future. The paucity of social roles and the dominance of familiar and predictably timed routines, repeated day in and day out, provided residents with significant temporal reference points. Examples of these were clear expectations of what happens before and after meals and routines around the giving of daily pocket money and cigarettes. Routines facilitated future expectation, fundamentally organising the person's time into past, present and future.

However, they argue that the balance in these temporal markers is too much weighted in the present, resulting in the immediate fulfilment of the person's wishes at the expense of allowing and encouraging them to develop skills for flexibility, long-term planning and autonomous decision-making. This has implications for smokers residing in hostels that need further exploration.

The Role of Organisations

Psychiatric institutions are organisations with collections of services and groups of people that interact with each other. Any discussion about the problem of smoking rates in psychiatric institutions and attempts to improve this involves the notion of change. Central to the notion of change is the need to understand why change does not occur. Nisbet (1972) states, "there is not the slightest possibility of understanding the mechanisms of change unless we understand, or at least recognize seriously, the mechanisms of fixity and persistence" (p.6). Schon (1972) refers to this phenomenon as 'dynamic conservatism' in which organisations tend to offer services and behave in set ways rather than respond by modifying services according to changing needs. Schon (1972) further argues that a lack of co-ordination in service systems creates both horizontal and vertical fragmentation. "The result is that there exist almost no points at which public action might effectively move the system as a whole" (p.94). In this climate, agency discretion is used to work against change via control of access, duration of stay and control of the portion of the clients' 'life space' that the agency takes up, extending its service beyond the actual disability. In the extreme, the agency becomes the person's total environment. The fragmentation of staff in the psychiatric inpatient settings and its effects is a demonstration of Schon's (1972) ideas. Ogburn (1972) argues that the culture of organisations itself is innately resistant to change. He cites seven reasons for this, involving cultural and psychological aspects:

1. Difficulties of invention in that it is easier to use existing forms of behaviour than to create new ones;
2. Vested interests exist with power of particular groups being exerted to maintain the status quo;
3. The power of tradition;
4. Habit;
5. Social pressure by the group to conform to existing behaviours;
6. Forgetting the unpleasant thereby the past appears brighter than it actually was; and
7. **Psychological traits such as anxiety about the uncertainty of change.**

Architectural Determinism – A Smoking Environment

The work of Rudolf Moos (1976) on the physical characteristics of the milieu and its influence on the behaviours of its members is also relevant here. Moos (1976) argued that the physical and social environment cannot be understood independently of each other and that behaviour therefore cannot be studied apart from the environment in which it occurs. Moos theory of architectural determinism concludes that, "man-made physical environments may profoundly influence psychological states and social behaviour" (Moos and Insel, 1974, p.8). The reasons for behaviour and environmental congruence are argued to be due to a combination of learning theories (Wicker, 1974). This involves operant and classical learning by positive and negative reinforcement, involving stimulus and response interactions, repeated over time and in various situations. Behaviour settings theory sees people obtaining satisfactions from, for example, peer smoking to overcome boredom and provide companionship and autonomy. Social exchange theory, involves the selection of settings on the basis of reward or cost analysis. Finally, observational learning theory involves the person's behaviour being affected and influenced by observing and learning from the actions of others and the consequences of their actions. Peer smoking as a potential barrier to quitting needs investigation, given these processes.

The Role of Group Dynamics

An understanding of the concept of the group (Lewin, 1948) is also useful in understanding organisational culture and interactions between and interdependence among its members, in particular, peer smoking groups. Forsyth (1999) defines a group as, "two or more interdependent individuals who influence one another through social interaction" (p.6), involving shared social identity. Group conflict and oppression can be regarded as, "different manifestations of the same basic human predisposition to form group-based social hierarchies" (Sidanius and Pratto, 1999, p.38). The rules, procedures and actions of social institutions produce group-based social hierarchy. It can be conscious, deliberate, overt, unconscious, unintended and covert (Sidanius and Pratto, 1999). Theories of group dynamics are influenced by Skinner's (1953) behavioural approach, known as social exchange theory, in which rewards are maximised and costs are minimised as part of a negotiated process of interaction (Forsyth, 1999). Deviance has specific functions for groups. It is accepted as part of and as a requirement of group formation, expressed as a need for 'other' in order to define self. It also allows for displacement of hostilities onto a scapegoat in order to maintain group equilibrium and maintain boundaries (Dentler and Erikson, 1984). These processes may be relevant to psychiatric settings and smoking behaviour within those settings.

Smoking by Minority Groups as an Expression of Power

The notion of substance use by minority groups in order to experience personalised power, albeit brief and artificial has been convincingly argued by Barber, Punt and Albers (1988)who found that this was exactly what Aborigines on Palm Island were doing with their alcohol use. They suggested that the politics of empowerment would be more effective in lessening the problem of alcohol abuse than education about alcohol use. Roche and Ober (1997) examined the problem of smoking by Aborigines, a marginalised group that has smoking rates approximately twice that of the general population in Australia. They argued that smoking is adaptive in the same way as drinking alcohol, despite its adverse consequences, suggesting that it aids social cohesion and solidarity, acting as a symbol of exchange and as a symbol of coping and being in control. Parallels between these behaviours and that of smokers with mental illness is worth exploring.

A Canadian study by Stewart et al. (1996a, 1996b), looking at disadvantage and the link to low quit rates, concluded that day-to-day barriers to quality of life and empowerment were likely to act as barriers to quitting. Therefore, long-term goals were perceived as irrelevant because immediate circumstances are overwhelming motivators to continue smoking as the mechanism to cope with those circumstances. More generally, social determinants have been identified as playing a prominent role in the production and maintenance of health and disadvantage. Marmot has undertaken extensive research and advised the WHO and UK National Health Service about this problem over many years.

Cigarettes and Violence in Institutional Settings

In settings where cigarettes are an item of value to the members and where others control access to those valued items, there is potential for conflict. Such may be the case in psychiatric settings where staff have a role in making decisions about distribution and access to cigarettes by clients. Morrison (1990a) states that, "patient-staff conflict over the enforcement of rules and denying of requests is identified as a major cause of assaults"(p.17). Rolfe (1995) reviewed the phenomenon of violence towards nursing staff in psychiatric settings but neglected to examine the role of smoking despite this being of much concern as expressed in all psychiatric research on smoking bans (Lawn and Pols, 2005).

Others have argued that violence in psychiatric settings is a product of the socio-cultural field, not just a symptom of the person's illness (Stanton and Schwartz, 1954). Lion (1972) argues that, "the patient's aggressive behaviour represents a defensive stance against overwhelming feelings of helplessness and fragility" (p.3) in psychiatric settings. A Belgian study reported verbal and physical assaults in closed wards over an eleven-month period in 1996-7 by Nijman and Rector (1999). They discovered that the lack of psychological space involving the lack of privacy and ability to get rest in these settings triggered aggression. Katz and Kirkland (1990) studied violent and peaceful psychiatric wards and concluded that staff behaviour was a major influence on the level of violence. In wards where there was strong and supportive leadership, there was less violence. Where staff spent more time with patients, the level of violence declined, whereas increased levels of violence were noted in wards where nursing staff spent more time in the glassed nurses' station, this being how staff communicated their fear of violence by patients. The role of environment, systems, structures and relationships, was also recognised to contribute to violence. Rolfe's (1995) own study of forty-nine assaults in a 110 bed psychiatric setting over a six-month period found that 53-90% of these assaults occurred in the context of staff-patient interactions, with the patients' mental state relevant to only 10% of all incidents. Blair (1991) noted that taking something away from a patient, such as cigarettes, led to an increased risk of assault towards the limit setter.

Smoking by Psychiatric Nurses

Within psychiatric inpatient settings, nurses provide a high proportion of the direct care and contact with patients. Therefore, they are in a unique position to act as role models and to make a significant impact on clients' smoking behaviour and the associated risk of suffering tobacco-related diseases by directly supporting and participating in pharmacological and psychosocial interventions. Recent research has claimed substantial evidence exists that psychiatric nurses can be effective in promoting smoking cessation (Sarna, 1999; Wewers, Ahijevych and Sarna, 1998).

Despite the potential for positive input by psychiatric nurses, the high rate of smoking by patients continues to be an insidious problem in psychiatric settings. The rate of substance use by nurses, in particular, the rate of smoking by psychiatric nurses continues to be high compared with nursing in other health-related fields. The reasons for this are unclear, though some have suggested that this may be largely due to accessibility, the emphasis on medication use and work-related stress (Griffith, 1999; Plant, Plant and Foster, 1991; Rowe and Clark, 2000; Tagliacozzo, Sci and Vaughn, 1982; Trinkoff and Storr, 1998; Collins, Gollnisch and Morsheimer, 1999). Features of the institution and its impact on how nurses think about and resolve ethical dilemmas involving smoking have been proposed as reasons for their lack of effective responses to smoking by patients in their care (Lawn and Condon, 2006). These forces could equally apply to other professional groups that interact with patients in psychiatric institutions.

STATEMENT OF THE PROBLEM

The knowledge that smoking and passive smoking is a serious health hazard is well established (Doll and Hill, 1950, 1964; Lopez, 2000; Office of Environmental Health Hazard Assessment, 1997; Royal College of Physicians of London, 1962, 1971, 1977, 2000; U. S. Department of Health and Human Services, 1964, 1984, 1988, 1989). Low quit rates for psychiatric populations suggest that there may be barriers to quitting for these groups that have been overlooked. Many reasons for this have been proposed including those associated with shared neurobiology of mental illness and nicotine dependence, self-medication of symptoms, psychosocial coping responses, environmental factors, psychological factors and systemic factors.

Research in the area has increased, especially within the fields of medicine, psychiatry and psychology. In spite of this, there has been a general absence of social research on smoking and mental illness, with a few exceptions (Esterberg and Compton, 2005; Lawn, 2001; Levin, 2001). The current literature does not explain why some people with a mental illness succeed in quitting smoking whereas others fail, despite having similar psychiatric diagnoses, severity of symptoms and levels of nicotine dependence. Anecdotal evidence suggests that many people with mental illness wish to quit smoking but cannot within the existing clinical, social and organisational milieux which appear to contain disincentives and barriers to quitting. Several ethical dilemmas arise for mental health professionals continually seeing patients' quality of life challenged as a consequence of their smoking. These dilemmas include: the cycle of smoking-related poverty; stigma and social exclusion; issues of fairness and equity of treatment and access to services. There are also social justice issues to do with how these groups are viewed and therefore how they have their needs defined, recognised and then met as citizens.

AIMS AND OBJECTIVES

This research began as a simple attempt by us as mental health service staff to understand why people with mental illness find quitting difficult, bourne out of frustration at watching the high number of patients smoking and the impact on their lives generally. What began simply as good reflective practice developed into a realisation that people with mental illness smoke for a range on reasons involving not only the person but also the circumstances in which they found themselves and in which they sought help; each interacting in a complex web that served to perpetuate and reinforce their smoking. Hence, this research had a number of diverse aims and objectives. These were:

- To describe in a holistic way the phenomena of concurrent smoking and mental illness within psychiatric institutions from the perspective of patients and staff.
- To interpret and understand this phenomena by looking at the person, the setting and the system, viewed through multiple theoretical lenses.
- To contribute to strategies for health professionals, based on this understanding, that will enhance their knowledge and skills in providing support to people with a mental illness who may wish to quit smoking.
- To identify focus areas for policy development with regard to cigarette smoking within psychiatric settings generally.

DESIGN

This research comprised three distinct studies that were triangulated in order to provide a thorough description and understanding of the smoking behaviours of institutionalised psychiatric populations in the public mental health system. This included both inpatient hospital wards and community hostels. Qualitative semi-structured open-ended interviews were performed with people with mental illness to explore their smoking behaviours, their perceptions of smoking as it related to their illness, nicotine dependence and the cultural contexts in which their smoking developed and occurred. Mental health service staff who worked in the settings were also interviewed to gain their perspective on the issue. An extensive participant observation of the settings was then performed as part of triangulating the interview data with an ethnographic approach and to enhance the overall validity of the data.

Using a grounded theory research design for data analysis (Glaser and Strauss, 1967; Strauss and Corbin, 1990), themes emerged linking mental illness, smoking behaviours and systems of care. The combined ethnographic and grounded theory approach was used because of its suitability for exploring, relatively uncharted waters, or to gain a fresh perspective in a familiar problem, looking at not only what was occurring but why.

METHODS

Ethics approval for the research was obtained from the Flinders Clinical Research Ethics Committee and the Royal Adelaide Hospital Ethics Committee. Information sheets and consent forms were provided for all participants for interviews. General information sheets were displayed in the settings where observiations occurred and the researcher attended ward meetings involving patients and staff to explain the research purpose to them. In settings where patients' consent could not be obtained, such as the locked ward where patients were acutely unwell, consent to proceed was obtained from representative consumer groups and advocacy groups. Non-participation and the right to withdraw at any time without prejudice to treatment or status was offered and assured for all participants. All client interviewees were cleared by their psychiatrist prior to their participation. An independent auditor oversaw the conduct of the data collection and analysis process from its inception to its completion, finding that a clear audit trail had been established. All interviews were coded by the primary researcher and an independent psychiatrist with 85% or better intercoder reliability achieved.

Confidentiality was a significant concern for the researcher and the ethics committees, given that the research involved voluntary and involuntary clients, stigmatised groups and potential taboo issues. Friedrichs and Ludtke (1975) suggest that there are political consequences of studies such as this that a likely to illustrate the mechanisms of discrimination, the relationships between participants, and subtle and obvious forms of social control. Clear feedback to all participants was therefore a significant consideration.

Safety issues for self and others were apparent. The primary researcher was bound by her own status as an employee of a mental health service to adhere to policies regarding safety in the settings being observed. The researcher also had a duty of care to report any abuses and safety concerns to the appropriate bodies. This included such incidents as illicit drug dealing and consumption within the grounds of the hospital, sexual harassment or abuse by clients towards other clients and threats of violence. Passive smoking considerations for the primary researcher also needed to be addressed when in the company of participants who were smoking and when in settings where smoking was occurring.

Qualitative interviews were performed with 24 currently smoking patients of a community mental health team within the Southern Adelaide Health Service catchment area (total client population = 340). All of these participants had experienced hospital admissions in the context of treatment for their mental illness. Six consumers who had successfully quit for 6 months or more, who had experienced their mental illness for at least 10 years, and who had previously smoked for at least 10 years, were also interviewed. All consumer participants were purposively approached by their community mental health case manager who then notified the researcher of their agreement to be interviewed. Interviews occurred in participants' homes or at the community mental health service if this was requested by them or mandated due to existing safety protocols applied to them. Equal number so women and men were interviewed with varying diagnoses (Schizophrenia n=6, Depression n=6, Bipoloar Affective Disorder n=6, Borderline Personality Disorder n=6). Futher details of methods for data collection from client interviews can be found elsewhere (Lawn, 2001; Lawn, Pols and Barber, 2002; Lawn and Abrams, 2002). The following questions guided interviews with consumers:

- Basic demographic details of diagnosis, years smoked, amount smoked per day, cigarette strength, highest educational level reached, source of income, accommodation status, marital status
- Belief in level of control over smoking and quitting
- Past Quit Attempts and what happened
- Quitting methods tried
- What it is like being a smoker
- Who is responsible for smoking and quitting
- Response of doctor and case manager to their smoking
- Hospital experience as a smoker
- View of smoking policies and potential bans
- Reasons for commencing smoking
- Reasons for continuing smoking
- Experience of having a mental illness
- What happens to their smoking when they become unwell
- Role of families regarding smoking

Qualitative interviews were performed with 26 staff of community and inpatient services from a range of the following professions: nursing, psychiatry, social work, occupational therapy, and psychology, each with at least 2 years experience of working in the sector. Staff participants were purposefully approached by the researcher and were either currently smokers, ex-smokers or non-smokers with similar numbers of men and women being interviewed. Interviews took place at worksites or other agreed locations, as per the participant's request. Privacy was assured with pseudonymns used for all participants. Where a staff member may have been identifiable to those familiar with the settings, such as a Clinical Nurse Consultant in a particular type of setting, the status of the participant was not identified; they were referred to as 'nurse'. The following questions guided interviews with staff:

- Description of mental health service experience
- Their own smoking history, why they smoking, and smoking while at work
- Being a non-smoker while at work – what this is like
- What occurs in their work setting re smoking
- Their views on patients smoking and staff smoking while at work
- What informs their decisions about how they act re smoking in the workplace
- What do they think would happen if there was a smoking ban
- Mental illness and smoking – any links perceived and why/why not
- View of their own and other professions' response to smoking issue
- How do they respond to patients who demand help to get cigarettes, what determines their decision
- Level of involvement in supply of cigarettes to patients, and how they decide

Futher details of methods for data collection from staff interviews can be found elsewhere (Lawn, 2001, 2004; Lawn and Condon, 2006).

PARTICIPANT OBSERVATION OF THE CLIENTS AND STAFF

Participant observation is useful when little is known about the phenomenon, when differences exist between the view of insiders as opposed to outsiders, when the phenomenon is obscured from the view of outsiders and when it is hidden from public view (Jorgensen, 1989). All of these conditions were thought to exist in psychiatric settings. It allows greater understanding of the context, therefore providing a more holistic approach to the data and allows an inductive approach by experiencing first hand the phenomenon. It provides the opportunity to see things that may otherwise escape conscious and routine awareness among participants because it is taken for granted. It provides an opportunity to learn about things people may be unwilling to talk about in interviews, such as taboo topics and provides the opportunity to move beyond individual perceptions. It also allows the researcher use direct experience as a resource in order to understand and interpret phenomena (Patton, 1980).

The everyday life of mental health patients and staff could therefore be best understood by observing the natural environment in which they interact. The advantages of participant observation identified by Friedrichs and Ludtke (1975) were particularly relevant for studying mental health patients, that is, it did not depend on the verbal capabilities of the interviewees and it aided the comprehension of situations and understandings that were difficult to get out through questioning alone. The sensitivities and cognitive difficulties of many people experiencing mental illness were therefore accounted for in this type of methodology. It also gave an opportunity to describe the extent of passive smoking by patients and staff; patterns and intensity of smoking to assist the management of patients, differences in the settings and to verify occupational health and safety concerns made by staff.

Participant observation is also cited as a good support methodology for qualitative interviews, its purpose being to better understand the relationship between behaviour and culture, and to further validate the qualitative data. Therefore the role of participant observation in hypothesis testing of ideas and themes from the interviews was apparent. For this research, analysis of the qualitative interviews and the trustworthiness of the results confirmed by the audit process, clearly established a thematic framework that could then be standardised and applied to an observation schedule to be used for the participant observation phase.

The Pilot Period

A one-month pilot study preceded the main participant observation period. It was performed by the primary researcher to gain familiarity with the settings and rapport with the participants. This habituation of the environment served to improve the validity and reliability of observations by allowing the observed to become familiar with the researcher's presence and go about their usual day in their usual manner without staging activities or behaviours for the researcher. The pilot period was also used to identify and resolve any problems and barriers to access, to test a series of observation sheets that had been devised from interview data from the previous phases and to make any adjustments accordingly. Regular meetings with an independent auditor occurred throughout the total participant observation period. At the conclusion of data collection, the audit report confirmed that the research was conducted ethically, according to clearly described and justified methods and that a clear audit trail was established. The decision to enlist the auditor was made to strengthen the validity of the data, as suggested for this methodology (Guba, 1981; Rodgers and Cowles, 1983; Rodwell and Byers, 1997; Rose and Webb, 1998).

Description of the Settings

Participant observation occurred at a stand-alone public psychiatric hospital within metropolitan South Australia over a period of six months in the second half of 2000 and early 2001. At that time the hospital has a population of approximately 350 consumers, 450 nurses and 300 other professional and service staff. It comprised a series of open, locked and extended care wards staffed by multi-disciplinary teams from the professions of psychiatry, general medicine, nursing, social work, psychology and occupational therapy, as well as ancilliary and administrative staff and volunteers. Several of the hospital's buildings are heritage listed by the National Trust. The hospital displays many features of a 'total institution' (Goffman, 1961a) with many of the consumers having the majority of their needs met within the hospital system of care. the grounds comprise expansive shady lawn areas under tall pines and gum trees, nestled within the inner city suburbs. The hospital is bounded at its main entrance by a low wall, its taller counterpart having been dismantled in 1964 with the process of deinstitutionalisation. Remnants of the moat, previously used to prevent escape, still exist outside the entrance to the main building. All wards have an outside area, designated for smoking and recreation, where both patients and staff congregate. This has become the social hub of each ward and was the primary place for performing participant observation. Staff and consumers involved in the pevious interview phases of the study identified with the psychiatric hospital as their main designated inpatient facility. Each type of inpatient ward was visited multiple times, at different times in the day and different days of the week. Two community hostels within the hospital's catchment area were also visited in the same way as part of the participant observation methodology.

Participant observation also occurred in two hostels within the region. The first of these had a resident population of twenty-four with predominantly older residents between the ages of 45-80 years. The second hostel had a resident population of twenty-four with predominantly younger men and women between the ages of twenty-five to fifty years. Both hostels were characterised by set routines and rules of behaviour, set meals, shared day areas, shared bathrooms and toilets and few single rooms, most residents sharing bedrooms with one to five others. Bedrooms were often sparse and cramped with only a few personal belongings of residents visible. Many residents had few belongings. Both hostels had outside covered areas with seating where the predominant activity appeared to be smoking. Both hostels housed male and female residents, the first with predominantly female residents and the second with predominantly male residents. The hostel staff were non-professionals, with minimal nursing or mental health training. Local GPs visited the hostels regularly, at set times to see residents for medical review and to administer psychiatric treatments. Most residents had an assigned key worker from the community mental health clinic, with a clinic doctor or psychiatrist overseeing the psychiatric medication needs. During the day residents either remained at the hostel or went out to the nearby shops and streets. Some attended rehabilitation activities or sheltered workshops. These hostels were chosen because they were typical of hostels that house mental health patients, as per the researcher's knowledge and experience.

The Observation Sheets

Predetermined standardised observation sheets were used, based on the themes that emerged from the qualitative interviews with patients and staff during the earlier phase of the project. Ideas for the structure of their were gained from adaptation of observation instruments used for evaluation of teacher-student interactions (Simon and Boyer, 1974). An extensive descriptive of each setting and interactions and detailed commentary and reflective notes were kept to support and illustrate the meaning and impact of what the researcher observed, including the researcher's own feelings and reactions to observations. As suggested by Jorgensen (1989) all observations were recorded at the time they occurred or as soon as possible after, with details of date, place, time, main activity and players being recorded. A variety of observations were used:

- Unobtrusive measures - measures of physical aspects of the environment, such as wear and tear in specific areas and use of ashtrays, as noted by Patton's (1980) reference to the study by Wolf and Tymitz measuring wear on rugs to indicate popularity of particular areas of the National Museum of Natural History Smithsonian Institute.
- Sequential measures of interactions between participants - looking at roles, types of behaviours and responses, source, direction of behaviours, modes of communication and their functions and the circumstances under which certain behaviours occurred.
- Descriptive measures - detailing the type of encounters and social milieu of the settings in which they are observed, the composition of the group, their language and behaviours.
- Frequency measures - counting of particular types of events and interactions over set periods of time as a proportion of time spent on overall roles for staff and overall activity for patients. This included counting the consumption of cigarettes for participants over set periods. Measures also reflected the proportion of people engaged in certain activities and the proportion of time they spent in those activities.
- Dummy observation and recording was also used, that is, giving the appearance of actively observing and recording at times when this was not the case and likewise, appearing not to be observing and recording when this was, in fact, the case. This procedure was performed in order to improve the validity and reliability of observations and to avoid "staged" activity by participants.

Participants

The participants comprised inpatient staff and patients present in the nominated wards, as mentioned above, at the time of the researcher's presence at the hospital. It also included participants present in the grounds of the hospital. These participants were potentially from other wards and were observed as part of the social milieu of the hospital grounds. At the hostels, participants included staff and residents.

Gaining Entry and Recruitment of Participants

Permission to enter each site was gained from the relevant authorities prior to entry. These included the service directors and the head nurse at each ward, given their gatekeeper role. Joint ward meetings between staff and patients were identified as a useful forum for explaining the purpose of the study and the researcher's presence. Experience of previously working in this setting and entering it to interview staff enhanced the preparation for entering to observe the participants. The primary researcher's prior work experience in the open, locked and extended care settings gave her the advantage, once in the setting, of gaining greater access and making the role of participant observer more convincing to other members. It also allowed the researcher to travel along the continuum from complete observer to complete participant with skill and comfort, therefore enriching the significance of the observations (Leedy, 1997). Acceptance of the researcher by the participants was particularly relevant in the locked wards and for the culture of the nursing staff role as a 'closed shop' to outsiders. Jorgensen (1989) suggests that participants need to see some gain from the research. For this study, staff were keen to participate because they saw the research as an attempt to address their grievances about the system of care and their working conditions. For patients, there was the potential to influence or improve the treatment they received. Gaining entry to the community hostel setting followed a similar process, with official letters requesting entree permission and detailing the terms and aims of the research, followed by face to face meetings with hostel managers.

Data Collection

Extensive journal notes were kept, recording observations, interactions and reflections from each setting and each visit, either as the settings were being observed or as soon as possible after this took place. The researcher was present in each setting in varying lengths of time as observer and participant, dependent on the setting, the needs of staff and consumers and the circumstances on the day. Settings were visited at random with no predetermined order in mind, occurring in blocks of three to five hours, at various times during the day and evening, Monday to Sunday, dependent on times and days agreed by the managers and the researcher's availability. This allowed for constant comparative observation of the different settings as well as repeated observation of the individual settings. The number of visits to each setting was determined as the participant observation proceeded. Decisions to perform further visits were made on the basis of patterns emerging and needing to be checked out. Decisions to cease further visits were made once the repetition of patterns of behaviour and observation of environmental aspects occurred four or more times. For example, at the first visit a series of general observations were made. These observations were either observed with enhanced understanding or refuted at the second visit. The third visit was an opportunity to confirm the presence of particular aspects observed in earlier visits, and further visits were done to verify previous observations. Where unexpected observations were made, these were noted, with hypotheses made and tested by further observations and reflections and discussions with participants, the auditor and research supervisors.

Data Analysis

As described by the ethnographic method, data collection and data analysis tended to occur simultaneously using the constant comparative method of checking and cross referencing the data (Leedy, 1997). Journal notes, memos, supervision notes and artefacts were organised and arranged according to each setting. They were chronologically ordered so that all the data pertaining to each setting could then be read and re-read several times and coded for recurrent themes and patterns and any leads followed up. As with the earlier interview phases, an independent psychiatrist acted as second coder of the data with inter-coder reliability established for 85%. The methods used to determine overarching themes for each setting are discussed in the results section. The researcher made repeated observations and descriptions of each setting. From these, a narrative account of each setting was made as a preliminary entrée into the analysis of the data. Quantitative data was analysed using descriptive and inferential statistics.

RESULTS FROM PATIENT INTERVIEWS

Patient interviews yielded extensive data about the phenomenon of smoking and mental illness and this is reported in more detail elsewhere (Lawn, 2001; Lawn, Pols and Barber, 2002). Data specifically relating to delivery of care and mental health institutions will be reported here within the following two themes:

The Inpatient Setting
Cigarettes as an Instrument of Control

The Inpatient Setting

Several comments where made about the hospital environment and the system of care by mental health services generally. The impression gained from all participants was that, if people went into hospital as non-smokers, in all probability they would leave as smokers. They saw the peer pressure to smoke and the lack of other activities to occupy them as key causal factors in this.

(Mark)
Sometimes I never used to smoke. It was just good being around other people but they all used to smoke so I just joined in. It was a real social thing. Sometimes it was better than the treatment. Some of the nurses used to come out and have a smoke and talk to you. They'd be talking to you just as a friend, not like when you were talking to the doctor...Seeing them smoking there and talking seemed less intimidating. It helped step over the barrier of us and them.

In one extreme instance, one person recounted her observation of staff treatment of another patient with schizophrenia and brain injury who was prone to wandering from the ward. She stated that staff had encouraged this consumer to commence smoking to give him something to do so that he would not pester them. He was also encouraged to smoke to ensure that he would not wander too far from the ward or abscond, due to the need to come back every hour or so for his next cigarette.

Most participants said that their psychiatrist rarely mentioned their smoking. If they did, they gave it a negative, judgemental connotation or openly accepted consumers' smoking. The assumption gained by these smokers was that their doctor was clearly demarcating the area of their responsibility for treatment and smoking cessation was not included in that area. Community mental health service case managers were also described to be accepting of smoking by these participants and often assisted these smokers to budget for cigarettes. All participants felt that their doctors condoned their smoking, believing that they needed to smoke, that there were other priorities related to illness and treatment, and that they were incapable of quitting because of their illness. The perception of these smokers was that doctors believed that advice on smoking just wasn't relevant to their role as treatment providers.

(Jenny- Talking about her doctor)
He doesn't really talk about it. I have a smoke before I go in there to prepare me to sit there for an hour and I think he's aware of that...but generally it's not a topic we discuss because we're talking about other issues.

(Mark)
The psychiatrist doesn't encourage me to quit because she's a smoker herself. I bring it up sometimes; she says there's nothing wrong with it and that I probably need to smoke for my illness.

Several smokers said that they smoked more once they went to the open ward, due to the absence of staff to limit their consumption, and because the culture of interaction with other patients was more social in the open setting. David's comments highlight a particular problem with the way staff monitored cigarette distribution, with implications for conditioned smoking and the establishment of nicotine dependence.

(David)
Hospital is really boring. The staff and the doctors never mention it, but when you go out the door you get bombarded by people smoking. In the lock up section you have to wait and ask for smoked and that's hard, that freedom being taken away...Like I've been there when I've wanted two cigarettes for one half an hour time period and not one for another three hours and you're taking cigarettes when you don't really feel like one because you know that you're not going to have one for the next period. You have to smoke by their rules. It's like a bit of social control. You can't predict that everyone's going to want a smoke every half and hour because not everyone's like that...I can't afford to have the smokes but I can't afford not to have them. It's a case of weighing up the immediate instead of the long-term and I just don't think that far into the future. I don't see much hope in it.

(Julie - On being in hospital)
Oh, I smoke one after the other, that's what everyone does because you just get so bored; there's just nothing to do. I definitely smoke more in hospital...And also because you've just got no responsibilities, nothing to worry about when you go there. You're in your own little world. You're just walking around and go and have a cigarette all the time because there's just nothing else to do.

The ways in which smoking was accepted, reinforced, and used as a tool in treatment and symptoms management in inpatient setting was also noted by these participants. Smoking was used by staff in these settings as a therapeutic tool to build rapport, facilitate assessment processes, and to manage patients' demands generally.

(Sylvia)
One night in hospital when I couldn't sleep, one of the nurses could see that I wasn't quite right and I went down to her and said I couldn't sleep and could he give me something and she said, "Would you like a cigarette?" and I said, "Oh, I'd love one." She knew what I needed, even though it wasn't allowed. I went to sleep then.

(Anne)
The first time I went to (Private hospital), my primary nurse, she was a smoker, so when it was my turn during the course of the day to sort of sit down with her, she'd always have a smoke...We'd just go out and sit in the garden and it was fine. It helped build up the relationship.

(Julie)
All the therapy's done amongst the patients, not the bloody nurses or doctors. You just go to them when you need something. Smoking's just a way of keeping the patients out of their hair sometimes, it seemed.

For many of these people, smoking was cited as an activity when there was just nothing else to do while in hospital. The poverty of organised activities or encouragement by staff to participate in what was available, and the dominant focus on pharmacological treatments, was noted. Many participant observed staff smoking for stress relief while on their breaks from ward duties, saying this put staff in the position of acting as role models for patients' smoking.

(Jack) It's very boring because of the environment. There's just nothing to do. You don't see the staff unless they come down for a smoke and even then they don't usually talk to you.

Cigarettes as an Instrument of Control

The experience of having a psychiatric diagnosis and the perceived stigma associated with this became part of the everyday experience of those interviewed. The unpredictability of the course of the illness and its destructive effects on relationships, financial security and self-worth came to affect the very core of these people's being. The most striking feature of their decision to continue smoking was the sense of freedom it gave in the presence of overwhelming powerlessness to predict their future and lack of freedom in deciding that future. Smoking appeared to become a search for more autonomy.

(Rod)
I'm told by the doctors that I have to take medication. I get detention slapped on me and get locked up. A lot of the things I get told but I can choose to smoke and drink. So when there's not many choices, to have something you can choose to do is pretty good you see.

(Jenny)
At least I've got a smoke.

James' comments give clues to the unique experience and significance of this source of freedom in the presence of a psychotic illness:-

(James)
Smoking gives me a feeling of freedom that I just don't have with other parts of my life. I can choose when I have my next smoke but I can't choose not feeling stressed or intimidated by my thoughts. I can't choose not to take medication because of the consequences of this.

This perceived lack of freedom was most pronounced while the smokers were being treated in inpatient psychiatric facilities. This role of smoking was inadvertently reinforced by the system of care and the staff administering that care. Talking about her experiences in the locked ward, Jenny's comments and her choice of words, referring to the smoking area as 'a cage' (as it was referred to by staff also), demonstrate the depth of deprivation she felt:

(Jenny)
The whole experience of being locked in a cage for five minutes to have a cigarette, it's just a horrible experience. I didn't like it at all...it's like you get out of this cage and get into the other cage but at least I'm having a smoke and they can't control that bit.

Mark's experience of the open ward was similar:

(Mark)
I just wanted to get back to my house and freedom. Like they let me out and let me go to town, but it wasn't the same. They used to get you up at 8 am and have breakfast, then have a shower and then what do you do for the rest of the day...Every day the same; set meals, medication. A routine I had no say in. At home you can smoke when you want and as often as you want.

Smokers with a diagnosis of borderline personality disorder expressed clear protest against the authority of others, especially service providers. Smoking was one means of asserting themselves, of being self-determining, when other aspects of their lives seemed out of their control, or when they perceived having no say in determining their future. These smokers smoked in an attempt to regain power and control in their relationships with others.

Their comments demonstrate how cigarettes were relied upon to mediate and facilitate interactions and treatment between staff and consumers.

(Kathy)
When you're locked up and treated like animals in a cage, you choose to smoke because there's not much else that you can choose. If you fight back then they throw you in seclusion…When other things are so restricting on you, it's one thing you can decide to do to nark them, to show them that they're really not controlling you. Like if you're surrounded by rules and you feel you're never part of making any of them, you feel powerless; you feel very powerless…Like times I was in the hospital in the past, if they (the staff) gave me that sort of stuff (judging her and trying to control her smoking) I'd just bounce off the walls and laugh at them. I'd give it back to them. When you're just confronted by people who are just labelling and judging and trying to take control. The doctor I've got now tries to give me some control with the management plans and things. The smoking is just there in the background going up and down with the level of control…Every time I go to see my doctor I have to have a smoke before I see her because it gets you so stressed and agitated to have to talk about your illness in their territory and on their terms.

All participants related stories of cigarettes being used, by staff, as tools to reward or punish consumers in order to control their behaviour. John's comments on how this felt exemplify the dehumanising effects of this that he felt. It also exemplifies the likely consequences for people who experience involuntary admission to a mental hospital:

(John – When asked about being in the locked ward and being permitted to smoke every hour) I thought it was a fairly good thing for me and others. Sometimes the smokes were almost used like blackmail so that, if you didn't do the right thing, the cigarettes were denied you. So if you're someone who usually smokes a cigarette every twenty minutes or so you'd be frantic. It takes away your sense of being a person.

These participants spoke at length about the use of cigarettes, by staff, for behaviour control. The descriptions and interpretations of staff behaviour, made by these participants, clearly show the use of cigarettes to manipulate and modify consumers' behaviour.

(Kathy - On the acute locked ward)
It's worse because you're actually hanging out because there's literally nothing to do…They treat the patients differently too. They're a bit more short tempered because, in the locked ward, a lot of the staff don't want to hang around while everyone has a smoke. Whereas, in the open ward, you can come and go. The other thing is how they manipulate you. Like the other day in (the locked ward) they kept saying, "If we don't stop hanging around the nurses station, then at smoke time we just won't give the smokes out." So that's real manipulation in some ways. It's like putting kids in front of the TV to keep them quiet. It's almost like they're using smokes as medication.

(Sandra - Who said she experienced intense suicidal thoughts when in hospital)
I've had several times when I've been in there and the nurses have told me that if I'm good and behave and try to settle down, that I can have a smoke. It makes me feel mad (angry). I think feeling like this helps me to get better.

(Joan)
I've been to [the locked ward] twice. At the time I just thought, "This is it. I've been locked up for life. That's it!" I had these dreadful fears that I wouldn't be leaving. We could smoke in [the locked ward], oh, yes, but they (the nurses) had the cigarette lighters and I felt so embarrassed going to ask for my cigarette to be lit, but you know they were trying to get me going and if you're really depressed you won't do a thing...At [the locked ward], they treated me very nicely. I don't remember how much I smoked but I think I was able to have one whenever I was able to have one...I was just too unwell. So I don't even remember whether I wanted more than they gave me. I know I was craving for them. They (the nurses) were very very good because they let us out in the quadrangle. In fact, I was scared there because of the other people there. (Whispers) It was like a jail there you know. I used to feel guilty for asking for a smoke when they were busy and they'd go, "click," and light your cigarette as if you were inconveniencing them or as if it was a way of controlling your behaviour to keep you out of their way.

RESULTS FROM STAFF INTERVIEWS

Staff responses can be grouped into seven main themes that emerged from the data:

- Staff smoking behaviour and interactions with patients
- Staff attitudes towards smoking by patients
- How staff determine priorities
- Ethical response to patients' smoking
- Smoking as a tool within their work environment
- Accountability for change
- The culture of smoking within the settings

Staff Smoking Behaviour and Interactions with Patients

All staff interviewed commented on the prevalence of smoking by staff and several staff noted the history of staff smoking within mental health services. Although only two of the four inpatient nurses interviewed were current smokers, comments about the high level of nursing staff smoking were common and the statistics represented in this sample may not have accounted for currently smoking nurses who chose not to participate in this study. One inpatient nurse estimated that 75% of current nursing staff of locked wards were smokers. Each direct quote from staff indicates their discipline, setting and smoking status.

(Grace –psychiatric nurse / community / ex-smoker)
One clear picture in my mind was in third year, 1978...when you went into the staff meeting in the morning, everyone smoked. There'd be about 2 people in the staff of twenty to thirty people who didn't smoke. All the staff smoked.

One nurse who had worked in the hospital for thirty-five years recounted his experience of smoking. The future legal implications will be discussed elsewhere.

(Terry – psychiatric nurse / inpatient / extended care wards / smoker)
It was actually work that started me smoking...I was a non-smoker when I started psych nursing. Back in those days the tobacco was supplied by the hospital in bulk in big brown paper bags, and nurses, especially in the K ward (locked) because of the patients inability to roll their own cigarettes, we used to spend hours just sitting there rolling up cigarettes in bulk, and because the patients were incapable of lighting their own or handling matches safely, quite often it was expected that nurses would light the cigarettes for them and then hand them the lit cigarette. That's how I started smoking.

Many inpatient staff spoke about how the hospital environment exerted pressure on them to smoke, indicating that smoking served similar social and emotional purposes for them as it did for patients. These included smoking to facilitate communication between peers, to relieve boredom and alleviate stress. Staff also noted differences in their smoking behaviour dependent on whether they were working in the community or inpatient setting.

(Sasha - occupational therapist / inpatient / ex-smoker)
So I took up smoking because it was the only way that I could get nursing staff to spend any time with me apart from direct confrontational arguments. I'd go out the back and have a fag with them, and that's where they were anyway. They were smoking more than the patients. They were inside and the staff were outside smoking. The only way I could get any informal conversation going at all was to be smoking with them.

(Jane - social worker / community / ex-smoker)
When I'm away from the hospital I have not wanted to smoke at all, for about 3 or 4 months. It was strange, almost like the hospital culture was rubbing off on me. The time I worked at the locked ward, I hadn't smoked for 2 years or 18 months...I smoked continuously for the first 2 months that I worked in the locked ward.

Smoking activity was described as part of the relationship between staff, especially direct peers. It was incorporated into their daily interactions with other staff. Staff ex-smokers identified these peer benefits of smoking.

(Sam - occupational therapist / community / ex-smoker)
Sometimes I'll go out here and sit with the smokers, and have a coffee and sit with them while they're smoking and I'd find that I'd be privy to information that I would otherwise not be privy to. It was like a debrief for the end of the day...all the staff get-togethers and Christmas parties, and it would be all the party people, the smokers, who would stay on.

Several staff had been smokers in the past and these staff said they could identify strongly with the patients' struggles to giving up smoking and smoking for stress relief. Many staff identified with patients' need to smoke, based on their own use of cigarettes or, where they were ex-smokers, their memory of their own former smoking. Non-smokers could also empathise with both patients and staff who were smokers

(Marg – psychiatric nurse / inpatient ward / smoker)
(Regarding condoning patients' smoking) To tell you honestly, it's probably my own nicotine addiction...When I'm stressed about something, I usually have a cigarette and pace.

(Jean - social worker / inpatient / non-smoker)
And the environment must be so reinforcing for staff also...everything in their daily work environment says it's OK to smoke, that this is how you get time out and how you resolve stress.

(Janet – psychiatric nurse / inpatient / locked ward / non-smoker)
In a ward like this where it's fairly full on all the time for staff, it's a good way of getting away from it all just for 5 minutes. It's relaxing before you have to go back in again. I know quite a few who only smoke at work and never do much at home...It's part of the culture of the place.

The use of cigarettes to establish and maintain rapport with the consumers and to gather information from them while they were in hospital was clearly described, with acceptance, by the large majority of inpatient staff interviewed. This was so regardless of their professional discipline and whether they were smokers or not. Cigarettes were openly incorporated into everyday interactions between staff and consumers and non-smoking staff were described by some as less communal.

(Alison - career medical officer / inpatient / non-smoker)
The nursing staff regularly have a smoke with them as part of the treatment and care. Having a smoke with them has some therapeutic benefit sometimes.

(Sue – social worker / community / smoker)
(On smoking with patients and the relationship with them)
It probably improves it...Like people are certainly very comfortable about the fact that I'm a smoker like them, and they prefer that, and they often ask if, once they are transferred out, whether their new worker will also be a smoker, It's one of the very first questions they ask me.

Some staff struggled with this way of relating to patients. They spoke of the pressure involved in being required to step into the patients' smoking culture in order to establish rapport and to gain access. Many staff did not identify this as a problem for them, or as a health concern while others showed that it was an ethical dilemma for them.

(Jane - social worker / community / ex-smoker)

And when I was working in the long-term wards, my ability to empathise and almost openly to model smoking behaviour at different points in time in my career when I didn't have different tools. And realistically, by the nature of the clients that I worked with in extended care, who were really hard to work with and really hard to engage with. And part of working with really difficult clients is trying to find an entry point where you can develop rapport with them. And what was more easy than sitting around with them and having a smoke? It was easy to do this in the community also, but even more so in the hospital ward...you were almost conducting group work over an informal cigarette.

Ultimately, staff comments demonstrate that most staff recognised, accepted and often did not challenge smoking activity within their work environment so that smoking continued unchecked. A description of staff attitudes to patients' smoking will help build an understanding of how and why this recognition and acceptance was present.

Staff Attitudes towards Smoking by Patients

Most staff, especially inpatient staff, spoke about their overwhelming acceptance of patients' smoking based on the belief that patients 'need' to smoke. They believed in and condoned the role of cigarettes in helping patients, especially as it related to symptom management, anxiety, agitation and illness relapse prevention. Their comments demonstrate that they often failed to recognise the symptoms of nicotine withdrawal by patients and therefore interpreted this as escalation of illness symptoms requiring relief with cigarettes.

(Sue - social worker / community / smoker)

There've been people here who are just so determined to get cigarettes that workers have just said, "OK. It's not worth it." Buying them smokes seemed to almost prevent an admission. It's the reality of needing that's the issue...It's the same for psychotic experiences; it seems real to them and that needs to be respected.

(Marg – psychiatric nurse / inpatient / smoker)

We've had people agitated and escalating and we have desperately found cigarettes. All of the nursing staff have given cigarettes to give this person...If it's going to reduce the negative impacts of their illness, then surely it's helpful.

Staff believed that the presence of cigarettes allowed patients to participate more fully in other activities, to provide stress relief and to overcome the sedating effects of their illness medications. The level of acceptance of patients' smoking by staff reflected a willingness to allow whatever helps to provide comfort, as defined by the patients, in the face of often difficult to treat illness. In this sense, staff were not using their health care expertise and knowledge of addiction, dependence and withdrawal to assist patients. They accounted for these symptoms by comprehending them as symptoms of the patients' mental illness.

(Sue – social worker / community / smoker)
It's hard to tell them not to use cigarettes when the fact is that they are trying to deal with symptoms that feel out of control...a lot of people we see have lost a lot of social skills through having an illness and therefore rely more heavily on the smokes and don't have as many skills to get past the dependence on smoking.

(Jill – psychiatric nurse / community / ex-smoker)
I think a lot of people with schizophrenia are quite introverted and with paranoid schizophrenia, quite a loner where you face problems where you don't fit into society as a normal person would. So you're often in your own little world... You're often just sitting. You can't concentrate on TV. You don't want to talk to a lot of other people because there's so much going on in your own mind and if there's not then you're probably sedated with the medications you're on which slows you down. So what do you do? You smoke cigarettes.

(Kathryn – psychologist / community / ex-smoker)
It helps people cope with their feelings...I would never tell anyone they should give up smoking.

The patients' level of functioning and degree of illness effects were considered to be important determinants of the person's level of need for cigarettes. Staff variously condoned patients' smoking according to this, especially those staff in extended care settings. Patients in these settings were characterised by having chronic mental illness. They lived at the hospital, in supported care, or received intensive community input over an extended period. For these patients, assistance to stop smoking was given low priority because smoking was perceived to be a central part of their daily experience and illness management.

(Brian - psychologist / community / non-smoker)
(Regarding a co-worker's heavy involvement in ensuring the cigarette supply for a consumert) He [the consumer] was four years in extended care, and for God's sake, four years in extended care is enough to change anyone. I suspect that all he did for so long was line up for his smokes so it just became his reason for living almost. It was one of the few things he could actually do; was light a cigarette.

These staff saw themselves as having greater responsibility for assisting patients to obtain cigarettes, arguing for their needs on humanitarian and benevolent grounds, or from strictly institutional grounds. In this respect, the management of symptoms and avoidance of adverse social and financial consequences of patients' need for cigarettes, by ensuring the supply of cigarettes, were given greatest attention by staff. These consequences included the social stigma of begging and looking for butts on the street and the financial burden of pawning goods for cigarettes.

(Terry – psychiatric nurse / inpatient / smoker)
(Explaining the process of handing out cigarettes as part of the daily routine)
The illness is best managed with the rigid structure because once you start to vary from the routine, they tend to become easily confused, because of their cognitive function problems, and disorientated about what the routine is going to be.

(Bob - consultant psychiatrist / inpatient)
I focus very much on the disfiguration such as the nicotine stained teeth and fingers, etc. I'll even get the dentist to do a scourge (scour) of everyone's teeth to try and make their appearance seem more normal and acceptable in the wider community...They're more noticeable in the community if they look different.

Several staff believed that smoking performed a number of existential roles for patients. These included the role of smoking to fill the vacuum of daily existence and to compensate for the effects of isolation and loneliness by providing patients with companionship and a sense of belonging when around other smokers. Staff expressed deep sadness, pity and concern for patients. Most staff felt powerless to effect genuine improvement for 'their' patients, several staff perceiving patients to be 'a lost cause', as people who smoke in the face of incurable illness and should therefore be left to smoke.

(Sue - social worker / community / smoking)
I think smoking becomes their friend and it doesn't matter to them what else happens with their social skills...It's a real problem if you can't even order a cup of coffee or take yourself off for a walk somewhere because you feel you can't approach other people. So you think, "What the hell do you do with your life?" You just sit home and smoke.

(Kathryn – psychologist / community / ex-smoker)
What else have they got in their life? It's a comfort, it's nurturing...They've got no money and no friends...They don't know anyone who goes on bloody holidays...It's something they see on TV. It's displaced from them. It's over there somewhere.

((John – consultant psychiatrist / inpatient / ex-smoker)
In my heart of hearts, with patients with schizophrenia, I feel that they haven't got much left for them, so good luck to them, if they want to smoke, let them.

In general, inpatient staff tended to express attitudes that reflected the belief in smoking as one of the patients' few pleasures, whereas community staff comments reflected a tendency to give the consumer more responsibility for their choices. Staff in the locked settings directly placed the pleasure of having a cigarette in the context of patients being deprived of other pleasures and basic freedoms in those environments.

(Janet – psychiatric nurse / inpatient / non-smoker)
(On the locked ward) When they're in here, they've go so little anyway, that's one of the pleasures that they've got.

Many staff of both inpatient and community settings openly accepted the role of cigarettes as a core need for patients and therefore played an active role in helping them to obtain cigarettes and ensuring an ongoing supply. Staff incorporated cigarettes as core items in budgets for patients in their dealings with the Public Trustee for patients on Administration Orders for the management of their finances. Community staff tended to take the approach of allowing the person a period of problem-solving on their own if they came to staff requesting financial assistance to buy more cigarettes, rather than assisting immediately. Overall, however, staff emphasised that patients needed to smoke and staff either advocated harm minimisation as the more realistic option to quitting, advocated for cigarettes, or expressed their opposition to smoking but continued to incorporate the supply of cigarettes as part of their interaction with patients. A health promotion approach with the aim of smoking cessation, as a universal part of health settings, was absent in comments made by the majority of staff.

How Staff Determine Priorities

Staff described how they determined their priorities and how and whether they broached the issue of smoking with patients, according to three main areas of decision-making: prioritising of risks to patients' mental health and well-being, prioritising of professional roles by staff, and perceptions of who is responsible for action to assist patients to quit.

Staff in the inpatient and community settings were unanimous in the belief that there exists a time and place for talking with patients about their smoking. They agreed that it was not appropriate to raise the topic of quitting or cutting down when the person was acutely unwell, that this would hinder their recovery, that it would be like enforcing a 'double dose' of suffering. Inpatient staff also saw the role of assisting people to quit as a community responsibility. The nature of the hospital setting posed unique concerns. The ward milieu in which patients lived and interacted in close proximity to each other, often while in a disturbed or unsettled state, was noted. Patients' abilities to resolve conflict and to manage their emotions were seen to be challenged under these circumstances. This was particularly so for those who were detained against their will. Under these circumstances, smoking was given lesser priority than concern than the treatment of the person's mental illness and concern for the safety of the group. Immediate deteriorating physical health and consumer intimidation of other patients in order to get cigarettes were the only exceptions that prompted staff to intervene to limit consumers' smoking. Nicotine dependence was also treated differently to other drug dependence.

(Marg - psychiatric nurse / inpatient / open ward / smoker)
What they do here is going to impact on their ability to stay in an open ward, and on all the other clients as well. If they get toey at home and smack the wall because they haven't got a cigarette, that's one thing. If they get toey here and smack the wall; number one, they're likely to end up in the closed ward; number two, there are likely to be other people around because basically it's a small community here at any one point in time and whatever one person does is likely to impact on others...and if it's going to actually increase the anxiety for other people and end up with three of them transferred to the locked ward then I have a problem with that. Once they go to the locked ward, you have taken away everything...They can't even choose when they have a cigarette or if they're going to have one. They have no choice left at all. It's completely taken away, and I can't condone that just over a couple of cigarettes...Once they're here, my aim is to keep them on an open ward and to get them as well as soon as I can, to get them back to the community where they belong, and then the choice is theirs. While they're acutely unwell, and probably agitated, what right do I have to agitate them further by telling them they can't have a cigarette. And to me, I would consider that to be abusive.

(Jane - social worker / community / smoker)
You don't want a client at that level of personal distress that they are risking their own personal safety for a cigarette. And people's judgements are so impaired and when you're prioritising what you're there to do, you don't give a rats about their addiction at that time. The addiction is by far the lesser of the evils that you're dealing with at the time. It's just so low on the list of priorities.

In the hierarchy of time and resource management, addressing the smoking problem received low priority except when workers were diligent in assisting patients with the supply of cigarettes. Doctors said that they did not have the luxury of time to spend talking to patients about smoking and quitting. Others saw no therapeutic value in challenging the person's smoking; doing so was in fact seen as undermining their role with the patient and the success of treatment.

(Alison - career medical officer / inpatient / non-smoker)
My priorities are simple and that's getting the patient well enough to go home. I think the rapport is just as important. If I haven't got rapport then my job is just so much harder. If I'm going to lose that rapport by continually suggesting or saying that they can't smoke I don't believe that's the right thing to do for the patient at the time. It's a case of not doing more harm, of maleficence.

The type of setting largely determined how staff prioritised smoking and assistance with quitting. In the locked ward, nursing staff focused on the short-term goal of getting patients to open wards. Some staff, notably social workers, expressed total frustration at working within a medical system that appeared to have double standards regarding smoking by patients while they were receiving treatment.

(Kim - social worker / inpatient / non-smoker)
We treat everybody else's addiction. If they're somebody who comes in if they're withdrawing from alcohol, we immediately put them on a diazepam regime. If somebody comes in and they're withdrawing from nicotine, well it's just tough luck. We really should be treating their withdrawal as well...It's a bit of a contradiction isn't it. The doctors are happy to categorise it as a mental illness but not happy to recognise that it also needs treatment...They won't even write nicobate patches scripts...They just say, "Speak to the social worker."

The open ward staff described their role with patients as fragmented and not likely to be as consistent as more long-term follow up in the community. The provision of assistance with ensuring the continued supply of cigarettes for patients who wanted to smoke, assistance with quitting or to help get the person ready to quit was seen as the role of the community workers who did not necessarily share this view. Hence, tensions between inpatient and community staff often ensued over who was responsible for ensuring the supply of cigarettes to patients while they were hospitalised. The comments of many inpatient staff suggest that they saw action on policy decisions about smoking within the hospital as someone else's responsibility. In particular, doctors said they could do little while the barrier of a predominantly pro-smoking nursing staff existed. Nurses spoke of following the lead from medical staff.

(Bob – consultant psychiatrist / inpatient / non-smoker)
(On smoking) It's something that's largely nursing reinforced, and from a medical side, I've got to convince my nursing staff to give up first.

(Janet – psychiatric nurse / inpatient / non-smoker)
(Regarding doctors and the smoking issue) They tend to lump everything on to the nursing staff, rather than buy into it themselves.

The majority of comments by all staff, about others in the multi-disciplinary teams in which they worked, showed a significant degree of frustration regarding the smoking issue. Some staff coped with this by blaming other professions or placing responsibility for change onto others, as mentioned in the previous section. A few staff chose to distance themselves from the debate altogether

(Janet – psychiatric nurse / inpatient / non-smoker)
If they want to smoke, that's fine by me. I haven't really thought about it that much. I just never think about it.

Ethical Response to Patients' Smoking

In their role as health care service providers, staff made decisions about their ethical stance on the issue of smoking generally and smoking by patients, according to various ethical principles. This determined their actions and inaction within the system of care. Staff made several rationalisations about patients' smoking. These can be grouped into three main areas of ethical decision-making:

The right to smoke- self-determination
Free and informed choice to smoke
The hierarchy and priority of concerns and harms

When asked what they thought about patients' smoking, most staff interviewed spoke of their belief in patients' right to smoke. Staff were mindful of imposing their own value judgements on patients and mindful of the power imbalance in their relationship with patients. Staff were particularly concerned for those patients hospitalised against their will, in hostels and under Administration Orders for financial management. Staff identified strongly with the role of smoking as giving the patient greater opportunity for autonomous activity, as already highlighted in their comments on patients' 'need' to smoke. Staff spoke of the need to compensate patients for a perceived lack of choices within the system of care. Ultimately, most staff appeared genuinely to struggle to work out their own ethical stance.

(Sam - occupational therapist / community / ex-smoker)
They smoke out of hospital, so why should it suddenly mean they be made to not smoke in hospital. When we've taken away everything else, all other rights. Are we going to take that away as well?

A small number of staff questioned those who claimed to be making value free judgements as misguided in their ethical thinking. They argued that actions are never value free. These staff said that they regularly strove to assist their patients to quit smoking.

(Grace – psychiatric nurse / community / ex-smoker)
If we had safe cigarettes tomorrow, I suppose my argument would end, but they're not safe and they never have been and the politics of smoking is just disgusting. I'm sure the human rights arguments came from the tobacco companies...Often people, in the pursuit of what they perceive as their human rights, present spurious arguments. You can't argue with, "Well, I like it and I'm going to do it." You can't argue with that if the person knows the risks and they choose, but misinformation, you can argue with, and I tend to give people articles and cartoons.

(Jane - social worker / community / ex-smoker)
It's also easy to rationalise by saying it's their quality of life, it's their only pleasure. We don't have to question it or push very hard for it. It's like sometimes it just comes out of the too hard basket so it's easier to just say it's us granting them their self-determination and therefore we don't have to do anything about it...People will explain anything as duty of care if they thought they wanted to justify it.

Staff also spoke of patients' smoking as an informed choice made freely without restriction and based their full knowledge of the harms and costs of smoking. Some staff used this reasoning even when they also acknowledged that choice was not fully informed. Staff did not see a duty of care to intervene with these patients regarding their 'choice' to smoke despite the harms. However, staff used the duty of care argument when seeking guardianship orders for treatment and financial management with regard to other 'choices' made by patients that were deemed to be harmful to their health. Staff also used this argument when patients' spending on cigarettes occurred at the expense of meeting core commitments like accommodation costs or food.

Only two staff clearly argued that smoking was not an informed choice by patients. One person spoke of the interaction of mental illness with smoking and the other person spoke of the role of addiction influencing the smoker's decision-making capacity. This was separate from staff comments and beliefs about patients' need to smoke, to be discussed elsewhere.

(Terry – psychiatric nurse / inpatient / smoker)
This ward helps them limit because it recognises that it is not informed consent to smoke. Other workers are like fence sitters who just say it's their right to smoke rather than buying into the debate. It's very much individualised here according to the person's capacity.

(Bob - consultant psychiatrist / inpatient / non-smoker)
Anything that has a primary addiction habit means it is not a level playing field. It is not a free choice, and I don't pretend that it is. Therefore, we as professionals must assist. Therefore they are not making an informed choice because of the clearly addictive nature of the stuff.

The third form of reasoning used by staff in deciding their ethical stance on patients' smoking was to propose a hierarchy of ethical concerns that guided them in prioritising harms and duty of care towards patients. Related to the staff prioritising of their actions, as discussed in the previous sub-theme, many staff perceived smoking as less visibly damaging than more immediate problems faced by patients.

(Terry – psychiatric nurse / inpatient / smoker)
I accept that it affects their health in a derogatory way, however, I think the greater priority is the immediate client and staff safety. And if withholding cigarettes is going to increase client irritability and the potential for aggression or violence, I think the long-term decline in their health is the lesser of evils, because of the potential that the immediate violence can cause. And I've seen the results of that, and that has an immediate and devastating effect on people's lives....

One staff participant made several angry comments about the prevalence of debate on the smoking issue in contrast to debate about other practices occurring within the hospital setting. Her hierarchy of concerns was clear and smoking was low on her list. Her comments point to other ethical concerns within mental health services and to the conditions in which staff and patients spend their day.

(Sasha - occupational therapist / inpatient / ex-smoker)
(If there was a smoking ban in the hospital) I think we'd distress an awful lot of people unnecessarily, and a whole lot of staff would be distressed also, and some would leave. That would be close to bordering on cruel. How could we say that we are doing that for their health, but feeding them such low quality food, and housing them absolutely inadequately? And if we're talking about care, maybe we should be talking about actually how often someone manages to get a shower in [extended care ward], or how often a really unwell woman has been left to menstruate without pads, those type of things. If we're so concerned about physical care, has anyone cleaned those guy's teeth in the last four years. I find it hypocritical that we'll give them a drug that will reduce their bone density, but we'll go on about their smoking...It amazes me that you can't even get a bloody condom in this hospital for free.

The majority of staff, regardless of the professional alliances or practice setting, spoke openly about smoking reinforcement and acceptance within the mental health system. They proposed various reasons for their actions that appeared to be based on their beliefs and attitudes towards mental illness, mental health patients and the system of care. This in turn informed how they acted or did not act to assist patients with their smoking and quitting.

Cigarettes as a Tool within Their Work Environment

In the previous themes, staff comments have indicated that they believe patients use cigarettes for a variety of reasons. Likewise, staff have also indicated that they use cigarettes to perform a number of roles with consumers.

(Janet – psychiatric nurse / inpatient /non-smoker)
It's a good way of establishing rapport with a patient and getting good relationships so that you can get a working relationship with them. When they first come in and they really don't' want to be there, it's a good opportunity to sit there and they're more relaxed so they're more likely to talk to you, so you've got a better idea of what's going on.

This theme describes the most dominant theme to emerge from interviews with staff, that is, the use of cigarettes as a management tool to manage patients' perceived mental illness symptoms and behaviour. In the same way that patients said they used cigarettes to manage the symptoms of their illness, staff condoned and reinforced this same process stating that they used cigarettes to reward and punish patients in order to assert control over their behaviour. They did this in response to occupational health and safety concerns regarding verbal and /or physical threats made towards them by patients. This was especially evident in comments by staff from inpatient locked and extended care settings. All of these measures were described as having developed over time and become an entrenched part of the daily interactions between staff and patients. The effects of nicotine withdrawal were not mentioned.

Several staff spoke about the historical development of this use of cigarettes, citing several decades of official hospital policy of providing a tobacco ration for consumers in expectation of behaviour and treatment compliance. Terry's previous comments, referring to the 1960's, about nursing staff duties to roll and distribute and light cigarettes for clients have already been noted.

(Grace – psychiatric nurse / community / ex-smoker)
(Speaking of her time working in the hospital in the early 1970's) And cigarettes were a currency. If you wanted the patients to do something, you could give them a cigarette and they'd probably do it. In fact, I can remember my first ward, the charge sister saying, "Go and run this errand and I'll give you a cigarette. Go and make you bed and I'll give you a cigarette...." It was how you got things done...If you wanted to talk to someone about something, you'd kind of offer them a cigarette and at least you got their attention for the time it took to smoke a cigarette. It was a salesman kind of ploy.

(Peter – psychologist / community / ex-smoker)
(Of the hospital and smoking in the 1970's) Smoking was seen as something that was therapeutic, and that was the last thing that you would deprive people of if you wanted to keep them unstressed, or pleasant, or non-aggressive, or whatever.

One staff participant described the consequences of the power exercised by staff over patients, claiming that the system of care leads to situations of abuse of power.

(Paul – psychiatric nurse / inpatient / ex-smoker)
Like, back in the 1970's there was a lot of abuse. I worked in a lot of security hospitals where people [staff] who wouldn't hurt a fly, once they're exposed to that environment, you see people change, and it's quite true what they say about power corrupting, very much.

All staff spoke about an inherent structure that existed within the mental health system that created and perpetuated power imbalances between staff and patients, placing staff in the dominant role. Staff were not necessarily happy with that role. Several staff noted the effect the setting and of having locked doors separating staff and patients and the 'us and them' situation that this created.

(Grace – psychiatric nurse / community / ex-smoker)
(talking about the locked ward at the hospital) It didn't have a positive feeling at all. The ceiling was too low; the sound was deadening; and it had the feeling of being in a waiting room all your life...The smoking area is really a cage like you put animals in. When I was acting ADON (Acting Director of Nursing), I remember one day I went into the cage, and there were several smoking staff in there at the time and the interaction was that a group of staff had a conversation and the patients were kind of, "sit down and shut up." It was perhaps not quite to the extent that that's what they were told, but it was quite clear that the dominant activity going on there was staff having a smoke and talking to each other...

(Paul – psychiatric nurse / inpatient / ex-smoker)
If they didn't smoke, they wouldn't come back to the door every half an hour either. There's something about having a closed door between us that makes the difference. It's a real power thing. It's a typical us and them situation. The staff retreat to be behind the closed door...It seems to be institutionalised. I mean, even if you didn't follow that procedure, just merely by being here and being exposed to the way the ward operates, the policy, and the staff; staff tend to adopt a certain mentality of control, just because of the environment. It's easy to give people cigarettes. It's easier than not giving them.

(Kim – social worker / inpatient / non-smoker)
Simply having the door as the barrier; that becomes part of the reward/punishment stuff. It's not that the person has deliberately used it in that way; it's just the fact that it's a locked door. It's very disempowering. But it's not just that; it's the sense of a locked ward where all your belongings are taken away from you. Your smokes are taken off you. Your laces and belts and jewellery are taken off you, actually encouraging you to come to the door every five minutes if you want something.

The extended care wards were identified by staff as areas where staff control over patients was very pronounced. This was based on cigarette distribution to patients being overseen by nursing staff as part of routine policy on the wards.

(Sue – social worker / community / smoker)
There seems to be even more paternalism in the extended care wards. People are handed out cigarettes as if they had no self-discipline. Almost all extended care nursing staff do control cigarettes on the ward and you do see them, yeah, packaging them all up in lots of 5 and 10 with all the names written on them. "Here's your cigarettes. Don't ask for any more until tonight or when the next lot comes, or whatever". Most people get them dished out 2 or 3 times a day in a package already made up and that's amazing. It's been like it as long as I've known.

Several comments were made by staff about the giving and withholding of cigarettes as part of everyday staff - patient interactions in order to influence patients' behaviour.

(Kate - trainee psychiatrist / inpatient / smoker)
When you're in the locked ward where there has to be supervised smoking, it does give you some bargaining power in terms of, "I'll talk to you now. Sit down and we'll have an interview and then you can have a smoke."

(Sasha - occupational therapist / inpatient / ex-smoker)
I've seen nursing staff who will bow their head and tote their forelock and hide the cigarettes in the top drawer and measure them out, because they can. It's a control thing. And if they haven't got the skills to relate to someone like a bloody human being, and have to do it by measuring out the smokes, and when they arrive in the paddy wagon, it's like, "Just see the doctor and then we'll take you out for a smoke."

(Janet – psychiatric nurse / inpatient / non-smoker)
(On the locked ward) Why should we be so like prison wardens and say, "No, you can't have one [a cigarette]?" I think a lot of the time it's power games with some nurses…like, "I'm the nurse and I'm looking after you and I can tell you what to do," kind of thing. That's the feeling I get from a lot of the nurses…I remember an incident once when we had some exams here for the doctors and they were bribing patients to agree to sit in and be used in the exam, like, "We'll give you 20 extra cigarettes if you agree to do this." I just thought it was amusing…If they're going to do something, then they should get some benefit from it, if that's the reward they want.

(Sue – social worker / community / smoker)
(On the hospital) In such a controlled environment and because of the punishment system and the reward system, there tends to be a fair bit of that in the locked wards where, "You'll get a cigarette when you behave".

This use of reward was particularly noted in the extended care wards where the distributing of cigarettes was described as a core part of nurses' duties to maintain the order of the setting.

(Terry – psychiatric nurse / inpatient / smoker)
Because the majority of the ward are heavy smokers, the patients here tend to watch each other, so if one gets an extra smoke then the rest will want it, and staff here have learnt very quickly that it's unfair to do something for one and not the other because they have to do the same for everyone, and it becomes a very expensive exercise after a while. So generally the staff don't, except the rare occasions if the patient does something like a favour or something like that, then we slip them a 'good one' [better brand].

Many inpatient staff described their work environment as a place where staff control over patients was continually tested, in that they continually needed to assert their authority over potentially violent patients and deal with potentially out of control situations. The inpatient nursing staff, in particular, highlighted their fear of assault by patients. They saw the use of cigarettes as directly improving the safety of the work environment, even though smoking was not officially sanctioned as part of hospital occupational health and safety policy in this respect.

(Terry – psychiatric nurse / inpatient / smoker)
Both from a nurses and client management perspective, if you can keep the ward running smoothly and minimising the amount of aggression, by allowing them to smoke, then allowing them to smoke facilitates that. By all means, I'd rather have a smooth running ward than go home with a broken arm.

(Jill – psychiatric nurse / community / ex-smoker)
It's just too complex to think about really. I just treat it as a day to day thing. It's just in the too hard basket. Smoking is an easy solution and sometimes it's the only one there readily available when someone is about to snot you one...Letting them smoke is the easy option.

(Janet – psychiatric nurse / inpatient / non-smoker)
I think that because in the inpatient setting you've got so many patients in close proximity to one another, that if one gets agitated because they haven't got their cigarettes, then it could just upset all the other people around them, or they could just go around pestering or being a nuisance to other patients, saying, "Can I have a cigarette?" So in the inpatient setting we try to ensure that they have cigarettes to keep them settled. And I think the consequences of not giving them a cigarette can be a lot worse than giving them. Like, I've seen patients hit because they've been pestering other patients for a cigarette because they haven't got any...(If there was a smoking ban) I think there would be more medication given; I definitely think a greater amount of PRN would be given, especially for agitation, and things like that. And there'd be a lot more incidents and violence as well.

At a more routine, day to day level, many inpatient staff commented on how staff control the supply of cigarettes (and lighters in some settings) to patients as a way of keeping the peace, to ensure the smooth running of the setting, to reduce fire risks and in the best interests of the patients for their protection and the protection of others. This idea is further illustrated in the section describing the culture of smoking with the settings. Of note, most staff descriptions of inpatient routines and rules about smoking clearly placed the nursing staff in the direct role of control over cigarette supply and distribution to patients.

(Alison – career medical officer / inpatient / non-smoking)
The nurses don't normally try to limit too much unless there's a problem with other patients and with staff and then they try to limit it to one every couple of hours. They keep the cigarettes locked up in that case and hand them out one by one. The problem they find when they hand them out in packets is that the other patients who smoke are congregating with that patient, almost demanding at times to get smokes from them so one of the things they try to do is to keep the cigarettes in the nursing station...especially if you've got a patient who is fairly timid and they'll just hand over their whole packet with the stand over tactics of some of the other patients, and that's impossible to really monitor all the time.

(John – consultant psychiatrist / inpatient / smoker)
You don't want patient X to be exploited so why not try to manage the exploitation. That's what the nurses are there for.

(Kate – trainee psychiatrist / inpatient / smoker)
When the patients come in and ask for their cigarettes, it means it's one extra contact that they might not have had with the nursing staff, otherwise you might never see them...So it gives them a reason for having to make contact with the nurses. Like, I've been in areas where the nurses would go out the back to smoke with the patients and that way they would get some information...It's fairly acceptable practice, and all the nurses do that.

(Terry – psychiatric nurse / inpatient / smoker)
(On the extended care ward where nurses keep patients' cigarettes in named pigeonholes within the nursing area and distribute them to patients) Most people here don't carry their own smokes on them. There's one or two that can. The nurses decide who can by first of all considering the risk factor that they're not going to be a fire danger to the ward, that they can comply with the rules about not smoking indoors, or in their rooms, but also not vulnerable to being stood over by those who are persistent in the know about cigarettes from others. Some people, because they're incapable of handling money, effectively have canteen accounts...They're allowed to purchase up to $2 or $3 in items on a daily basis. It's a vulnerable situation, of being vulnerable to being ripped off by others if they had the money on them, due to stand over behaviour and so on.

(Terry – psychiatric nurse / inpatient / smoker)
(On the supply of cigarettes to patients in the locked ward if they haven't had the opportunity to buy their own) It's to keep some semblance of behavioural order, I suppose. It's certainly a big factor in those environments and also the resentment of seeing other clients who might have heir own smokes when they don't have any themselves, that can provoke them to some extent. So yes, it can help keep the peace in those environments.

This perceived need to keep peace and order extended to the wider community, with staff identifying further consequences of denying patients cigarettes in the hospital setting.

(Terry – psychiatric nurse / inpatient / smoker)
(Regarding a smoking ban) I think people from the hospital would start going around knocking on doors, or walking around the streets looking for butts, or accosting people in the street...That would certainly increase; and the criminality aspects.

Only one staff participant challenged the notion of staff overseeing the distribution of cigarettes and lighters to patients in order to improve safety on the ward.

(Paul – psychiatric nurse / inpatient / ex-smoker)
One of the reasons why we hold the cigarettes and tobacco here is because they say it's a safety issue...I don't know. Like I worked at [the gaol] for 4 years and certainly all the inmates there had their own cigarettes and lighters and they didn't go around setting fire to

their cells or things like that...(If they had their cigarettes to carry on them?) Oh, I think they'd feel a bit more in control, rather than everything being taken away from them.

In inpatient settings, staff said that the key-locked nurses station door provided a significant barrier between them and patients, as well as protection from potentially violent or difficult patient behaviour. One staff participant commented on how the current system and its structures operate to disempower patients. He made suggestions about how this could be changed and gave evidence for these suggestions.

(John - consultant psychiatrist / inpatient)
I've had an interesting experience with the locked ward. as an example of disempowering people, there was a time about two years ago or so when the hospital nurses went on strike and they all went out. It was quite amazing and so a lot of us decided, regardless of what the rights of the nurses were, you couldn't leave the patients without any care, so we volunteered to provide that. Another doctor and I spent the first afternoon looking after people in [the locked ward]...We simultaneously decided that this was ridiculous so we just opened the door and said to the patients, "Well, there you are, just take one when you want one," and I swear to you the smoking went down. The other interesting thing was they didn't come intruding into the nurses space...they didn't feel as intimidated by the barrier.

One staff participant argued that the smoking policy change of banning smoking indoors had a significant and noticeable effect of the power differential between staff and patients in the inpatient locked setting.

(Jill – psychiatric nurse / community / ex-smoker)
It changed when the rules changed which meant that you could only smoke outside which meant you had to open all the doors up, which meant you had to have a certain amount of staff in the courtyard with the clients. That's when it became a really noticeable issue of control between the client saying, "I want a cigarette", and the staff having to say, "Well, we can't go out right now". It created tension. So it was a staffing issue around smoking rather than a safety issue of the ward in general.

Overall, smoking was overwhelmingly accepted as part of the work setting by all disciplines involved in interviews.

Accountability for Change

Each profession responded differently to the smoking issue within the inpatient settings. One social worker saw the nursing staff as being scape-goated by the doctors. She saw the doctors as ultimately responsible for leading decisions about smoking policy.

(Jane – community / ex-smoker)
I think for doctors to say that their biggest barrier is the nurses is an easy cop out. They [the nurses] are such an easy target and when they're trying to get people to give up smoking, blaming the nursing staff is a quick solution...passing off blame is rife.

All social workers said they felt pressure from the system of care and from other professions, especially from the nurses who they said pressured them to collude with the process of ensuring the supply of cigarettes to patients. Social workers described this as feeling like a process of entrapment in which their professional and personal values were being compromised.

Social workers expressed a high degree of anger, despair and anxiety about their own profession. They felt disillusioned with the system of care for clients and with the smoking issue. They were well aware of the dilemmas posed by the problem of smoking; most social workers said they made adaptations accordingly.

(Jane - community / ex-smoker)

I'd moved from the point, on the one hand, of hating the fact that, as a paid clinician, I was spending my time going to the shop and buying fucking smokes for people and often that would take an hour and a half of every day with the bank run for a number of people. And I was developing a relationship with the woman at the bloody smokes shop because I was there so often...I found that very degrading but then I'd combat that ethically by saying this is seen as a client need and this is what I'm called up for, that's great, you know. Who am I to be sanctimonious about that I should only be a clinician? ...On the flip side of the coin, you had clients who were so diempowered and had had so much removed from them that, to be able to go to the shop and get them a bloody chocolate bar and a packet of smokes that they wanted, was so enabling and allowed me to work with them in such a different way from what the doctors and nursing staff did because I didn't have the same power kick...but I actually resented the time I had to spend doing that.

Like their social work counterparts, the inpatient nursing staff made several comments about doctors' non-involvement in the smoking issue and pressure from doctors for nurses to 'just fix it'. Nurses said they felt much pressure in their roles, often simply because of their close proximity to patients and the smoking and their role in providing direct care. Inpatient nurses who were not smokers said they reluctantly performed their role in handing out cigarettes to patients, finding ways around pressure from the system of care to perform this duty, rather than challenging it outright.

(Paul- inpatient / ex-smoker)

I give out cigarettes only when I have to, only because I'm following ward policy. I try not to...I won't stay out there. I'll only light one person's cigarette and then I'll ask them to all get a light off each other. I won't hang around out there, mainly for my own health because of the passive smoking.

(Janet – inpatient / non-smoker)

I hate it. I absolutely hate it being out with the patients while they're smoking. So I stand in the doorway or keep away.

Doctors made very few comments about other professions in the context of smoking; most made no comments. Those doctors who did comment directed their comments at the nursing staff.

(Alison – inpatient / non-smoker)
It's easier for me than the nursing staff to stand back from it because I don't smoke. Most of the nursing staff smoke and they find it beneficial. Most of them find they can go out with the patients and have a smoke…I've seen them with a patient of mine who's been very irritable, walked out and was going to storm off, and the nurses would say, "Let's just go outside and have a cigee (cigarette)," and they've settled down, and they often do. Whereas, I wouldn't have been able to do that in that manner…I can't go out with them and have a cigarette.

Doctors' comments about their own profession demonstrated that clients' smoking was largely an irrelevant issue for them, the mental illness having a far greater priority. They abrogated responsibility for involvement by defining the smoking problem as not part of their role. It was the least experienced doctor who made comments that showed the greatest questioning of professional values with regard to patient care and smoking.

(Kate – inpatient / smoker)
In mental health it's such that you've asked it so many times [whether patients smoke or not]…you become complacent. [Does it worry you?] Yes it does…I'm trying to keep checking on myself about my values and how I'm becoming part of the culture of just accepting it.

Of all staff interviewed, psychologists made the least comments about their own and other professions. They saw themselves as completely autonomous and separate from other professions and the day-to-day care of patients, preferring the role of 'specialist' who provided therapy to usually willing patients and consultation to other professions.

The lack of occupational therapy services and staffing at the inpatient setting had forced the two occupational therapists there to limit their role and work with particular individuals rather than install group programs. Their services were seen as outside the system of care and constantly under threat from further funding cuts. They felt powerless and saw other staff in this way also. They presented themselves as mere observers of all that was wrong with the system, with little or no effect on it or the smoking within it.

Overall, each profession made general comments about patient care that reflected their roles and responsibilities within the multi-disciplinary team. However, debate about the smoking issue, rather than being a team approach to the problem, tended to fuel inter-disciplinary professional rivalries, especially in inpatient settings. Most comments reflected a high degree of powerlessness, despondency and acceptance by all staff within the mental health system. The high prevalence of smoking by patients seemed too hard for staff to address and few saw it as their responsibility; the consequence being that no-one took responsibility. This warrants an investigation into the systemic culture of the settings in which the staff worked.

The Culture of Smoking

Many comments were made about the hospital culture by both inpatient and community staff. Most participants in this study had trained in or had recent experience of working in inpatient wards and used the hospital setting as their point of reference to describe the overall culture of mental health services. In this sense the power exerted by the inpatient setting in shaping both inpatient and community mental health culture was significant, with many facets of hospital life transferred over to the community setting. Three aspects of the culture of inpatient psychiatric settings will be described, as highlighted by inpatient and community staff:

- The environment of the hospital
- The barter system, and
- Reinforcement and acceptance of smoking

Several staff participants recounted their knowledge of smoking policy in the hospital in the past, with many highlighting that there were plenty of opportunities to smoke and plenty of smokers, staff and patients. In this respect, they described an historical level of acceptance of smoking as a shared activity by both staff and patients, of unwritten rules that all were aware of.

(Peter - psychologist / community / ex-smoker)
(As a student at the hospital in the 1970's) I couldn't actually pick out who were the patients and who were the staff. Almost everyone smoked...they literally hid behind a cloud of smoke.

Staff described the physical structure and layout of the hospital wards and the organisational structure of routines around doctors' and nurses' duties as contributing greatly to the elevation of the role of smoking and its core place in daily activity within the setting. This was particularly evident in comments about locked wards, but was equally applied to open wards where each external area immediately outside the ward was called 'the smoking area'. Each of these areas was described as a centre for interactions between patients. This was also seen as a focal point for staff and patient interactions, as was the nurses station door.

(Kim - social worker / inpatient / non-smoker)
You often get people who come in who just automatically come up to the door asking for cigarette, and you say, "but you don't smoke," and they say, "oh, that's right." Because it relieves the boredom, they go out there and see all the others doing it.

One nurse described the effect that such a system and its structures had on his approach to his work.

(Paul – psychiatric nurse / inpatient / ex-smoker)
I've worked in a lot of hospitals around the country and security hospitals and things; mainly locked settings. No community. I'm institutionalised. It's quite a culture.
There's a lot of similarities to be drawn between the prison system and the closed wards here; the seclusion rooms are like isolation cells; locked doors; staff with keys; there's a great similarity. That's why I can roam between a prison system and a closed setting somewhere with little difficulty...you can run on autopilot.

A psychologist described how his experience of the inpatient setting influenced his views about the system of care and the patients:

(Peter – psychologist / community / ex-smoker)
(Reflecting on the inpatient environment and the clients there) It's like a gaol. They've learned to survive and some of them may be lost in their world of hallucinations and so on but the majority of people in the hospital didn't seem to be doing that. They just seem to have this knack of not being stressed out by not doing anything...They smoked like cows in a paddock munching on grass every so often.

The impact of these arrangements for staff and patients, with regard to smoking, was of much concern to many staff participants. Of particular note was the perceived sense of powerlessness, expressed by staff, to have any meaningful influence on improving the current situation. Mirroring the patients' conditioned social behaviour, staff said they found it easier to deal with just what was in front of them on a day to day basis.

(Paul - psychiatric nurse / inpatient / ex-smoker)
And they know the routine. It's just, "Oh, we're in [locked ward]," (Knock, knock, knock on the nurses' station glass door) It's just an instant thing. They turn off to it and so do the staff.

(Sasha - occupational therapist / inpatient / ex-smoker)
I think the demoralisation and the lack of skills amongst staff, and the lack of support for staff working in this environment, is what perpetuates that system where little is done to overcome the problems of the hospital culture where staff continue to be fully aware of the stand over tactics, and the violence that occurs in order to get cigarettes.

One aspect of the hospital culture, described at length by staff participants, was the extensive informal barter system used by patients involving cigarettes as tradable commodities. Again, staff spoke about the historical beginnings of this practice. A tobacco ration was, in fact, a formal part of hospital policy for patients throughout the nineteenth century in psychiatric settings. According to Peter, this practice continued up until the 1970's and only changed when people with a psychiatric illness became eligible for government pensions and benefits for the first time and therefore could buy their own cigarettes. Hence, the source of supply changed but the practice continued as an understood activity within the system of care.

(Peter - psychologist / community / ex-smoker)
(Previously inpatient in 1970's)
By having a tobacco ration, in effect, people took up smoking because they got a ration. It was like being in gaol. If you give up this something, that's still a tradable commodity. If you didn't smoke, you still got a ration. You could barter with other people.

Several staff described their full knowledge of the current informal system of barter with and for cigarettes, often with amusement, but always with acceptance of its practice. This acceptance was true of all staff interviewed from all professional disciplines. Many staff made direct reference to the setting parallelling a gaol culture where levels of hierarchy and understood rules of interaction and survival exist between 'inmates', one of these being that 'you don't rat on your mates' to the staff.

(Ros - social worker / inpatient open ward / ex-smoker)
They know how to trade with each other. It's quite a little community with the trading. And it's also an emotional thing where they'll give someone a hug and say, "Hi, (and give them all these positives) and by the way do you have a smoke?" And they have a system where people genuinely haven't had cigarettes and then they've traded and you'll find they'll usually repay in kind when their next payday comes and they can buy a packet.

(Terry – psychiatric nurse / inpatient / smoker)
One of our clients has quite a little business going. He purchases his own cigarettes on a daily basis and then sells them to other clients at a slight profit...They have $2 or $3 a day pocket money, no more, and whatever money they've got left over, they're then able to buy any extra cigarettes that they might need.

(Bob - consultant psychiatrist / inpatient / non-smoker)
Occasionally we have entrepreneurial people who charge considerably more than the cost of the cigarettes, or they'll actually use cigarettes in order to get sexual favours...But it's a case of knowing that it's happening because a lot of these people are reticent to tell staff about other patients' behaviour because it's part of the culture that exists that you don't tell. It has it's own social rules...Smoking still accounts for the main form of language amongst the mentally ill.

The barter and sale in other drugs was also fully known by staff. They said they felt ineffective in preventing it's occurrence, other than token attempts to contact police when they sighted known dealers in action on hospital grounds. A number of patients of extended care wards and other inpatient wards were known by staff to be dealers.

(Terry – psychiatric nurse / inpatient / smoker)
There's quite a healthy little skirt (drug dealers living nearby) around the hospital that do this (come into the hospital to deal in illicit drugs), and the oval over the other side of the hospital grounds has quite a little conglomerate of people that gather there doing their deals.

Several mechanisms were reported for the reinforcement and acceptance of smoking by patients and staff within inpatient settings. This too had a history according to staff participants. The structure of brief breaks for staff on duty in order to promote equity between smokers and non-smokers is one example of this. Staff also believed that patients had nothing else to do and should be allowed to smoke as a result. Staff said that they found observing patients' smoking behaviour was an effective assessment tool for observing their level of interaction and degree of paranoia or other mental illness symptoms, assessing them as more isolative and paranoid if they avoided interacting with other patients in the smoking area. Admission of patients to the inpatient setting was seen, by all staff interviewed, as the surest initiation into smoking for patients if they had entered as non-smokers.

From the comments made by staff, several points are the same, similar, or bear direct relationships to comments made by patients who were interviewed. The high order of priority given to cigarettes and the central role of smoking in helping staff to cope with and to manage the mental health service environment is of particular note. To further validate the comments of patients and staff and to elicit more detailed information on the dynamics of interactions involving smoking, participant observation of the settings was seen to be necessary. Distinctions between the settings were also implied by patients and staff and these needed to be tested and understood more fully.

RESULTS FROM PARTICIPANT OBSERVATION

Description of the Settings

Participant observation occurred at a public stand-alone psychiatric facility within a metropolitan area of Australia. The metropolitan area served by the hospital comprised a population of approximately one million people. The hospital had a current population of approximately three-hundred and fifty patients and a staff population of four-hundred and fifty nurses and three-hundred professional and service staff. It comprised a series of open, locked and extended care wards staffed by multi-disciplinary teams with staff drawn from the professions of psychiatry, general medicine, nursing, social work, psychology, occupational therapy, administrative and ancillary services and volunteers. The hospital had a significant history with several of the buildings being declared by the National Trust for preservation. The hospital displayed many features of a 'total institution' (Goffman, 1961a, 1961b, 1961c) with many of the patients having the majority of their needs met within the hospital grounds and subject to set routines and schedules imposed by the system of care. In the past, the hospital also had workshops, orchards and market gardens within its grounds, now lying idle or sold off for housing as it is increasingly encroached upon by the surrounding suburb. At the time of participant observation, the remaining grounds comprised expansive shady lawn areas under tall pines and gums. There was a sense of sanctuary within the hospital grounds in contrast to a number of secluded areas within these grounds, better known these days for their drug dealing activity and sexual exchanges. The various buildings were mainly one and two storeys with gargoyle statues still keeping watch on some of the corners of the older buildings. The hospital was bounded at its entrance side by a low wall; its taller counterpart having been removed in 1964 with the process of deinstitutionalisation. Remnants of the mote, used to prevent escape, still existed outside the entrance to the main building. Regarding the various wards, all had an outside area, designated for smoking and recreation, where both patients and staff congregated. This had become the social hub of each ward and this was the primary place for performing the participant observation. Up until May 2001, the hospital canteen held a license to sell tobacco and provided free cigarettes to indigent patients in the locked wards.

Number of Visits Performed in each Settings

Acute Locked Ward	4
Extended Care Locked Ward	5
Acute Open Ward	9
Extended Care Open Ward	8
Canteen/Grounds of Hospital	5
Community Hostel (1)	6
Community hostel (2)	6

Communicating Findings

Results from the participant observation phase are presented in the following ways: firstly, snapshots are given in the form of vignettes that describe a typical day in the life of the people in each setting, the aim being to present a holistic description of the everyday experiences of staff and patients in the settings. Each vignette is followed by a description of the dominant characteristics of that setting and participants within it, that is, the most prominent cultural patterns that emerged in relation to smoking. These dominant characteristics were determined by coding the data collected from each observation period in that setting, then drawing together all the data from that setting into chronological order and recoding the data from this larger data set and constantly comparing the data. The dominant characteristics reported were routinely apparent during all visits. A description of quantitative data from the observation sheets is then provided. In the final section, all aspects of the participant observation are drawn together as a series of themes that describe the overall picture of life in these settings.

The Acute Locked Ward: (Beds = 10)

Afternoon in the nurses' station sitting room leading into the work area overlooking the patients' day room. The patients' area, with its absence of décor except for foam seats in the centre of the room and a television attached high up in one corner, is in stark contrast to the cramped and narrow nurses' area, crowded with desks and other office furniture and several years collections of cartoons and memos stuck haphazardly on every piece of available wall space. It's hard to decide who is in the fish bowl, the staff or patients; who is the watcher and who is being watched, as each is separated from the other by a series of waist high glassed panels and doors that allow for complete vision by all to all daytime areas. The nurses have just finished supervising lunch. Keys sound to unlock the series of doors that lead all back through to the day room. A male nurse comes through from the adjoining door, ready with the ice-cream container of cigarette packets, ready at the nurses' station door. He stands with the door ajar and calls out in a loud voice: "Who wants a smoke?" He calls again just in case some of the patients didn't hear the first time. Next to him, stuck on the glass, is the smoking policy for the ward and details about the hazards of smoking and passive smoking. As quickly as he has reached the door from one direction, the patients have come through and some are already lined up waiting for their cigarette. The smokers' cage is a small concrete-floored room of approximately two metres by three metres, attached to the ward with wire mesh on the two exterior walls to give access to the open air and therefore fulfilling the smoking policy requirements of no smoking indoors. It becomes quickly crowded with eight of the ten patients and two staff members, all smoking. One nurse squats on the concrete floor of the cage, rolling herself a smoke, engaging in calm conversation with one of the patients. It's an opportunity to relate to some of the patients and get to know them better. Others stand concentrating on the ritual, tolerating each others' company momentarily, nervous and suspicious, relieved to finally have something to do. The two non-smokers wander aimlessly in the day area unattended.

As the afternoon wears on, the staff busy themselves with answering phones and doing paperwork. They take turns at sitting in the patient day area, reading the paper, coming in to the nurses' station for respite periodically. Patients pace aimlessly in the day area, occasionally coming near the glass to look in to see what the staff are doing. Staff tend to remove themselves into the second room away from patients' view; clients tend repeatedly to approach the glass to glare silently through at staff or bang on the nurses' station door for attention when they see a staff member in the work station. There doesn't appear to be a happy medium; the barrier is fixed. The staff continue with their tasks, sometimes offering calm reassurance, sometimes ignoring, knowing that the requests for cigarettes will be denied as it's not smoke time yet. In the day room, a client lies on the foam couch in the middle of the room sleeping, a blanket half falling on the floor next to him. Others pace and hover. Few patients exchange words with each other. Many stare suspiciously, walking guardedly within the small empty space of the day room. The main entertainment is watching the nurses move around from behind the glass. The grassed enclosure that serves as an exercise yard opens to the fresh air but is not used today; the door remains locked. Through the wire mesh of the cage and the nurses' station glass, the blue sky is clearly visible.

In the seclusion corridor, a young female patient cries out and bangs defiantly on the locked door leading into nurses' sitting room, the Venetian blinds drawn from the nurses' side to give them some respite from her gaze. The nurse calls out gruffly, "Have patience, I can't do everything at once." The patient wails, paces, staggers, acts confused as the nurse reassures her finally, "Have a bit of a rest and then I'll take you out for a smoke." A short time passes and the secluded client becomes restless again, "I have rights you know." The nurses retort, "We have rights too, not to be yelled at." Two nurses stand quietly, imposing, speaking softly to the patient at the doorway. The desired effect is achieved; she settles briefly. They re-enter the staff area, shutting the door quickly behind them and agree that this case warrants giving her a cigarette to pacify her, sooner rather than later. She is taken through the doors and assisted to smoke, then returned to the seclusion corridor. All is calm. Meanwhile, another nurse hurries to the nearby shop to purchase cigarettes for his patient. He's on his tea break and happy to oblige. Outside in the 'sheep run', the security corridor between the locked wards, a casual agency nurse sits alone, relieved to be having a break away from the milieu, smoking hard on a cigarette.

Dominant Characteristics of the Acute Locked Ward

Smoking as a Core Activity

Of the total number of patients present in the acute locked ward, most or all were observed to participate in the smoking routine at each designated smoking time. All cigarette packets were kept together, labelled and ready near the nurses' station door leading directly to the patient area. Patients often knocked on the locked nurses' station door or stood next to it waiting for some response from staff. Staff often went about their duties within the nurses' station in spite of this, often only responding when the person's behaviour appeared to escalate. Patients frequently needed to be told to wait when they requested cigarettes outside of the designated smoke time. Staff smokers were frequently observed to join in the smoking routine with patients during these designated smoking times. Verbal and physical aggression by patients, towards staff and other patients in the context of cigarette supply and the smoking routine, was commonly reported by staff and observed.

A Low Stimulus Environment

Apart from set meal times and set smoking times, other structured activities were absent. The clients' television was switched on at various times, although few patients were observed to be watching it; most paced or wandered back and forth in the day area or sat, usually alone, or slept, especially throughout the afternoon. Nurses variously took turns at spending time in the patients' day area, some reading the newspaper, doing a cross word puzzle, or playing simple card games with a patient. The workload of nursing staff was observed to be unpredictable; sometimes they were very busy making phone calls and organising around particular requests, and at other times experiencing extended periods with few duties other than being present on the ward. Reading and sitting talking with other staff was common. Most staff took the opportunity to have their lunch break away from the ward altogether. Doctors usually only entered the patients' area to perform detention reviews and clinical reviews, otherwise they made notes and performed other duties in the staff areas often away from clients' direct vision or away from the ward altogether.

The Nurses' Station Door

The nurses' station door acted as the most common point of interaction between staff and patients, with shared smoking in the smoking cage being the second most frequent interaction point. Meal times were the third most frequent interaction periods, this being when medications were also routinely distributed. Individual nursing care duties involving personal care for patients was also a routine part of the day, as were detention reviews where nurses accompanied doctors into the patients' area. The nurses' station door was the point where most requests were made and most interaction was initiated between staff and patients once they were on the ward. It was also therefore a common point from which refusals or limit setting by staff and protests by patients occurred. The promise of cigarettes was often made by staff in order to manage patients' mood and behaviour. Conversely, patients were regularly heard to threaten to 'act out' when denied cigarettes outside the designated times. During the observation period, no reference to the use of NRT was made, and none was observed to be offered or used.

The Extended Care Locked Ward : (Beds = 11)

It's 7.25am. The nurses have congregated in the nurses' station for handover. The room is extremely cramped, with staff standing huddled together, those without seats leaning against the wall and the doorway. The dull lighting hides the ageing paint and evidence of disrepair. The last of the night staff have just gone. A couple of patients in the corridor tap tap on the small, high glass window separating the staff and patients. No response given except for a silent glance. "They know the rule – requests only at the designated time." The glass dulls their voices. They gesture for cigarettes in almost playful defiance, testing the limits. "They know that smoke time is not for another five minutes. The limit setting and consistency is important in helping them with their cognitive disorganisation."

Out in the entry area, now a makeshift space for the medication trolley, one nurse takes ironic delight in showing me the stair case leading to a now disused part of the building; the vinyl covered steps scarred with the many butts that were stamped out as patients and staff from another era entered the building, the black dots appearing less and less as they ascended. He recounts vivid scenes of smoke filled rooms. "Everyone smoked". The burn holes on the floor underneath each window are large and profuse where once there were large ashtrays. Renovations have been a long time coming here. He recounts the day management came for a tour during a rain storm, to find "buckets here and there catching the leaks and possum piss running down the walls…They don't come here very often. We've been waiting years for the plumbing to be fixed."

Smoke time every hour, on the half hour. Everyone cues ready as usual, some chatting and more sociable, others quiet and withdrawn. They all know the routine. Most have been here a number of times before from the open wards and are known to the staff. Their faces express an odd mixture of disappointment at being here again and jovial camaraderie. Some are watching and waiting. Most are in their late twenties and thirties. They pass through the doors one by one once everyone is assembled, cigarette in hand, after the nurse has attentively handed them out one by one from the makeshift lunchbox, making sure each patient has their own cigarettes according to the names on each box. One patient doesn't have any. Today is payday but the revenue department is not open yet. It's too early. The nurse provides him with one so he doesn't miss out. He has been good this morning and the nurse perceives that he needs a smoke as much as the others. In the courtyard, we enjoy the morning air and light conversation. Everyone is satisfied.

The staff take the opportunity to talk about their concerns as they smoke and watch the patients. It's time out for everyone. They are disgruntled with the social worker refusing to do a bank run for smokes money for the patients now that the case aide's contract will not be renewed. "Isn't that her role after all. For what else do these patients need in reality." One nurse tells me how this environment is much less severe than the prison system where people sometimes go a whole week without cigarettes. Another nurse talks about a young female patient, how she has been transformed in the system of care here, how in the past she was rewarded with food to comfort and settle her excessive, often unmanageable behaviour. Attractive then, she is now obese and hardly recognisable as her former self. She returns here often, rarely out for a day before some act of self-harm brings her back to familiar surroundings again.

It's late morning now. It's going to be a scorcher today. The day room is filled with both patients and staff, passing time. It's too hot to go outside. Here and there patients lean against the wall, sit on the floor, or lie down on one of the foam couches. Smoke time. The nurse positions herself at the door to the smokers' cage, a shady room buttressing the outside with wire mesh and railed seats all the way round the edges. She holds the lunch box of cigarette packets under her arm, lighter attached at one corner with a string. She tells them in her organised voice to line up along the line, marked with tape stuck on the grubby carpet on an angle to the door. They do so without argument, one behind the other, waiting for all to assemble before the door is opened. She calls out and reminds them to 'Get in line", as they increasingly crowd her. Another nurse comes to her aid with another lighter, one each side of the line. They create a smooth production line through the door, lighting cigarettes as they go. The usual nurse sits out there with them, smoking and supervising. Another nurse takes the opportunity to duck out the back to have a quiet smoke on his own. I ask a nurse why this ward is particularly sociable with staff spending much of their time during the day in direct contact with patients. "I suppose we try to make the best of it seems we're all in here together. Then everyone is better off." In the smokers' cage, the nurse is lecturing one patient about the risks of sharing butts and transmitting diseases. Others sit more quietly, concentrating on their smoking ritual.

It's afternoon and hot. Lunch is over. The cutlery has been counted and is all accounted for. The patients and staff have moved back to the day area. One nurse decides to spend some time outside with her patients under the trees in the enclosed yard. She takes their smokes with her; a bonus smoke to help set the recreation time. Lunch was stodgy today. One nurse shows his disgust. "The dietician should be sacked. Do they realise the level of bowel cancer and other physical illnesses in these people." The chooks [chickens] appreciate the left-overs. Inside, two nurses sit planning and reading up on their notes. They're organising the shopping list for the afternoon in preparation for the weekend ahead. There is much discussion about where the best prices for smokes and coke are, and what shops are a rip off. One nurse rings the supermarket to check their specials for the day. In the day room, one patient maintains her stance not to eat or drink. Her goal: "To die". She continues to join the smokers' queue throughout the day.

Dominant Characteristics of the Extended Care Locked Ward

Togetherness

The style of interaction between the staff and patients was the most noticeable feature of this setting. Both staff and patients shared a very high rate of smoking and smoking together during the set smoking periods. Staff in this setting spent much time in the patients' area and in direct contact with them, often playing pool or in light conversation. Staff routinely joined in during meal times also. At these times, the uniforms worn by staff were arguably the only feature that clearly distinguished them from the patients; as one staff member put it, "We're as institutionalised as the patients". Humour was common between them and the group cohesion, ritualised routines and regimentation was striking.

The Centrality of Smoking

The regimentation and routines involving smoking appeared to form the foundation from which all other activities and routines were measured and prescribed. Meals, ward rounds, movements between the day-time area and the night-time area were always preceded or followed by a smoking period. Cigarettes packets were individually labelled, budgeted for and bought by staff from the canteen on campus, and meted out at set times and lit by staff. An important role for each nurse was to ensure that their patients had sufficient funds from their pension, managed via the revenue department, for the purchase of enough cigarettes to meet their immediate needs. All patients were observed to be smokers and were totally reliant on staff to ensure their supply of cigarettes whilst in the ward.

Together but Separate

Under these circumstances, daily care was described by staff as a process of behaviour modification, the goal being to help patients learn that there are consequences for actions. This interaction occurred in the context of a parenting role, with many of the patients known to these staff over a long period of years. However, this was tempered, at all times, by the potential for violence by patients, and the conscious process of providing maximum security care with all its attendant keys, locked doors and regimentation. The starkness and poverty of the décor was oddly balanced by the chooks that roamed the internal enclosure. In response, the patients 'played the game' and largely co-operated with the institutional rules and routines, their goal being to be seen to be behaving in order to gain the freedom of the hospital grounds once more. The revolving door cycle of patients returning to the ward was regarded as inevitable. Hence, coexistence by staff and patients in this ward was always flavoured with an 'us and them' ambience to all activities and interactions between staff and patients. The sociability and communal feel on the ward served to reduce the incidence of violence and to help alleviate stress levels for both staff and patients, as they each dealt with the incarceration. Within this context, staff also felt separate from their colleagues in other wards and particularly suspicious of management whom they perceived as having little understanding of the realities of care in the context of incarceration. One staff member explained the ward's uniqueness in this way, "We'll have them even though all others have rejected them." Staff enjoyed their exclusiveness, their high walls allowing them a peculiar type of autonomy within a system that they saw as largely foreign to them. For example, they recounted with delight, the day that they managed to get a donkey inside their enclosure without the knowledge of the rest of the hospital. This ward truly felt like an asylum enclosed within the larger system.

The Open Ward : (Beds = 24)

Early morning driving into the hospital grounds past the open ward enclosure set aside for the early morning risers prior to the main entrance door being unlocked for the day. It's a crisp and clear morning. A group of six patients and a night-staff member congregate, smoking, inside the open door leading into the activity room that doubles as a staff meeting room for ward rounds. They've learnt that the fire alarms don't go off if they blow the smoke towards the open door. On the wall the sign reads, "This room is a declared non-smoking area." Someone has blocked out the 'non' with paint some time ago by the look of the faded colours.

Late morning outside the main entrance door to the ward, numerous patients congregate; some in small groups, some more isolative, suspicious, openly voicing or mumbling paranoid ideas, sitting away at a safe distance; sitting against the wall, lying on the grass, or sitting at the table and chairs next to the door. All are smoking. Some sit, others stand and pace up and down the path leading to the ward. It's a day like every other day. The boredom is numbing. Mealtime gives brief relief. The radio blares out across the whole area. No-one is listening to it. One patient is intrusive and suspicious. He sets the mood for the area. The other patients keep their distance. They feel uneasy needing to be in the same area in order to smoke. The reminder of his unsettledness isn't helping them. They focus on the smoking and draw hard. Inside, the staff are constantly on the move, getting requested items for their patients, answering phones, running errands, or writing notes. The smokers among them come out to join the patients for a smoke when they have a free moment. A patient comes in to use the nurses station phone to give a relative a call to negotiate them bringing in some clothes for her. Another patient, having just had a shower, sits at the desk as his nurse helps him comb through his long matted hair. The environment is reassuring as they chat amongst themselves.

One patient returns from her walk around the grounds; it's her fifth for the afternoon, she says. She sits and lights a cigarette and is momentarily occupied and relieved. Another patient joins us, looking perplexed, "I've got to try not to keep sleeping all day." He lights another cigarette and stares out across the lawn. Inside, clients sit on the worn and grubby lounge chairs lined up in the small foyer adjacent to the door, watching the activity as nurses and patients come and go. Occasionally, one gets up to have a cigarette outside. It's a continual rotation of sites throughout the afternoon. The music blares on in the background.

Early evening now, and the smokers' area is busy with people as they wait for teatime to come. The sun has set and a light shower falls as people huddle under the narrow eaves next to the front door to the ward. The music is still loudly playing. A nurse has popped out to join the group and grabs a quick smoke before teatime. A new arrival under escort, comes despondently up the path to the ward, bag in hand. He goes in with his nurse, dropping his bag at the nurses station door and comes outside to have a smoke and make small talk with us, as if practising a polite initiation in this unfamiliar group with whom he will be spending the next few weeks. He nervously asks for a light and takes a deep breath.

Dominant Characteristics of the Open Ward

Boredom
The high level of perceived boredom experienced by patients was the most striking feature of this setting. Although there were opportunities to participate in or initiate other activities, such as playing pool, going for walks, joining in token occupational therapy art groups, and so on, the majority of patients in the open wards sat outside in the smoking area immediately in front of the ward, went to the canteen, or roamed the grounds to fill in their inpatient days. The expectation that they would eventually leave and return to their community homes was played out as a process of waiting and making the most of the company while they were there. As time and treatment proceeded and these patients began to recover from the mental illness relapses that brought them into the hospital, they became

more sociable and sometimes more restless. Smoking served to fill in the time. Sharing cigarettes served as an icebreaker to initiate newcomers, or when patients sought out the company of others to relieve their boredom.

The Nurses' Station Door

The use of the nurses' station door as a formal barrier between staff and patients was observed in each open ward, being closed when confidential staff discussions were in progress or when staff were absent, hence preventing tampering or theft of confidential notes and belongings. The degree to which this barrier took on a combatant feel varied between each individual open ward. This appeared to be due to the physical design of the different wards, as much as the group ethos of the staff within each different open ward. In some wards, the nurses' station door was kept open at most times when staff were in the nurses' station. This allowed for more open interaction with patients and attending to their individual needs. However, in other wards, the nurses' station door was always kept shut whether staff were present or not. These wards were characterised by quick entries and exits of staff. The barrier served to keep patients out and distant from staff. In one such ward, the physical design of the nurses' station, with its high windows and corner position made it appear more like a fortress. A couple of boxes of matches were conspicuously placed on the window sill outside the door so that patients could help themselves, and not need to bother staff with any requests.

The Primacy of the Here and Now

The focus on immediate treatment, illness symptom management and day-to-day monitoring of patients' mental state was also a noticeable priority in the open wards. What happened beyond the internal walls of the ward was perceived variously as beyond the control or influence of staff and therefore not their business or responsibility. The immediate priority of ensuring that patients had access to their finances and hence, an uninterrupted supply of cigarettes, was stressed in day to day planning with and for patients. All else could wait until the patient was discharged, to be resolved once they were back in the community.

Extended Care Open Wards : (Beds = 24)

Early morning. It's 7am. Upon arriving at the ward, the nurses' station door is quickly and firmly shut behind us. We're in a fishbowl again. The nurses move into the second room to talk away from view of the patients. From time to time, a client approaches the outer door, knocking incessantly. Staff respond with delay, ignoring, or providing a quick, brief response, then return their focus to the 'handover'. Staff express their level of powerlessness on the smoking issue. I'm advised not to tell the patients that I'm a social worker for fear that they will hound me for money for cigarettes if I do. I leave the nurses inside with their heater, put on my gloves, shut the door and go out to meet the patients.

In the smoking area next to the front door to the ward, the grass is littered with more than three-hundred butts. A cleaner is busy sweeping the concrete. The dust and ash flies up. The patients sit silently on the lined up metal seats along the window next to the door of the ward, smoking one after the other; most are in their thirties. They don't appear to feel the cold. My teeth chatter as I tuck my hands into my sleeves for warmth. No one speaks, except to say hello, then contemplative silence or blank looks again. They look at the ground or stare down the path out into the grounds. There is a chorus of coughing. One man verges on choking before his spits on the concrete in front of us. Nearby, an occasional sparrow comes down onto the table to peck at any crumbs left from the day before. I strike up a conversation with a male patient. He proceeds to explain the ward routine to me. Asking for a piece of paper, he proceeds to write in rote fashion the various meals and organised activities for the week. His face is vacant and emotionless. His eyes seem like bottomless pits of despair.

A patient from the adjacent ward comes over from his smoking area across the way. "Please give me a smoke love? I'll give you $3 dollars for it." He realises I'm not a smoker and moves away, picking up butts next to the ashtray on the ground as he goes. He gets no response, not even a glimpse, from the other patients. The staff are nowhere to be seen out here.

Dominant Characteristics of the Extended Care Open Ward

Us and Them

The physical and emotional distance between staff and patients was the most striking feature of their interaction in the extended care open wards. Staff clearly saw themselves as providing paternalistic and regimented care to dependent patients. Staff rarely interacted with patients, other than at the nurses' station door or when in the smoking area themselves. Smoking as a transaction involving basic human contact was therefore elevated in significance for patients. Staff regularly talked about the patients in the third person, despite the patients being present at such time. Structure and routine and predictability were the order of the day. Hence, many patients were left to sit outside or to roam the grounds, returning to the ward for meals and bed. Many patients in these wards had their cigarette supply controlled by staff, with a daily allowance from the revenue department and cigarettes rationed from individually labelled pigeon holes in the staff area.

Life in a Vacuum

The lack of interaction between the patients was also noticeable. Although they often shared the same living and smoking spaces, most rarely spoke to one another in conversation, except to ask for a cigarette or a light. The level of distress or paranoia from illness symptoms combined was noted. The perceived vacuum existence for many of the patients observed while near the ward, was also noted. Satisfying the nicotine addiction and ensuring the next cigarette seemed to be of greatest priority to these patients. There were few friends here, each patient observed to be ultimately watching out for themselves and watching their backs; often silent, offering few signs of recognition to those nearby and staring out the corner of their eyes as others approached. Requests for cigarettes by other patients were usually denied, as all were on strict budgets. They seemed afraid to relate, as these clients had shared living space for years in some cases and they knew who could be trusted to pay back and who could not.

The Acceptance of Smoking

The attitudes of staff towards smoking, their level of acceptance and the proportion of staff smokers on the particular ward (especially where they were in leadership positions), appeared to influence how the ward staff as a whole perceived and responded to patients' smoking. In wards where most nursing staff smoked, there appeared to be a higher level of client smoking and a greater belief in patients' need for cigarettes and inability to quit. Patients in these wards were also charged reduced boarding fees if they were a smoker.

The Canteen, Grounds, and Outside the Revenue Department

All roads lead to Rome. Like ants, the patients come from each corner and crevice of the surrounding buildings. Sitting on a park bench along the stone wall bounding the open lawn on one side; the canteen on another side, several tall trees providing much shade to the tables and chairs at the other end and just beyond them, the revenue department. Further off, the gated entrance to the administration buildings. It's approaching 9am. Outside the big wooden door of the revenue department, patients begin to line up ready for opening time. More patients emerge one by one in all directions from the various corners and cracks between the buildings. Payday means cigarettes. Some are lying on the grass, others crouch against the wall or sit on the concrete and smoke while they wait, others wait patiently and watch in expectation or borrow a smoke and promise to pay back once they get paid. Everyone is co-operative for this very important task for the day. Not long to wait now!

As the morning progresses, the canteen area of tables and chairs becomes a hive of activity and sociability as patients sit in groups, chatting. They come and go, calling out greetings to each other from across the way, or sitting for extended periods at the tables smoking and talking, catching up with their fellow patients. "How have you been?" "How long is it since you were last here?" "A couple of years ago." "See ya. I'm off to see so and so in ….. ward now." Occasionally, a staff member passes through on their way to another part of the hospital or to grab something from the canteen. The chatter quietens or stops as the patients watch the staff pass through. Sometimes they hiss and mumble. The staff do not stay, but hurry on their way. This is not staff territory.

One by one, the patients check me out to make sure I'm not a staff member before they will offer further conversation. Two patients sit at a distance. They sneer and mumble. Eventually, one comes up to me to ask what I'm doing. We tentatively shake hands and our conversation begins. He speaks of his lack of hope and feelings of powerlessness and dependence on the hospital and of the disappointment of being here again. A lady sitting quietly nearby, watching all this time, finally summons up a question for me, "Are you the police?" She pauses for a few moments and then has another try, "Have you ever lived in Canberra [national capital and centre of political activity]?" I reply in the negative to both questions. Later in the morning, a patient who tells me she has been here for more than thirty years, comes over and joins me. She insists that I share her coke with her. She respects that I'm a non-smoker and says, "I wish I was." We chat about how nice the surroundings are; "It's freer here. The ward is depressing; it's staff territory." Then she gathers up her bags and is on her way, but not before handing me an apple. Under the trees, the garden workmen sit at the tables and chairs having their morning break. A female patient comes from nowhere, wearing a combination of bright, mismatched clothing, plastic bags and extra clothes in hand, and immediately asks them politely for a smoke. One is given without hesitation and she is scurrying on her way again as quickly as she came.

It's lunchtime now; the canteen is deserted except for those patients who don't like the menu for today – fish. The ladies serving in the canteen know all the regulars. It's a daily ritual. A large glass screen with holes in it separates them from the customers. They are curt, impatient, emotionless. Outside, I'm joined by an Aboriginal man who has seen me buy a can of coke from the canteen and has seen me put my change in my pocket. He says, "By the way, have you got twenty cents for a phone call?" and soon followed with, "Can I have some of your coke, please?" Another male client approaches us and asks the man for a light. He fumbles through his pockets, at which the other man becomes abusive and starts threatening to kick him. They make aggressive gestures to each other before the other man leaves. "It's a jungle out here," he mumbles.

Dominant Characteristics of the Canteen and Grounds

Territorial Activity

The communal atmosphere and the sense of the canteen being patients' territory, as opposed to the ward which was perceived by the clients as staff territory was in striking contrast in both the clients' descriptions and actions in the settings. The table and chairs outside the canteen served as a meeting place where patients could talk freely without staff presence. They congregated regularly as part of their social interaction away from the ward. Staff rarely entered these communal meeting places. When they did, they came and went quickly and sometimes awkwardly, only sometimes acknowledging the clients and usually not speaking at all. In response, the chatter between patients would stop abruptly as a staff member approached, accompanied by suspicious jeers and derogatory mumbles until the staff were gone again. In line with these unspoken territorial rules, patients did not enter into staff administration areas. Large iron locked gates bared entry on the weekends, and despite them being open during the week for anyone to pass through, patients did not enter into this territory.

A Market Place

Smoking was a constant activity in the background, and served to mark the sociability of the occasion in these settings. Observing patients who were not smoking was a rare occurrence. Joining together to smoke was observed to be how these patients clearly strengthened their group cohesion in these settings. However, this also meant that cigarettes were a much sought after commodity, competitively vied for like a commodity in short supply. Under these circumstances the full range of talents and abuses were able to emerge and to flourish, dependent on the skills and personalities of the people involved. A market economy of barter and negotiation was routinely observed, with exchange items including clothing, food, money, other personal belongings, threats and intimidation. Although no direct observations were made of patients exchanging cigarettes for sex, staff spoke of this as 'common knowledge'. Hospital patients were also noted to be providing very healthy business to a nearby pawn shop.

The First Community Hostel: (Beds=40)

Break of day at the hostel. It's 7.30am. It's cool and mild. The smoking area is deserted. The chairs are lined up ready for today's activity. The seven ashtrays have been emptied the previous night and are lined up ready for today's deposits, though already they have received the offerings from those who couldn't sleep. The ten kilogram coffee tin, now a makeshift ashtray, sits amongst them ready to help cope with the load of butts envisaged for the day. The concrete has been swept early, the table sparkles. Inside the sounds from the kitchen as the cook busily prepares breakfast. An occasional sound of showers and running water as the residents slowly emerge from their beds.

A middle-aged man comes out in his pyjamas, half down on one side and surveys the smokers' table and sifts through the ashtrays for butts. No luck yet today; they're all smoked down to the filters. Straight back inside. The usual three elderly ladies come out together. They light up their smokes and make small talk. "I like your jumper." "It's Tuesday today, isn't it?" The middle-aged man rushes back out now, stands over the ladies and immediately asks them for a smoke. The second lady says, "I'm not meant to give them to you," but she relents. He makes conversation with them as they all smoke together. Two male residents come out and take up positions alongside the ladies. The staff member comes out. "You didn't give him one did you? He's not meant to ask for them. I'll get his in a minute. You mustn't give them away. He gets his own money for smokes." The tall lady replies. "No, we didn't give him one," as they all look like the cat that swallowed the bird. The staff member shakes her head and returns a cigarette to her to make up for the one she gave away. When the staff member is gone, they all confer and stress to the second lady that she only gets five cigarettes and they have to last her for the morning. She immediately gives this cigarette to the man. "Now you only have four left." The three women leave and the three men stay. The middle-aged man breaks wind loudly as he smokes his second cigarette. He stands pressured, restless, already lining up his next cigarette as he finishes his second. He persists with one man and then the other, over and over again asking, "You got a smoke? You got a smoke?" They remain silent. He returns inside to try his luck later.

The staff member moves busily here and there, getting breakfast organised and supervising the showering, as she is the only one on duty so far. One lady has been incontinent again. A mop and bucket appear instantly. The smell of cigarettes and toast and the sound of residents being directed here and there fills the morning air. The three ladies have returned to have a smoke. A small lady has sat down and begins patiently to roll a cigarette. The middle-aged man is outside again. He stands silently over her, insistently. He has apparently cornered her inside. The coughing is horrendous from all. She tells him to sit but he says no, preferring to stand, shuffling his feet in expectation. She hands him a smoke and proceeds to roll herself one. Through the sliding door, a lady in the adjoining room sits patiently as the staff member attends to her personal care. The staff member hands her the three cigarettes she is rationed for the morning. Her eyes beam as she holds them tightly between her fingers. "OK sweetheart, enjoy." The middle-aged man has, in the space of thirty minutes, managed to bott [cadge] five cigarettes so far. He persists again as he stands over one lady, holding a half-smoked cigarette behind his back. She yells back at him after his third plea, "No." He eventually leaves. Before she finishes her first cigarette, she lights the second from it. The third follows in similar style. No more now till late afternoon, unless someone responds to her pleas beforehand.

It's 9am now. Another lady is showered, dressed and she's off to the bank and then local shops to buy more cigarettes. She returns in minimum time. She says she plans to sit and smoke for most of the day. "I'm sixty soon. I've done my jobs for the day, so I can do what I want to now." A younger man sits quietly at one end of the table, in the corner as he does most days, smoking, silently observing the antics of the middle aged man and the others. He's passing time. A young man in his early twenties quickly comes out to the smokers' area. " Do you want some coke for a smoke, please, do you want some?" "No," the old lady replies gruffly. He immediately moves to the next person and gets the same response. He goes to the butts and lights what seems like nothing left of a cigarette and sucks quickly on it. He persists with the ladies. "It's nice and cold. You can have as much as you want? Please?" he asks each person who comes out. There are nine smokers now. The elderly lady who had given one away previously says, "I'll get into trouble if I give you one". He leaves abruptly again. Another elderly lady returns from her brief walk, through the cloud of smokers. She's an ex-smoker and rarely sits in this area now due to her asthma. She huffs and puffs as she goes. The ladies congregate again in peaceful, polite conversation. They share a light and smoke, attempting the small social graces. The young man comes again, holding out his coke. This time, he's successful with the lady who rolled her own beforehand. They all sit or stand around smoking, concentrating, saying little to one another.

The Second Community Hostel: (Beds=40)

Mid-morning at the hostel, coming up the driveway, the area is strewn with clients sitting on the plastic seats or on the curbing, or standing, pacing aimlessly and all smoking. Most are in their twenties and thirties. They have many more years of this existence. I have the overwhelming sense of this not being a home, rather a place for people to exist in parallel, together but separate, as few words are exchanged with each other, only the occasional vacant look or stare. Talking to a young female resident, "It's really hard here because everyone smokes. I find I've got less to look forward to the longer I'm here. I spend most of the day doing the circuit of the hostel, pacing through the building and up and down the drive, over and over, smoking." This is a common activity for many residents.

Late afternoon now and we're sitting under the large veranda at one of the many tables and chairs. Ashtrays are strewn throughout the area although the blackened concrete, strewn with cigarette butts, suggests that few people use them. Twelve residents sit or stand as a fragmented group; few talk to each other. Next to me, one man looks beseechingly and attempts the social graces. He deserves whatever conversation I can offer him. He talks about his dreams of meeting a lady and having a life together. He's been here for five years now. He manages a half smile through his blackened, crumbling teeth. His fingers are stained from many years of smoking. Life here appears to have a dampened pace. "It's just good to have someone to talk to. You know you can get pretty lonely, even when there are other people around. Will you be coming here to visit me again?" A staff member is shuffling through the storage cupboard next to us, cigarette hanging out the side of his mouth for the duration. At regular intervals, he shares the cigarette, exchanges puffs with one of the female residents. It's a ritual requiring few words.

Evening now: single rooms, individual televisions and four walls. Residents emerge occasionally to have a smoke. It provides intermittent relief in the later hours of the day and into the night. Beyond the front gate, the suburb sleeps.

Dominant Characteristics of the Community Hostels

Quality of Life

The impoverished lifestyle of the residents of the community hostels was the most noticeable feature of these settings. Their day seemed to be filled with little more than eating, sleeping and smoking. Their actions seemed to be beyond a mere loss of hope; they spoke and acted as if they were powerless to participate in any future other than the banal existence in which they currently found themselves. Each day seemed the same, with activities and expectations having shrunk to wondering when and where the next cigarette was coming from. Long-term goals were spoken of as if they were dreams, with the reality of the present totally dominant.

Asylum in the Community

These community hostels bore a striking resemblance to the extended care open wards. They shared the same routines and regimentation and lack of other meaningful activity, so that smoking together formed one of the few meaningful exchanges between residents. The staff were often scarce, except when they were also coming out to the smoking area for a smoke. Cigarette supplies were kept by staff and strictly controlled and meted out to those residents who were deemed to be 'at risk' if allowed to carry their own cigarettes. Standover intimidation and trade involving cigarettes was rife in the hostels. Smoking leftover butts was common. It was more a case of who got to the ashtrays first rather than which residents chose this level of self-degradation. Dependence on government benefits, coupled with hostel fees that used up the vast proportion of these benefits, meant that these residents, like their inpatient counterparts, were usually extremely poor. Cigarettes were scarce and prized commodities.

Quantitative Results from Observation Sheets

Smoking Area Observations

The researcher sat in the smoking area and recorded the number of cigarettes consumed, the number of people smoking at each 10 minute interval, whether they were patients or staff and the number of those present who were not smoking at the time (passive smokers). The ten minute interval recording occurred over a continuous 3 hour period (Total=18 ten minute intervals). Ten minutes was determined to be the approximate time that it takes to smoke a cigarette. During any ten-minute period, each person was only counted once. This was determined by what activity they were predominantly doing during the 10 minute period. A smoker was deemed to be a person who was actively smoking their own cigarette, or sharing a cigarette with another person. A passive smoker was deemed to be a person who was not actively smoking. They could therefore be a non-smoker or a smoker who was not smoking at the time of observations. These results did not acknowledge the occurrence of smoking outside the observed areas and did not analyse the composition of the smoking area group in relation to the total population of the setting. They also did not account for the smoking behaviours of individuals and their repeated presence in the smoking area; for example, some people were present and smoking during the entire 18 intervals of time.

The aim of the observations was to check on self-report data of roles and behaviours and interactions between staff and patients. From this point, the further aim was to discover patterns of similarity and difference between the settings. This included patterns of overall cigarette consumption, passive smoking and peer smoking. Results from each of the settings are given individually then comparatively. A Poisson distribution test has been performed to further describe the data and confirm relationships within and between the variables.

THE ACUTE OPEN WARD SMOKING AREA

The acute open ward was visited 9 times to record data in the area immediately outside the entrance door to the ward. This area was where patients sat or stood to be outside the ward for a change of scenery, to smoke or to get fresh air, or to talk to other patients away from staff. The acute open ward visits occurred between the hours of 6.30am and 10.30pm, across all seven days of the week. Each recording period was 3 hours, totalling 27 hours of recording and 162 recording intervals (10 minutes each). The total number of cigarettes consumed for the 9 visits was 752, being consumed by a total of 708 smokers. The total number of people in the smokers' area for the 9 visits was 821, 760 of these being patients and 61 of these being staff. Of the 821 people in the smokers' area, 113 of them were not smoking at the time. This occurred for 68 of the 162 smoking intervals recorded.

Observations of Smoking for the Acute Open Ward Smoking Area

The Acute Open Ward (9 visits)	N
Cigarettes consumed	752
Smokers / Total	708
Group in the Area / Total	821
Patients in the Area	760
Staff in the Area	61
Passive Smokers / Total	113
Occasions- Passive Smokers Present	68
Intervals Recorded	162

From these figures, it is apparent that patients used the observed area very regularly, in order to smoke. Passive smokers were present almost half the time that smokers were also present. The sociability of this outside area of the ward is noted in the description of the ward environment. More than 1 in 6 patients present in the area were passive smokers while they were in the area. All staff members observed in the area were smoking at the time of observations.

THE EXTENDED CARE OPEN WARD SMOKING AREA

The extended care open wards were visited 8 times, as per the criteria described for the open ward. Designation of patients to particular wards was based on their level of mental illness, chronicity and prospects of rehabilitation back to community living. The long-stay ward housed patients who were expected to be resident at the hospital for between 2 and 5 years. The rehabilitation focus ward housed patients who were expected to be resident at the hospital for between 3 and 12 months. Each of the extended care wards was visited 4 times between the hours of 6.30am and 8.30pm. These two types of extended care wards were selected to provide a picture of the range of extended care settings. Aged Care asylum wards were not observed.

Observations of Smoking for the Extended Care Open Wards Smoking Area

Extended Care Open Ward (8 visits)	N
Cigarettes consumed	454
Smokers / Total	391
Group in the Area / Total	553
Patients in the Area	510
Staff in the Area	43
Passive Smokers / Total	162
Occasions- Passive Smokers Present	85
Intervals Recorded	144

Distinguishing between the different types of extended care open wards, by separating out the results of observations, yields further patterns.

Observations of Smoking for the Extended Care Open Wards
Separation of Long-stay and Rehabilitation Wards

Observations	Long-stay Ward (4 visits)	Rehab- Focus Ward (4 visits)
Cigarettes consumed	188	266
Smokers / Total	145	246
Group in the Area / Total	220	333
Patients in the Area	214	296
Staff in the Area	6	37
Passive Smokers / Total	75	87
Occasions- Passive Smokers Present	33	52
Intervals Recorded	72	72

In the long stay extended care ward (2-5 years), most patients' cigarette supply was closely monitored and rationed by staff. Therefore they had limited access to cigarettes. Patients also tended to sit separate to one another in this area, due possibly to their heightened level of paranoia and symptom distress. Therefore direct contact leading to passive smoking potential was less likely than their more sociable counterparts in the rehabilitation-focus extended care ward. This latter setting was more focused on structured rehabilitation, with patients often participating in ward activities together. These patients were more able and more communal than in other extended care open wards, and therefore more interactive, with a greater potential to sit together, and with more control over their own cigarette supply. The total number of patients for each of these wards was the same (N=24). Staff in the rehabilitation focus ward appear to socialise significantly more often with patients in the smoking area that their long-stay ward counterparts. All staff in the observed areas were smoking at the time.

THE LOCKED WARDS

The locked wards were visited 9 times to record data in the area designated as the smoking area for the ward. Both wards contained a small smoking room as part of the internal structure of the building, with wire mesh on the outer wall to allow smoke to escape to the outside air. These smoking 'cages' were a compromise to allow smoking in an area of convenience, given the nature of the settings as locked and the policy ban on smoking within the interior of the buildings. The extended care locked ward also had a large internal garden area open to the sky, bounded on all four sides by the ward building, that was used for smoking by the group at certain times in the day. The acute locked ward had a small outside grassed area bounded by a security fence, however this was rarely used by patients or staff. Both wards had strict routines regarding the dispensing of cigarettes to patients. The acute locked ward distributed cigarettes hourly for patients who had their own supply and 6 times per day, supplied through canteen donated funds, at set intervals for those who had none. The extended care locked ward dispensed cigarettes to patients every hour. Therefore, the researcher could not use the 10-minute interval method of recording smoking activities for these settings. Instead, the smoking activities at each designated smoking period were recorded. Results from both settings are given in total and then individually in separate tables as follows:

Observations from the Locked Wards Smoking Areas

The Locked Wards (8 visits)	N
Cigarettes consumed	468
Smokers / Total	452
Group in the Area / Total	474
Patients in the Area	336
Staff in the Area	136
Passive Smokers / Total	22
Occasions- Passive Smokers Present	18
Intervals Recorded	39

Observations from Acute and Extended Care Locked Wards

Observations	Acute Locked Ward (4 visits)	Extended Care Locked Ward (5 visits)
Cigarettes consumed	216	252
Smokers / Total	216	236
Group in the Area / Total	230	244
Patients in the Area	174	162
Staff in the Area	56	80
Passive Smokers / Total	14	8
Occasions-Passive Smokers Present	11	7
Intervals Recorded	24	15

From this data the routine of patients and staff being together in the smoking area is apparent. The designated purpose of the area as a smoking area needs to be acknowledged, hence the dominant activity for both patients and staff at these times is smoking. Of note in the extended care locked ward is that the total population of patients (N=11) smoked at all designated smoking periods and that most staff smoked at these times also (N= 5-6). Of further note in the extended care locked setting, the number of cigarettes consumed was more than the number of smokers present, despite the policy of one cigarette per person at smoking times. This is explained by the observation of some staff smoking more than one cigarette at some of these times and the granting of a further cigarette to patients at certain times, especially in the early morning when the group smoked in the garden area of the ward. Staff who were non-smokers did not tend to nominate for the duty of supervising patients during smoking periods.

THE COMMUNITY HOSTELS

Two community hostels were visited 12 times in total to record data in the area immediately outside the entrance door to the hostel, nominated for smoking and daytime outside seating and recreation. Visits occurred between the hours of 6.30am and 10pm, over seven days. Combined results are given followed by separate table for each hostel as follows:

Observations from the Hostels' Smoking Areas

The Community Hostels (12 visits)	N
Cigarettes consumed	878
Smokers / Total	799
Group in the Area / Total	901
Residents in the Area	862
Staff in the Area	39
Passive Smokers / Total	104
Occasions- Passive Smokers Present	69
Intervals Recorded	216

Observations from Hostel One and Hostel Two

Observations	Hostel One (6 visits)	Hostel Two (6 visits)
Cigarettes consumed	361	517
Smokers / Total	322	475
Group in the Area / Total	371	530
Residents in the Area	363	499
Staff in the Area	8	31
Passive Smokers / Total	49	55
Occasions- Passive Smokers Present	34	35
Intervals Recorded	108	108

The first hostel housed both younger and older residents, with predominantly older residents. Its environment was highly regimented by staff, with several residents required to ask staff for their cigarette ration for the day. The second hostel observed housed residents who were predominantly under 50 years of age. Many of these residents were away from the hostel during the day and returned to the hostel for the evening meal. Of note was the higher number of cigarettes consumed compared to the number of smokers during the observations that occurred in the early morning at each site. The role of nicotine withdrawal, given that this was early in the day when residents were first waking, may have played a role here. Some residents were given their morning ration of, for example, 3 or 5 cigarettes for the morning and chose to smoke them as quickly as they could. The consistent and repeated use of the smoking areas by several residents throughout the day was noted, as was the high level of staff smoking interaction in the smoking area of the second hostel. The frequency and high number of passive smokers was also noted, with several residents observed to sit next to smokers in order to inhale their cigarette smoke, presumably when they had run out of their own supply. Differences between each hostel were noted, with the number of cigarettes consumed and the number of smokers being higher at the second hostel. This may be due the resident population at this site being generally younger and more able to move in and out of the area. In the first hostel, many residents were frail and spent much of their day sitting indoors.

Differences between the Settings

General patterns from the above tables were further analysed by making comparisons based on percentage scores for specific variables as they occurred in the different settings. These are shown in the following tables and figures.

**Percentage of Patients in the Smoking Area According to the Total
Number of the Group in the Smoking Area and The Setting**

Setting No.	Setting Type	Number of the Group	Number of Patients Present	% of Patients in the Group
1	Acute Open Ward	821	760	92.57
2	Ext.Care Rehab. Ward	333	296	88.89
3	Ext. Care Long-stay Ward	220	214	97.27
4	Ext. Care Wards (both)	553	510	92.22
5	First Hostel	371	363	97.84
6	Second Hostel	530	499	94.15
7	Hostels (both)	901	862	95.67
8	Acute Locked Ward	230	174	75.65
9	Ext. Care Locked Ward	244	164	67.21
10	Locked Wards (both)	474	338	71.31

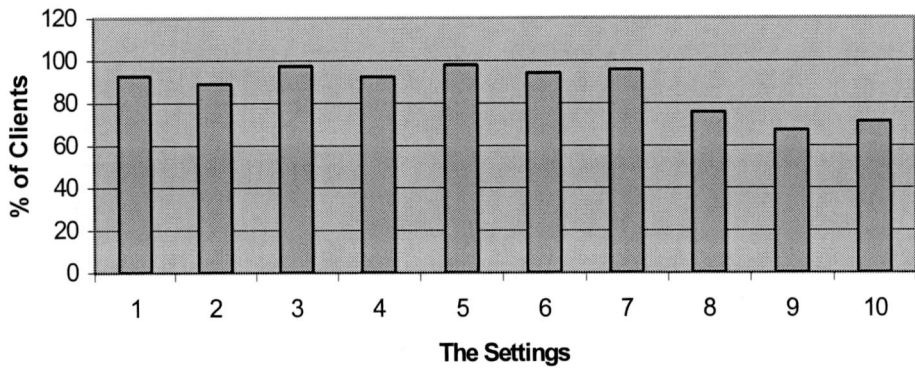

Figure 1. Patients in the Group as a Percentage of the Total Group

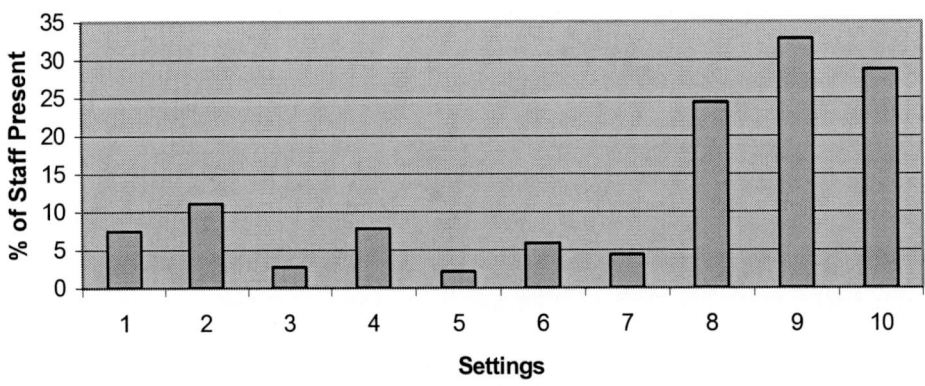

Figure 2. Staff in the Group as a Percentage of the Total Group

From these figures, it can be seen that significantly more staff are present in the smoking area within the locked wards (setting numbers 8-10) that in the open wards (setting numbers

1-4). This is most likely due to their role in supervising smoking in the locked settings. Also, very low percentages of staff were observed to be present in the long-stay extended care open ward. This confirms other observations made of staff leaving patients very much to their own devices in this setting. Differences in the level of disability and sociability of the patient group in the different extended care wards have already been noted. These results confirm those observations.

The community hostels had similar very low percentages of staff presence in the smoking areas (setting numbers 5-7). The low ratio of staff to residents in these settings, especially in the early morning and later afternoon, may also account for this low figure. Differences between the hostel may be associated with the ethos of the individual hostels and their general make-up of residents, the first hostel housing largely older residents and possessing a more paternalistic ethos and separation between staff and residents than the second hostel.

Differences in the observed smoking activity in the different settings can be shown by looking at differences in the percentage of smokers present in the settings as shown by the following table and figure.

Percentage of Smokers in the Group According to the Total Number of the Group and The Setting

Setting No.	Setting Type	Number of Smokers Present	Number of the Total Group	% of Smokers Present
1	Acute Open Ward	708	821	86.24
2	Ext.Care Rehab. Ward	246	333	73.87
3	Ext. Care Long-stay Ward	145	220	65.9
4	Ext. Care Wards (both)	391	553	70.71
5	First Hostel	332	371	89.49
6	Second Hostel	475	530	89.62
7	Hostels (both)	807	901	89.57
8	Acute Locked Ward	216	230	93.91
9	Ext. Care Locked Ward	236	244	96.72
10	Locked Wards (both)	452	474	95.36

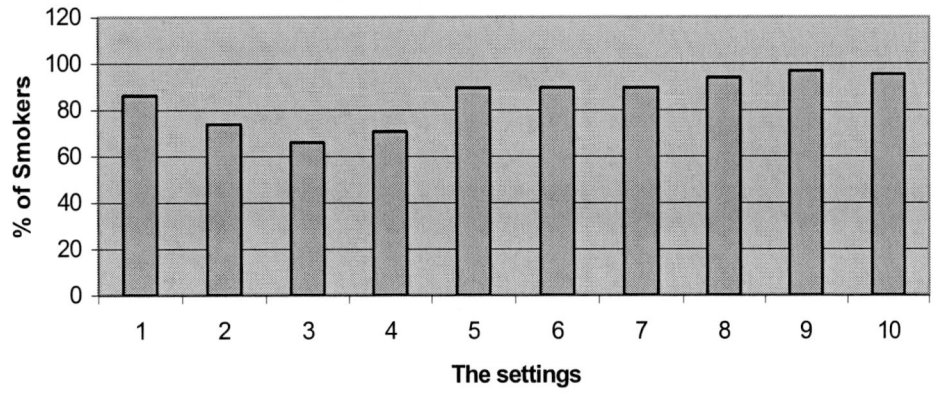

Figure 3. Percentage of Smokers in the Group for the Settings

These results indicate high percentages of smoking activity in the locked wards (setting numbers 8-10) and confirm the general observations made throughout the participant observation of the settings. In these settings, all patients were smoking due to the observed period and the observed area being specifically for smoking. Therefore the interpretation of the figures needs to acknowledge this difference between observations made in this setting compared to other settings where the observed areas had the potential to be used for activities other than smoking. Even given this distinction, the overall percentages for all settings are high, indicating that most people took the opportunity to smoke while in these areas.

Another facet of the smoking area observations was the degree of passive smoking activity in the different settings. Questions arose from the observations of the settings and the levels of disability and access to funds to purchase cigarettes, and the potential impact of these circumstances on the rates of passive smoking. The following table and figure summarises these results.

Percentage of Passive Smokers According to the Total Number of the Group and Setting

Setting No.	Setting Type	Number of the Group	Number of Passive Smokers	% Passive Smokers in Group
1	Acute Open Ward	724	94	12.98
2	Ext.Care Rehab. Ward	333	87	26.13
3	Ext. Care Long-stay Ward	220	75	34.09
4	Ext. Care Wards (both)	553	162	29.29
5	First Hostel	371	49	13.21
6	Second Hostel	530	55	10.38
7	Hostels (both)	901	104	11.54
8	Acute Locked Ward	216	14	6.48
9	Ext. Care Locked Ward	236	8	3.39
10	Locked Wards (both)	452	22	4.87

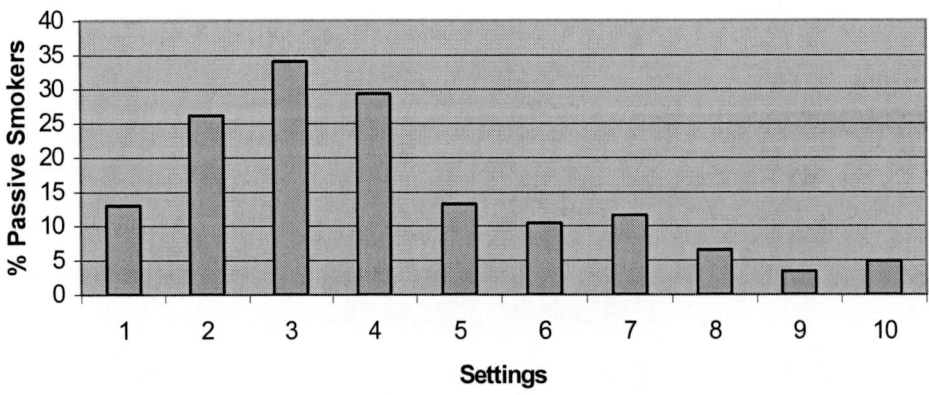

Figure 4. Passive Smokers as a Percentage of the Total Group

These figures confirm other observations during the period of participant observation, that is, that passive smoking was highest in the extended open care settings (setting numbers 2-4). The reasons for the higher percentage of passive smokers in the extended care open settings can be attributed to the rationing of cigarettes and the shortage of funds to purchase cigarettes by patients in these settings. As observations confirm, many patients in these settings deliberately sat next to other patients who were smoking when they did not have cigarettes of their own. Similar figures should have been expected from the hostels where rationing and shortage of funds by residents was likewise noted. However, this is not shown to be the case (setting numbers 5-7) and would need further investigation. The very low rates of passive smoking in the locked wards (setting numbers 8-10) is to be expected, as all of the patients were smoking at the times observed due to this being the designated activity at the time and non-smoking clients were generally not allowed in the area. However, this means that all of the passive smokers were staff in the area to supervise patients' smoking. The acute locked ward possessed almost twice as many passive smoking staff as the extended care locked ward. The reasons for this are unclear, although other observations of these two settings demonstrate that the environment of the acute setting revealed more of an 'us and them' air compared to the extended care setting where staff described themselves as being as institutionalised as the patients, with higher rates of smoking as a group than their acute ward counterparts. This suggests an enculturation of long-stay staff into the smoking routine. In the open ward, patients usually had access to money in order to purchase cigarettes, or had relatives (or community key workers) who were able to ensure the supply of cigarettes to them. Their rates of passive smoking can be related to their observed sociability of the observed area.

Once the results of observations were gathered and tabled as percentages, further questions arose from the data. The Poisson test, or Z test was therefore applied, measuring potential differences between the periods of time using a simple count principle, with any difference determined as significant if a score of $\geq \pm 1.96$ was achieved. This was based on the principle of the expected value for two counts of the same activity, for example smoking, being zero. Any difference between the two counts could then be analysed using the following formula to obtain a z score. This particular formula was chosen due to the small sample size and sampling method. It was useful to assist in the inference of results and was not meant to be taken as exact (Armitage and Berry, 1996).

$$Z = \frac{(x1-x2)}{\sqrt{x1+x2}}$$

One would expect the number of cigarettes smoked in each ten-minute interval to be the same as the number of smokers present in each ten-minute interval, that is, for the expected value to be the same. However, this was not the case in the settings, especially in the mornings. The following table summarises the results using the Poisson test. The locked settings are not included due to their rule of one cigarette per smoking occasion.

Cigarettes Smoked Compared with the Number of Smokers and The Settings

Setting Type	x1	x2	z
Acute Open Ward	666	628	1.06
Ext.Care Rehab. Ward	266	246	0.88
Ext. Care Long-stay Ward	188	145	2.36
Ext. Care Wards (both)	454	391	2.17
First Hostel	361	322	1.49
Second Hostel	517	475	1.33
Hostels (both)	878	797	1.98

x1 = number of cigarettes smoked
x2 = number of smokers present
$Z = \geq \pm 1.96$ (significant).

The higher rate of smoking by the smokers present in the extended care long-stay open ward was found to be significant with z=2.36. When figures were combined for the extended care open wards, this figures remained significant with z= 2.17. When the figures for the hostels were combined, they were also found to be significant with z= 1.98. In the absence of cigarette rationing and unlimited funds, these figures were expected to be even higher for the hostels and extended care settings. In the open ward, this smoking behaviour was not found to be significant.

Data from observations made in the morning, prior to lunch at 1pm, were compared with data from observations made in the afternoon and evening, after 1pm, to see if patients smoking patterns are different at different periods in the day. In order to achieve equivalent periods of time to then analyse data from the open ward setting, one of the nine three hour observation occasions was randomly selected out, leaving eight three hour periods, four in the am period and four in the pm period. Observation data for the locked settings, the extended care wards, and the hostels did not require any adjustments as equal numbers of am and pm observations were achieved. The results are as follows:

Morning and Afternoon Smoking in the Acute Open Ward

The Acute Open Ward	am	pm	z
Cigarettes Consumed	360	306	2.09
Smokers / Total	329	299	1.20
Group in the Area / Total	386	338	1.78
Patients in the Area	362	307	2.13
Staff in the Area	24	31	-0.94
Passive Smokers	57	39	1.84
Occasions – Passive Smokers	33	23	1.34
Intervals Recorded	72	72	

Smokers in the acute open ward smoked more cigarettes in the morning and this was found to be significant (z=2.09). These findings support findings from client interviews and from observations made of the setting throughout the participant observation. Patients stated that they smoked more in the morning to overcome the nicotine withdrawal experienced as a consequence of sleeping. Several patients, especially those with schizophrenia, described having several cigarettes first thing in the morning to raise the level of nicotine in their system. This is confirmed by the Poisson test. As expected, given this result, the number of smokers in the area in the morning was significantly higher than compared to the numbers for the afternoon. Although not significant, the score for passive smoking is high (z=1.84) and heading in the right direction, with 12.98% of the group being passive smokers in this setting, according to the previous percentages table.

Morning and Afternoon Smoking in the Extended Care Open Ward

The Extended Care Open Ward	am	pm	z
Cigarettes Consumed	236	218	0.84
Smokers / Total	190	201	-0.56
Group in the Area / Total	266	287	-0.89
Patients in the Area	259	261	-0.09
Staff in the Area	17	26	-1.37
Passive Smokers	76	86	-0.78
Occasions – Passive Smokers	38	37	0.11
Intervals Recorded	72	72	

No variable showed significant differences between morning and afternoon in the extended care open ward setting. Given that cigarettes were rationed and in short supply due to these patients' lack of funds to smoke at will, this result is not surprising. The long-term nature of their residence at the hospital would suggest that they had learned to ration out the supplies of cigarettes they did possess. This is supported by observations made in which very few of these patients were observed to oblige others in their requests for cigarettes. Overall, the sense was gained that these patients closely guarded their supply and made it last for the day, and this is what account for the lack of significance of differences between the morning and afternoon.

Morning and Afternoon Smoking in the Community Hostels

The Community Hostels	am	pm	z
Cigarettes Consumed	452	426	0.88
Smokers / Total	389	408	-0.67
Group in the Area / Total	443	458	-0.50
Residents in the Area	425	437	-0.41
Staff in the Area	18	21	-0.48
Passive Smokers	54	50	0.39
Occasions – Passive Smokers	40	29	1.32
Intervals Recorded	108	108	

Similar to the extended care open wards, no significant differences were found between the morning and afternoon smoking behaviours of residents at the hostels. This is assumed to be the result of similar conditions related to rationing and finances, and learned coping. In these settings, some residents were given a set number of cigarettes by staff in the morning and a set number of cigarettes in the afternoon. Several residents at the first hostel actively sought cigarettes from other residents throughout the day, with varying degrees of success.

Intimidation of other residents for cigarettes was observed during visits to occur more frequently and more persistently in the early and mid-morning.

DISCUSSION

The following six themes provide a summary of the most dominant ideas to emerge from the qualitative and quantitative data collected during the interview and participant observation phases. The complex nature of interactions and behaviours in the context of smoking, combined with a long history of their cultural development, meant that many behaviour patterns were interconnected and difficult to unravel from each other. A final overarching theme describing the culture of smoking is then discussed to further synethise the data.

Theme (1) A Systemic Problem

The entrenched nature of smoking activity within all settings was an overwhelming feature. Smoking was a tool serving many purposes for the different groups observed. It was woven into the central fabric of daily life encompassing therapeutic, social, political and economic exchange in all settings. It occurred within a foundation of beliefs and attitudes that served to perpetuate powerlessness and inaction, so that each group tended to pass responsibility for action onto others while the social, legal, ethical and occupational health and safety aspects of the smoking problem remained untouched and unchallenged. Smoking therefore acted as a symbolic currency within a dysfunctional system.

Staff openly acknowledged the occurrence of barter and standover tactics between patients, as well as begging, scavenging for butts and harassment of shoppers for cigarettes in the local streets and shopping areas. Staff responded with the provision of medication and large ashtrays, while the social context remained unchanged. They either saw themselves as powerless in the face of 'the problem', or not responsible for it or for initiating change. Some staff pleaded for assistance but continued to act out the dominant reinforcing culture of smoking, in the absence of any preferred replacement culture. Other staff remained passive within it, focusing on the day to day tasks at hand. The effect of this system on the clients seemed devastating, with many spending their day in a vacuum, 'waiting for nothing'.

The structure of the work within the settings created its own dilemmas for staff, especially in the locked settings where there was a noticeable absence of meaningful rehabilitation activities and resources for this. Other wards were similar though. During quiet times staff were tied to the immediate environment, unable to leave or to get absorbed in any activity that required much concentration or time due to the nature of the setting requiring them to be constantly in limbo ready to react to patients' demands. Under such circumstances, smoking provided a convenient, readily available source of activity to relieve the monotony of the setting and many staff took up this option.

Theme (2) Smoking as a Tool - An Instrument of Treatment

Within each setting, smoking was observed as a tool, fulfilling a variety of purposes for the smokers, both patients and staff and the institution. The most common purpose for patients appeared to be the use of smoking to fill in time and break up the monotony of the day. Within the hospital wards, as well as at the hostels, the act of smoking formed part of a continual rotation of activity, sites and scenery in the absence of other stimulation. Smoking was used to compartmentalise the long slow day into more tolerable pieces. Mealtimes complemented the smoking activity as a central activity for patients to look forward to and to give some order to the day. Conversely, staff were also aware of the role of smoking and relied on it to act as 'babysitter' in the absence of other activities within the hospital. Both staff and patients readily succumbed to the utter boredom of the settings.

The primary function of smoking to satisfy the person's addiction to nicotine was accepted as given by participants, with people in all settings observed to be smoking en masse and in greater quantity in the early morning when the craving and withdrawal following periods of sleep were evident. Secondary, or latent, functions of smoking are also of great interest here. Within a system built around routines, smoking provided a central structure to all other routines and processes. This was especially evident in the locked wards where all other activity appeared to be dependent on the timing of the smoking routine, which occurred rigidly each hour. The only other routine to provide such a structure was mealtime. For clients, the smoking routine acted as a vehicle for human contact with other patients and with staff. Nursing staff in all settings busied themselves each day with the important task of ensuring the supply of cigarettes to patients, with 'smoke runs' to the local shops forming one of their many core duties.

In these settings where few rewards and pleasures were apparent, smoking provided an easy, readily accessible source of gratification within the vacuum of daily existence. The exchange of cigarettes between patients, for money, food, drugs, sex, or other favours, was spoken of as common knowledge by staff and patients and was observed as part of the daily life of the setting. Cigarettes provided the currency for which most other activities and interactions were exchanged between staff and patients, and patients and patients. Within a system dominated by routines and external controls, the ability to smoke provided one of the few opportunities to act autonomously and feel 'normal'. Within the locked wards, especially, smoking provided 'time out' from the pressures and rigidity of the setting, for both patients and staff. This was confirmed by nursing staff self-report data. During the smoking times, staff and patients in these settings appeared to call a truce from the usually combatant air within the setting, both gaining some relief from it by smoking. However, cigarettes were also clearly and consistently used as reward by staff to manage patients' behaviour, to pacify distressed or disruptive clients, to foster compliance and co-operation, and to foster conformity to the system and its rules and routines. Staff in one locked ward spoke openly about the allocation of twenty cigarettes per patient per day, this incorporating the seventeen cigarettes that they would consume each hour at smoke time between 6.30am (first smoking time for the day) and 11.30pm (last smoking time for the day), with the remaining three cigarettes used to reward good behaviour. This also provided an important means of assessing the person's readiness to progress to an open ward. Patients quickly learned these rules of engagement with staff. Staff, demonstrating the importance of smoking within the hospital setting provided several anecdotal scenarios. One nurse in a locked ward where cigarettes were dispensed each hour, recounted an incident of assault of a staff member by a patient in order to instigate a transfer to the other locked ward where cigarettes were offered every half hour.

For nursing staff particularly, being involved in the distribution of and act of smoking with patients provided them with fundamental opportunities to interact and establish rapport with clients. Smoking allowed nursing staff to assess patients' mental state and progress. As smokers, they were privy to information that they would not otherwise hear from patients. Hostel staff noted the same benefits of involvement in the smoking ritual with residents. Though never overtly incorporated into policy and procedure, in reality, many nurses had grown to rely on this interaction and many expressed their sense of inadequacy in their professional capacity when they gave up smoking, realising that they would have to find new ways to perform these tasks, that did not involve smoking.

Theme (3) Smoking as a Social Currency

The smoking area of each setting was observed to be a hive of activity and social stimulation that was not apparent in other areas within the settings. It was where people came together to talk, or merely to be with others, to gain some sense of human connectedness, especially in the long-stay open wards. In the open wards, the smoking area was often the first point of reference for new arrivals and served as a type of initiation into the ward and the group. Smoking provided a comfortable and safe means of initiating conversation, meeting others for the first time, portraying oneself as non-threatening and alleviating ones own nervousness about being with others. Staff openly encouraged this peer interaction and used it to aid their assessments of the person's level of paranoia, withdrawal, inhibition, irritability and other components of sociability with others. In the locked wards, smoking with others was perceived as a 'normalising' activity. The act of smoking and sharing cigarettes, or going to the shops together to buy cigarettes, gave people the opportunity to share and relate to others in a democratic way, whether they were staff or patients. Within this context, patients who were non-smokers were seen to receive less attention from staff, to be less interactive and to stand back from the group, suggesting that their needs were not being given as much attention because of their non-smoking status.

However, there existed the usual pitfalls that one would expect in any society where the currency is in demand and supply is curtailed by lack of resources or access. Within the hostels and the extended care open wards, an hierarchical social structure was evident between those who possessed cigarettes and those who were forced to beg, trade or threaten others for cigarettes. The group clearly knew who within its ranks was reliable at paying back for borrowed smokes and who was not, who needed to be looked after within the group by giving them cigarettes and who was a threat if their requests were refused. Within the wards and grounds of the hospital, this daily ritual of determining where one was placed in the hierarchy was played out, sometimes with open acts of violence between patients. Similar interactions were observed at the hostels. This reliance on cigarettes as social currency, involving the co-existence of smoking and socialisation within the one area, had a number of pitfalls. People found themselves in close proximity to others who were at times quite unwell or distressed and this was seen to aggravate their own illness symptoms and level of distress.

Further to this, the demoralising effects on the person and their sense of value and purpose, of begging on a regular basis, was clearly observed.

Theme (4) Attitudes of Staff

Throughout the settings, the overwhelming prevailing attitude towards patients and their smoking was that there was little that could be done to change the current situation, that there was little hope of them giving up smoking, that the situation was unresolvable. Therefore, no attempt was made to alter the daily routines and rituals around smoking. In the extended care wards, staff largely left patients to sit in the smoking areas among their peers or roam the grounds, while staff remained indoors. In the hostels, the situation was the same because "everyone smokes here." Ultimately, staff felt powerless to change the situation. Neither did staff feel it was their responsibility to act on the smoking issue, reflecting the ethos of the system of care.

The attitudes of many staff involved a weighing up of harms. They assumed that the patient's mental illness would always be present and that there was little hope of genuine recovery. The stigma of mental illness was perceived as a lifelong influence on the person. Few staff believed that patients could quit successfully. This was in contrast to the majority of patients who stated that they did want to quit but felt unable to, lacking the power to do so given the overwhelming reinforcement to smoke while at the hospital and in the community, as well as feeling unsupported in their efforts when they did try to quit.

Theme (5) Us and Them

In all settings, the fundamental and unresolved dilemma of incarceration versus care underpinned the often combatant and coercive nature of interactions between the participants. The threat of detention and seclusion that could deprive basic freedoms, down to the counting of cutlery in locked settings, were characteristic of this dilemma. For much of the time in the hospital environment, staff physically separated themselves from patients. Whatever happened outside the boundary of the ward was perceived as none of their concern or responsibility. Many wards were physically structured to create barriers between staff and patients, the most obvious being the use of keys throughout the hospital and the often-closed nurses' station door. This door was frequently held ajar by staff as they spoke to patients so that they could keep one foot inside and one foot outside and could readily close it if needed. During quiet times, staff frequently retreated into the staff area away from patients' gazes, to seek some relief from the combatant environment and the incessant banging on the nurses station door. In the hostels, many patients paced up and down the driveway but did not go outside the gate that separated them from their community. Staff frequently used the analogy of the prison system to describe their work situation and patients and hostel residents referred to themselves as 'inmates'.

Fragmentation into 'us and them' occurred at all levels and between all participants : staff to patient, ward to ward, patient to patient, staff to staff, discipline to discipline and hospital to community. Each ward setting possessed its own unique variation on the dominant culture of paternalism, and each compared itself to other wards, painting itself in a more favourable light than its counterparts. Each hostel was a hidden ward within the community. Management was perceived to be ignorant of the daily experience and needs of patients and staff, rarely visiting the wards. Doctors came and went, keeping their interaction within a tight range, the smoking issue being, "of no concern to them." Within this context, the exercise of power could be clearly seen, cigarettes acting as a prized commodity and source of influence and control over the behaviour of others. By controlling the supply of cigarettes, staff ultimately exercised power over patients. Patients variously made small attempts to regain some of this power by identifying strongly with their peers, defying staff requests, or engaging in barter and intimidation for cigarettes.

Theme (6) The Absence of a Clinical Approach to Smoking

Many of the decisions made by staff about the care of patients in the inpatient and community settings involved significant mistaken attribution of smoking as therapeutic. Staff failed to distinguish between illness relapse and agitation due to illness symptoms and nicotine withdrawal symptoms. At no time when patients were displaying agitation did staff equate this with withdrawal from nicotine. It was always perceived as symptoms of their mental illness. Patients also misinterpreted the situation in this way. Alternatives to finding cigarettes to alleviate the agitation were not usually explored by staff or patients. No formal policy and commitment to the use of NRT existed at the time of participant observation. The generally held belief was that patients would refuse NRT, preferring to smoke. The risks and dilemmas involved in monitoring compliance with NRT within the hospital grounds was perceived to create further unwanted problems for staff and patients. It just seemed too hard. The current system of 'letting them smoke' remained as the preferred option.

Like their patient counterparts, most staff believed that patients who smoked needed cigarettes in order to manage their mental illness symptoms and that not having cigarettes on hand would worsen their mental state. Like their patient counterparts, staff also used cigarettes to cope with the environment in which they found themselves and the pressures of their role. In the locked settings, these staff clearly became bound up in the smoking sequence and the rote nature of smoking activity in the settings.

The Culture of Smoking

Bronfenbrenner's (1979) ecological framework of micro, meso, exo and macro layers is used here to provide a comprehensive, theoretical perspective for understanding the culture of smoking within mental health settings. Within this framework, the micro level involves the immediate personal environment in which the person lives, the meso level involves the interrelations among two or more settings in which the person participates, the exo level involves community settings which impact indirectly upon the person because of their membership within it, and the macro level which involves the society or culture as a whole. He made two significant and relevant points when devising his framework. He stressed that the best way to understand something is to try to change it, that this would clarify the different levels of resistance to change and the degree of embeddedness of a particular behaviour or activity. Bronfenbrenner also stressed that change in one system was likely to promote change in other systems. These two points are critical in understanding the current research, in particular, the barriers to quitting experienced by smokers with a mental illness and by those who attempt to assist them to quit. Building on Bronfenbrenner's framework, the current research has found that several aspects of relationships between patients and staff within mental health settings appear to be central to understanding the culture of smoking They include the attitudes and values that determine communication styles and actions between the participants within the system, the nature of group organisation and organisational culture, power relationships and the physical and social environment in which the system exists. These aspects filter through each of Bronfenbrenner's system layers, via a complex two-way process of learning and transfer between the layers. It is these aspects of the system that both patients and staff identified as perpetuating the culture of smoking.

Applying the ecological framework to the current research, immediate relationships between patient and patient, and patients and staff exist in the microsystem. The supply and use of cigarettes by patients and staff and the activity of smoking, barter and intimidation all occur in this microsystem. The interrelations among inpatient patients and the community, as well as community-living patients and their mental health service, the hospital and the wider community are examples of relationships within the mesosystem. Quit services, general health services, police and media, consumer groups, mental health legislation and the community's relations with the mental health institutions represent relationships within the exosystem. At the macrosystem level, belief systems and ideologies that influence the culture as a whole are apparent. These beliefs filter down through each of the three lower-order systems. They include society's fear of mental illness, notions of stigma and deviance. Beliefs about institutionalisation and patterns of group organisation and bureaucracy also occur at this level of the system, with each reinforcing the culture of smoking in the system as a whole.

Culture is defined here as consisting of, "conventional patterns of thought and behaviour, including values, beliefs, rules of conduct, political organisation, economic activity and the like, which are passed on from one generation to the next" (Hatch, 1985, p.178). The culture of an organisation determines how it defines itself, how it solves problems, how it perceives its members and how it responds to change. In this respect, culture involves various players, with various roles and rules for behaviour, interaction and communication, informed by beliefs and attitudes, set in the context of established rites, structures, artefacts and ideologies that together serve to perpetuate the culture (Jones and May, 1992).

Smoking as a Primary Activity (The Players)

Results of all three studies confirmed that smoking was a primary activity in mental health settings, forming a central part of the daily experience of all the players. An extensive history of smoking in the settings was apparent. The extensive use of areas outside each inpatient ward and community hostel for smoking, the lengths taken by patients and staff to ensure the supply of cigarettes as a core need, as well as the smoking sequence in the locked wards were examples of the primacy of smoking activity in the settings.

Smoking as a Multifaceted Tool (The Roles)

All participants described the social, personal and temporal habits of smoking in much the same way as non-mentally ill smokers described them, that is, to fill in time, to relieve boredom, to move from one activity to the next, for stress relief, to aid concentration, for relaxation and as part of socialising with others (Carter, Borland and Chapman, 2001). However, the participants appeared to use cigarettes and smoking behaviours as part of a much more complex set of social rules for interactions and learned responses in dealing with mental illness. The use of cigarettes for clinical purposes, for power and control, ensuring safety and for social and economic exchange have been noted.

Us and Them (The Rules of Communication)

This chapter has described multiple examples of how smoking was used by patients and staff as a source of power and control. Beyond the effects of the drug itself, the role of cigarettes in mediating social interactions has been noted. The use of cigarettes by patients in order to feel a sense of control over their illness symptoms and to gain a sense of autonomy within a system of care in which they felt a loss of personal identity (Lawn, Pols and Barber, 2002). The involvement of staff in the supply of cigarettes to patients and the consequences of this for transactions of power between them was described earlier. The inter-disciplinary rivalries and tensions, fuelled by the system's reliance on a continuous supply of cigarettes to patients in the hospital setting, have been noted. As a consequence of this, no united focus on overcoming the smoking problem was apparent; the high level of smoking was likely to continue unabated. The smoking sequence in the acute locked settings was akin to the calling of a truce, during which patients and staff laid down their fear and mistrust of each other and joined together to have a smoke in the smokers' cage. This was a unique finding of the research.

The terminology of 'the cage' and 'the fishbowl', with patients and staff describing themselves as 'inmates' seemed to perpetuate an environment in which combatant interactions were the norm. In support of this idea, Barrett (1996) notes the important role of language in defining social relationships within psychiatric settings. The physical environment of the settings, with glassed, locked doors between patients and staff also appeared to promote a divisive, combatant air between patients and staff. The design of the acute locked setting mirrored Bentham's prototype panopticon from which it only took a single gaze to see all areas (Roach-Anleu, 1999). The banality of the settings and the lack of other meaningful activity was also noted by patients and staff to have a negative effect on the sense of control and power they felt. For patients, it appeared to diminish their sense of control. For staff it gave them greater control but paradoxically appeared to induce an 'us and them' air in the settings. This ultimately drew many staff into a culture that fostered powerlessness in the longer term. The comments made about 'running on autopilot' and being 'as institutionalised as the patients' were examples of this effect.

Systemic Issues (The Structures, Ideologies and Artefacts)

The smoking areas outside each ward and the smokers' cages in the locked wards appeared as control points for social interaction and exchange in the settings. The current system was described in the context of its historical cultural antecedents. Staff possessed full knowledge of cigarettes being used by patients in exchange for food, sex and other drugs. Staff were also fully aware of the standover and barter for cigarettes by patients and the use of cigarettes for reward by staff. Confusion, ambivalence and powerlessness were noted in comments made by staff when speaking about their ethical responses to the smoking issue. Their sense of professional demoralisation was evident. Each professional group appeared to be struggling to preserve its own patch in the face of this situation, with many staff appearing to blame staff from other professions for inaction on the smoking problem. The animosity this created between the disciplines only served to alienate them further from each other. Patients stood by, watched and smoked.

Cultural Transfer - Hospital to Community (Rules of Communication)

Staff made many comments about the community hostels as mirroring the inpatient long-stay wards. Most of the staff interviewed had trained in the hospital setting. Their attitudes and beliefs about patients appeared to be negatively influenced by that experience. Comparison of the hostels with inpatient wards revealed few perceived differences in the activities involving smoking. Trade, barter and intimidation by patients and reinforcement by staff were apparent and common to both settings. An attitude of 'let them smoke' prevailed.

A Hierarchy of Values (Attitudes and Beliefs)

Staff interviews provided unique data on the personal, clinical, social and professional attitudes and values held by staff that determined their ethical responses to smoking and mental illness. An absence of concern for the physical health consequences of smoking was noted for the majority of patient and staff participants. The lack of focus on legal concerns was also prominent in all three phases of the research. Patients made no mention of it. Only a small number of staff made reference to passive smoking and occupational health and safety in the context of smoking. No mention was made of the legal consequences of colluding with the supply of cigarettes to patients or the reinforcement of smoking within the hospital setting. Multiple occasions of passive smoking by non-smokers was observed, especially non-smoking patients. This was also observed for staff who were required to monitor patients' smoking in the locked settings.

Attitudes and Values

The culture of smoking in the mental health setting appeared to be influenced by underlying attitudes and values held by the participants of this study. The historical context of this has been explored previously. These beliefs and attitudes were determined at the macrosystem level and involved notions of deviance and stigma. They encompassed beliefs and values about the mentally ill that seemed to influence all layers of the system and determined responses by patients and staff. Inherent in the notion of deviance is social control. "Whenever we use such terms as persuade, restrain, discipline, coerce, penalise, reward, direct, manage or regulate to describe aspects of the activities of individuals or groups, organisations or societies, we are talking about the exercise of social control over peoples' bodies, minds, and behaviour" (Edwards, 1988, p.1). All of these facets of social control were evident in the settings observed for this study.

Organisational Culture and Group Dynamics

The culture of an organisation is central to how one understands social relationships between its members (Jones and May, 1992). At the microsystem and mesosystem levels, observation of the mental health settings revealed complex subgroup arrangements, each with its own sub-culture based on specific shared meanings and symbols. The separation of mental health settings into patient and staff and separation of staff into professional disciplines were examples of this phenomenon. The hierarchical organisation within and between the professions was a further influence on the day to day interactions, relationships and transfer of meaning and culture. At the exosystem and macrosystem level, the structural relationship between the psychiatric hospital and the larger society also appeared to influence the culture of the settings, with rules, policies and official ideology tending to reflect, reinforce and reproduce the dominant culture (Jones and May, 1992). The Guardianship Act and The Mental Health Act are examples of overt shared meanings and symbols. An extensive literature exists on the role of the psychiatric institutions over time, in particular, descriptions of the social, political and economic purposes they have served for the wider community (Dwyer, 1987; Rhodes, 1991; Shlomowitz, 1990).

Central to the notion of change is the need to understand why change does not occur. Schon's (1972) concept of 'dynamic conservatism' is demonstrated by these findings, in particular, the fragmentation of the professional disciplines and the impact of this on smoking within the settings. Ogburn's (1972) explanation of why organisations are resistant to change is also evident here, that is, staff and patients tended to use existing forms of behaviour management, out of habit, rather than create new ones. The use of cigarettes by staff to manage patients in mental health settings acted as the mechanism for many of the rules of interaction, and procedures and actions taken in the settings. Their use took all the forms suggested by Sidanius and Pratto (1999), involving a high level of passive and active co-operation by the groups with lower status in the hierarchy, often by their deferential behaviour towards those with higher status in the system. The passive line up of patients at the nurses' station door to receive cigarettes is an expression of this process.

The system of exchange and barter of cigarettes throughout the settings is an example of Skinner's (1953) social exchange theory as an activity in subcultures (see also Forsyth, 1999). Sykes' (1958) descriptions of prisoners' social arrangements in response to the system, with its detail on the pecking order involving exchange of goods such as cigarettes, clothing, food and gestures of deference between prisoners, was similar to that observed in the mental health settings.

A further factor in group dynamics is the notion of secondary adjustments that exist within institutions. These involve, "practices that do not directly challenge staff but allow inmates to obtain forbidden satisfactions or to obtain permitted ones by forbidden means" (Goffman, 1963, p.53). With this comes a kind of code or informal social control by the group to prevent informing staff. This mechanism was evident in the trade and stand-over for cigarettes, a practice that was fully known by staff and largely ignored. It involved a shared code of conduct by patients, such as the way that the hostel residents refused to tell the staff member that one of the male residents had been begging for cigarettes.

Power Relationships

Within the mental health settings cigarettes appeared to perform a central role in how individuals and groups asserted power and control French and Raven (1959) argue that the inherent mechanism of rewards heightens power when the rewards are valued, when the group relies on the power holder for the resources and when the power holder seems credible. In a system in which cigarettes were valued by patients and staff, where clients relied on staff for the supply of cigarettes and where patients were dependent on the system for their care and treatment, cigarettes clearly became a central force in power relationships. Cultural power via, "control over the means of value creation, interpretation and maintenance" (Jessop, 1972, p.58), comprising economic, political and social power, is also useful in understanding smoking within the settings. Economic power involved the distribution of ward cigarettes as well as the trade and stand-over for cigarettes in the hospital grounds. Political power was exemplified by the Mental Health Act that enabled detention and involuntary treatment. Social power could be seen in the deference shown to psychiatrists. Observations suggest that cigarettes were variously used by patients and staff to assert power. The comments on freedom and protest made by clients were attempts to assert power and to combat the power of others over them. The notion of substance use by minority groups in order to experience personalised power (Barber, et al., 1988; Roche and Ober, 1997), has been demonstrated by these findings.

The Physical and Social Environment in which the System Exists

Several physical and social aspects of the settings appeared to contribute to and reflect beliefs about the mentally ill across all four layers of the ecological system. The culture of smoking in the settings appeared to be communicated within and between the various groups of players by fear.

There is an extensive literature on the rates of assault upon nurses in psychiatric settings. According to the literature, up to 80% of nurses have experienced assault (Baxter, Hafner and Holme, 1992), with assaults accounting for 70% of all work-related injury for nurses (Lawson, 1992). Morrison (1990a) concluded that organisational norms that emphasise control of patients' behaviour via the enforcement of rules and denial of requests promote a 'tradition of toughness'; that they promote violence (see also Harrington, 1974; Morrison, 1990b). Burrows (1994) found that restricted movement, inhospitable décor, inadequate activities and lack of information led to increased rates of assault. Both staff and patients, especially those in the locked wards, identified the presence of these problems.

CONCLUSION

This chapter has described the culture of smoking within mental health settings using a sociological framework. The various components of that culture, as they apply to the results of this study, have been given. The forces at work in perpetuating a smoking culture have been outlined. Bronfenbrenner's ecological systems framework was applied to summarise how the culture of smoking has developed and is perpetuated. Theories. that contribute to further understanding the relationships within and between Bronfenbrenner's system layers will now be outlined.

Impoverished Learning Environments

The nature of the physical environment in which smoking interactions occurred between patients and staff was also shown to encourage smoking and discourage quitting. Mentally ill smokers in this study appeared to be well aware of the risks of their smoking. Their tendency to minimise the risks appeared to be due to their loss of hope of recovery, their sense of stigma and perceived powerlessness. They chose to smoke, knowing the risks, because they did not view the alternative as improving their situation. Staff generally held similar beliefs about patients. All patients interviewed for this study and many of the patients observed said that they would quit if they felt they could, a view supported by other research (Doherty, 2006; Lawn and Abrams, 2002; McCreadie, 2003). Solutions therefore need to address the impact of the environment on its members and the relationships and values that are fostered as a result of this (Moos and Insel, 1974; Moos, 1976). The introduction of more meaningful alternative activities is also indicated.

Clinical Use of Smoking

This research has highlighted the complicated role played by staff within mental health settings where many patients are involuntary participants. Nurses in particular performed complicated roles with patients. They acting as custodian, carer, cigarette source, counsellor, educator, behaviour modifier and gaoler (see Sykes, 1958 for parallels within the prison system). Smoking appeared to provide the means by which these role conflicts were eased for nursing staff. The latent consequence of this was that smoking was condoned, so much so that it was increasingly relied upon to facilitate interaction. Nursing staff who did not smoke commented on their perceived loss of this care option once they stopped smoking. The promotion of clinical alternatives for staff is indicated so that they do not rely on smoking to manage patients.

Challenging the Culture of Smoking

In the inpatient and community settings, many examples of smoking reinforcement and conditioned smoking were apparent for patients and staff. This appeared to be a group-based phenomenon within the cultural milieu. It was not limited to individual experiences. The majority of staff appeared to accept patients' smoking, seeing it as a central part of the dominant culture of the settings. Staff relied heavily on medications to treat and manage patients. One consequence of this was that, when medications were not adequate, staff were left with few other effective alternatives to assist patients with their symptoms and distress other than to let them smoke or to smoke with them to give them a sense of comfort and support. In the same way that many patients said that they had learned to rely smoking to self-medicate, it appears that staff had acquired the belief in these benefits of smoking for patients, perceiving it as unusual if patients were not smokers. Other studies have found similar beliefs held by staff (Jochelson and Majrowski, 2006; Stubbs, haw and Garner, 2004). The findings suggest that these systemic patterns of learning and reinforcement need to be challenged and replaced within treatment environments.

Nicotine Withdrawal

No clear policy to guide interventions with patients wishing to quit or to provide NRT to patients was apparent. Throughout the participant observation period, no doctor was observed to make the diagnosis of nicotine withdrawal for agitated patients who were in their care. This was especially so for patients in locked wards where they were subjected to repeated, enforced nicotine withdrawal. The effect of the culture was so strong that doctors omitted to recognise the pharmacology of nicotine. They accepted an explanation that fitted in with cultural beliefs rather than one provided by their professional training. The number of cigarettes supplied as part of the smoking sequence in locked wards would not have been sufficient to address patients' nicotine withdrawal symptoms (Schein, 1995). It arguably incited patients who continued to seek and demand cigarettes outside the designated time, further increasing the threat of violence in the settings. A commitment by doctors to diagnose nicotine withdrawal and to treat it accordingly with NRT is needed. Fundamental support by the hospital to provide NRT, as it does other pharmacological treatments, would also be part of this process. Support for more effective interventions and strategies at a day to day level of clinical care are also indicated.

A Community Response is Needed

In the hostels, as with other mental health settings, limited social roles and predictable routines were important in promoting the use of cigarettes as temporal reference points, that is, markers for orientating the person to time, place and person. These predominantly orientated the person to the present or to a few hours into the future (Suto and Frank, 1994), resulting in the immediate fulfilment of the person's wishes. It discouraged them from developing skills for flexibility, long-term planning and goal-setting and autonomous decision-making. This has further consequences for smoking reinforcement and the planning needed to quit smoking. A community response that addresses the negative effects of institutionalisation and encompasses the mentally ill as more fully participating members, with equal access to resources and supports, is suggested.

Occupational Health, Safety and Welfare Issues

When attempting to address concerns about smoking and occupational health and safety for staff, psychiatric institutions and prisons share similar dilemmas. They are, "the workplace of some people and the living space of other" (Biggins and Wares, 1993, p.327). Balancing any rights of patients to smoke in their living space with the rights of staff to a smoke-free work environment becomes difficult, especially in the locked settings where staff have designated roles in supervising patients while they are in the smokers' cage. A number of examples from the current research suggested that occupational health and safety for staff may have been compromised, with the potential for legal claims in some situations (Lawn, 2005).

Moving Forward

Imposing smoking bans as a solution to the culture of smoking within mental health settings has been considered, tried and studied. Overall, the results are mixed. Unintended negative consequences of such a policy change are evident in each study. Introducing smoking bans is possible but would need to be a clearly and carefully planned process involving all parties affected by a ban with an emphasis on consistency, coordination and full clinical and administrative support (Lawn and Pols, 2005; Seymour, 2001).

As an important step, the current study has demonstrated staff's reliance on smoking to assist with the clinical management of patients. Within psychiatric inpatient settings nurses, and to a lesser degree other staff, provide a high proportion of the direct care and contact with patients. Therefore, they are in a unique position to act as role models and to make a significant impact on patients' smoking behaviour and the associated risk of suffering tobacco-related diseases by directly supporting and participating in pharmacological and psychosocial interventions. Supporting nurses and other staff to clarify their values and the ethical principles on which they make decisions and act would seem important as well as promoting a learning environment where there is active dialogue amongst staff so that they can navigate through the dilemmas posed by their role (Lawn and Condon, 2006).

LIMITATIONS OF THE RESEARCH

This study has a number of limitations that need to be acknowledged. Firstly, the potential for participant selection bias was apparent, given the purposive sampling used and the voluntariness of participation. The absence of in-depth interviews with inpatients, especially those in long-stay wards, was a significant limitation of this study.

The potential for differences in systems of care also exists. These participants talked about, and were observed in, one institution in one state within Australia, though similar practices have been observed elsewhere (Lawn, 2004).

Cultural bias (Patton, 1980) and the potential for "observer drift" (Robson, 1993, p.224) were recognised by the researcher and acknowledged. Inter-observer agreement checks to minimise this potential problem (Robson, 1993) were performed. To combat these potential problems, the researcher trialed observations and regularly debriefed with supervisors. She also kept copious reflective, descriptive notes about the observations. She was disciplined in recording these notes as soon after the observations as practicable. The use of standardised observation sheets, based on the results of the fully audited qualitative data prior to entering the field also helped to overcome potential threats to validity and reliability and to enhance replicability. Field observations were limited to particular groups and areas and to particular times in the day. This was acknowledged and overcome by multiple periods of time spent in each of the settings, with varied timing of visits to incorporate the potential for observing the maximum variety of participants and interaction conditions.

The researcher was attuned to the potential for affective changes due to immersion in the settings being observed. As described by Schwartz and Schwartz (1955), these influences can be subtle but are an inevitable product of becoming involved in the emotional life of the participants. Regular debriefing with supervisors and diligent reflective notes were kept to combat this potential influence on the observation data.

ACKNOWLEDGMENTS

We would like to sincerely thank all those who participated in this research and the mental health services for allowing us to enter their unique world. The courage of patients in sharing their stories and the commitment and openness of staff was greatly appreciated.

Dr Pols has been acknowledged as co-author in appreciation for his mentorship, enthusiasm, generosity and contribution to the coding and analysis of data, and critical input to the original research and supervision of the initial PhD. Prof Jim Barber is also acknowledged for his support during the initial PhD research as co-supervisor to the primary author. Several others provided critical comment and support, including Ms Judith Condon (School of Nursing/Flinders University) and Ms Shaun Byrne (formerly from Southern Mental Health), who audited the research, Dr Lawrence Johnson (Department of Philosophy/Flinders University) for his role as reviewer for the ethics committee, and Dr Peter Blanksby (School of Social Work and Social Administration/Flinders University) and Dr Adrian Esterman (Department of Epidemiology/Flinders University) who provided invaluable comments and suggestions regarding the quantitative analysis of data. Mr John Harley (The Public Advocate) and Mr Owen Ames (Legal Services Commission) provided comments on legal and ethical aspects of the research findings. Dr Maria Zadoroznyj (School of Sociology/Flinders University) and Professor Sharyn Roach-Anleu (School of Sociology/Flinders University) gave confirming support for the direction of the research findings.

REFERENCES

Addington, J., el-Guebaly, N., Duchak, V., and Hodgins, D. (1997). Readiness to Stop Smoking in Schizophrenia. *Canadian Journal of Psychiatry,* 42 : 1, pp.49-52.

Addington, J. and Duchak, V. (1997). Reasons for substance Use in Schizophrenia. *Acta Psychiatrica Scandinavica,* 96, 329-333.

Adler, L. E., Hoffer, L. D., Wiser, A., and Freedman, R. (1993). Normalization of Auditory Physiology by Cigarette Smoking in Schizophrenic Patients. *American Journal of Psychiatry,* 150: 12, 1856-1861.

Aguilar, M. C., Gurpegui, M., Diaz, F. J. and de Leon, J. (2005). Nicotine Dependence and Symptoms of Schizophrenia. *British Journal of Psychiatry,* 186, 215-221.

American Psychiatric Association (2000). DSM-IV-TR: *Diagnostic and Statistical Manual of Mental Disorders.* Washington, DC, American Psychiatric Association.

Anda, R. F., Williamson, D. F., Escobedo, L. G., Mast, E. E., Giovino, G. A., and Remington, P.L. (1990). *Depression and the Dynamics of Smoking. Journal of the American Medical Association,* 264:12, pp.1541-5.

Armitage, P. and Berry, G. (1996). *Statistical Methods in Medical Research, Third Edition,* Oxford, Blackwell Scientific.

Barber, J. G., Punt, J., and Albers, J. (1988) - Alcohol and Power on Palm Island. *Australian Journal of Social Issue,* 23: 2, 87-101.

Barrett, R. J. (1996). The Psychiatric Team and the Social Definition of Schizophrenia: *An Anthropological Study or Person and Illness.* Cambridge, Cambridge University Press.

Baxter, E., Hafner, R. J., and Holme, G. (1992). Assaults By Patients: The Experience and Attitudes of Psychiatric Hospital Nurses. *Australian and New Zealand Journal of Psychiatry,* 26, 567-573.

Bellack, A. S. and DiClemente, C. C. (1999). Treating Substance Abuse Among Patients With Schizophrenia. *Psychiatric Services,* 50:1, 75-80.

Benezzi, F. (1989). Severe Mania Following Abrupt Nicotine Withdrawal, [letter]. *American Journal of Psychiatry,* 146:12, 1641.

Biggins, D. and Wares, H. (1993). Developing Policy for a Smoke-Free Work Environment in a Prison. Part 2. Policy Development. *Journal of Occupational Health and Safety – Australia and New Zealand,* 9:4, 325-330.

Blair, D. T. (1991). Assaultive Behaviour: Does Provocation Begin in the Front Office? *Journal of Psychosocial Nursing,* 29:5, 21-26.

Blanchard, J. J., Brown, S. A., Horan, W. P., and Sherwood, A. R. (2000). Substance Use Disorders in Schizophrenia: A Review, Integration, and a Proposed Model. *Clinical Psychology Review,* 20:2, 207-234.

Brayne, C. (2000). Smoking and the Brain: No Good Evidence Exists that Smoking Protects Against Dementia. *British Medical Journal,* 320:7242, 1087-1088.

Breslau, N. and Johnson, E. O. (2000). Predicting Smoking Cessation and Major Depression in Nicotine-Dependent Smokers. *American Journal of Public Health*, 90:7, 1122-1127.

Bronfenbrenner, U. (1979). The Ecology of Human Development: Experiments by Nature and Design, Cambridge, MA, Harvard University Press.

Brown, C. (2004). Tobacco and Mental Health: A Literature Review. Edinburgh: ASH Scotland. Available at: http://www.ashscotland.org.uk/ash/files/ tobacco%20and %20mental%20health.pdf (accessed 30 Aug 2006).

Brown, G. R. and Anderson, B. (1991). Psychiatric Morbidity in Adult Inpatients with Childhood Histories of Sexual and Physical Abuse. *American Journal of Psychiatry,* 148; 55-61.

Brown, R. A., Lewinsohn, P. M., Seeley, J. R., and Wagner, E. F. (1996). Cigarette Smoking, Major Depression, and Other Psychiatric Disorders Among Adolescents. *Journal of The American Academy of Child and Adolescent Psychiatry,* 35, 1602-1610.

Brown, S., Birtwhistle, J., Roe, L., and Thompson, C. (1999). The Unhealthy Lifestyle of People with Schizophrenia. *Psychological Medicine,* 29, 697-701.

Bulbena, A., and Berrios, G. E. (1993). Cognitive Function in the Affective Disorders: A Prospective Study. *Psychopathology,* 26, 6-12.

Burrows, S. (1994). Nurse-Aid Management of Psychiatric Emergencies. *British Journal of Nursing,* 3: 3, 121-125.

Carmody, T. P. (1989). Affect Regulation, Nicotine Addiction, and Smoking Cessation. *Journal of Psychoactive Drugs,* 2 : 3, 331-342.

Carosella, A.M., Ossip-Klein, D.J., and Owens, C.A. (1999). Smoking attitudes, beliefs, and readiness to change among acute and long term care inpatients with psychiatric diagnoses. *Addictive Behaviors, 24*(3), 331-344.

Carter, S., Borland, R., and Chapman, S. (2001). Finding the Strength to Kill Your Best Friend – Smokers Talk About Smoking and Quitting, Sydney, *Australian Smoking Cessation Consortium and GlaxoSmithKline Consumer Healthcare.*

Carton, S., Jouvent, R., and Widlocher, D. (1994). Nicotine Dependence and Motives for Smoking in Depression. *Journal of Substance Abuse,* 6:1, 67-76.

Coghlan, R., Lawrence, D., Holman, C.D.J. and Jablensky, A.V. (2001). *Duty of Care: Physical Illness in People with Mental Illness.* Perth, The University of Western Australia.

Collins, R.L., Gollnisch, G. and Morsheimer, E.T. (1999). Substance Use among a Regional Sample of Female Nurses. *Drug and Alcohol Dependence,* 55, 145-155.

Covey, L. S., Glassman, A. H., and Stetner, F. (1990). Depression and Depressive Symptoms in Smoking Cessation. *Comprehensive Psychiatry,* 31, 350-354.

Covey, L. S., Glassman, A. H., and Stetner, F. (1997). Major Depression Following Smoking Cessation. *American Journal of Psychiatry,* 154:2, 263-265.

Davidson, S., Judd, F. Jolley, D., Hocking, B., Thompson, S., and Hyland, B. (2001). Cardiovascular Risk Factors for People with Mental Illness. *Australian and New Zealand Journal of Psychiatry,* 35: 2, 196-202.

Decina, P., Caracci, G., Sandyk, R., Berman, W., Mukherjee, S., and Scapicchio, P. (1990). Cigarette Smoking and Neuroleptic-Induced Parkinsonism. *Biological Psychiatry,* 28, 502-508.

Dentler, R. A. and Erikson, K. T. (1984). The Functions of Deviance in Groups. Chapter Seven in D. H. Kelly (Ed.) Deviant Behaviour: *A Textbook in the Sociology of Deviance,* Second Edition, New York, St. Martin's Press, 90-103.

Doherty, K. (2006). Giving Up The Habit. *Mental Health Today,* May 2006, 27-29.

Doll, R. and Hill, A. B. (1950). Smoking and Carcinoma of the Lung. *The British Medical Journal,* 2, 739-748.

Doll, R. and Hill, A. B. (1964). Mortality in Relation to Smoking: Ten Years' Observations of British Doctors. *The British Medical Journal,* 2, 1399-1410.

Dulitt, R. A., Fyer, M. R., Haas, G. L., Sullivan, T., and Francis, A. J. (1990). Substance Use in Borderline Personality Disorder. *American Journal of Psychiatry,* 147, 1002-1007.

Dwyer, E. (1987). Homes for the Mad: *Life Inside Two Nineteenth Century Asylums,* New Brunswick, Rutgers University Press.

Edwards, A. R. (1988). Regulation and Repression: *The Study of Social Control, Sydney,* Allen and Unwin.

Escobedo, L., Kirch, D. G., and Anda, F. F. (1996). *Depression and Smoking Initiation Among US Latinos. Addiction,* 9: 1, 113-119.

Escobedo, L. G., Reddy, M., and Giovino, G. A. (1998). The Relationship Between Depressive Symptoms and Cigarette Smoking in US Adolescents. Addiction, 93: 3, 433-440.

Esterberg, M. L. and Compton, M. T. (2005). Smoking Behaviour in Persons with a Schizophrenia-Spectrum Disorder: A Qualitative Investigation of the Transtheoretical Model. *Social Science and Medicine,* 61, 293-303.

Fergusson, D. M., Lynskey, M. T., and Horwood, J. (1996). Comorbidity Between Depressive Disorders and Nicotine Dependence in a Cohort of 16-Year Olds. *Arch. General Psychiatry,* 53, 1043-7.

Forchuk C., Norman, R., Malla, A., Vos, A., and Martin, L. (1997). Smoking and Schizophrenia. *Journal of Psychiatric and Mental Health Nursing,* 4, 355-359.

Forsyth, D. R. (1999). *Group Dynamics,* Third Edition, Belmont, USA, Brooks/Cole, Wadsworth.

Foucault, M. (1977). Discipline and Punish: *The Birth of the Prison,* Harmondsworth, UK, Penguin Books. .

Friedrichs, J. and Ludtke, H. (1975). Participant Observation : *Theory and Practice,* Westmead, England, Saxon House / Lexington Books.

George, T. P. and Krystal, J. H. (2000). Comorbidity of Psychiatric and Substance Abuse Disorders. *Current Opinion in Psychiatry,* 13: 3, 327-331.

Glaser, B. G. and Strauss, A. L. (1967). *The Discovery of Grounded Theory: Strategies for Qualitative Research,* New York, Aldine Publishing Company.

Glassman, A. H. (1992). Cigarette Smoking, Major Depression, and Schizophrenia.Clinical Neuropharmacology, 15, Supplement 1, Part A, 560A-561A.

Glassman, A. H. (1993). Cigarette Smoking: Implications for Psychiatric Illness, *American Journal of Psychiatry,* 150, 546-553.

Glynn, S. M. and Sussman, S. (1990). Why Patients Smoke. (letter) *Hospital and Community Psychiatry,* 41: 9, 1027-1028.

Goff, D. C., Henderson, D. C., and Amico, E. (1992). Cigarette Smoking in Schizophrenia: Relationship to Psychopathology and Medication Side Effects. *American Journal of Psychiatry,* 149: 9, 1189-1194.

Goffman, E. (1961a). Asylums: Essays on the Social Situation of Mental Patients and Other Inmates, New York, Anchor Books/Doubleday.

Goffman, E. (1961b). On the Characteristics of Total Institutions: The Inmate World. Chapter Two in D. R. Cressey (Ed.) *The Prison: Studies in Institutional Organisation and Change,* New York, Holt, Rinehart, and Winston, Inc.,15-67.

Goffman, E. (1961c). On the Characteristics of Total Institutions: Staff - Inmate Relations. Chapter Three in D. R. Cressey (Ed.) *The Prison: Studies in Institutional Organisation and Change,* New York Holt, Rinehart, and Winston, Inc., 68-106.

Goffman, E. (1963). Stigma: Notes on the Management of Spoiled Identity, Harmondsworth, Penguin.

Gold, M. S. and Miller, N. S. (1994). The Biology of Addiction and Psychiatric Disorders. Chapter Three in N. S. Miller (Ed) *Treating Coexisting Psychiatric and Addictive Disorders: A Practical Guide, Minnesota, Hazelden,* 35-49.

Gonzalez-Pinto, A., Gutierrez, M., Ezcurra, J., Aizpuru, F., Mosquera, F., Lopez, P., and de Leon, J. (1998). Tobacco Smoking and Bipolar Disorder. *Journal of Clinical Psychiatry,* 59: 5, 225-228.

Goodman, E., and Capitman, J. (2000). Depressive Symptoms and Cigarette Smoking Among Teens. *Pediatrics,* 106: 4, Part 1 of 2, 748-755.

Greeman, M. and McClellan, T. A. (1991). Negative Effects of a Smoking Ban on an Inpatient Psychiatry Service. *Hospital and Community Psychiatry,* 42: 4, 408-412.

Griffith, J. (1999). Substance Abuse Disorders in Nurses. *Nurses Forum,* 34: 4, 19-28.

Guba, E. G. (1981). Criteria for Assessing the Trustworthiness of Naturalistic Inquiries. Education, Communication and *.Technology Journal.* 29: 2, 75-91.

Hall, S. M., Munoz, R. F., Reus, V. I., Sees, K. L., Duncan, C. Humfleet, G. L., and Hartz, D. T. (1996). Mood Management and Nicotine Gum in smoking Treatment: A Therapeutic Contact and Placebo-Controlled Study. *Journal of Consulting and Clinical Psychology,* 65: 5, 1003-1009.

Harrington, A. J. (1974). Hospital Violence. *Nursing Mirror,* 135: 3, 12-13.

Hatch, E. (1985). Culture. In A Kuper and J. Kuper (Eds.) *The Social Science Encyclopedia.* London, Routledge and Kegan Paul, *178-179.*

Hatzitaskos, P., Soldatos, C. R., Kokkevi, A., and Stefanis, C. N. (1999). Substance Abuse Patterns and Their Association With Psychopathology and Type of Hostility in Male Patients with Borderline and Antisocial Personality Disorder. *Comprehensive Psychiatry,* 40: 4, 278-282.

Haywood, T. W., Kravitz, H. M., Grossman, L. S., Cavanaugh, J. L. Jr., Davis, J. M., and Lewis, D. A. (1995). Predicting the 'Revolving Door' Phenomenon Among Patients with Schizophrenic, Schizoaffective, and Affective Disorders. *American Journal of Psychiatry,* 152, 856-861.

Hennekens, C. H., Hennekens, A. R., Hollar, D. and Casey, D. E. (2005). Schizophrenia and Increased Risks of Cardiovascular Disease. *American Heart Journal,* 150, 1115-1121.

Herran, A., de Santiago A., Sandoya, M., Fernandez, M.J., Diez-Manrique, J.F., and Vazquez-Barquero, J.L. (2000). Determinants of smoking behaviour in outpatients with schizophrenia. *Schizophrenia Research,* 41, 373-381.

Himelhoch, S., Lehman, A., Kreyenbuhl, J., Daumit, G., Brown, C. and Dixon, L. (2004). Prevalence of Chronic Obstructive Pulmonary Disease among those with Serious Mental Illness. *American Journal of Psychiatry,* 161, 2317-2319.

Holmberg, S. K. and Kane, C. (1999). Health and Self-Care Practices of Persons With Schizophrenia. *Psychiatric Services,* 50, 827-829.

Hughes, J. R., Hatsukami, D. K., Mitchell, J. E., and Dahlgren, L. A. (1986). Prevalence of Smoking Among Psychiatric Outpatients. American Journal of Psychiatry, 143, 993-997.

Jarvis, M. J. (2004). Why People Smoke. *British Medical Journal,* 328, 277-279.

Jessop, R. D. (1972). Social Order, Reform and Revolution: *A Power, Exchange and Institutionalisation Perspective.* London, MacMillan.

Johnson, J. G., Cohen, P., Dohrenwend, B. P., Link, B. G., and Brook, J. S. (1999). A Longitudinal Investigation of Social Causation and Social Selection Processes Involved in the Association Between Socioeconomic Status and Psychiatric Disorders. *Abnormal Psychology,* 108: 3, 490-499.

Jones, A. and May, J. (1992). Working in Human Service Organisations: A Critical Introduction, Melbourne, Longman Cheshire.

Jorgensen, D. L. (1989). *Participant Observation: A Methodology for Human Studies,* Newbury Park, California, Sage Publications.

Kandel, D. B. and Davies, M. (1986). Adult Sequelae of Adolescent Depressive Symptoms. *Arch. General Psychiatry, 4*3, 255-262.

Kaplan, M. S. and Weiler, R. E. (1997). Social Patterns of Smoking Behaviour: Trends and Practice Implications. Social Work, 22: 1, 47-52.

Katz, P. and Kirkland, F. R. (1990). Violence and Social Structure on Mental Hospital Wards. Psychiatry, 53, 262-277.

Kelly, C. and McCreadie, R. G. (1999). Smoking Habits, Current Symptoms, and Premorbid Characteristics of Schizophrenic Patients in Nithdale, Scotland. *American Journal of Psychiatry,* 156, 1751-1757.

Kendler, K. S., Neale, M. C., MacLean, C. J., Heath, A. C., Eaves, L. J., and Kessler, R.C. (1993). Smoking and Major Depression: A Causal Analysis. *Arch. General Psychiatry,* 50: 1, 36-43.

Khantzian, E. J. (1985). The Self-Medication Hypothesis of Addictive Disorders: Focus On Heroin and Cocaine Dependence. *American Journal of Psychiatry,* 142:11, 1259-1265.

Kinnunen, T., Doherty, K., Militello, F. S., and Garvey, A. J. (1996). Depression and Smoking Cessation: Characteristics of Depressed Smokers and Effects of Nicotine Replacement. *Journal of Consulting and Clinical Psychology,* 64:4, 791-798.

Kisely, S., smith, M. Lawrence, D. and Maaten, S. (2005). Mortality in Individuals who have had Psychiatric Treatment: Population-Based Study in Nova Scotia. *British Journal of Psychiatry,* 187, 552-558.

Koob, G. F. (1992). Drugs of Abuse: Anatomy, Pharmacology and Function of Reward Pathways. *Trends in Pharmacological Science,* 13, 177-184.

Kumari, V. and Postma, P. (2005). Nicotine Use in Schizophrenia: The Self-Medication hypotheses. *Neuroscience and Biobehavioural Reviews,* 29, 1021-1034.

Laakso, A., Vilkman, H., Kajander, J., Bergman, J., Haaparanta, M. Solin, O., and Hietala. J. (2000). Prediction of Detached Personality in Healthy Subjects by Low Dopamine Transporter Binding. *The American Journal of Psychiatry,* 157: 2, 290-292.

Lasser, K., Boyd, J. W., Woolhandler, S., Himmelstein, D. U., McCormick, D., and Bor, D. H. (2000). Smoking and Mental Illness: A Population-Based Prevalence Study. *Journal of the American Medical Association,* 284: 20, 2606-2610.

Lawn, S.J. (2001) Systemic Barriers to Quitting Smoking Among Institutionalised Public Mental Health Service Populations. Unpublished PhD Thesis, Flinders University of South Australia, Adelaide, South Australia.

Lawn, S. (2001a) Australians With Mental Illness Who Smoke. *British Journal of Psychiatry,* 178, 85.

Lawn, S.J. and Abram, L. (2002). Quitline Workers and Mental Health Services: A Rewarding Partnership. 12th Annual TheMHS Conference Proceedings, TheMHS Conference Inc of Australia and New Zealand, 2002.

Lawn, S. J., Pols, R. G., and Barber, J. G. (2002). Smoking and Quitting: A Qualitative Study of Community-Living Psychiatric Clients. *Social Science and Medicine,* 54, 93- 104.

Lawn, S.J. and Pols, R.G. (2003). Nicotine Withdrawal: Pathway to Aggression and Assault in the Locked Psychiatric Ward. *Australasian Psychiatry,* 11:2, 199-203.

Lawn, S.J. (2004). Systemic Barriers to Quitting Smoking Among Institutionalised Public Mental Health Service Populations: A Comparison of Two Australian Sites. *International Journal of Social Psychiatry,* 50, 204-215.

Lawn, S. J. and Pols, R. G. (2005) Smoking Bans In Psychiatric Inpatient Settings? A Review of the Research, *Australian and New Zealand Journal of Psychiatry,* 39, 874-893.

Lawn, S. J. (2005) Cigarette Smoking in Psychiatric Settings: Occupational Health, Safety, Welfare and Legal Concerns, *Australian and New Zealand Journal of Psychiatry,* 39, 894-899.

Lawn, S. and Condon, J. (2006) Psychiatric Nurses' Ethical Stance on Cigarette Smoking by Patients: Determinants and Dilemmas in their Role in Supporting Cessation. *International Journal of Mental Health Nursing,* 15, 111-118.

Lawson, J. R. (1992). Patient Assault as an Occupational Health and Safety Issue for Psychiatric Nurses and Some Preventative Strategies: *A Discussion Paper.* The Lamp, 49: 1, 23-29.

Leedy, P. D. (1997). Practical Research : Planning and Design, Sixth Edition, New Jersey, Prentice Hall Inc.

de Leon, J., Dadvand, M., Canuso, C., White, A. O. (1995). Schizophrenia and Smoking: An Epidemiological Survey in a State Hospital. *American Journal of Psychiatry,* 152: 3, 453-455.

Levin, T. (2001). A Psychiatric Resident's Journey Through the Closed Ward. *Psychiatric Bulletin,* 27:3, 539-547.

Lewin, K. (1948). Resolving Social Conflicts: Selected Papers on Group Dynamics, New York, Harper. .

Lion, J. R. (1987). Training for Battle: Thoughts on Managing Aggressive Patients. *Hospital and Community Psychiatry,* 38: 8, 882-884.

Lohr, J. B. and Flynn, K. (1992). Smoking and Schizophrenia. *Schizophrenia Research,* 8:2, 93-102.

Lopez, A. (2000). Investigating Australia's Burden of Disease. *Medical Journal of Australia,* 172, 572-573.

McCreadie, R. G. (2003). Diet, Smoking and Cardiovascular Risk in People with Schizophrenia: Descriptive Study. *British Journal of Psychiatry,* 183, 534-539.

McEvoy, J. P. and Brown, S. (1999). Smoking in First-episode Patients with Schizophrenia. *The American Journal of Psychiatry,* 156: 7, 1120-1121.

McNeill, A. (2001). *Smoking and Mental Health: A Review of the Literature.* London, SmokeFree London Programme, London Region National Health Service.

Miller, M., Hemenway, D., and Rimm, E. (2000). Cigarettes and Suicide: A Prospective Study of 50,000 Men. *American Journal of Public Health,* 90: 5, 768-773.

Miller, W. R. (1990). Spirituality: the Silent Dimension in Addiction Research. The 1990 Leonard Ball Oration, *Drug and Alcohol Review,* 9, 259-266.

Moos, R. H. (1976). The Human Context: Environmental Determinants of Behaviour, New York, Wiley.

Moos, R. H. and Insel, P. M. (1974) (Eds.). *Issues in Social Ecology: Human Milieus,* Palo Alto, California, National Press Books.

Morrison, E. F. (1990a). The Tradition of Toughness: A Study of Non-Professional Nursing Care in Psychiatric Settings. IMAGE: *Journal of Nursing Scholarship,* 22: 1, 32-38.

Morrison, E. F. (1990b). Violent Psychiatric Inpatients in a Public Hospital. *Scholarly Inquiry For Nursing Practice: An International Journal,* 4: 1, 65-82.

Mortensen, P. B. and Juel, K. (1993). Mortality and Causes of Death in First Admission Schizophrenic Patients. *British Journal of Psychiatry,* 163, 183-189.

Nace, E. P. (1990) – "Substance Use Disorder and Personality Disorders: *Comorbidity,"* *Psychiatric Hospital,* 20, 65-69.

Nijman, H. L. I. and Rector, G. (1999). Crowding and Aggression on Inpatient Psychiatric Wards. *Psychiatric Services,* 50:6, 830-831.

Nisbet, R. (1972). Introduction: The Problem of Social Change. Chapter One in R. Nisbet (Ed.) *Social Change,* Oxford, Basil Blackwell , 1-45.

Office of Environmental Health Hazard Assessment (1997). Health Effects of Exposure to Environmental Tobacco Smoke, Sacramento, California Environmental Protection Agency.

Ogburn, W. F. (1972). *Fixity and Persistence in Society.* Chapter Two in R. Nisbet (Ed.) Social Change, Oxford, Basil Blackwell, 46-71.

Parrott, A. (2000). Smoking and Adverse Childhood Experiences. *Journal of the American Medical Association,* 283: 15, 1958-1960.

Patton, M. Q. (1980). *Qualitative Evaluation Methods,* Beverley Hills, California, Sage Publications Inc.

Plant, M. L., Plant, M. A., and Foster, J. (1991). Alcohol, Tobacco and Illicit Drug Use Amongst Nurses: A Scottish Study. Drug and Alcohol Dependence, 28, 195-202.

Poirier, M., Canceil, O., Bayle, F., Millet, B., Bourdel, M., Moatti, C., Olie, J., and Attar-Levy, (2002). *Prevalence of smoking in psychiatric patients. Progress in Neuro-Psychopharmacology and Biological Psychiatry,* 26, 529-537.

Pontieri, F. E., Tanda. G., Orzi, F., and DiChiara, G. (1996). Effects of Nicotine on the Nucleus Accumbens and Similarity to Those of Addictive Drugs. *Nature,* 382, 255-257.

Prochaska, J. J., Gill, P. and Hall, S. M. (2004). Treatment of Tobacco Use in an Inpatient Psychiatric Setting. *Psychiatric Services,* 55, 1265-1270.

Rhodes, L. A. (1991). Emptying Beds: The Work of an Emergency Psychiatric Unit. Berkeley, University of California Press.

Roach Anleu, S. L. (1999). *Deviance, Conformity and Control, Third Edition,* Melbourne, Longman.

Robertson, G. and Taylor, P. (1985). Some Cognitive Correlates of Affective Disorders. Psychological. *Medicine.* 15, 297-309.

Robson, C. (1993). Real World Research: A Resource for Social Scientists and Practitioners, Oxford, Blackwell.

Roche, A. M. and Ober, C. (1997). Rethinking Smoking Among Aboriginal Australians: The Harm Minimisation-Abstinence Conundrum", *Health Promotion Journal of Australia,* 7: 2, 128-133.

Rodgers, B. L. and Cowles, K. V. (1993). The Qualitative Research Audit Trail: A Complex Collection of Documentation. *Research on Nursing and Health,* 16, 219-226.

Rodwell, K. and Byers, K. V. (1997). Auditing Constructive Inquiry: Perspectives of Two Stakeholders. *Qualitative Inquiry,* 3: 1, 116-135.

Rolfe, A. (1995). An Examination of Contextual Influences on the Incidence of Staff Assault in Psychiatric Settings, Master of Nursing Studies by Coursework, Flinders University of South Australia, Adelaide, South Australia.

Rose, K. and Webb, C. (1998). Analyzing Data: Maintaining Rigor in a Qualitative Study. *Qualitative Health Research,* 8: 4, 556-562.

Rowe, K. and Clark, J. M. (2000). The Incidence of Smoking Amongst Nurses: A Review of the Literature. *Journal of Advanced Nursing,* 31: 5, 1046-1053.

Royal College of Physicians (1962). *Smoking and Health,* Tunbridge Wells, Kent, Pitman Medical.

Royal College of Physicians (1971). *Smoking and Health Now,* Second Report, Tunbridge Wells, Kent, Pitman Medical, 144-147.

Royal College of Physicians (1977). *Smoking or Health,* Third Report, Tunbridge Wells, Kent, Pitman Medical.

Royal College of Physicians (2000). *Nicotine Addiction in Britain,* London, Tobacco Advisory Group, Royal College of Physicians.

Sabo, A. N. (1997). Etiological Significance of Associations Between Childhood Trauma and Borderline Personality Disorder: Conceptual and Clinical Implications. *Journal of Personality Disorders,* 11, 50-70.

Salokangas, R. K. R., Vilkman, H., Ilonen, T., Taiminene, T., Bergman, J., Haaparanta, M., Solin, O., Alanen, A., Syvalahti, E., and Hietala, J. (2000). High Levels of Dopamine in the Basal Ganglia of Cigarette Smokers. *The American Journal of Psychiatry,* 157: 4, 632-634.

Sandyk, R. (1993). Cigarette Smoking: Effects on Cognitive Functions and Drug-Induced Parkinsonism in Chronic Schizophrenia. *International Journal of Neuroscience,* 70, 193-197.

Sandyk, R. and Kay, S. R. (1991). Tobacco Addiction as a Marker of Age of Onset of Schizophrenia. *International Journal of Neuroscience,* 57, 259-263.

Sarna, L. (1999). Hope and Vision Prevention: Tobacco Control and Cancer Nursing. *Cancer Nursing,* 22:1, 21-28.

Schachter, S. (1973). Nesbitt's Paradox. In W. Dunn (Ed.) *Smoking Behaviour: Motives And Incentives,* New York, Wiley.

Schein, J.R. (1995). Cigarette Smoking and Clinically Significant Drug Interactions. *The Annals of Pharmacotherapy,* 29, 1139-1148.

Schon, D. A. (1972). *The Social System and Social Chang.* Chapter Four in R. Nisbet (Ed.) Social Change, Oxford, Basil Blackwell, 83-100.

Schwandt, T. and Halpern, E. (1988). Linking Auditing and Metaevaluation: Enhancing Quality in Applied Inquiry, Newbury Park, California, Sage.

Schwartz, M. S. and Schwartz, C. G. (1955). Problems in Participant Observation. *The American Journal of Sociology,* 60, 343-353.

Seymour, L. (2001). Where Do We Go From Here? Tobacco Control Policies Within Psychiatric and Long-Stay Units: *Guidance on Development and Implementation.* Health Development Agency, London.

Shiffman, S., Hickcox, M., Paty, J. A., Gnys, M., Kassel, J. D., and Richards, T. J. (1996). Progression From a Smoking Lapse to Relapse: Prediction From Abstinence Violation Effects, Nicotine Dependence, and Lapse Characteristics. *Journal of Consulting and Clinical Psychology,* 64: 5, 993-1002.

Shlomowitz, E. A. (1990). *The Treatment of Mental Illness in South Australia 1852-1884: From Care to Custody,* Unpublished doctoral dissertation, Flinders University of South Australia, Adelaide, Australia.

Sidanius J. and Pratto, F. (1999). Social Dominance: An Intergroup Theory of Social Hierarchy and Oppression, Cambridge, Cambridge University Press.

Simon, A. and Boyer, E. G. (1974) (Eds.). *Mirrors for Behaviour III: An Anthology of Observation Instruments,* Third Edition. Wyncote, Pennsylvania, Communication Materials Centre.

Skinner, B. F. (1953). *Science and Human Behaviour.* New York, MacMillan.

Sonne, S. C., Brady, K. T., and Morton, A. (1994). Substance Abuse and Bipolar Affective Disorder. *Journal of Nervous and Mental Disorders,* 182: 6, 349-352.

Soyka, M., Albus, M., Kathmann, N., Finelli, A., Hofstetter, S., Holzbach, R., Immler, B., and Sand, P. (1993). Prevalence pf Alcohol and Drug Abuse in Schizophrenia Inpatients. *European Archives of Psychiatry and Clinical Neuroscience,* 242, 362-372.

Stage, K. B., Glassman, A. H., and Covey, L. A. (1996). Depression After Smoking Cessation: Case Reports. *Journal of Clinical Psychiatry,* 57: 10,467-469.

Stanton, A. and Schwartz, M. (1954). *The Mental Hospital,* New York, Basic Books.

Stefanis C. N. and Kokkevi, A. (1986). *Depression and Drug Use. Psychopathology,* 19 (suppl.2), 124-131.

Stewart, M. J., Brosky, G., Gillis, A. Jackson, S., G., Johnston, G., Kirkland, S. (1996). Disadvantaged Women and Smoking. *Canadian Journal of Public Health,* 87: 4, 257-260.

Stewart, M. J., Gillis, A. Brosky, G., Johnston, G., Kirkland, S., Leigh, G., Persaud, V., Rootman, I., Jackson, S., and Pawliw-Fry, B. (1996). Smoking Among Disadvantaged Women: Causes and Cessation. *Canadian Journal of Nursing,* 28: 1, 41-60.

Strakowski, S. M. and DelBello, M. P. (2000). The Co-occurrence of Bipolar and Substance Use Disorders. *Clinical Psychology Review,* 20: 2, 191-206.

Strauss, A. and Corbin, J. (1990). Basics of qualitative Research: Grounded Theory Procedures and Techniques, London, Sage.

Stubbs, J., Haw, C. and Garner, L. (2004). Survey of Staff Attitudes to Smoking in a Large Psychiatric Hospital. *Psychiatric Bulletin,* 24, 204-207.

Suto, M. and Frank, G. (1994). Future Time Perspective and Daily Occupations of Persons with Schizophrenia in a Board and Care Home. *The American Journal of Occupational Therapy,* 48: 1, 7-18.

Sykes, G. M. (1958). The Society of Captives: A Study of a Maximum Security Prison, Princeton, New Jersey, Princeton University Press.

Taiminen, T. J., Salokangas, R. K. R., Saarijarvi, S., Nieme, H., Lehto, H., Ahola, V., and Syvalahti, E. (1998). *Smoking and Cognitive Deficits in Schizophrenia: A Pilot Study. Addictive Behaviours,* 23: 2, 263-266.

Tagliacozzo, R., Sci, N., and Vaughn, S. (1982). Stress and Smoking in Hospital Nurses. *American Journal of Public Health,* 72: 5, 441-448.

Tidey, J. W., Rohsenow, D. J., Kaplan, G. B. and Swift, R. M. (2005). Cigarette Smoking Topography in Smokers with Schizophrenia and Matched Non-Psychiatric Controls. *Drug and Alcohol Dependence,* 80, 259-265.

Tiihonen, J. Vilkman, H., Rasanen, P., Ryynanen, O-P., Hakko, H., Bergman, J., Hamalainen, T., Laakso, A., Haaparant-Solin, M., Solin, O., Kuoppamaki, M., Syvalahti, E., and Hietala, J. (1998). Striatal Presynaptic Dopamine Function in Type 1 Alcoholics Measured with Positron Emission Tomography. *Molecular Psychiatry,* 4, 156-161.

Trinkoff, A. and Storr, C. (1998). Substance Use Among Nurses: Differences Between Specialities. *Journal of Addictions Nursing,* 10, 77-83.

Trull, T. J., Sher, K. J., Minks-Brown, C., Durbin, J., and Burr, R. (2000). Borderline Personality Disorder and Substance Use Disorders: A Review and Integration. *Clinical Psychology Review,* 20: 2, 235-253.

Tsoh, J. Y., Humfleet, G. L., Munoz, R. F., Reus, V. I., Hartz, D. T., and Hall, S. M. (2000). Development of Major Depression After Treatment for Smoking Cessation. *The American Journal of Psychiatry,* 157: 3, 368-374.

US Department of Health and Human Services (1964). Smoking and Health: Report of the Advisory Committee to the Surgeon General of the Public Health Service, Washington, DC, US Department of Health and Human Services, Government Printing Office.

US Department of Health and Human Services (1984). The Health Consequences of Smoking: Cardiovascular Disease: A Report of the US Surgeon General, Rockville, Maryland, Us Department of Health and Human Services, Office on Smoking and Health, DHHS Publication No. (PHS) 84-50204.

US Department of Health and Human Services (1988). The Health Consequences of Smoking: Nicotine and Addiction : A Report of the US Surgeon General, Rockville, Maryland, US Department of Health and Human Services, Office on Smoking and Health, DHHS Publication No. (CDC) 88-8406.

US Department of Health and Human Services (1989). Reducing the Health Consequences of Smoking – 25 Years of Progress: A Report of the US Surgeon General, Rockville, Maryland, US Department of Health and Human Services, Public Health Service, Centers for Disease Control, Center for Chronic Disease Prevention and Health Promotion, Office on Smoking and Health,. DHHS Publication No. (CDC) 89-8411.

Watt, J. and Hocking, B. (1996). Mental Illness and Smoking Cessation: An Urgent Public Health Issue. Symposium - Introduction and Abstracts, Melbourne, Quit Victoria / Schizophrenia Australia.

Wewers, M.E., Ahijevych, K.L. and Sarna, L. (1998). Smoking Cessation Interventions in Nursing Practice. *Nursing Clinics of North America,* 33, 61-74.

Wilhelm, K., Arnold, K., Niven, H. and Richmond, R. (2004). Grey Lungs and Blue Moods: Smoking Cessation in the Context of Lifetime Depression History. *Australian and New Zealand Journal of Psychiatry,* 38, 896-905.

Wicker, A. W. (1974). Processes Which Mediate Behaviour-Environment Congruence. Part 10, No.5, in R. H. Moos and P. M. Insel (1974) (Eds.) *Issues in Social Ecology: Human Milieus,* Palo Alto, California, National Press Books.

Worthington, J., Fava, M., Agustin, C., Alpert, J., Nierenberg, A. A., Pava J., and Rosenbaum, J. F. (1996). Consumption of Alcohol, Nicotine, and Caffeine Among Depressed Outpatients: Relationship With Response to Treatment. *Psychosomatics,* 37, 518-522.

Wu, L. and Anthony, J. C. (1999). Tobacco Smoking and Depressed Mood in Late Childhood and Early Adolescence. *American Journal of Public Health,* 89, 1837-1840.

Yassa, R., Korpassy, A. and Ally, J. (1987). Nicotine Exposure and Tardive Dyskinesia, *Biological Psychiatry,* 22, 67-72.

Ziedonis, D. M. and George, T. P. (1997).Schizophrenia and Nicotine Use: Report of a Pilot Smoking Cessation Program and Review of Neurobiological and Clinical Issues. *Schizophrenia Bulletin,* 23: 2, 247-254.

Ziedonis, D. M., Kosten, J. R., Glazer, W. M., and Frances, R. J. (1994). Nicotine Dependence and Schizophrenia. *Hospital and Community Psychiatry,* 45, 204-206.

In: Smoking Cessation: Theory, Interventions and Prevention   ISBN: 978-1-60021-591-9
Editor: Jerome E. Landow   © 2008 Nova Science Publishers, Inc.

Chapter 2

COLLEGE SMOKING PREVENTION AND CESSATION: ENGAGING STUDENTS IN THE SEARCH FOR SOLUTIONS

*Catherine Chambliss[1], Brett Hartl[1],
Chris Hartl[1] and Amy Hartl[2]*

[1] Ursinus College, Collegeville, Pennsylvania, USA
[2] Spring-Ford High School, Royersford, Pennsylvania, USA

ABSTRACT

Cigarette smoking imperils roughly 6000 additional individuals in this country each day (that many youngsters light up for the first time daily); over 400,000 die annually as a result of having made the decision to smoke tobacco. The more we know about the factors influencing the decision to smoke, and the more we amass evidence in support of the decision to refrain, our power to effect positive change will be enhanced.

Given the imperfect efficacy of smoking cessation programs, prevention needs to be a top priority. Since many young people begin to smoke as a means of enhancing their social image, it may be helpful for them to learn more about the actual magnitude of negative stereotyping of smokers. Perhaps if they are better informed about the social hazards of smoking, they will be more likely to make the decision to refrain. Failing that, at least this information should make them less likely to smoke in public. This in itself should be beneficial, because reductions in public smoking should reduce pro-smoking norms.

A research project consisting of several studies conducted over a five year period was developed to increase campus awareness of the risks associated with campus smoking. In order to shift student norms, a large number of undergraduates, including several student leaders, participated actively in the research process. The studies assessed the reasons students smoke, the reasons many refrain, the social costs associated with public smoking, the impact of environmental manipulations on smoking behavior, and the effects of participation in campus smoking cessation programs. Several of the studies explored how students and teachers in high schools, colleges, law and medical schools view adolescents who smoke cigarettes. The results revealed pervasive, harsh negative stereotypes of smokers. Campus discussion of these findings increased students' awareness of the potential social, academic, and career repercussions of choosing to smoke.

Collectively, these studies were accompanied by an 8% reduction in the percentage of students reporting regular use of cigarettes (from 34% in 1999 to 26% in 2004). Since student involvement in this research project seems to have helped to interrupt a rising trajectory in undergraduate smoking on campus, this chapter will review the results of the studies comprising this project and explore various strategies for engaging students in smoking prevention and cessation programs.

PREFACE

This chapter integrates the findings from twenty studies on the problem of high school and college student cigarette smoking that have been conducted in collaboration with a wonderfully talented group of undergraduate students at Ursinus College. The research groups have included former, in-transition, and nonsmoker students. This summary report of the results of these various studies may assist others interested in responding to the expanding problem of campus tobacco use, and may suggest ways of getting students involved in this issue. Use of similar surveys and interventions may help others to increase their own campus' awareness of this threat. These types of efforts may also help them to counter the national trend on their own campus, perhaps making their institution a healthy exception to the rule.

The studies summarized here were designed to address the following four objectives: (I) to obtain information about the reasons for the recent upsurge in college student smoking, including both internal and external factors, and to quantify depictions of smoking behavior in recent films (including assessment of the personality characteristics of film characters who smoke) (II) to quantify current campus attitudes toward smokers (among students and faculty, including current smokers, former smokers, and nonsmokers, using both an American and a cross-cultural sample), (III) to determine the efficacy of a standard smoking cessation treatment method when delivered on a college campus, using both a group format and an individualized method of presentation strategy, and (IV) to assess the utility of interventions aimed at restoring antismoking norms on campus, by exploring the impact of an unobtrusive environmental intervention on the level of public smoking outside campus buildings, and assessing whether public smoking restrictions have unintended detrimental effects on young smokers (by inadvertently increasing the appeal and reinforcing properties of tobacco, thereby increasing the risk of nicotine addiction).

PERSONAL RATIONALE FOR THIS RESEARCH

A while back, the senior author of this chapter was asked to bring a prop related to her recent research projects to a faculty conference. It seemed easy enough: she'd bring a pack of cigarettes. But she had never purchased cigarettes before that week. When she bought them at the supermarket, it was a very foreign experience. She felt the strange need to apologize to the cashier and to let her know she wasn't actually a smoker. She was very reluctant to buy them in the first place, because it bothered her to contribute even trivially to the profits of tobacco companies. She ended up returning them to the store after the conference (she considered saying "Hey, when I got these home I read the label and it says that these are no good for you!"). There; her bias is clear.

She was lucky enough to come of age at a time and in a place where the successful smart people she longed to emulate didn't smoke. (Of course they did other dumb things, and she dutifully followed suit, but that's another story). So for her it was an easy choice; there was no external temptation to start smoking. Plus, inhaling cigarette smoke always made her feel queasy, so the internal, subjective experience of smoking was also unappealing.

The week before that faculty conference, when she was carrying a pack of cigarettes around, was unexpectedly disturbing. When she opened her purse, and saw a red pack of cigarettes inside, it seemed much more like an adult's purse. That's because her mother's purse always had a pack of cigarettes in it. Rummaging in a purse containing cigarettes evoked a flood of feelings. She was nine years old again, really concerned about her mother's smoking, yet somehow comforted by the familiar smell of tobacco.

About twenty years ago, her mother died of lung cancer. That grim disease was made all the grimmer by the response of others to her dying. "Well, she smoked", "She was a smoker, right?," they said. Although they never shared this sentiment so directly with her mother, their beliefs about her mother's responsibility for her own terminal illness doubtless colored their reactions to her mother. Interestingly, some people seem to show much more compassion for those who commit suicide. The misfortune of smokers who get sick is somehow dismissed; they are held fully responsible for their plight, perhaps thereby reassuring the healthy of their own invulnerability. Their blaming stance, mingled with the author's own anger about losing her mother, left the author deeply resentful toward tobacco companies and their manipulation of consumers.

The lead author of this chapter is currently a professor of psychology at Ursinus College. When she noticed that the rates of cigarette smoking among students there seemed to be creeping upward in the 1990s, she decided to see if she could interest undergraduates in a research program addressing the issue. As she and her students started the program, she remembered that she'd done some research on smoking reduction techniques. In fact, 30 years ago, as part of her masters' thesis, she'd actually conducted a smoking cessation program for 150 people. It was a standard misattribution study, looking at something called the negative placebo effect, which involves patients' getting worse while on placebos. This is believed to happen when people credit a placebo with reducing their symptoms, notice they still have symptoms, and then conclude that their underlying problem is worsening because even with the placebo they're a wreck.

She was interested in whether taking placebic medication during smoking cessation might backfire like this. Would people taking a placebo described as reducing appetite, irritability, and tension actually do worse than those in other experimental conditions? As it turned out, there was so much variability in the data that she didn't get much of a significant placebo effect, positive or negative. However, she found it interesting that some of her participants refused to turn in their placebos at the end of the study, swearing that they were terrifically effective, even after they had been debriefed about how the pills were pharmacologically inert sugar.

At the time she was not especially interested in smoking cessation treatment per se; it just provided her with a readily accessible population of clients she could use to explore attribution effects. Back then, she thought that smoking was obviously on its way out...so much so that when she was approached by a publisher to expand the work of her thesis into a book, she declined, thinking it would do her no good to specialize in treating a problem that would soon be obsolete. With these sadly incorrect expectations, it took her a couple of years before she acknowledged that more and more of her brightest students were not only smoking, but were developing this habit after arriving at college. More and more were congregating outside of buildings before classes, creating a cloud that all must pass through. Who would have ever thought that cigarette smoking would have made a comeback on American campuses, given all that we now know about its risks?

Recent research indicating an upsurge in college students' smoking is at odds with the popular assumption that the problem of smoking among the young is waning, thanks to more systematic health education initiatives. It is possible that the factors underlying smoking in today's college students may be quite different from those previously delineated by researchers. Additional research focusing on the specific features of this age group seemed warranted. With college student smoking currently on the rise, it also seemed important to evaluate the opinions of those people who see the students regularly—their peers and professors. It is hoped that more accurate information about these opinions may help students to make more responsible and wise decisions concerning tobacco use.

INTRODUCTION

Approximately 435,000 Americans die each year due to smoking related factors (Hobson, 2006; U.S. Department of Health and Human Services, 1989; Hanson and Venturelli, 1998; Lewis et al., 1998). The number of deaths from tobacco smoking exceeds those attributable to AIDS, alcohol, cocaine, heroin, homicide, suicide, motor vehicle crashes, and fires combined (Garfinkel, 1997; Dziuban, Moskal, and West, 1999). Although approximately 70% of smokers indicate that they want to quit, only 34% attempt to quit, and of those a mere 2.5% are successful in beating the addiction. Anecdotal reports attest to the challenges involved in smoking cessation. Many individuals who were cross-addicted to multiple substances report that cigarette smoking cessation was more difficult for them than quitting alcohol, cocaine, and heroin use.

Tobacco is notorious for its high cost, addictive nature, and health risks. However, smoking still remains prevalent among adolescents and college students. Since 1991, although there has been a decrease in the number of adults who smoke, the number of adolescents who smoke cigarettes has increased. Research indicates that young Americans typically begin smoking before the age of 18 years, with very few starting after the age of 22. Although the legal age to purchase cigarettes is eighteen, 87% of smokers begin smoking before this legal age (Dziuban, Moskal, and West, 1999).

Although for the first time an overall decline in teen-age smoking rates was observed between 1997 and 1999, this trend was not found among older adolescents. An August 24, 2000 Center for Disease Control report noted that although the rate of "current" smoking (at least one day a month) declined nearly 2% between 1997 and 1999 for all teenagers, the declines weren't found across all gender, age, or race groups. Additionally, the decreases only returned certain groups of students to where they were in the 1980s. The biggest declines were among ninth grade students, but this group had experienced substantial increases in the past decade. Even with the decline among 9th graders, the current smoking rate of nearly 35% equals the rate in 1995, and is still 7% over the rate in 1991.

Among older students and females, smoking rates have not declined significantly. For example, among females, smoking rates have remained virtually the same between 1997 and 1999. Over 70% of young people have tried smoking at least once, which is comparable to a decade ago. However, for "frequent" smoking (at least 20 days a month), rates for all genders and races jumped 4% during the decade. Some are concerned that more students than ever have already begun to use tobacco more frequently and are faced with a nicotine addiction problem.

While rates of cigarette smoking among middle-aged and older American adults have waned since the 1970s (Garfinkel, 1997), older adolescents and young adults continue to smoke at an alarming rate. In fact, Wechsler et al. (1998) found that there was a 28% rise in college students' smoking between 1993 and 1997. Several other recent studies have found college student smoking to be a problem that began to increase in the 1990s (Johnston, O'Malley, and Bachman, 1996; Hines, Fretz, and Nollen, 1998; Moore, 1998; Price et al., 1998). Despite the known risks, prevalence rates have been rising in some age groups. Among adolescents, the rate rose from 20% in 1991 to 36% in 1998; among young adults the rate increased from 22% in 1993 to 32% in 2000. Wechsler et al. (1998) noted that the rise in college student smoking in the late 1990s might be a result of the rise in high school student smoking in the early 1990s.

While Wechsler et al. found that few (11%) of students tried their first cigarette after age 19, 28% began to smoke regularly at age 19 or beyond (Wechsler et al., 1998). This suggests that many individuals may move from an experimental phase of occasional use (Duryea and Martin, 1981; Emmons et al., 1998; Page, 1998) to a much more pernicious steady pattern of cigarette consumption during their college years. Some see this as creating a mandate for colleges and universities to enact campus smoking policies that are conducive students' making health-promoting decisions. Establishment of policies that reinforce antismoking norms on campus may also help students make better choices regarding tobacco use.

This increasing rate of smoking on campuses is puzzling, given the current student generation's ongoing exposure to antismoking educational programs throughout their early years. Given the ubiquitous provision of health classes designed to deter smoking, along with highly publicized antismoking messages in both the print and electronic media, it seems surprising that roughly one-quarter to one-third of college students engage in this risky behavior. Even more disturbing is the realization that this estimate only takes into account those who smoke cigarettes; it excludes those young adults who smoke cigars, marijuana, or use smokeless tobacco.

Interestingly, much student smoking is occurring in social contexts that are often hostile toward this behavior; social norms tend to favor nonsmoking. Clark (1978) found that both nonsmokers and ex-smokers perceived smokers negatively, and others have found a negative stigma associated with smoking (Gilbert, 1979; Chaudary, 1997).

There has been much speculation about the causes of the smoking increase recently observed among the young adult population. Past researchers have inferred that cigarette advertisements make an enormous contribution to early smoking initiation (Reid, 1985; Potts, Gillies, and Herbert, 1986; Department of Health and Human Services, 1994; Zinser, Kloosterman, and Williams, 1994; Moore, 1998). Adolescents and young adults often spend considerable time in contexts that are saturated with pro-smoking messages (Schooler, Feighery, and Flora, 1996). Magazine advertisements for tobacco products frequently portray exciting, adventurous scenes depicting smokers as glamorous and appealing (Zinser, Kloosterman, and Williams, 1991; Hines et al., 1998; Moore, 1998).

A study by Zinser et al. (1991) discovered that both college student smokers and nonsmokers rated cigarette advertisements as more adventurous in comparison with advertisements for other products. Magazine ad content analyses validated the notion that advertisements were developed by the smoking industry to depict smokers as attractive, athletic, and lively (Altman et al., 1987; Altman, et al., 1996; Zinser et al., 1991). Such beliefs may promote smoking experimentation, especially among those at a developmental stage where preoccupation with social image is common. Many fall prey to the underlying suggestion that smoking will enhance allure (Zinser et al., 1991). Past research has revealed that the top-selling cigarette brands that are smoked by the younger population are also the most heavily advertised (Moore, 1998; King et al., 1998).

College students' reasons for smoking may be different from those underlying both early adolescents' and older adults' smoking. However, relatively little research has focused specifically upon those who initiated smoking during their college years. Past research has delineated several differences between young adolescent smoking and adult smoking. In adolescence, social motives are the primary source of smoking initiation; this behavior is frequently begun to project an image of toughness, sociability, precociousness, and extraversion (Chassin, Presson, and Sherman, 1990). According to Moore (1998). Young people commonly smoke in order to look mature or attractive, to keep slim, or to feel independent. Additionally, most children between the ages of 12 and 14 who smoke regularly say all or most of their friends smoke, and a third of pupils agree it is hard not to smoke if most of your friends do (Moore, 1998).

For adolescent smokers, the social benefits accompanying this behavior possibly outweigh the health risks (Leventhal and Cleary, 1980). Smoking may seem a smart choice if adolescents believe they will be seen as sophisticated, attractive, and socially successful by peers (Barton, Chassin, and Presson, 1982). Among adolescents smoking is often associated with toughness and precocity; male teenagers are especially likely to value these correlates of smoking.

In contrast, adult regular smokers have been found to be less socially connected and more depressed (Glassman et al., 1988; Glassman et al. 1990; Hemenway, Solnick, and Colditz, 1993). The social desirability of smoking seems to have little influence on the older adult's decision to maintain this habit. Instead, Chassin et al. (1990) discovered that stress management and reduction of negative affect contribute significantly to adults' continuance of smoking. Smoking behavior may additionally serve as a means for self-medicating depression and enhancing pleasurable relaxation (Austin, Brosh, Dous, Iannella, Outten, Rowles, and Chambliss, 2003: Gilbert, 1979; Clausen, 1987). Additional research clarifying the specific factors prompting college students' initiation and subsequent maintenance of cigarette smoking may help in the design of better prevention programs.

Maintaining antismoking norms on campuses is also probably important for the containment of this current trend. It is imperative for colleges and universities to determine what is prompting smoking behavior among future leaders, to attempt to reduce these factors, to provide counteractive preventive measures, and to assist smokers who are ready to relinquish the habit. The series of campus investigations summarized in the following chapter describe one small liberal arts college's struggles to address these issues. The Ursinus College psychology department has worked for nearly ten years to increase campus awareness of the problems associated with student smoking, and to assist students in making fully informed choices about whether or not to smoke cigarettes. A peer-mentoring model was employed, in order to maximize influence within the constraints of a sorely limited budget. Students collaborated on twenty research projects, which both increased their own understanding of the issues, and enabled them to transmit their findings to peers on campus and, through research conference presentations and publications, to a broader academic audience.

Because promoting the desire to quit and facilitating cessation are important in reducing college student smoking, finding appropriate strategies to motivate students to stop smoking and to help them quit is vital. While Wechsler et al. (1998) acknowledged that college may be a propitious time to teach smokers how and why to quit, little research on cessation attempts aimed specifically at college students had been published before the Ursinus students conducted their experimental examination of customized smoking cessation programs. Their work, summarized in the discussion of studies in section III, was designed in part to address this omission in the literature.

Each of the studies summarized here helps to clarify some aspect of the problem of college student smoking. They provide useful starting points from which future research may proceed. While each study was conducted on a small scale, some intriguing results were obtained. These studies reveal that people hold strong opinions regarding smoking and that college student smoking is perceived by many to be a major issue on college campuses today. The studies that follow were conducted to enhance our understanding of this problem and the various options available to remedy it.

SECTION I

Why do today's high school and college students smoke?
What contributes to the choice to abstain?
Subjective Determinants of Student Cigarette Smoking
Personality Correlates of Student Substance Use
Situational Determinants of Substance Use
Cultural Pressures to Smoke: Media Images of Smokers

The goal of this section is to examine findings from eight studies aimed at specifying both internal and external factors that may be influencing college students' decision to smoke cigarettes. In order to examine some of the internal reasons for the recent upsurge in college students' smoking, the first two studies involved surveys inquiring about the subjective effects of smoking tobacco. Next, research explored the factors associated with students' choice to abstain. The next few studies discussed in this section assessed the personality correlates of substance use among high school and college students. Some of them looked at gender and nationality group differences in substance use, and include speculation about what these differences may reveal about the motives for using psychoactive substances among college students. The final study in this section explored the depiction of cigarette smoking in recent films, and the typical ways in which characters that smoke cigarettes are viewed by audiences.

Bartlett, Brackin, Chubb, Covatta, Ferguson, Hinckley, Hodges, Liberati, Tornetta, and Chambliss (1999) administered a survey to 324 undergraduates to assess the importance of different subjective states in maintaining cigarette smoking behavior. The responses of the smokers in this sample were selectively examined. Their subjective smoking experience was assessed through sixteen Likert-format items (1=Never, 2=Rarely, 3=Often, and 4=Very Frequently). Participants were asked to rate "When you smoke a cigarette, how does it make you feel?" on the following dimensions: relaxed, content, trusting, anxious, jittery, attractive, sophisticated, immature, alert, competent, secure, intelligent, inadequate, physically fit, energized, and less hungry. These items were selected in order to investigate the importance of four hypothesized motivational factors underlying smoking: relaxation effects, image effects, competence effects, and stimulant effects.

To measure the motivational role of relaxation effects, scores were grouped and averaged for the following affective items: high levels of relaxation, contentment and trust, and low levels of anxiety and jitteriness. In order to assess the importance of image effects, scores were averaged and grouped for the following items: high levels of attractiveness, sophistication, and maturity. In order to assess the importance of competence effects, scores were grouped and averaged for the following items: high levels of alertness, competence, security, intelligence, and adequacy. In order to assess the importance of stimulant effects, scores were grouped and averaged for the following items: high levels of physical fitness, and energy, and low levels of hunger.

In order to determine if differences existed among the four personal smoking motivation factors, paired sample t-tests were performed on the smokers' factor scores. Significant differences were found between stimulant effects and the other three factors, all $p < .001$. Relaxation effects, image effects, and competence effects were all rated higher than stimulant effects. Smokers reported almost never feeling intelligent, physically fit, or trusting while smoking.

To examine gender differences in personal motivation for smoking, between-group t-tests on the four motivational factor scores were performed, comparing male and female smokers. No significant differences emerged.

To determine if a relationship existed between family income and current student smoking status, a Pearson correlation was calculated, using both smokers and nonsmokers. The correlation was found to be significant ($r = .23$; $p < .001$). In order to explore the joint influence of family income and parental smoking on college student smoking behavior, a median split was performed, yielding low and high family income groups of smokers (low family incomes were below \$80,000, high incomes were over \$80,000). In high income families of current student smokers, 69.7% of fathers and 82.4% of mothers were nonsmokers. Approximately twice as many fathers as mothers were smokers in families in this income range. In low income families, 73.3% of the fathers and 73.3% of the mothers were nonsmokers. Equal numbers of mothers and fathers in these lower income families smoked.

The results of this study suggest that there are three main factors motivating college student to smoke. Ratings of the four personal motivation factors underlying college students smoking placed them in the following descending order of importance: relaxation effects, image effects, competence effects, and stimulant effects. While the strong association between smoking and desired relaxation was not surprising, the highly influential role of social image in college student smoking was unexpected. Although research on younger smokers has clearly documented the importance of peer pressure in fostering smoking, older smokers were presumed to be more immune to these influences. The current findings suggest that concern about appearing sophisticated, mature, and attractive figure prominently in the decision of college students to smoke. College-age students appear to be in a transitory state concerning reasons for smoking; while they enjoy the benefit of relaxation like the older adult population, image is still a crucial factor in smoking motivation, much as it is for the adolescent.

Equally unexpected were the findings suggesting that few college students smoke in order to experience stimulant effects. These smokers report that they rarely experience the appetite suppression effects commonly associated with nicotine, infrequently feel energized by smoking, and almost never feel physically fit while smoking. This reality stands in sharp contrast to the lively, invigorating image of the smoking experience ubiquitously depicted in advertisements. Apparently these stimulant effects are less pronounced than commonly assumed, or misattributive processes may operate which prevent college smokers from recognizing the association between their intake of nicotine and these physiological effects. The energizing effects of smoking are evidently short-lived; smokers did not report enjoying stimulant effects on a regular basis. Similarly, cognitive enhancement was not commonly reported; the majority of smokers almost never experienced heightened intellectual ability while smoking.

Although the scores on the competence factor fell in the intermediate range, inspection of the individual items comprising this factor revealed interesting variability. Smokers reported almost never feeling intelligent while smoking, yet said they quite frequently felt adequate during the process.

Contrary to expectation, female smokers were not more likely to report appetite suppression effects in conjunction with smoking. This is inconsistent with other studies, which have suggested that many women smoke as a way of curbing appetite in order to maintain a desirable body weight.

Unlike much previous research, this study failed to observe a negative relationship between socioeconomic status and smoking behavior, and in fact found smoking to be more common among students from higher income families. This finding was not explained by higher rates of parental smoking in the wealthier families. The majority of parents in all families were nonsmokers. Smoking among some college students may represent a form of rebellion against affluent nonsmoking parents. This possibility received partial support from the finding that within the higher income family group, fewer than 19% of the mothers smoked. In comparison, within low income families, almost 29% of the mothers smoked. However, the fathers in the higher income families were about as likely to smoke as their low income counterparts. If for some college students smoking represents a way of asserting autonomy by engaging in behavior at odds with parental values, the offspring of wealthier nonsmoking mothers may quite unexpectedly be at higher risk. Future studies using larger samples of college students drawn from a broader range of institutions might clarify this possibility.

Cigarette smoking is generally assumed to be associated with several desirable subjective states. The current findings challenge some of these assumptions about the positive effects of smoking. Disseminating this type of information might further deromanticize this habit and dissuade potential smokers from starting.

**Table 1. Means and Standard Deviations for Items Describing
Smokers' Positive Smoking Experiences**

	Mean	SD
Relaxation Effects	2.32	0.85
Image Effects	2.17	0.72
Competence Effects	2.24	0.66
Stimulant Effects	1.73	0.73

A paper by Austin, Brosh, and Chambliss (2002) extended the Bartlett et al.(1999) study by including a sample of high school students. They discussed the paradoxical findings obtained when the self-reported motivations of student smokers were assessed. Relaxation was the primary motivator for smoking reported across the developmental periods studied, despite the fact that nicotine is actually a stimulant. Nonsmokers reported lower levels of stress than both occasional and regular smokers. Regular smokers reported increased levels of stress and irritability when refraining from smoking.

The source of positive affect experienced while smoking usually results from the reversal of abstinence/ withdrawal effects. Therefore, addicted smokers who seem visibly calmer after relieving their withdrawal symptoms provide a very misleading example to others and create the false impression that smoking has intrinsic relaxing effects.

Students with low self-esteem were significantly more likely to report concerns about image as a reason for smoking. However, peer reports indicated that smokers were perceived less favorably than nonsmokers. These findings suggest that adolescents with low self esteem might especially benefit from more accurate information about the actual stigma and social hazards associated with public smoking.

In studies assessing the reasons high school and college students give for refraining from smoking, fairly consistent patterns emerged (Venuti, Conroy, Landis, and Chambliss, 2000; Venuti and Chambliss,2000). Health concerns were the most salient reasons reported for not smoking across age, gender, and nationality groups. Interestingly, in these samples, financial concerns were the least significant factor in determining young people's decision to refrain from smoking.

PERSONALITY CORRELATES OF SMOKING

Several studies with students have explored the personality correlates of various types of substance use (Austin, Brosh, Dous, Iannella, Outten, Rowles, and Chambliss, 2003; Austin, Brosh, Iannella, Outten, Rowles, Dous and Chambliss, 2003; Chambliss, 2004; Chambliss, Austin, Brosh, Ianella, Outten and Rowles, 2005). Personality factors have long been presumed to influence substance use. Representative work from the last five decades has established a modest but fairly consistent association between certain personality characteristics and substance use. Early on, Eysenck (1967) predicted that extraversion would mediate sensitivity to various psychoactive substances. Zuckerman (1979, 1994) found that individuals with higher sensation seeking needs tend to become users earlier in life and are more prone to becoming regular users. Brennan, Walfish, and Aubuchon also found a link between impulsivity/sensation seeking and alcohol consumption (1986). Research by Wood, Cochran, Pfefferbaum, and Arneklev (1995) found that adolescents only used alcohol 10% of the time "when friends were doing it", and suggested that an individual's thrill seeking and impulsivity promote the likelihood of substance use. Other researchers have found that nonconformity and deviance are associated with multiple substance use (Wechsler, Dowdall, Davenport, and Castillo, 1995).

After reviewing three decades of research on young adults' alcohol use, Baer (2002) concluded that students with a history of deviant behavior tend to use alcohol earlier and consume more during college, and that students who are more rebellious and less committed to traditional values have a higher tendency to consume alcohol. Understanding the personality trait predictors of substance use might aid in the development of more effective prevention programs and help to elucidate the mechanisms underlying substance abuse.

Stewart and Zeithlin (1995) found anxious individuals were more likely to use both alcohol and cigarette smoking as a coping strategy. Comeau, Stewart, and Loba (2001) examined how anxiety and sensation seeking relate to adolescents' use of alcohol, cigarettes, and marijuana, and found that all of the personality factors they examined were associated with substance use patterns. Sensation seeking was related to use of alcohol for enhancement reasons, while anxiety sensitivity was associated with alcohol and marijuana use motivated by conformity desires. Personality factors were more strongly associated with alcohol use than marijuana and cigarette use (Comeau et al., 2001). Wagner (2001) found both sensation seeking and anxiety sensitivity to predict substance use. While sensation seeking was positively linked to alcohol and drug use, this work revealed a negative correlation between anxiety sensitivity and substance use (Wagner, 2001).

Smokers and nonsmokers have been found to vary on several dimensions. Smokers have been found to be more anger-prone, extraverted, and likely to manifest Type A characteristics (Geist and Herrmann, 1990; Gilbert, 1988; Seltzer and Oeschli, 1985). PET scan research by Potkin (2004) suggests that hostile tendencies make individuals more susceptible to nicotine effects on brain regions that play a major role in controlling emotional and social responses. This may help to account for some of the observed personality differences between smokers and nonsmokers.

However, some researchers investigating the link between personality and substance use have met with frustration. For example, Rutledge and Sher (2001) failed to find the link they had hypothesized between alcohol use and neuroticism/negative emotionality and extraversion/sociability, although they did obtain some evidence that behavioral undercontrol was predictive of heavy drinking. Zuckerman (1987) suggests that social attitudes toward substances mediate the relationship between personality and use. He notes that as social acceptance of substance use increases, the relationship between sensation seeking and substance use decreases. Therefore, a substance that is considered risky and less widely sanctioned would present a stronger relationship between sensation seeking and substance use. Since personality factors probably interact with variables such as gender and age in shaping substance habits, it is important to investigate the impact of multiple factors simultaneously. Further examination of the relationship between substance use and basic personality factors operating in conjunction with demographic variables may help to clarify some of the contradictions encountered in previous research.

Many who expect a relationship between personality types and substance use preferences also predict that those using different substances require different treatment approaches.

Clinicians have long debated whether type of substance used should dictate differential treatment, and whether substance users should be grouped homogenously on the basis of their choice of substance. Empirical findings indicate greater similarities than differences between alcohol-dependent and drug-dependent patients, when adequate statistical controls are exercised for critical demographics variables such as age, race, and sex (Carroll and Chambliss, 1990; Carroll, 1982; Carroll, Malloy, Roscioli, Pindjack, and Clifford, 1982). This work suggests that common factors are likely to underlie the various types of substance use.

Those who emphasize self medication motivation for substance use predict that users will select the substance whose psychoactive properties best address their idiosyncratic need(s). For example, since alcohol is a powerful central nervous system depressant and calmative, its appeal might be expected to be different from that of stimulants or hallucinogens. Those with a higher need for stimulation should seek out substances likely to impart this effect. Variation on personality measures presumably reflects differences in such underlying needs. For instance, extraverts have long been understood to have greater preferences for external stimulation, while introverts seem to actively avoid the excessive cortical arousal such stimulation produces for them.

To the extent that adolescent substance use is a means of self medicating, personality differences should predict type of substance used, because personality characteristics are associated with particular symptom tendencies (e.g., anxiety among those high in neuroticism versus boredom in those high in extraversion). Alternatively, if more generalized sensation seeking underlies most adolescent substance use, personality variables distinct from those related to risk taking and rebellion should be unrelated to substance use.

The Ursinus investigations (Austin, Brosh, Dous, Iannella, Outten, Rowles and Chambliss, 2003; Austin, Brosh, Iannella, Outten, Rowles, Dous and Chambliss, 2003; Chambliss, 2004; Chambliss, Austin, Brosh, Ianella, Outten and Rowles, 2005) explored the association between the five basic personality dimensions revealed by years of factor analytic research and three types of substance use by surveying high school and college students. The MMFFP Scale was selected as a measure of these five personality factors because it provides an efficient assessment of the five factors repeatedly found to be most basic in accounting for personality variability across multiple populations (Costa and McCrae, 1997; McCrae and Costa, 1989). Developed by Saucier (1992), this test assesses the five empirically derived core dimensions of personality: openness, conscientiousness, extreme agreeableness, and neuroticism often (summarized by the acronym OCEAN). Each of these variables is assumed to shape how the individual experiences and responds to the environment. Differences on these five dimensions might well influence the perceived attractiveness of different substances as well as involvement in social situations where these substances are made available.

One of the Ursinus studies obtained responses from 180 college students (81 males, 99 females) from a small liberal arts college from a suburban area in the Northeast United States and 141 high school students (68 males, 73 females) attending a public school in the same area. One hundred seventy-two female students and 149 male students, with a combined mean age of 17.31 years, completed the survey. The survey was administered to college students enrolled in an introductory psychology course, and high school students enrolled in health education classes.

The survey consisted of the Mini Markers Five Factors Personality Scale (MMFFP, Saucier, 1992) and items assessing the subject's reported substance abuse behavior and demographic variables. The MMFFP consists of 40 alphabetized self-descriptive personality characteristics that respondents endorse using a 10-point Likert scale; it yields summary scores on five basic personality traits (openness, conscientiousness, extreme agreeableness, and neuroticism). The frequency of the participant's cigarette, alcohol, and marijuana use was assessed using self report items developed by Wechsler et al.(1998). On these scales 1 denotes never having used, 2=used, but not in the past 12 months, 3=used, but not in the past 30 days, 4=used in the past 30 days, and 5=used on a daily basis.

During the previous month, 59% of the students reported having used alcohol, one quarter reported smoking tobacco, and one quarter reported using marijuana. Reported daily use of the three substances was 9%, 12%, and 7%, respectively. While only 17% of these students had never tried alcohol, half reported never using cigarettes and half declared no history of marijuana use.

Directionally adjusted items were totaled to create summary scores for openness, conscientiousness, extraversion, agreeableness, and neuroticism. A median split was performed on the summary scores for each of the five personality factors to create high and low level groups for each of the five traits.

Multivariate analyses of variance were used to evaluate sex and personality effects for each of the five factors assessed. A 2 x 2 MANOVA (sex: male and female; extraversion: low and high) on each of the three types of self-reported substance use (cigarette, alcohol, and marijuana) revealed a significant extraversion main effect for alcohol use (high: x=3.43, s.d.=1.18, n=160 versus low: x= 3.02, s.d.=1.31, n=161; F=5.48, df 1/313, p<.05) . Significant differences in marijuana use for the high and low extraversion groups were also found (high: x=2.30, s.d.=1.40, n=160 versus low: x= 1.98, s.d.=1.33, n=161; F=3.97, df 1/313, p<.05).

A significant conscientiousness main effect was obtained on the alcohol use measure (high: x=3.15, s.d=1.26, n=172 versus low: x=3.32, s.d.=1.25, n=149; F=4.99, df=1/317, p<.05). Conscientiousness and sex yielded a significant interaction effect on the measure of alcohol use (F=9.40, df=1/317, p<.01). Although no significant main effects emerged for openness, agreeableness, or neuroticism, a trend in the data suggested a possible neuroticism by sex interaction on the measure of alcohol use (F=2.97, df=1/317, p<.08).

Consistent with previous research, several of our studies have found a link between extraversion and reported use of both alcohol and marijuana. Extraverts' customary preference for social situations that are standard settings for alcohol use during the high school and college years is likely to increase their access to these substances and their exposure to norms favoring use. Additionally, their affinity for external stimulation and sensation seeking probably increase the appeal of illegal substance use. The absence of a significant relationship between extraversion and cigarette use may be due in part to tobacco's legality.

The observed relationship between conscientiousness and alcohol use was not surprising; less conscientious students reported that they drank more. However, separate consideration of the reports of men and women indicated an unexpected exception to this regularity. For males, high conscientiousness was associated with significantly greater alcohol consumption. This could be due to conscientious male students' feeling greater pressure to perform well in school and extracurricular activities, and consequently using alcohol as a socially sanctioned way to release resultant tension. Highly conscientious female students may find that their use of alcohol for this purpose is not as strongly supported by peers. Alternatively, these findings may be artifactual, reflecting more honest self reporting of alcohol use on the part of the more conscientious men. However, if this accounts for their higher scores, one would need to explain why highly conscientious females do not offer similarly honest accounts of their own behavior.

The failure to find an association between conscientiousness and marijuana use suggests that adolescents who see themselves as highly conscientious may not see this as being incongruent with certain types of illegal substance use. Many of these ordinarily conscientious adolescents may challenge the authority that defines marijuana use as illegal, and may thereby rationalize their use as consistent with their self-perceived responsibility.

Although more neurotic students did not make heavier use of alcohol and marijuana, as might be predicted by those emphasizing the role of self medication in motivating adolescent substance use, a trend in the results suggests the possibility of an interesting interaction between sex and neuroticism in shaping alcohol use. For females, high neuroticism was somewhat associated with greater use of alcohol use, while for males the opposite was true. This suggests that the motivation for alcohol use during the adolescent period may be different for women and men. Females who are high in neuroticism seem to be more likely than their highly neurotic male peers to consume alcohol as a means of alleviating their anxiety. Male adolescents' drinking may be less a form of self medication and more a function of thrill seeking. Less neurotic males, presumably being less anxiety prone, might be more inclined to seek high stimulation and endure the hazards associated with engaging in illegal underage drinking. Alternatively, the observed differences may be due to the disparate impact of neuroticism on popularity among males and females. If anxiety is more socially acceptable in females than in males, neuroticism would exact a different toll on the popularity of female and male adolescents. Consequently, highly neurotic females may be more likely than highly neurotic males to be popular, and therefore they might be more apt to participate in social activities that promote alcohol use.

Those concerned about reducing underage use of alcohol as a means of self medicating anxiety symptoms might wish to focus their energies especially on highly anxious adolescent females. However, since the greatest alcohol use was found among less neurotic males, ongoing attention to high sensation seeking adolescent males is certainly justified. The absence of a significant relationships between neuroticism and marijuana use challenges the notion that highly anxious adolescents are at greater risk of using this substance in order to alleviate suffering due to neurotic worrying.

Among high school students, agreeableness scores predicted cigarette smoking. Among college students, basic personality factors did not predict cigarette smoking in the initial studies we conducted, however in 2005 we found that students who were either high in neuroticism or low in self esteem were more likely to smoke. For the sample as a whole, not surprisingly, more conscientious students were less likely to report use of all substances, including cigarettes.

Since these findings were based on a correlational design, the causal influence of personality on substance use cannot be assumed. It is possible that substance use affects personality, or at least the tendency to endorse some of the items on personality measures. For example, the observation that high school smokers scored lower in agreeableness may reflect the fact that nicotine dependence increases smokers' frustration and irritability, and consequently depresses their scores on measures of agreeableness. Smokers' personalities may be adversely affected by cigarette use.

Additional factors complicate the interpretation of this type of study. Personality variables could well be associated systematically with differential willingness to admit to substance use. As a result, observed group differences in these studies could always be challenged as artifactual.

However, some recent neurophysiological research, which is less limited by this problem, has provided evidence supporting the validity of earlier studies describing personality differences between smokers and nonsmokers. Potkin et al. (2004) obtained PET scans following exposure to nicotine and found that nicotine triggered dramatic changes in activity in brain regions important for controlling emotion and social response in people rated as having more hostile tendencies (easier to anger, more impatient, and more irritable). In contrast, nicotine produced no effects in subjects characterized as cheerful and relaxed.

IS SMOKING IDEALIZED IN CURRENT FILMS?

The year 2000 saw the release of the film The Insider, an exposé detailing the deceptive practices of tobacco companies, and the efforts they made to suppress incriminating evidence. The success of this film testifies to the public's willingness to consider the economic and moral complexities associated with smoking. In an effort to clarify factors promting smoking among young adults, at Ursinus College, Hodges, Bartlett, Brackin, Chubb, Covatta, Ferguson, Hinckley, Liberati, Tornetta, and Chambliss (2000) explored the portrayal of smoking in films from the 1990s.

Other researchers have found that many films have portrayed smokers in a positive light, associating cigarette use with the characteristics of maturity, sophistication, and of high social class (Pechmann and Shih, 1999). In many films, little attention is paid to the negative consequences of smoking. Studies have found that audiences feel more positively toward smoking after seeing its glamorous, exciting, and adventurous depiction in film and advertisements.

Hazan, Lipton, and Glantz (1994) found that 80% of the recent film releases they assessed portray smoking in association with positive attributes such as youthfulness and attractiveness. Many of these films induce the audience to misperceive the reality of smoking. Despite the fact that lower socioeconomic status is associated with smoking in real life (Stronks et al., 1997), the socioeconomic status of smokers portrayed in films apparently increased during the 1990s. One study found that 57% of movie characters of high social standing smoke, yet only 19% of high socioeconomic status adults actually smoke (Hazan et al., 1994). During the 1980s, 17% of smokers in films were characterized as having a high socioeconomic status, while that figure rose to 30% in the 1990s. This inaccurate portrayal leads many views to have an unrealistic belief that smoking is widely accepted and encouraged by society (Pechmann and Shih, 1999).

Negative aspects of smoking, such as negative health consequences and concern about second hand smoke, are usually ignored in films (Shogren, 1997). Negative social or health effects are portrayed in less than 15% of films. Research has found that smoking scenes in films often lead viewers to believe that smoking is attractive and increased their willingness to smoke (Pechmann and Shih, 1999). Scenes containing characters of high social status that smoke may alter the viewers' attitudes toward smokers.

Hodges, Bartlett, Brackin, Chubb, Covatta, Ferguson, Hinckley, Liberati, Tornetta, and Chambliss (2000) obtained a list of the twenty top grossing movies from the years 1996, 1997, 1998 and 1999. From this list five movies from each year were randomly selected. A group of trained raters evaluated the movies for relevant characteristics. Included in this analysis were movie genre, approximate running time, and total number of cigarettes seen on film. Demographics were recorded for first, second, and third leading characters, including age, gender, and smoking status. When asked "How is the character generally portrayed?", raters evaluated each person on the following traits: selfish/considerate, cruel/kind, rebellious/compliant, crude/sophisticated, poor/wealthy, insecure/confident, angry/happy, unattractive/attractive, tense/relaxed, immature/mature, unintelligent/intelligent, and unpopular/popular.

Seventy-five percent of the 1996-1999 movies sampled depicted cigarette smoking. However, only approximately 20% of the leading characters in the movies sampled (85% of whom were male) smoked cigarettes. Of the second and third main characters, 26% in each category smoked. Among secondary main characters, more males smoked (63%) than females, and among tertiary main characters smoking was equal for males and females. Only 5% of the movies sampled featured three or more main characters who smoked.

A one-way ANOVA was used to compare the four years' of films in terms of the total number of cigarette smoking episodes portrayed in each film. No significant differences were found. Comparisons of personality ratings for smoking and nonsmoking characters showed significant differences on two variables. Nonsmokers appearing more considerate and less selfish ($p<.01$). Though not significant, there was also a trend for nonsmokers to be viewed as more kind and less cruel ($p=.09$).

The Hodges, Bartlett, Brackin, Chubb, Covatta,Ferguson, Hinckley, Liberati, Tornetta, and Chambliss (2000) findings indicate that the majority of movies sampled expose members of the audience to role models who smoke cigarettes. Given the growing consensus regarding the negative health effects of smoking, and findings demonstrating that positive portrayals of smoking in advertisements induce people to start smoking, the high frequency of smoking observed in the movies sampled is somewhat alarming. Routine witnessing of movie characters' smoking may subtly alter attitudes toward this behavior; increased acceptance of smoking may be a consequence of this steady exposure because affinity tends to increase with familiarity.

However, the present analyses also showed that only a minority of the leading characters were smokers, which may attenuate these negative effects. Perhaps the movie industry may be refraining from including smoking in the characterization of leading men in order to reduce negative influences on viewers. Consistent with this, only a small minority of films included three or more main characters who smoked cigarettes.

The type of role a smoker plays influences the impact of the film character's smoking status on the viewer. When highly charismatic, attractive, compelling characters are seen smoking cigarettes, the audience may be more likely to view smoking positively. In contrast, when unsavory, antisocial, unscrupulous characters are shown smoking, this may serve as a deterrent to the audience's smoking. The Ursinus study found a tendency for the negative personality attributes of selfishness, cruelty, and inconsiderateness to be linked with smoking behavior in the movies sampled. This negative portrayal of film smokers may actually serve to decrease the perceived attractiveness of smoking to viewers. Future research should explore the generalizability of this finding, and assess this hypothesized impact on the audience.

Although smoking prevalence in movies increased through the early 90's, this study indicates a leveling off toward the end of the decade. Perhaps the use of tobacco in films may decrease as a result of the increased awareness of the harmful effects of misleading images of smoking and decreased acceptance of smoking.

SUMMARY OF RESULTS

Most college students who smoke report experiencing relaxation effects while smoking, and say they feel more sophisticated while engaged in this behavior. We were surprised that concerns about image figured so prominently in the motivation of college-age smokers, because members of focus groups we had conducted had denied this. We also expected stimulant and cognitive enhancement effects to be more important than they were; apparently smokers are not aware of any energizing effects of smoking. While personality factors and media influences contribute to the decision to smoke cigarettes, maintenance of smoking behavior seems to depend heavily upon students' interest in relaxation and favorable self presentation. These findings were encouraging, because they suggest two lines of attack in trying to reduce student smoking: First, help smokers develop alternative ways of relaxing and feeling sophisticated. Second, bolster antismoking norms on campus, so that would-be smokers realize that this behavior will tarnish rather than enhance their image.

SECTION II

Why students should quit: Prejudice against smokers
What are smokers risking, other than their health?
How pervasive is the social stigma associated with smoking?
The Relative Stigma Associated with Smoking, Obesity, and Criminality
High School, College, and Professional School Student and Faculty members' views of current smokers, former smokers, and nonsmokers

The goal of this section is to examine current campus attitudes toward smokers (among high school and college students and faculty, including current smokers, former smokers, and nonsmokers). Clarifying the picture that students are painting for others when they make the decision to smoke cigarettes in public may help students to make more informed decisions about smoking. Since concerns about self presentation seem to figure prominently in much social behavior, accurate understanding of how being seen as a smoker may contaminate others' reactions to them may induce some students to think twice before engaging in pervasive public smoking. Even if this fails to motivate students to quit smoking altogether, it may reduce their tobacco use somewhat, and contribute to stronger antismoking norms by confining the behavior to less public venues.

Several studies conducted at Ursinus in collaboration with undergraduate students (Srebro, Hodges, Authier, and Chambliss,1999; Hodges, Chubb, Liberati, Covatta, Brackin, Bartlett, Tornetta, Ferguson, Hinckley, and Chambliss, 1999, Venuti, Conroy, Bucy, Landis and Chambliss, 2002; Venuti, Conroy, Bucy, Landis, and Chambliss, 2002; Brosh, Austin, and Chambliss, 2002; Outten, Rowles, and Chambliss, 2004; Baker, Katona, Shull, Brosh, and Chambliss, 2004; Chambliss, 2004; Chambliss, Shull, Baker, Burton, Nesbit, Weir, Wilson, Katona, and Brosh, 2006) have explored the social hazards of cigarette smoking in academic contexts. Students' and teachers' attitudes about student smokers have been assessed by obtaining ratings of hypothetical student smokers, nonsmokers, and former smokers in high schools, colleges, and professional schools (medical and law schools).

In a paper entitled "Social Rejection of Unhealthy Pleasures: Views of Cigarette Smoking in Academic Institutions," Chambliss (2006) summarized data collected over a five year period from students and teachers describing the stigma associated with smoking. Since wider dissemination of information about the pervasive social hazards associated with cigarette smoking may help deter this behavior, this study extended earlier work documenting that smokers are perceived in a much more negative way on a variety of dimensions than are their nonsmoking counterparts (Bleda and Sandman,1977; Brosh, Austin and Chambliss, 2003; Chambliss, 2004; Dermer and Jacobsen,1986; Goldstein,1991).

Research comparing the stigma associated with smoking, criminality, and obesity, and found that smokers were viewed more negatively than those who are clinically overweight on several dimensions (Venuti, Conroy, Bucy, Landis, and Chambliss, 2002). One of the only studies on stigma reporting discrepant results was based on a survey of Australian students (Lee, 1989). Although negative attitudes toward smokers have consistently been observed in studies conducted on American campuses, Lee (1989) found that Australian students rated smokers as more successful, sociable, sophisticated, modern, liberated, and hardworking than nonsmokers. Cultural differences may have accounted for these contradictory findings. In the U.S., the minority of individuals who smoke increasingly find themselves the victims of negative stereotypes and targets of restrictive policies.

Despite this reality, most young smokers are currently unconcerned about the potential social and occupational repercussions of their decision to smoke. They are often oblivious to the increasing condemnation of smokers, and fail to realize that overt discrimination against those who smoke is increasingly sanctioned (Venuti et al., 2000; Gibson, 1997; Hines, Fretz, and Nollen, 1998; Srebro, Hodges, Authier, and Chambliss,1999; Douglas, Allen, Arian, Crawford, Headen, Spigner, Tassler, and Ureda, 2001). Adolescents and young adults confronting this choice tend to underestimate the social risks they are running when they smoke; college students who smoke reported negligible awareness of discrimination against smokers on the part of employers, teachers, and fellow students (Venuti et al., 2002). Given the ubiquity of negative stereotypes of smokers on American campuses, students should be more informed about the possible negative social and academic repercussions of the choice to smoke. Research clarifying the attitudes of students and faculty members in education settings may help students to develop a more valid picture of the full social ramifications of their decision to smoke cigarettes.

A questionnaire assessing perceptions of a hypothetical student smoker, a former smoker, and a nonsmoker, as well as personal smoking habits, was administered to student and teacher participants. Student respondents were 103 high school students (age $M= 16.96$, $SD=.74$) enrolled in health education classes at a public school in a suburban area in the northeastern USA, 151 college students (age $M=18.90$, $SD=1.05$) enrolled in introductory psychology courses at a nearby small liberal arts college in the same area, and 68 professional school students (age $M= 26.97$, $SD=8.90$) enrolled in a law or medical school in the area. The sample included 44 male and 58 female high school students, 73 male and 76 female college students, and 33 male and 35 female students attending law or medical school who were administered the anonymous survey during class.

Faculty respondents were 35 high school instructors (age M= 42.37, SD=7.59) from a public school in a suburban area in the northeastern USA, 34 college instructors (age M= 45.01, SD=8.70) from a small liberal arts college in the same area, and 24 professional school faculty members (age M= 48.95, SD=9.25) from the law or medical school. The sample included 13 male and 22 female high school instructors, 12 male and 22 female college instructors, and 11 male and 13 female law or medical school instructors who were administered the anonymous survey through campus mail.

The majority of the three student samples were nonsmokers; 18.6% of these high school students, 28% of these college students, and 17.6% of the professional school students surveyed engaged in smoking behavior classified as habitual and regular. Similarly, the majority of the three faculty samples were nonsmokers; 10.5% of these high school faculty, 7.5% of these college faculty, and 16.6% of the professional school faculty surveyed engaged in smoking behavior classified as habitual and regular.

The subjects rated each of three hypothetical situations – smoker, nonsmoker, and former smoker – on six 5-point Likert-format items (anchors: 1=extremely low, 2=somewhat low, 3=neutral, 4=somewhat high, 5=extremely high). They described their impression of an average student in each of these three categories along dimensions of intelligence, artistic creativity, independence, conscientiousness, ambition, and hostility. The order of presentation of the hypothetical cases was counterbalanced.

Several of the preliminary studies evaluating the stigma associated with student smoking used a summary character rating which included the dimensions of both intelligence and judgment, which arguably overlap. Critiques of this work have suggested that because the judgment of youngsters who smoke is so widely challenged, this redundancy in the summary measure may have skewed results. To avoid this weakness, the 2006 study used a summary measure omitting the specific judgment dimension.

Directionally adjusted items were totaled for each participant to create a summary character rating for each of the three student cases (nonsmoker, former smoker, and current smoker). In order to assess the stigma associated with smoking, for each respondent the summary rating of the smoker was subtracted from that of the nonsmoker, and a constant of 10 was added to avoid negative numbers in subsequent analyses. Similarly, the residual stigma associated with being a former smoker was measured by subtracting the summary score for the former smoker from the nonsmoker score (a constant of 10 was added to these scores as well). This provided comparative ratings of hypothetical student smokers (stigma) and former smokers (residual stigma) relative to the ratings of nonsmoking controls.

A 2 x 6 multiple analysis of variance (MANOVA) was conducted to determine the association between the participant's own smoking status (smoker and nonsmoker) and the six academic levels (high school student, college student, professional school student, high school faculty, college faculty, and professional school faculty) on the stigma and residual stigma measures. Significant differences were found between the two smoker groups on the dependent measures, Wilks' lambda =.98, F =2,389)=4.15, p<.01. The multivariate eta squared based on Wilks' lambda was .02. Table 2 contains the means and standard deviations on the dependent variables for the two groups.

Analyses of variance (ANOVA) on each dependent variable were conducted as follow-up tests to the MANOVA. Using the Bonferroni method, each ANOVA was tested at the .025 level. The ANOVA on both the stigma scores, $F(1,390)=7.40$, $p<.01$, eta squared = .02, and the residual stigma scores, $F(1,390)=5.14$, $p<.025$, eta squared = .01, was significant. Nonsmokers' ratings yielded higher stigma and residual stigma scores than smokers.

The MANOVA also revealed a significant difference among the student and faculty groups, Wilks' lambda =.93, $\underline{F}$ =10,778)=3.04, $p<.001$. The multivariate eta squared for this analysis was .04. Table 2 contains the means and standard deviations on the dependent variables for the six groups. The follow-up ANOVA on the stigma scores was significant, $F(5,390)= 4.68$, $p<.001$, eta squared = .06, while the ANOVA on the residual stigma scores was nonsignificant, $F(5,390)= 1.63$, $p=.15$.

Post hoc analyses to the univariate ANOVA for the stigma scores consisted of conducting pairwise comparisons to find which academic status groups differed. Each pairwise comparison was tested at the .025 divided by 15 or .002 level. High school students' ratings yielded higher stigma scores than college students, college faculty members, and professional school faculty members. College teachers' and professional school teachers' ratings yielded lower stigma scores than professional school students, but not college students. In addition, high school teachers' ratings yielded higher stigma scores than professional school teachers. No significant interaction effects were observed.

Table 2. Mean Stigma and Residual Stigma Scores of 489 High School, College, and Professional School Student and Faculty Member Smokers and Nonsmokers

	Stigma		Residual Stigma	
	Mean	SD	Mean	SD
Smokers	12.31	4.14	9.63	2.29
Nonsmokers	15.77	5.75	11.17	3.30

Table 3. Mean Stigma and Residual Stigma Scores of 489 High School, College, and Professional School Students and Faculty Members

	Stigma		Residual Stigma	
	Mean	SD	Mean	SD
High School Students	16.81	6.09	12.13	3.44
College Students	14.28	4.85	10.33	2.98
Professional Students	16.88	5.61	11.03	2.45
High School Faculty	15.87	5.10	11.63	3.29
College Faculty	11.26	4.19	10.06	4.67
Professional Faculty	10.08	4.92	10.04	2.29

In order to evaluate whether there was disproportionate smoking among the academic groups, chi square analyses were performed for both student and faculty member groups. Among students, a significant difference was obtained (chi square=6.08, df=2, $p<.05$); a higher percentage of college student than high school or professional school participants smoked. Among the faculty groups, no significant differences emerged.

Consistent with previous research, these findings show that perceptions of student smokers are more negative than those of nonsmoker students, and that smoking cessation partially restores a student's image in the eyes of peers and faculty members. These results corroborate earlier findings showing that current smokers, both students and faculty alike, downgrade ratings of hypothetical student smokers relative to nonsmokers less than nonsmokers, suggesting that they stigmatize smokers less. The difference pronounced ratings of nonsmokers and former smokers (residual stigma) was also less among participants who currently smoke than those who do not smoke. This suggests that current smokers are less likely to penalize a student for a history of tobacco use.

Differences in relative ratings among the academic groups only partially supported the hypothesis that stigma associated with smoking decreases linearly as students progress through school. High school students' ratings of student smokers relative to nonsmokers yielded the highest stigma scores, which were significantly greater than those of college students, college faculty members, and professional school faculty members. However, professional school students' ratings of smokers were every bit as negative as those of high school students.

High school teachers were more disparaging of student smokers relative to their nonsmoking peers than professional school instructors. This finding is consistent with previous research indicating that high school teachers are especially critical of student smoking (Brosh, Austin, and Chambliss, 2003). College and professional school teachers' ratings yielded the lowest stigma scores, which were substantially less than the professional school students' scores.

There are several possible reasons why high school students expressed especially strong negative attitudes about current student smokers. In addition to being unhealthful, smoking is illegal for most high school students. Probably as a result, a smaller proportion of high school students than college students smoke cigarettes. Consequently, high school students who smoke are violating multiple norms, which may result in greater stigma being directed against them by their peers. Smoking among professional school students was also rare, which may help to account for why members of this group also reported highly negative perceptions of smokers. It is impossible to determine from the present study's design whether norms against student smoking in academic settings produce stigma, which in turn deters smoking, or if the infrequency of smoking supports norms more critical of smokers. Because in this study the college student participants were disproportionately more likely to smoke, it is possible that this confound accounted for this group's apparent forgiving stance toward smokers.

This possible artifact cannot explain the observed differences among the faculty groups, because smoking rates were fairly similar for the three groups. This suggests that the differences between professional school faculty members' ratings and high school teachers' ratings are not simply a function of the respondents' own smoking choices. Since smoking prevention is commonly an institutional priority for high schools, it may be that high school teachers resent students who smoke because their behavior represents an institutional failure. This offers a plausible explanation of high school teachers' greater condemnation of student smokers. However, although professional schools are less likely to make antismoking indoctrination a formal educational objective, medical school curricula typically include negative messages about smoking. Accordingly, since half of the professional school professors in this sample taught in the medical school, it was surprising to find this group so uncritical of smokers. Future research including a larger, more representative sample of law and medical school professors might permit further assessment of possible attitudinal differences between these groups.

It is also possible that the illegality of smoking among high school students affects high school teachers' perceptions. As students get older, perhaps their teachers are more likely to respect them for making autonomous choices, including the legal choice to smoke. Perhaps as a result of a combination of these factors, as students progress through educational levels, smokers may encounter less discrimination in school from teachers.

It is also possible that differences in social desirability responding, "political correctness" sensitivity, and legal sophistication among the faculty groups may have contributed to these results. Since half of the professional faculty consisted of law school professors, this group may have been more likely to refrain from endorsing items in a manner suggesting discriminatory attitudes. Such reluctance to acknowledge prejudicial attitudes toward student smokers may have accounted for the especially low stigma and residual stigma scores received by the professional faculty members. Supporting this notion is the fact that when the constant of 10 is removed from these scores, the professional school teachers' stigma and residual stigma scores drop to zero.

Lastly, the possibility that there are genuine differences among high school, college, and professional student smokers cannot be dismissed. High school smokers may truly be dramatically less intelligent, independent, ambitious, etc. than their peers, while professional school students who smoke may typically be no different from their nonsmoking counterparts. Consequently, the faculty members may have been accurately rating the average student smoker they are likely to encounter at their school. Arguing against this notion are the students' evaluations, which, if taken as valid descriptors, would imply that professional school smokers actually display less desirable qualities than their nonsmoking peers.

These results provide support for the notion that many members of educational communities tend to view students who smoke more negatively than students who refrain from smoking. The disparaging ratings of student smokers, provided by both students and faculty members, suggest that students who choose to smoke publicly may be seen prejudicially and could expose themselves to discriminatory behavior. These findings suggest that in many academic settings (particularly high schools), it may be wise to conceal one's current or former use of cigarettes in order to avoid negative stereotyping.

Extending the work of previous researchers, this study also indicated that students who quit smoking partially restore their image; while smoking cessation failed to erase stigma, it did appear to alleviate it. However, since some residual stigma was in evidence, the implication is clear that it is best for an individual never to start smoking.

Chambliss, Shull, Baker, Burton, Nesbit, Weir, Wilson, Katona, and Brosh (2006) used the same paradigm to compare the ratings of hypothetical student smokers and nonsmokers on specific individual attributes (intelligence, artistic creativity, independence, conscientiousness, ambition, and hostility). The following excerpt originally appeared in the *Journal of Alcohol and Drug Education.*

In order to assess how perceptions of individual personality characteristics differed between students and faculty, these groups were separated before within subject t-tests were performed on the individual item ratings of smokers and nonsmokers. Table 4 summarizes the results of these analyses for the student respondents. Significant differences in ratings of smokers and nonsmokers emerged on every individual dimension assessed. In every case students who smoke were evaluated less favorably than their nonsmoking peers.

Table 4. Ratings of Personality Characteristics of Student Smokers and Nonsmokers from High School, College, and Professional School Students (N=392)

	Smoker		Nonsmoker		t	df	p<
	Mean	SD	Mean	SD			
Intelligence	2.61	.76	3.89	.88	20.03	391	.001
Independence	2.92	.90	3.70	.93	10.37	324	.001
Conscientious	2.47	.87	3.85	.90	17.77	325	.001
Ambition	2.55	.77	3.90	.92	18.35	326	.001
Artistic creativity	2.90	.73	3.40	.80	7.82	325	.001
Hostility	3.13	.72	2.87	1.07	3.27	326	.01

Within-subject t-tests comparing faculty members' ratings of students who smoke and those who do not revealed significant differences on every dimension but artistic creativity (table 5).

Table 5. Ratings of Personality Characteristics of Student Smokers and Nonsmokers from High School, College, and Professional School Faculty Members (N=95)

	Smoker		Nonsmoker		t	df	p<
	Mean	SD	Mean	SD			
Intelligence	2.83	.71	3.39	.96	3.98	93	.001
Independence	2.82	.85	3.37	.88	3.93	93	.001
Conscientious	2.67	.74	3.46	.90	5.43	93	.001
Ambition	2.77	.63	3.29	.82	4.17	92	.001
Artistic creativity	3.03	.58	3.11	.54	1.00	93	ns

An investigation of high school and college students' perceptions of current smokers, former smokers, and nonsmokers by Brosh, Austin, and Chambliss (2003) was based upon work supported by a grant from the 2002 Ursinus Summer Fellows Program. This study assessed the generality of previous findings showing negative attitudes toward smokers by including both an adolescent and young adult sample, and explored whether smoking cessation reverses the negative social stigma associated with smoking, in order to replicate Goldstein (1991). The following is an excerpt from an article that originally appeared in *Perceptual and Motor Skills*.

A questionnaire assessing perceptions of hypothetical male and female current smokers, a former smoker, and a nonsmoker, as well as personal smoking habits, was administered to 108 high school and 115 college students. Participants were asked to describe their impression of an average student in each of these four categories along the following dimensions: intelligence, hostility, judgment, artistic creativity, independence, conscientiousness, ambition, and consideration

In order to determine if differences exist among perceptions of current male and female smokers, nonsmokers, and former smokers, paired sample t-tests were performed on summary character ratings of the four hypothetical target cases (see table 6 and 7). The nonsmoker was rated most favorably, followed by the former smoker. Male and female smokers were rated similarly.

Table 6. Mean summary ratings of hypothetical targets mong 217 high school and college students

Perceptions	Mean	SD
Male smoker	30.65	3.94
Female smoker	30.46	3.55
Former Smoker	35.00	3.13
Nonsmoker	43.43	5.30

Table 7. Within-subject t-test results of comparisons of summary ratings of four hypothetical cases among 217 high school and college students

Perceptions	t	df	P
Nonsmoker vs. Male smoker	25.13	210	.001
Nonsmoker vs. Female smoker	26.92	210	.001
Nonsmoker vs. Former smoker	27.31	214	.001
Former smoker vs. Male smoker	12.06	208	.001
Former smoker vs. Female smoker	13.61	215	.001
Male smoker vs. Female Smoker	00.75	211	.457

Within subject t-tests on each individual character item revealed that nonsmokers were viewed more positively than both current and former smokers on every dimension (ambition, artistic creativity, conscientiousness, considerate, hostility, independence, intelligence, and judgment). Former smokers were evaluated more favorably than current smokers on all dimensions except for hostility, where no significant difference was found between ratings of former smokers and current female smokers. Within subject t-tests showed significant differences between perceptions of male smokers and female smokers on only three of the eight character dimensions. Male smokers were seen as more hostile, artistic, and independent than their female counterparts.

In addition to the hypothetical cases, impressions of the prevalence of smoking and expectations of typical behavior towards smokers were assessed through MANOVA. High school students agreed more with the statement, "the majority of students at my school smoke cigarettes," than did college students (high school: x=2.65, sd=.88, n=104; college: x=2.40, sd=.92, n=111; F=9.74, df=1, p<.01). High school students perceived there to be greater discrimination by teachers than college students did (high school: x=2.32, sd=1.02, n=104; college: x=1.87, sd=.85, n=111; F=13.60, df=1, p<.01).

These findings corroborate those of earlier studies, suggesting that the decision to smoke severely handicaps an individual socially. The adolescent sample expressed views paralleling the adult group, suggesting that individuals absorb critical ideas about those who smoke early. This study also supports the notion that those who quit smoking at least partially restore their image; while smoking cessation failed to reverse stigma, it did appear to attenuate it. Finally, this 2003 study showed that more high school than college students believe the majority of the students at their school smoke and that teachers discriminate against smokers.

Chambliss (2004) summarized additional research on educators' views of student smokers in high schools, colleges, and law and medical schools, supported by a sabbatical grant from Ursinus College. The following is an excerpt from an article originally appearing in *Perceptual and Motor Skills*. A questionnaire assessing perceptions of a hypothetical student smoker, a former smoker, and a nonsmoker, as well as personal smoking habits, was administered to 35 high school, 35 college, and 30 professional school faculty members. To assess possible differences among perceptual ratings of current student smokers, nonsmokers, and former smokers, paired sample *t* tests were performed on means of summed ratings of the three hypothetical target cases (see table 8). The smoker was rated less favorably than the nonsmoker and former smoker.

Table 8. Mean Summary Ratings of Hypothetical Students By 88 High School College and Professional School Faculty Members And Within-subject *t* Ratios

Perception	Mean	SD
Smoker	23.69	3.31
Former Smoker	26.48	3.80
Nonsmoker	27.27	4.42
Comparison	*t*	*df*
Nonsmoker vs. smoker	5.34*	87
Former smoker vs. smoker	5.16*	87
Nonsmoker vs. former smoker	1.23	87

Note.—p<.001.

Within subject *t* tests on each individual characteristic showed nonsmokers and former smokers were viewed more positively than current smokers on every dimension except artistic creativity (ambition, conscientiousness, hostility, independence, intelligence, and judgment). Nonsmokers were evaluated more favorably than former smokers on only one dimension, artistic creativity; no differences emerged on other dimensions.

Oneway ANOVA indicated a significant difference in summary ratings of student nonsmokers among the three faculty groups (F=12.98, *df*=2/77, *p*<.001); to compensate for these variations, difference scores were calculated to provide a comparison of each faculty member's perception of nonsmoker students at their school and current and former smoker students at their school. For each respondent, summary ratings of smokers were subtracted from summary ratings of nonsmokers in order to assess the stigma associated with student smoking. Similarly, summary ratings of former smokers were subtracted from summary ratings of nonsmokers in order to measure the residual stigma associated with being a former smoker. Oneway ANOVA revealed significant differences among high school, college, and professional school faculty members on the stigma measure (F=14.60, *df*=2/85, *p*<.001), but not on the residual stigma measure. High school instructors' stigma scores were higher than those of college and professional school faculty.

The Chambliss (2004) results are consistent with the other reported findings and suggest that students who smoke may be viewed critically by their teachers. The results also indicate that students who quit smoking can successfully restore their image in the eyes of faculty members; respondents' perceptions did not significantly differentiate between nonsmokers and former smokers on most attributes.

SUMMARY OF RESULTS

Considered collectively, these findings show that the majority of the faculty, staff, and students surveyed see smokers in a very negative light. Even smokers perceive other smokers to be generally unattractive. The prejudice against those who smoke is real.

Perceptions of student smokers are more negative than those of nonsmoker students, among both students and teachers at the high school, college, and professional school levels. It was also noted that college and professional school teachers perceived student smokers less negatively than the other groups. Importantly, several of these studies found that smoking cessation appears to restore a student's image in the eyes of faculty members, especially at the college and professional school levels. Among their peers, smoking cessation ameliorates the stigma associated with smoking, although substantial residual stigma seems to persist among high school students.

Generational factors may have accounted for why students evaluated smokers more negatively than instructors. Members of the student cohort were born after a consensus about the harmful effects of cigarette smoking had emerged. It seems likely that their lifelong exposure to negative messages about smoking contributed to their more disparaging attitudes.

These findings have several implications for substance use education programs. In trying to deter cigarette smoking, it may be helpful to publicize its social hazards more zealously. Informing students about their peers' and teachers' negative reactions to those who smoke may improve students' decision making about this form of substance use. The finding that smoking cessation often effectively reverses discrimination might also be fruitfully incorporated into treatment programs. These results may assist those wishing to quit in maintaining their motivation to face the formidable challenges involved in cessation.

SECTION III

Traditional Individual Treatments:
Campus Cessation Programs
How can we help individual students quit smoking?
Which treatments work?
Group format program effects
Individualized format program effects

This section explores the outcomes of two campus smoking cessation programs. The first study in this section determined the efficacy of a standard smoking cessation treatment method when delivered to students recruited via college bulletin boards.

The second study describes the results of providing a reformulated treatment opportunity, which was more customized to the needs and convenience of individual students.

A 1999 paper entitled "Attempts to Reduce Cigarette Smoking Among College Students", authored by Kane, Hodges, Srebro, Fruhwirth, and Chambliss, endeavored to use a small groups approach to reduce college student smoking through behavioral mehtods. Despite much positive publicity, several researchers have failed to obtain evidence supporting reliance on nicotine replacement strategies for long term smoking cessation. For example, Lewis, Piasecki, Fiore, Anderson, and Baker (1998) reported the results of a randomized, double blind placebo controlled study comparing three treatments: nicotine patch plus counseling, placebo patch plus counseling, and minimal care intervention. Their objective was to assess if the nicotine patch plus counseling increased long term abstinence over placebo or minimal intervention programs, and to identify factors associated with long term cessation after the treatment was completed. The study involved 185 individuals and the participants were randomly assigned to one of the three treatment programs. After the initiation of the patch, a study nurse phoned the participants at 1, 3, 6, and 24 weeks to provide cognitive therapy counseling and motivational support to the individual. Patch compliance and smoking behavior were also evaluated at these times. At the end of the six month treatment program, rates of abstinence were 4.9% for the minimal intervention group, 6.5% for the placebo patch group, and 9.7% for the nicotine patch group. However, the study showed no significant differences in long term cessation rates.

Rosal, Ockene, Hurley, Kalan, and Hebert (1998) studied the efficacy of nicotine gum on patients who wanted to quit smoking. The Physician-Delivered Smoking Intervention Study consisted of 299 participants (42% male, 58% female). Participants were counseled and offered strategies on smoking cessation. Those participants willing to quit smoking were offered the nicotine gum. The results showed that at the end of the study there was no significant difference in the rate of abstinence between those who had accepted the gum (24%) and those who did not accept the gum (20%) at 6-month follow up. The researchers also found that longer and multiple attempts at smoking cessation were better predictors for cessation than stated desire and social support to quit.

Cinciripini, Lapitsky, Wallfisch, Mace Nezami, and Van Vuakis (1994) studied multicomponent behavioral therapy conjointly with scheduled smoking reduction. Scheduled smoking reduction was defined as a three week process with the participant gradually reducing their nicotine intake and thus easing withdrawal symptoms after the individual stopped smoking. In this treatment, the intake of nicotine is regulated by time as opposed to the individual's urges or personal situations associated with cigarette consumption. The results of the researchers' study showed a forty-four percent abstinence rate compared to an eighteen percent abstinence rate with a nonscheduled, reduced smoking group at one year follow up.

The Kane et al. (1999) study investigated the effectiveness of a scheduled smoking reduction treatment plan, as defined above, in combination with a multicomponent behavioral program (including coping with withdrawal symptoms and relapse prevention strategies) in helping smokers who volunteered for a smoking cessation program, drawn from a small, liberal arts undergraduate institution.

College students volunteered to participate in a three-week smoking cessation program, which was advertised throughout campus. The program was offered both in a group setting at a counseling center in a campus building, and also in an individualized, confidential format with a student-researcher meeting with participants at their convenience. The individual format was provided to accommodate the needs of those who were either unable or unwilling to attend the program when offered at a counseling center in a campus building.

At the start of the program, an informed consent form outlining the basis of the study was signed by each participant. The participants then completed a survey on determinants of smoking, familial patterns, and feelings while smoking. A student researcher interviewed each participant to evaluate current smoking consumption and assess reasons the individuals wanted to quit. The participants were given two brochures published by the American Cancer Society to read on their own as they felt necessary. The first pamphlet, entitled "Commit to Quit" (1998), discussed three questions for smokers to ask themselves as they prepare to quit smoking. The next pamphlet, entitled "Smart Move! A Stop Smoking Guide", outlined the positive benefits of quitting, former smoker success stories, and guides to remaining abstinent. A comprehensive plan to quit smoking developed by Glaxo Wellcome (1997) was handed out to the participants; this guide was prepared by Michael Fiore, MD, Director of the Center for Tobacco Research and Intervention at the University of Wisconsin Medical School. This packet consisted of strategies to quit smoking, ways to cope with withdrawal symptoms, cognitive reasoning skills helping one deal with smoking trigger situations, and a self reward system. Participants were guided through the packet and asked to share some of this information; it was highly encouraged that participants later fill out this packet for self-motivation. In addition, the American Lung Association's Quit Smoking Action Plan (1998) was given to participants, providing them with a plan to prepare for smoking cessation, nicotine replacement options, and information about possible prescription medications available to aid in smoking cessation. This also provided information pertaining to support groups available on smoking cessation. It was at this point that the participants were informed that they could phone the psychology student aiding them in their smoking cessation whenever they needed any extra support. A list of common nicotine withdrawal symptoms and withdrawal symptom coping strategies (Morton, 1989) was given to the participants. These coping strategies were grouped into relaxation, distraction, rethinking, problem solving, self-support, and protection methods. Each section was discussed with the participants to help them determine those methods that they were most likely to use and to permit them to ask any questions regarding these strategies. Following this, participants received a short list of the positive benefits one gains when one quits smoking. A brief discussion of information gleaned from a review of the literature took place. Next, any questions about the material given out or facts stated by the researcher were answered. A smoking-intake weekly monitoring chart was given to the participants to complete during the first week of the program. On this log, they were asked to state the brand of cigarette consumed and length. In addition to this, participants were asked to write in the log each time they smoked, indicate the time of day, situation surrounding the smoking behavior, and number of cigarettes smoked within each situation.

No reduction in the baseline amount of cigarettes smoked was to occur during the first three days at the start of the program. During a mid-week discussion between the researcher and participant, participants were asked to begin scheduling their smoking for every four hours, beginning the fourth day of the first week.

At the end of the first week, another brief meeting was held between the participant and researcher. The completed smoking log was collected, and the log for the second week was distributed. Smokers were again asked to limit smoking to every four to five hours, depending on their individual abilities. Another mid-week discussion ensued to monitor the participants' progress. During this meeting, they were guided to smoke every five hours and limit the number of cigarettes smoked each time (i.e., no more than two cigarettes every five hours).

A final brief meeting was held before the last week of the program. The participants were encouraged to continue cutting back on cigarette consumption and to extend the amount of time between smoking, until no cigarettes were consumed.

A paired sample t-test was conducted to evaluate whether there was a significant difference between the number of cigarettes smoked during the baseline, scheduled smoking, and reduced/scheduled smoking days. The results, as shown in tables 9 and 10, indicate the mean number cigarettes smoked on baseline days (M=7.44, SD=5.05) was significantly higher than cigarettes smoked on scheduled smoking days (M=5.80, SD=4.25), t (8)=2.57, p<.05. Another paired samples t-test indicated that the mean number cigarettes smoked on baseline days (M=7.44, SD=5.05) was significantly higher than the number smoked on reduced/scheduled days (M=3.57, SD=3.58), t (8)=2.84, p=.05. Lastly, results from a paired samples t-test showed that the number smoked on scheduled smoking days (M=5.80, SD=4.25) was not significantly higher than number smoked on reduced/scheduled days (M=3.57, SD=3.58), t (8)=-1.69, p=0.13).

Table 9. Means and Standard Deviations for Three Smoking Cessation Phases

	Mean	SD
Baseline Days	7.44	5.05
Scheduled Smoking	5.80	4.25
Reduced and Scheduled	3.57	3.58

Table 10. Differences between Three Levels of Smoking Cessation Phases[a]

		Mean Change	SD	t	df	sig.
Pair 1	Baseline – Scheduled	1.64	1.92	2.57	8	0.03
Pair 2	Baseline – Reduced	3.88	4.09	5.84	8	0.02
Pair 3	Reduced-Scheduled	2.23	3.98	1.68	8	0.13

[a] All possible pairs were compared.

Despite the limited number of subjects recruited for this study, significant reductions in smoking were found during both the scheduled and reduced scheduled phases of the treatment. This type of cessation program appears to be effective in helping college students reduce their smoking or quit smoking. The small number of students volunteering indicated that there was little desire for college students to quit smoking, whether they participated in a group or individualized program. The results of this study were in concordance with the Cinciripini et al. (1994) study, which used a non-student population. In the future, it is recommended that this type of cessation program, along with innovative strategies for reaching out to college student smokers, may decrease the size of the student smoking population.

A paper entitled "Individualized Attempts to Reduce Cigarette Smoking Among College Students", by Kane, Hodges, Srebro, Authier, and Chambliss (2000), extended the work of Kane et al. (1999). Due to the difficulty in attracting large numbers of college-age smokers to a traditional counseling center for a group-based smoking cessation program, a more convenient and customized way of reaching these smokers was employed in a follow-up study. In this second study, participants contacted one of the researchers in order to arrange for an individualized cessation program. In the Kane et al. (2000) study, the literature on home based models of care was applied to the task of helping young adult and older adult students reduce their smoking. A reduced, scheduled smoking approach was coupled with withdrawal coping skills training to help a volunteer college students to quit smoking. Though few participants were involved, significant smoking reduction was observed following use of the individualized scheduled smoking program.

Since previous work demonstrated that it was very difficult to attract large numbers of college-age smokers to a traditional counseling center based smoking cessation program, despite repeated efforts at advertising the availability of this free program, an individualized treatment approach was developed. Based on the assumption that young smokers are at best ambivalent about modifying their smoking, a more convenient and customized way of reaching these less highly motivated individuals was developed.

In order to streamline the counseling center-based program used by Kane et al.(1999) to make it more suitable to the needs of busy participants, several modifications were made. Weekly one-on-one intensive smoking cessation sessions replaced the original three one-hour sessions over a three-week period. Participants were monitored through administration of logs they maintained tracking their smoking behavior (similar to those in the first smoking cessation program), and also with regular telephone calls from the staff involved in the treatment program.

The researchers also abandoned the group-administered smoking cessation program in favor of home based individualized treatment methods. This afforded increased confidentiality and helped to sustain students' motivation to quit smoking. The literature on individualized home based preventive treatments supports the use of this type of approach. Meyer and Gibbons (1997) found evidence of a decline in home based health care delivery starting after World War II; for example, house calls at that time were forty percent compared to 0.6 percent in 1980. Despite this trend, several researchers have discussed the advantages of home based treatment approaches. Campion (1997) noted that home based care spares clients the nuisance and inconvenience of trekking to the area where health care service is provided. Campion (1997) also notes that clients feel more assured in their own home setting than at the point of service treatment setting. Clients feel that home based care offers several advantages: caregivers who participate in home based programs provide greater empathy, increased commitment to the client, enhanced reassurance to the client, and reduce perceptions of isolation (Campion, 1997). In addition to these positive outcomes from home based care, programs based on this model allow the evaluator to assess the clients' function and compliance in a "real world setting".

There is a recent trend favoring heavier reliance upon home based care and prevention programs among those addressing the problem of HIV. Low risk gay men have been found to be more inclined to participate in small group intervention programs than high risk homosexual individuals (Hoff et al., 1997). Hoff and his colleagues performed an 18-month comparison study evaluating HIV/AIDS prevention programs targeting the gay community. The four programs assessed were outreach, home meetings, safer sex workshops and HIV antibody testing and counseling. Hoff and his colleagues found that outreach programs were able to address the needs of a large proportion of men (59% of 49 participants) at risk. It must be noted that the outreach program took place in gay bars, sex environments, and community events that enabled the target group to participate in HIV prevention programs without having to be present at group activities. The second most effective program was the home meeting prevention program, followed by safe sex (6 % with 12 participants). The HIV testing and counseling sites had few participants attend.

Further investigations into the efficacy of home based prevention programs involve high-risk prenatal care. Olds and his colleagues (1998) examined home based prevention programs aimed at women with high-risk health related behaviors during pregnancy. These behaviors included cigarette smoking, drinking, and substance abuse. The programs were aimed at prevention of poor pregnancy outcomes, the prevention of infant health and developmental problems, and improving the mothers' life course. Olds and his colleagues found that specific parental behaviors and social risk factors were potentially alterable; and if intervention was available developmental problems in children of high-risk mothers could be reduced. In 1977, the researchers began the Elmira trial; ironically, it was the same year that cigarette smoking was identified as a serious threat to the health and development of the fetus. Empirical evidence has shown that preventive home based programs targeting high risk women during pregnancy can improve the outcomes of pregnancy, improve the mother's ability to care for the child, and reduce welfare dependence (Olds et al. 1998).

It is important to note that for home based treatment to be effective, treatment providers must be well trained in the area of the target behavior. Continuity of care from the treatment providers and empathy toward those in treatment also play a significant role in the effectiveness of home based preventive programs (Campion, 1997; Olds et al., 1998.).

In the Kane et al. (2000) investigation, thirteen young adults volunteered to participate in a three-week smoking cessation program, which was advertised throughout campus. The program was offered in an individualized, confidential format with a student-researcher meeting with participants at their convenience. The individual format was provided to accommodate the needs of those who were either unable or unwilling to attend programs offered at a counseling center in a campus building.

At the start of the program, an informed consent form was signed by each participant outlining the basis of the study. The participants then completed a survey on determinants of smoking, familial patterns, and feelings while smoking. A student researcher interviewed each participant to evaluate current smoking consumption and assess reasons the individuals wanted to quit.

The participants were given two brochures published by the American Cancer Society to read on their own as they felt necessary. The first pamphlet, entitled "Commit to Quit" (1998), discussed three questions for smokers to ask themselves as they prepare to quit smoking. The next pamphlet, entitled "Smart Move! A Stop Smoking Guide", outlined the positive benefits of quitting, former smoker success stories, and guides to staying clean.

As in the earlier Kane et al. study, a comprehensive plan to quit smoking developed by Glaxo Wellcome (1997) was handed out to the participants; this guide was prepared by Michael Fiore, MD, Director of the Center for Tobacco Research and Intervention at the University of Wisconsin Medical School. This packet consisted of strategies to quit smoking, ways to cope with withdrawal symptoms, cognitive reasoning skills helping one deal with smoking trigger situations, and a self reward system. Participants were guided through the packet and asked to share some of this information; it was highly encouraged that participants later fill out this packet for self-motivation.

In addition, the American Lung Association's Quit Smoking Action Plan (1998) was given to participants, providing them with a plan to prepare for smoking cessation, nicotine replacement options, and information about possible prescription medications available to aid in smoking cessation. This also provided information pertaining to support groups available on smoking cessation. It was at this point that the participants were informed that they could phone the psychology student aiding them in their smoking cessation whenever they needed any extra support.

A list of common nicotine withdrawal symptoms and withdrawal symptom coping strategies (Morton, 1989) was given to the participants. These coping strategies were grouped into relaxation, distraction, rethinking, problem solving, self-support, and protection methods. Each section was discussed with the participants to help them determine those methods that they were most likely to use and to permit them to ask any questions regarding these strategies. Following this participants received a short list of the positive benefits one gains when one quits smoking.

A brief discussion of information gleaned from a review of the literature took place. Next, any questions about the material given out or facts stated by the researcher were answered. A smoking-intake weekly monitoring chart was given to the participants to complete during the first week of the program. On this log, they were asked to state the brand of cigarette consumed and length. In addition to this, participants were asked to write in the log each time they smoked, indicate the time of day, situation surrounding the smoking behavior, and number of cigarettes smoked within each situation.

No reduction in the baseline amount of cigarettes smoked was to occur during the first three days at the start of the program. During a mid-week discussion between the researcher and participant, participants were asked to begin scheduling their smoking for every four hours, beginning the fourth day of the first week.

At the end of the first week, another brief meeting was held between the participant and researcher. The completed smoking log was collected, and the log for the second week was distributed. Smokers were again asked to limit smoking to every four to five hours, depending on their individual abilities. Another mid-week discussion ensued to monitor the participants' progress. During this meeting, they were guided to smoke every five hours and limit the number of cigarettes smoked each time (i.e., no more than two cigarettes every five hours).

A final brief meeting was held before the last week of the program. The participants were encouraged to continue cutting back on cigarette consumption and to extend the amount of time between smoking episodes, until no cigarettes were consumed.

A paired sample t-test was conducted to evaluate whether there was a significant difference between the number of cigarettes smoked on baseline, scheduled smoking, and reduced/scheduled smoking days. The results indicate the mean number cigarettes smoked on baseline days (M=9.78, SD=5.34) was significantly higher than cigarettes smoked on scheduled smoking days (M=7.93, SD=4.70), t (12)=3.25, p<.01. Another paired samples t-test indicated that the mean number cigarettes smoked on baseline days (M=7.93, SD=5.34) was significantly higher than number smoked on reduced/scheduled days (M=5.97, SD=4.87), t (12)=3.50, p<.01. Lastly, results from a paired samples t-test showed that the number smoked on scheduled smoking days (M=7.93, SD=4.70) was significantly higher than number smoked on reduced/scheduled days (M=5.97, SD=4.87), t(12)=-2.12, p<.05).

Participants in this individualized scheduled smoking program experienced significant reductions in their smoking, both during the scheduled and reduced scheduled phases of the treatment. This type of cessation program appears to be a promising way of addressing the needs of young adult and adult smokers, many of whom are reluctant to participate in large, group-format, counseling-center based programs. Future extensions of this research should attempt to recruit larger numbers of participants, and include collection of one-year follow up data in order to assess maintenance of treatment gains over time. This and other types of smoking cessation programs may be helpful in trying to address the problem of campus smoking.

SUMMARY OF RESULTS

Ursinus College offered traditional workshops for smokers on campus, using empirically supported treatment methods such as behavioral monitoring and scheduled smoking, combined with supportive encouragement. Few students participated, although those who did reduced their use of tobacco. Next, a more customized approach was provided, with counselors meeting smokers when and where they chose, in order to reach a bigger audience. These smokers showed highly significant reductions in smoking during each of two treatment phases. In addition to reducing individuals' use of cigarettes, advertising the availability of these programs on campus helpfully affirms antismoking norms.

SECTION IV

Campus Environmental Interventions:
Reestablishing Antismoking Norms on Campus
How can antismoking norms be strengthened?
How can we reduce public smoking on campuses?
Use of Signs to Reduce public smoking
How Smoking Restrictions Can Backfire

This section describes less traditional approaches to reducing the problem of student smoking, aimed at influencing the campus on a systems level. The first study explored the effects of an unobtrusive environmental intervention on the level of public smoking outside campus buildings. This experiment involved posting simple signs aimed at making smokers more aware of their behavior while they congregate in public spaces outside classroom buildings. This intervention was intended to reduce the amount of time students spend smoking cigarettes in these highly visible settings, in order to reverse the implicit message that smoking is a normative and accepted form of student behavior. The second study examined the disturbing possibility that the increasingly common restrictions on public smoking may have untoward consequences for some smokers. This study assessed whether public smoking restrictions have unintended detrimental effects on young smokers, by inadvertently increasing the appeal and reinforcing properties of tobacco, thereby increasing the risk of nicotine addiction. The concern is that for some young smokers restrictions may actually serve to inflate subsequent cravings, and thereby inadvertently accelerate the development of an addictive cycle of nicotine use.

A 1999 paper, entitled "Use of a Visual Prompt to Reduce Public Cigarette Smoking on a College Campus", authored by Hodges, Srebro, Kane, Fruhwirth, and Chambliss attempted to influence student smoking with a simple environmental manipulation. In order to reduce smoking outside of public classroom buildings, paper signs reading "Think...Why Smoke?," designed to make smokers more conscious of their behavior, were composed and posted by the research team. Cigarette butts were collected during a baseline week prior to the posting of signs and for a week after signs were posted. A paired samples t-test showed that the mean number of whole cigarettes smoked on baseline days (M=92.33, SD=12.74) was significantly higher than the amount of cigarettes consumed on experimental days (M=59.67, SD=15.50), $t(2)$=-4.25, p=0.05. Comparison of the number of cigarettes smoked outside the buildings during the baseline and experimental weeks revealed a 35% reduction.

Use of this environmental manipulation was compelled by the fact that cigarette smoking is considered by many to be the largest single preventable cause of death in the U.S. (Compas et al., 1998; Price et al., 1998; Wechsler et al., 1998), causing roughly 435,000 premature deaths annually (Hobson, 2006; Lewis et al., 1998). After years of decline, cigarette smoking has resurged on many college campuses (Price et al., 1998; Wechsler et al., 1998). Despite decades of educational programs aimed at alerting young people to the risks associated with smoking, more college students are choosing to engage in the habit, often beginning to smoke after coming to live on campus.

Of particular concern is the apparent shift in norms regarding public smoking outside of classroom buildings. A simple, inexpensive intervention was used to discourage smoking by making smokers in public areas more self-conscious of their habit. By reducing smoking in public areas, it may be possible to restore antismoking norms on campuses, and discourage the initiation of smoking among students.

In previous years, most students who smoked in college arrived on campus with the habit. They typically came from families where their parents smoked, and had adopted the habit in middle school or high school, in the context of a peer group that smoked socially. In contrast, today many college-age smokers did not smoke prior to leaving home, and have parents that do not smoke (either because they successfully quit, or because they never started the habit). For these students, smoking is a way of defying parental norms and signifying independence. Many confess they start smoking because they felt uncomfortable being the sole nonsmoker in social situations; some even started because the smoke made them feel less sick if they were participating. Others see smoking as a way of managing the stresses associated with college. Most do not see their behavior as placing their health in future jeopardy, because they view this as a temporary habit that is under their control.

The irony is that while many college students are asserting their right to "experiment" with tobacco in much the same way that many of their parents' "experimented" with marijuana, the stigma associated with cigarette smoking among older adults (age 30 and up) is becoming increasingly pronounced. Students who casually begin smoking do not realize how this decision may have a negative impact on how they are viewed by members of the generation of older adults making professional school and employment decisions. Only 25% of older adults now smoke (Compas et al., 1998), and those who do smoke tend to be less economically successful and less well educated. Most of the older adults wielding power over the lives of today's college students do not themselves smoke.

These older adults tend to think of cigarette smokers in very unflattering terms. Having struggled themselves to give up this habit, watched others struggle, and/or watched others die of smoking-related illnesses, many of these individuals view those who started to smoke after the risks associated with this behavior and second hand smoke were well publicized as careless, unintelligent, and selfish. Prejudice against young smokers is evident in increasing discriminatory hiring practices and adoption of nicotine testing as an employment prerequisite in some states (e.g., the state of Washington). Although the ACLU and other groups are challenging such discrimination, the current work environment remains quite hostile to smokers. College students need to be made aware of how, given the current climate, their choice to smoke may jeopardize both their health and their future careers.

While the decision to smoke is a private one, and arguably adult students should have the right to make their own decisions about whether or not to begin this habit, proximity to public smoking may have a subtle but pernicious effect on this ostensibly autonomous decision-making. The social psychology literature is replete with examples of how simple exposure increases affinity for various products and ideas; familiarity breeds fondness (Zajonc, 1968; Brickman and D'Amato, 1975; Moreland and Zajonc, 1982). Considerable research on social influence and the impact of role models (Bandura and Walters, 1963) has established the potential for proximity to smokers to increase the probability of habit adoption.

Social contexts on campuses dominated by smokers may therefore increase the likelihood of some students' initiation of this behavior while in college. Most college-age smokers initially do not see themselves as "heavy smokers" in danger of becoming addicted to nicotine. Instead, when challenged, they dismiss their behavior as mere "social smoking", limited to specific situations, such as parties where alcohol is served and others are smoking. Unfortunately, a percentage of these "negligible" smokers will go on to develop dependence on nicotine, and will find it very difficult to reverse their decision.

Although most campuses have adopted smoke-free policies for buildings and residence halls, smoking behavior continues in public areas. Although restricting indoor smoking has been extremely beneficial, acceptance of outdoor smoking in central public areas remains a problem. Public gatherings of students smoking outside of public classroom buildings compel all students to pass through smoke-filled areas on their way to classes. Tolerance of this highly visible, public smoking implicitly condones it. Acceptance of public smoking on campus is potentially problematic because it may increase the likelihood of students' adopting the habit while on campus. The Hodges et al. (1999) study attempted to reduce public smoking outside of classroom buildings by posting signs designed to make smokers more conscious of their behavior. These signs were developed to counter the implicit pro-smoking message conveyed by gatherings of smokers outside classroom buildings, with a gentle antismoking message (Think. Why smoke?) designed to encourage students to reflect and to consider the antismoking attitudes of others. Finding ways of reversing the apparent shift to pro-smoking norms on campuses may ultimately reduce the number of new users on campus, although this study did not attempt to assess this long-term impact.

On the Friday preceding the start of the baseline observations, the designated smoking area outside of three large smoke-free public classroom buildings on a small college campus were cleared of all cigarette butts. This designated area was defined by a ten-foot radius originating at the center of the main entrance to the buildings, where ashtray receptacles were located. During the week of the baseline observations, buildings were visited in a standardized order between the hours of five and six o'clock in the evening. At this time, researchers collected cigarette butts from all of the designated areas. This occurred daily from Monday through Thursday during one week in early April. The number of butts was recorded in terms of length of remaining cigarette, in order to permit calculation of the number of whole cigarette equivalents smoked, as well as the simple number of butts left in the designated area.

The designated smoking area for each building was again cleared of cigarette butts on the Friday prior to the experimental manipulation. In addition, signs reading "Think...Why Smoke?" were placed near the doorway of the smoke-free public buildings. Researchers consistently visited these sites between five and six o'clock in the evening to collect cigarette butts on Monday through Thursday. After counting the number of cigarette butts, they were tallied and measured using the aforementioned method. Cigarette butts were also collected at one student residence site, in order to provide an informal estimate of whether the posting of signs around the public building sites actually reduced outdoor smoking or merely displaced this behavior.

Cigarette butts counted were broken into five categories: full cigarette left, three-quarters left, half left, one-quarter left, and only filter left. Using the tally sheet, the total numbers of cigarettes found at each site were entered according to the length. In order to calculate daily whole cigarettes smoked equivalents, the number of cigarette butts were weighted on a scale from 0.25 to 1.0. (cigarettes with three-quarters left were multiplied by 0.25.; those where half a cigarette was left were multiplied by 0.5; one-quarter of a cigarette left was weighted 0.75; when cigarettes were fully smoked, they were counted as 1.0.) No full cigarettes were found. A simple count of unweighted butts was also made.

A paired samples t-test was conducted to determine whether there was a difference in the amount of whole cigarettes smoked during baseline days and on the days after signs were placed outside of academic buildings. Table 11 and table 12 show the results of this analysis. The mean amount of cigarettes smoked on baseline days (M=92.33, SD=12.74) was significantly higher than the amount of cigarettes consumed on experimental days (M=59.67, SD=15.50; $t(2)$=4.25, p<.05). When the mean number of whole cigarettes smoked outside the buildings during the baseline week was compared with the mean number of whole cigarettes smoked outside the buildings during the intervention week, a 35% reduction was observed.

A second paired samples t-test was conducted on the unadjusted measure of cigarettes smoked (simple number of cigarette butts collected at each site) to assess the effects of the sign intervention. Table 13 shows the results of this analysis. The number of butts collected on baseline days was significantly higher than the number of butts collected on sign days (t=4.68, df=2, p<.05).

As an informal check on whether the signs were actually reducing smoking behavior or merely displacing it, the number of cigarette butts left at a representative student residence hall was counted. The mean daily number of butts collected during the week prior to the intervention was 57, and the mean number collected on days during the intervention week was 78. When length of cigarette butt was taken into account in order to permit an estimation of the number of whole cigarettes smoked, the baseline daily number of whole cigarettes smoked was 51 and the number of whole cigarettes smoked during days of the intervention week was 58.

There is no way of knowing whether this intervention actually reduced smoking or simply motivated smokers to relocate elsewhere. Inferred observations after the experimental period revealed no obvious development of alternative smoking sites. This intervention may have made smokers more self-conscious, and therefore encouraged them to avoid smoking in public places. While it would be most desirable to motivate them to refrain from smoking entirely, even just reducing public smoking may have a positive impact on campus norms.

This shift from public smoking could be a move in the positive direction for several reasons. It appears that smokers were affected by the signs; even if thoughts lasted only for the few minute walks to their rooms, some effect seems to have reached the smokers. This decrease in amount of cigarettes consumed over a one-week period is beneficial to the non-smokers on campus. With a decrease in smoking, there is less of annoyance upon entering these academic buildings; they do not have to worry about walking through smoke to get to class. For future studies, a longer baseline period may yield results that better mirror the pattern of campus smokers. Because the campus studied is small, a larger number of buildings may be needed as campus size increases.

Review of the data collected at the residential site presents an ambiguous picture. The adjusted (whole cigarettes) measure indicated a trivial increase in the number of cigarettes smoked during the intervention week. On the other hand, the nonadjusted measure (simple number of butts) showed an increase during the period that signs had been posted. While smoking behavior decreased outside the public classroom sites following the posting of the signs, the one residential site that was monitored showed an increase in smoking on the nonadjusted measure. This suggests that rather than simply reducing smoking behavior, posting of signs outside of public buildings may have reduced smoking for some, but led other students to relocate their smoking to a less public venue.

Although the experimental intervention was designed to discourage smoking, given the typical persistence of this habit, one week's exposure to the sign's message was not necessarily expected to motivate smokers to quit entirely. Although less desirable than cessation, relocating smoking to less public and less visible campus locations can be viewed as potentially beneficial, because of its potential effect on campus norms. Future research should examine the effects of longer interventions, assess displacement of smoking more completely, and monitor the long-term impact of these types of interventions on student attitudes and smoking behavior.

Table 11. Total Number of Cigarettes Smoked Daily at Three Public Sites

	Mean	N	SD
Baseline Week	92.33	3	12.74
Sign Week	59.67	3	15.50

Table 12. Total Cigarettes Smoked (Adjusted) PRE-POST

	Mean	SD	t	df	p<
Cigarettes smoked	32.67	13.32	4.25	2	.05

Table 13. Total Cigarette Butts (Non-Adjusted) PRE-POST

	Mean	SD	t	df	p<
Cigarette Butts	36.67	13.58	4.68	2	.05

Do smoking restrictions sometimes backfire?
For some, do restrictions increase risk of addiction?

A paper by Campbell, Bartlett, Liberati, Tornetta and Chambliss (2000) examined some of the potential unintended negative consequences of campus smoking restrictions. This study explored the possibility that restrictions might increase the risk of addiction among some young smokers by inadvertently enhancing the appeal of smoking.

Policies restricting smoking are among a number of possible reasons for the overall drop in smoking prevalence that the U.S. has experienced in recent decades. The dangers of cigarette smoke are now widely known and accepted. There are large numbers of smoking cessation programs and countless anti tobacco campaigns aimed at adults. Nicotine addiction is better understood and pharmaceuticals have been developed to curb nicotine withdrawal. In addition, restrictive smoking policies are widespread and steadily increasing. Schools, restaurants, shopping malls, movie theaters, air flights, and many work sites are only a few examples of public places that have initiated no-smoking policies. The hospital industry has enacted a nationwide ban on smoking (Longo et al., 1996). Jason and Lonak (1990) assessed over 600 corporations and found that a quarter had workplace smoking restriction policies in effect and another 35% were developing such policies. The policies they encountered ranged from limiting smoking to particular areas to a comprehensive ban on all worksite smoking.

Smoking restriction policies have been enacted for a variety of reasons. In educational and work settings, many assume that restricting smoking has a beneficial impact on task performance. Gibson (1997) summarized research indicating that various social and environmental stressors decrease various types of task performance. He also found that research consistently reveals performance decrements when nonsmokers are forced to be near smokers and second-hand smoke. In addition, several companies have effected smoking bans in order to improve their employees' health, by motivating smokers to quit and thereby reducing the overall prevalence of smoking among their employees.

Smoking restrictions have been associated with lower smoking prevalence, higher lifetime quit rates, more recent quit attempts, and lower daily cigarette consumption (Jeffrey et al, 1994; Brenner et al., 1997). One study found that a hospital smoking ban resulted in a decrease in cigarette consumption by an average of four cigarettes a day (Brigham et al., 1994). The same study reported that restricted smokers did not appear to smoke more cigarettes during non-work hours in an attempt to compensate for cigarettes not smoked at work (Brigham et al., 1994). Nonsmokers also benefit from this restriction because they are no longer subjected to second-hand smoke. The resulting benefits of smoking restrictions for both smokers and nonsmokers are promising, and most research supports the widespread implementation of these policies. It has also been shown that smokers and nonsmokers generally favor restrictive smoking policies in public places and usually abide by them. Studies have reported that between 90% and 95% of smokers and nonsmokers agree with restrictive smoking policies (Ashley, 1996; Brenner et al., 1997).

Gibson (1997) argues in favor of smoking restriction policies. "If we conceptualize today's smokers as members of a stigmatized outgroup, the current trend to restrict smoking in public places and in the workplace may benefit both smokers and nonsmokers. Nonsmokers receive the obvious health-related benefits associated with breathing cleaner air and smokers benefit from not worrying about their smoke offending nonsmoking coworkers. (Gibson, p.102)

Although some argue that smokers and nonsmokers should negotiate on an individual basis, several studies suggest that relying on "common courtesy" or assertive requests from nonsmokers is unproductive (Davis, Boyd, and Schoenborn, 1990; Gibson and Werner, 1992; Gibson and Werner, 1994). Since many health professionals believe that legislation restricting smoking and thereby separating smokers and nonsmokers will improve public health, many favor formalized policies restricting smoking.

However, the overall effects of smoking restrictions may not be entirely benign. Smokers may see bans on smoking in public areas as a challenge to their freedom and ability to control their own behavior. Such threats can produce reactance (Brehm and Brehm, 1981). Reactance could result in an actual increase in the smoking habit among many smokers, and strengthen the extent to which smokers define their identity in terms of their choice to smoke cigarettes.

No-smoking policies at work may place a particularly heavy burden on a small group of heavily addicted smokers. Borland and Owen conducted a study concerning perceived need to smoke during smoking restricted work hours. Nine percent of smokers reported a strong need to smoke at work and 26% reported a mild need (Borland and Owen, 1995). Workplace smoking bans have also been associated with increased ratings of common withdrawal symptoms (cravings/urges and concentration difficulties) among smokers during work hours (Brigham et al., 1994). Depending upon the severity of these symptoms, they may lead to a decrease in worker productivity.

The Campbell et al. (2000) study assessed the impact of smoking restrictions on the smoking behaviors and feelings of smokers was evaluated. Prevention of smoking during work and leisure experiences in smoke-free environments may increase the desire to smoke among some individuals. The Campbell et al. (2002) study was conducted in an attempt to uncover college students' psychological reactions to smoking restrictions, revolving around a possible perceived threat to their freedom.

The Campbell et al. (2000) study included participants from an introductory psychology course at a small liberal arts college located in southeastern Pennsylvania. Seventy-four students participated, including 39 females and 31 males. Seventeen of the participants were smokers. This was determined by a "yes" response to the question "Do you currently smoke cigarettes on a regular basis." The remaining participants were nonsmokers. Their ages ranged from 18 to 20 years.

The experimenters devised a 67-item 4-point Likert-type questionnaire divided into two sections. The first section, completed by all participants, consisted of forty-two items designed to measure participants' perceptions of smokers. The second section, completed only by smokers, consisted of 25 items measuring smokers' attitudes toward and behavioral effects of smoking restrictions.

The study was conducted prior to an introductory psychology course class period located in an auditorium setting. The questionnaire was distributed and collected by the researchers. The professor instructed the participants to complete the survey and advised them that they would receive class credit upon completion. No time restrictions were indicated.

The data indicated that nonsmokers viewed the majority of their fellow nonsmokers as intelligent (91%) while only 50% of the nonsmokers perceived smokers as being intelligent. Seventy eight percent of nonsmokers perceived other nonsmokers as sophisticated while only 37.4% of nonsmokers observed smokers as sophisticated. Ninety one percent of nonsmokers thought that other nonsmokers were considerate while 66% of nonsmokers viewed smokers as considerate. Nonsmokers also perceived smokers as less fit than nonsmokers (93% versus 64%). Almost all (96%) of the nonsmokers saw other nonsmokers as being mature, while only 67% of them perceived smokers as being mature.

Of the participants who were smokers, 71% try to conceal their habit from parents, faculty, staff, and others. However, no smokers reported only smoking in the presence of other smokers. Seventy one percent of the smokers say they never avoid situations because smoking is prohibited within them. Fifty seven percent of the smokers reported that they do favor smoking restrictions, but 71% smoke wherever and whenever it is permitted.

The majority (57%) of the smokers sampled did not smoke within 30 minutes of waking. However, 86% of them felt they were addicted to nicotine. Seventy one percent consistently reported finding smoking more satisfying after a period of restriction, however only 43% found smoking more relaxing after abstinence.

A majority of smokers (72%) did not experience an enhanced sense of freedom after leaving a smoke-free situation. They also did not feel constrained while in a smoke-free situation. Among smokers, 72% never or rarely craved cigarettes in a smoke-free situation. All smokers were at least sometimes less interested in smoking while in a smoke-free situation.

The findings of the Campbell et al. (2000) study corroborate those of other researchers who have found that perceptions of smokers are generally more negative than those of nonsmokers. Nonsmokers were nearly twice as likely to be seen as intelligent and sophisticated as smokers. While only two-thirds of students viewed smokers as considerate, physically fit, and mature, most (over 90%) saw these positive traits as descriptive of nonsmokers.

The majority of the smokers surveyed seemed responsive to others' negative attitudes toward smoking. Most concealed their smoking from their parents, although few went to the extreme of avoiding smoking in front of all nonsmokers. Most of these smokers supported restrictions on their smoking, and acknowledged that they tend to smoke whenever free to do so.

Most members of this sample of smokers see themselves as addicted, although only about a half engage in the "first thing in the day" smoking expected among those with strong addiction to nicotine. After periods of forced abstinence within smoking-restricted settings, the majority of smokers report chain smoking multiple cigarettes, and said they found cigarettes more satisfying (although not necessarily more relaxing). This supports the notion that for college students, smoking restrictions may enhance the appeal of cigarettes and lead to increased usage.

On the other hand, few smokers reported craving cigarettes while in smoking restricted settings. In fact, most experienced reduced interest in smoking while in these situations. These smokers did not seem to feel "liberated" upon leaving a restricted setting, so any apparent rebound elevation in smoking does not seem to be attributable to reactance or resentment toward smoke-free policies.

The small sample of smokers in this study severely limits the ability to generalize from these findings. On the other hand, this pilot study suggests the need for additional research examining ways in which college students may react to smoking restrictions differently from older adults. If compensatory increased smoking after abstinence is more of a risk with this age group, measures to reduce this problem may be worthwhile. The Campbell et al. (2000) findings suggest that while smoking restrictions may temporarily elevate the attractiveness of cigarettes and elicit increased smoking, they do not necessarily foster preoccupation with cigarettes, even among students who see themselves as addicted to nicotine.

SUMMARY OF RESULTS

The simple, cheap experimental intervention, which consisted of nothing more than posting paper signs reading "Think. Why do you smoke?" near public smoking areas, seems to have affected public smoking on campus. The challenging part of this naturalistic research was counting the hundreds of cigarette butts scattered in the smoking areas during the pretest and posttest weeks, in order to assess the impact of the signs. It turned out the signs apparently worked! There was a 35% reduction in public smoking after the signs went up. Although smokers may have merely relocated because the signs made them self-conscious, simply reducing the visibility of smoking on campus may help to reestablish and affirm antismoking norms. Every little bit counts.

The examination of potential boomerang effects following smoking restrictions was largely reassuring. The preliminary data suggests that although for a minority of young adult smokers restrictions may heighten the appeal of smoking, for most other students (including the nonsmoking majority) restrictions are more consistently beneficial. Since it is extremely important to minimize the risks of counterproductive interventions, further research describing when these unintended effects occur and how they can be minimized is urged.

SECTION V. CONCLUSION

Summary and Future Directions

This chapter has illustrated the use of student research as an indirect way of influencing community attitudes toward tobacco use. Publicity about student research projects may have helped to reinforce antismoking attitudes among some members of the campus. While preserving individual rights is extremely important, campuses also have an obligation to support choices that are in the best health interests of residents. Once a critical mass of a high school's, college's, or professional school's students routinely engage in public smoking, the campus begins to indoctrinate incoming students in a manner that may subtly increase their chances of choosing to smoke. Reversing this pressure is an important goal for faculty and administrators.

Implications for Stemming the Scourge of Student Smoking

Taken collectively, the twenty empirical studies conducted at Ursinus College suggest that a real potential exists to influence smoking behavior among high school and college students through the application of findings about these specific target populations. These findings illustrate an interesting paradox: although rates of college student smoking were growing, harsh and negative stereotypes of smokers are also on the rise. In other words, campus smoking was becoming more normative in a statistical sense during the 1990s, antismoking norms were simultaneously gaining support across high school, college, and professional school campuses. This suggests that one productive means of addressing the problem of smoking might involve encouraging wider discussions of the attitudes of the majority. Greater awareness of the growing stigma associated with smoking behavior may serve as a deterrent to smoking initiation and may help to motivate current smokers to quit. Appreciation of the real risks of discrimination on academic campuses might at least induce adolescents and young adults to refrain from smoking in public.

The two studies examining the efficacy of campus smoking cessation techniques illustrate our potential to reduce smoking by providing convenient treatment opportunities for students. There are apparently numerous successful means of assisting this college student population in their efforts to cease smoking. Scheduled smoking reduction appears to be a very effective yet inexpensive and minimally time consuming technique for reducing smoking. The issue here does not seem to be whether there is a reliable, effective treatment. Rather, it appears that while there are several methods for facilitating smoking cessation, a lingering problem involves inspiring college students to decide to quit smoking. The main challenge seems to be the limited number of students expressing an interest in ending their smoking behavior while on campus. Even when both individual and group treatments were offered free of charge, few college student smokers chose to attempt quitting. It may be that few college students acknowledge their need for help in changing their smoking behavior. Many may not yet be addicted to nicotine, or may not see themselves as addicted to nicotine.

The results of the experimental study assessing the impact of a brief environmental intervention demonstrate the potential utility of even simple, inexpensive strategies to affect smoking behavior on college campuses. Using the "Think…Why Smoke?" sign has appeared to reduce public smoking by encouraging students to examine their behavior more critically. Once this occurs, these students may decide also to reduce their private habitual smoking pattern with the goal of cessation.

Perhaps educating high school and college student smokers about others' reactions to such behavior might encourage them to consider quitting. If, as one of our studies suggests, college students feel they appear mature, attractive, and sophisticated by smoking, then explaining that both their smoking and non-smoking peers, along with many of their professors, do not view this behavior in this way may spark greater contemplation of quitting. In order to counter the beguiling depictions of smoking in advertisements, students may need to be more fully informed about what "real" people believe, and how being a smoker may make them a target of negative stereotypes and academic and employment discrimination. Aspiring students may be benefited by an enhanced awareness of how professional school faculty members question the judgment of students who smoke cigarettes. If students realize that public smoking can jeopardize their hard earned respect from faculty, they may think twice before lighting up.

One of the studies described in this review provides some basis for optimism about the problem of adolescent and young adult smoking; film depictions of smoking do not seem to be becoming universally more positive and compelling. While cigarette advertisements typically show smokers in exciting, glamorous, and adventurous contexts, the movie industry does not appear to be following suit. In fact, the findings from our film study show that in many recent films non-smoker lead characters appeared to be portrayed more positively than their smoker counterparts. Over time, this may help to ameliorate the smoking problem.

However it is of ongoing concern that in recent years the prevalence of smoking onscreen has increased, doubling since 1990 according to Kaufman (2003). Despite a 1998 national tobacco settlement with the states banning tobacco companies from paying to have their products appear in movies, a growing number of actors smoke in films. Unlike our study, a study by Dalton et al. (2003) observed few negative depictions of cigarette smoking in movies. Their finding that film smokers typically play rebellious or tough roles is disconcerting because adolescents often revere such characters.

Dalton et al. (2003) found that adolescents are significantly more likely to begin smoking if they watch movies featuring actors who smoke cigarettes, and adolescents whose parents don't smoke are the most likely to be affected by actors smoking onscreen. Dalton and her colleagues followed roughly 2,600 children aged 10 to 14 for two years Adolescents who watched the most movies with smoking were almost three times more likely to start smoking than those who watched the fewest number of movies with smoking. More than 50 percent of the adolescents who reported having tried smoking did so after seeing smoking in movies. Children of non-smokers were four times more likely to start smoking if they were in the group that saw many movies with smoking than those in the group that saw the fewest movies with smoking. Because the Dalton et al. study looked at young adolescents and early experimentation with smoking, it was unable to investigate the association between movie smoking and longer-term habitual smoking.

The Dalton et al. research offered some of the strongest evidence to date that smoking in movies encourages adolescents to start smoking; roughly half of the youngsters who started smoking apparently did so because they had seen smoking portrayed positively in the movies (Kaufman, 2003). Startlingly, the strength of the connection between movies and adolescent smoking was stronger than peer smoking. Furthermore, the impact of movie viewing was dose responsive; the more movies with smoking were viewed, the greater the likelihood that adolescents would start smoking themselves. These findings suggest that a reduction in movie depiction of smoking would likely result in a decrease in adolescents' initiation of smoking (Kaufman, 2003).

Though many tend to discount the role of social influences in college student smoking, the effects of these factors are probably not limited to younger age groups. Image motivation does seem to affect college student smokers to some extent. Actors who depict smokers as sophisticated and savvy urge even bright students to experiment with tobacco. Given their sensitivity to image concerns, increased antismoking media messages may urge college students to reexamine their unhealthy behavior or reconsider the decision to experiment. Offering salient information about the negative health risks associated with tobacco use, in conjunction with more negative depictions of smokers in film, may help reverse the troubling trend observed by Wechsler et al. (1998).

Outcome Assessment

One goal of conducting these collaborative studies with students at Ursinus College was to increase our college campus' awareness of the problem of student smoking. Increasing sensitivity to issues related to cigarette use and promulgation of discussion about the stigma associated with student smoking was expected to affect student behavior indirectly. Our outcome assessment yielded somewhat equivocal evidence about the impact of the Ursinus College campus Smoking Prevention and Cessation Project.

In order to assess whether this added attention to the problem made a difference, several types of evidence were considered. First, since college campus data was collected at regular intervals during this research period, it was possible to compare the rates of student smoking over time. A oneway ANOVA conducted on smoking rate data from four time periods of data collection revealed a significant difference among the time periods (F=9.79, df=3/7, p<.05). Post hoc t-tests indicated that smoking rates increased from the first (mean of 24% in 1998) to the second and third measurement periods (mean of 34% in 1999 and 33% in 2001), and then decreased at the final measurement period (mean of 26% in 2004). Overall, the percentage of students who smoked "regularly" went down following the period when these investigations were being conducted and disseminated on campus. The fact that there was an 8% reduction in the percentage of students reporting regular use of cigarettes from 1999 to 2004 (from 34% in 1999 to 26% in 2004) is somewhat encouraging. While this certainly fails to establish this research initiative as an effective means of reducing students' smoking rates on campuses, it is possible that conducting these studies may have interrupted a trajectory of rising use.

Another attempt to gauge the impact of these studies on the campus involved trying to tease apart experimental and habitual cigarette use. Comparison of reported smoking across the years of these investigation revealed that the percentage of college students who smoked "regularly" went down during the course of these studies, but the percent who acknowledged "any use in the past month" actually increased somewhat during the first two years of the project. However, although the percentage of students who had ever smoked rose following the first two years of these research efforts, the rate of occasional smoking then declined over the ensuing three years of the project.

The irony is that efforts to strengthen antismoking norms on campus (by informing students about the negative stereotypes of smokers, increasing their awareness through posting of signs in public places, restricting smoking behavior in public buildings, and encouraging wider campus discussion of the drawbacks associated with public smoking) may actually make smoking cigarettes more beguiling to those using this behavior as a way of flouting authority standards and demonstrating their independence and immunity to social pressure. There is a maddening risk that as campus norms become more intolerant of cigarette smoking, some students may actually elect to smoke to defy these norms, as a way of manifesting their individuality and ability to resist pressures to conform.

Without data from a control group, it is impossible to untangle the influence of these studies on campus behavior from unrelated historical trends. However, the prevalence of student smoking in front of several classroom buildings has declined strikingly. Since such public smoking implicitly supports this behavior, this change is particularly welcome. Another source of evidence for the positive impact of these studies consists of the anecdotal reports of the students involved in these collaborative studies. All of the student smokers involved in this research reported reexamining their choice, and the majority reduced or stopped their cigarette use. Perhaps the greatest value of these studies involved its personal impact on the lives of these men and women.

Each of these studies has implications for future research on this topic. First, high school and college students can be better educated about how their professors, who see them regularly and influence their futures, view student smoking. Next, high school and college students may benefit from learning that if they choose to smoke in public, they are generally not going to be perceived very positively by their peers (including smoking, formerly smoking, and non-smoking peers). Faculty and peers wield considerable social influence. If, along with learning about these attitudes, smokers are presented with antismoking messages (including stimuli such as the "Think…Why Smoke?" sign used in the study reported here), they may be prompted to contemplate their reasons for smoking, and they may begin to re-evaluate their desire to smoke. Once motivated to contemplate quitting, students can be offered free, convenient on-campus smoking cessation programs, including use of scheduled smoking techniques. Considered in combination, these studies may help to reshape student attitudes about the decision to smoke, and may play some role in helping to reduce college student smoking.

This chapter summarized the findings from twenty empirical investigations and discussed the value of student research as a means of reshaping campus attitudes toward tobacco use. We hope the work we've done at Ursinus might stimulate others to develop even more effective ways of addressing this pressing problem.

ACKNOWLEDGMENTS

This project was conducted in collaboration with the following outstanding students while they were attending Ursinus College. I am deeply indebted to them all for their extraordinary diligence, enthusiasm, and good humor throughout the various components of this project. Again, thanks to you all!

Megan Austin, Joanne Brosh, Allyssa Bartlett, Taryn Brackin, Paige Bucy, Michael Campbell, Jamie Chubb, Matthew Conroy, Sandra Covata, Elizabeth Ferguson, Adele Hinckley, Jilda Hodges, Cheryl Liberati, Jeanette Kane, Karen Srebro, Jonette Tornetta, John Paul Venuti, Pamela Landis, Charlene Authier, Mary Fruhwirth, Julie Anne Dous, Gina Iannella, Rebecca Outten, Margaret Rowles, Christopher Weir, Michael Nesbit, Christina Burton, Fallon Wilson, Kathleen Baker, Chris Katona, and Mary Shull

Please address correspondence and requests for reprints to Catherine Chambliss, Ph.D., Department of Psychology, Ursinus College, Collegeville, PA 19426-1000 or e-mail (cchambliss@ursinus.edu)

REFERENCES

Altman, D.G., Levine, D.W., Coeytaux, R., Slade, J., and Jaffe, R. (1996). Tobacco promotion and susceptibility to tobacco use among adolescents aged 12 through 17 years in a nationally representative sample. *American Journal of Public Health, 86* (11), 1590-1593.

Altman, D.G., Slater, M.D., Albright, C.L., and Maccoby, N. (1987). How an unhealthy product is sold: Cigarette advertising in magazines. 1960-1985. *Journal of Communication, 37* (4), 95-106.

American Lung Association. (1998). Quit smoking action plan. (National Publications). New York: New York.

Ashley, M.J. (1996). Support among smokers and nonsmokers for restrictions on smoking. *Journal of the American Medical Association, 11*, 283-287.

Austin, M., Brosh, J. and Chambliss, C. An Exploration of Paradox: High School and College Students' Self-Reported Motivations for Smoking. (2002). Resources in Education, ERIC/CASS,CG031872.

Austin, M., Brosh,J., Dous, J.A., Iannella, G., Outten, R., Rowles, P. and Chambliss, C.A. The relationship between personality and self reported substance use: Exploring the implications for high school and college educational programs, Resources in Education, ERIC/CASS, CG032168, 2003.

Authier, C., Hodges, J.,Srebro, K., and Chambliss, C. (1999). Faculty and Student Views of College Student Smokers. *Resources in Education*, ERIC/CASS, CG029394.

Baer, J.S. (2002). Student Factors: Understanding individual variation in college drinking. Special Issue: College drinking, what it is, and what to do about it: Review of the state of the science. *Journal of Studies on Alcohol, 14,* 40-53.

Baker, K., Katona, C., Brosh, J., Shull, M., and Chambliss, C. (2004). The vilification of smokers: High school and college students' perceptions of current smokers, former smokers, and nonsmokers. *Resources in Education*, ERIC/CASS, CG032693.

Bandura, A. and Walters, R.H. (1963). *Social Learning and Personality Development*. New York, Holt, Rinehart, and Winston.

Bartholow, B.D., Sher, K.J., Wood, M.D. (2000). Personality and substance use disorders: A prospective study. *Journal of Consulting and Clinical Psychology, 68*, 818-829.

Bartlett, A., Brackin, T., Chubb, J., Covata, S., Ferguson, L., Hinckley, A., Hodges, J., Liberati, C., Tornetta, J., and Chambliss, C. (1999). Factors influencing and motivating smoking among college students. *Resources in Education,* ERIC/CASS, ED440323

Bartlett, A., Brackin, T., Chubb, J., Covata, S., Ferguson, L., Hinckley, A., Hodges, J., Liberati, C., Tornetta, J., and Chambliss, C. (2000). Correcting Media Mis-education: The Portrayal of Smokers and Smoking in Top Grossing Films. *Resources in Education*, ERIC/CASS, CG029857.

Barton, J., Chassin, L., and Presson, C. C. (1982). Social image factors as motivators of smoking initiation in early and middle adolescence. *Child Development, 53*, 1499-1511.

Bleda, P. R. and Bleda, S.E. (1978). The effects of sex and smoking on reactions to spatial invasion at a shopping mall. *Journal of Social Psychology, 104*, 311-312.

Bleda, P. R. and Sandman, P.H. (1977). In smoke's way: Socioemotional reactions to another's smoking. *Journal of Applied Psychology, 52*, 452-458.

Borland, R., and Owen, N. (1995). Need to smoke in the context of workplace smoking bans. *Preventative Medicine, 24*, 56-60.

Brehm, S. S. and Brehm, J. W. (1981). *Psychological reactance: a theory of freedom and control.* NY: Academic Press.

Brennan, A.F., Walfish, S., and AuBuchon, P. (1986). Alcohol use and abuse in college students: I. A review of individual and personality correlates. *Int. Journal of Addiction, 21,* 475-493.

Brenner, H., Born, J., Novack, P., and Wanek, V. (1997). Smoking behavior and attitude toward smoking regulations and passive smoking in the workplace. *Preventative Medicine, 26,* 138-143.

Brickman, J.C. and D'Amato, B. (1975). Exposure effects in a free-choice situation. *Journal of Personality and Social Psychology, 32*, 415-20.

Brigham, J., Gross, J., Stitzer, M.L., and Felch L.J. (1994). Effects of a restricted work-site smoking policy on employees who smoke. *American Journal of Public Health, 84*, 773-778.

Brosh, J., Austin, M. and Chambliss, C. (2003). High school and college students' perceptions of current smokers, former smokers, and nonsmokers, *Perceptual and Motor Skills*, 97, 1200-1202, 2003.

Brynin, M. (1999). Smoking behaviour: predisposition or adaptation? *Journal of Adolescence,* 22, 635-646.

Burton, D., Sussman, S., Hansen, W.B., Johnson, C. A., and Flay, B.R. (1989). Image attributions and smoking among seventh-grade students. *Journal of Applied Psychology, 19,* 656-664.

Campbell, M., Bartlett, A., Liberati, C., Tornetta,J., Chambliss, C. (2000) Prejudice Against College Students Who Smoke Cigarettes, unpublished manuscript, Ursinus College, Collegeville, PA.

Campbell, M., Bartlett, A., Liberati, C., Tornetta, J., and Chambliss, C. (2000). Educational Discrimination Against Smokers: Evidence of Student and Faculty Prejudice. *Resources in Education,* ERIC/CASS, CG030121.

Campbell, R. L., Svenson, L. W., Jarvis, G. K. (1993). Age, gender, and location as factors in permission to smoke among university students. *Psychological Reports, 72,* 1231-1234.

Campion, E. W. (1997). Can house calls survive? *The New England Journal of Medicine, 337* (25), 1840-1841.

Carroll, J. F. X., Personality and psychopathology: A comparison of alcohol and drug-dependent persons. In J. Solomon and K.A. Keeley (Eds.) *Perspectives in Alcohol and Drug Abuse: Similarities And Differences,* Boston: John Wright PSG Inc., 1982, Ch. 4, 59-88.

Carroll, J. F. X., Malloy, T. E., Roscioli, D. L., Pindjack, G. M., and Clifford, J. S. (1982) Similarities and differences in self-concepts of alcohol and drug addicted women. *Journal of Studies on Alcohol,* 43(7), 725-738.

Centers for Disease Control and Prevention. (1995). Attitudes towards smoking policies in eight states- United States. *The Journal of the American Medical Association, 273,* 531-532.

Chambliss, C.A. (2004) High school, college, and professional school faculty members' perceptions of current smokers, former smokers, and nonsmokers. *Perceptual and Motor Skills, 99,* 629-632.

Chambliss, C., Austin, M., Brosh, J., Iannella, G., Outten, R., Rowles, M..(2005). The relationship between substance use and scores on the mini markers five factors personality scale in college and high school students. *Journal of Alcohol and Drug Education, 49,* 1, 21- 31.

Chambliss, C., Shull, M., Baker, K., Burton, C., Nesbit, M., Weir, C., Wilson, F., Katona, C. and Brosh, J. (2006). The social hazards of smoking in academic contexts: Students and teachers' attitudes about student smokers. *Journal of Alcohol and Drug Education,* 50, 3, 21-31.

Chambliss, C. and Murray, E. (1979). Cognitive Procedures for Smoking Reduction: Symptom Attribution Versus Efficacy Attribution. *Cognitive Therapy and Research,* 3 (1): 91-95.

Chassin, L., Presson, C.C., and Sherman, S.J. (1990). Social psychological contributions to the understanding and prevention of adolescent cigarette smoking. *Personality and Social Psychology Bulletin, 16,* 133-151.

Chassin, L., Presson, C.C., Rose, J.S., and Sherman, S.J. (1996). The natural history of cigarette smoking from adolescence to adulthood: Demographic predictors of continuity and change. *Health Psychology, 15* (6), 478-484.

Cinciripini, P. M., Lapitsky, L.G., Wallfisch, A., Mace, R., Nezami, E., and Van Vunakis, H. (1994). An evaluation of a multicomponent treatment program involving scheduled smoking and relapse prevention procedures: Initial findings. *Addictive Behaviors, 19,* 13-22.

Clark, R. R. (1978). Reactions to other people's cigarette smoking. *The International Journal of Addictions, 13 (8),* 1237-1244.

Clausen, J.A. (1987). Health and the life course: Some personal observations. *Journal of Health and Social Behavior, 28,* 337-344.

Cloninger, C.R. (1987). A systematic method for clinical description and classification of personality variants. *Archives of General Psychiatry,* 44, 573-588.

Cloninger, C.R., Przybeck, T., and Svrakic, D.M. (1991). The Tridimensional Personality Questionnaire: U.S. normative data. *Psychological Reports,* 69, 1047-1057.

Cloninger, C.R., Svrakic, D.M., and Przybeck, T. (1993). A psychobiological model of temperament and character. *Archives of General Psychiatry,* 50, 975-990.

Cloninger, C.R. and Svrakic, D.M. (1997). Integrative psychobiological approach to psychiatric assessment and treatment. *Psychiatry: Interpersonal and Biological Processes,* 60, 120-141.

Comeau, N., Stewart, S. H., and Loba, P. (2001). The relations of trait anxiety, anxiety sensitivity, and sensation seeking to adolescents' motivations for alcohol, cigarette, and marijuana use. *Addictive Behaviors, 26,* 803-825.

Compas, B. E., Haaga, D. A., Keefe, F. J., Leitenberg, H., and Williams, D. A. (1998). Sampling of empirically supported psychological treatments from health psychology: Smoking, chronic pain, cancer, and bulimia nervosa. *Journal of Consulting and Clinical Psychology, 66 (1),* 89-112.

Costa, P. T., Jr., and McCrae, R. R. (1997). Longitudinal stability of adult personality. *Handbook of personality psychology,* 269-291.

Dalton, M.A., Sargent, J.D., Beach, M.L., Titus-Ernstoff, L.,Gibson, J.J., Aherns, M.B.,Tickle, J.J., and Heatherton, T.F. (2003).Effect of viewing smoking in movies on adolescent smoking initiation: A cohort study. *Lancet ,* 362, 9380.

Davis, R. M., Boyd, G. M., and Schoenborn, C. A. (1990). "Common courtesy" and the elimination of passive smoking. *Journal of the American Medical Association,* 2208-2210.

Department of Health and Human Services. (1994). Preventing tobacco use among young people: A report of the surgeon general. Washington, DC: U.S. Government Printing Office.

Dermer, M. L. and Jacobsen, E. (1986). Some potential negative consequences of cigarette smoking: marketing research in reverse. *Journal of Applied Social Psychology, 16,* 702-725.

Douglas, L., Allen, P., Arian, G., Crawford, M. A., Headen, S., Spigner, C., Tassler, P., and Ureda, J. (2001). Teens' images of smoking and smokers. *Public Health Reports, 116,* 194-207.

Duryea, E. J. and Martin, G. L. (1981). The distortion effect in student perceptions of smoking prevalence. *Journal of School Health, 51,* 115-118.

Dziuban. C. D., Moskal, P. D., West, G. B. (1999) Examining the Use of Tobacco on College Campuses. *Journal of American College Health, 47*, p 260.

Emmons, K. M., Wechsler, H., Dowdall, G., and Abraham, M. (1998). Predictors of smoking among US college students. *American Journal of Public Health, 88* (1), 104-107.

Eysenck, H. (1967). The Biological Basis of Personality. Springfield:Charles C. Thomas.

Garfinkel, L. (1997). Trends in cigarette smoking in the United States. *Preventive Medicine, 26*, 447-450.

Geist, C. R. and Herrmann, S. M. (1990). A comparison of the psychological characteristics of smokers, exsmokers, and nonsmokers. *Journal of Clinical Psychology, 46*, 102-105.

Gibson, B. (1997). Smoker-nonsmoker conflict: Using a Social psychological framework to understand a current social controversy. *Journal of Social Issues*, 53, 1, 97-112.

Gibson, B. and Werner, C. M. (1992). The decision to attempt interpersonal control: the case of nonsmoker-smoker interaction. *Basic and Applied Social Psychology, 13*, 269-284.

Gibson, B. and Werner, C. M. (1994). The airport as a behavior setting: the role of legibility in communicating the setting program. *Journal of Personality and Social Psychology, 66*, 1049-1060.

Gilbert, D.G. (1979). Paradoxical tranquilizing and emotion-reducing effects of nicotine. *Psychological Bulletin, 86*, 643-661.

Gilbert, D.G. (1988). EEG and personality differences between smokers and nonsmokers. *Personality and Individual Differences, 9*, 659-665.

Glassman, A.H., Helzer, J.E., Covey, L.S., Cottler, L.B., Stetner, F., Tipp, J.E., and Johnson, J. (1990). Smoking, smoking cessation, and major depression. *Journal of the American Medical Association, 264*, 1546-1549.

Glassman, A.H., Stetner, F., Walsh, T.B., Raizman, P.S., Fleiss, J.L., Cooper, T.B., and Covey, L.S. (1988). Heavy smokers, smoking cessation, and clonidine: Results of a double-blind, randomized trial. *Journal of the American Medical Association, 259*, 2863-2866.

Glaxo Wellcome. (1997). Plan to succeed workbook. Research Triangle Park: North Carolina.

Goldstein, J. (1991). The stigmatization of smokers: an empirical investigation. *Journal of Drug Education, 21*, 167-182.

Hanson, G., and Venturelli, P. (1998). *Drugs and society. (5ᵗʰ ed.)* Boston, MA: Jones and Campbell.

Hazan, A.R., Lipton, H.L., and Glantz, S.A. (1994). Popular films do not reflect current tobacco use. *American Journal of Public Health, 84* (6), 998-1000.

Hemenway, D., Solnick, S.J., and Colditz, G.A. (1993). Smoking and suicide among nurses. *American Journal of Public Health, 83*, 249-251.

Hines, D., Fretz, A., and Nollen, N. L. (1998). Regular and occasional smoking by college students: Personality attributions of smokers and nonsmokers. *Psychological Reports, 83*, 1299-1206.

Hobson, K. (2006). Conquering craving. *U.S.News and World Report*, October 23, p.64.

Hodges, J., Srebro, K., Kane, J., Fruhwirth, M. and Chambliss, C. (1999). Use of a Visual Prompt to Reduce Public Cigarette Smoking on a College Campus, ERIC/CASS.

Hodges, J., Srebro, K., Authier, C., and Chambliss, C. (1999). Why Do Undergraduates Smoke? Subjective Effects of Cigarette Smoking. *Resources in Education*, ERIC/CASS, CG029396.

Hodges, J. (2000). Means of Influencing College Students' Health Related Behaviors, unpublished departmental honors thesis, Ursinus College.

Hoff, C. C., Kegeles, S. M., Acree, M., Stall, R., Paul, J., Ekstrand, M. and Coates, T. J. (1997). Looking for men in all the wrong places… HIV prevention small group programs do not reach high risk gay men. *AIDS, 11* (6), 829-831.

Jacobson, P. D., Wasserman, J., and Raube, K. (1992). *The political evolution of antismoking legislation.* Santa Monica, CA: Rand.

Jaffe, J.H. (1989). Drug dependence: Opiods, nonnarcotics, nicotine (tobacco), and caffeine. In H.I. Kaplan and B.J. Sadock (Eds.), Comprehensive textbook of psychiatry, 5th ed. Baltimore: Williams and Wilkins.

Janiszewski, C. (1993). Preattentive mere exposure effects. *Journal of Consumer Research, 20* (3), 376-417.

Jason, L. A. and Lonak, C. A. (1990). A survey of corporate smoking policies. *Evaluation and the Health Professions, 13,* 405-411.

Jeffrey, R., Kelder, S., Forster, J., French, S., Lando, H., Baxter, J. (1994). Restrictive smoking policies in the workplace: effects on smoking prevalence and cigarette consumption. *Preventive Medicine*, 23: 78-82.

Kane, J., Hodges, J., Srebro, K., Authier, C. and Chambliss, C. Individualized Attempts to Reduce Cigarette Smoking Among College Students. ERIC/CASS, CG029312, 1999.

Kane, J., Hodges, J., Srebro, K., Fruhwirth, M. and Chambliss, C. (1999) Attempts to reduce cigarette smoking among college students: A pilot study. Resources in Education, ERIC/CASS, ED430190.

Kaufman, M. Teens Who See Smoking in Movies More Likely to Light Up. *Washington Post*, June 10, 2003; p. A07

Lee, C. (1989). Stereotypes of smokers among health science students. *Addictive Behaviors, 14,* 327-333.

Leventhal , H. and Cleary, P. (1980). The smoking problems: A review of the research and theory in behavioral risk modification. *Psychological Bulletin, 88,* 370-405.

Lewis, S. F., Piasecki, T. M., Fiore, M. C., Anderson, J. E., and Baker, T. B. (1998). Transdermal nicotine replacement for the hospitalized patient: A randomized clinical trial. *Preventive Medicine, 27,* 296-303.

Longo, D., Brownson, R., Johnson, J., Hewett, J., Kruse, R., Novotny, T., and Logan, R. (1996). Hospital smoking bans and employee smoking behavior: results of a national survey. *The Journal of the American Medical Association., 275,* 1252-1257.

Malouff, J., Schutte, N. S., and Kenyon, A. (1991). Negative social effects of being a smoker. *Journal of Drug Education, 21,* 293-302.

McCrae, R. R, and Costa, P. T. (1989). The structure of personality traits: Wiggins' circumplex and the five-factor model. *Journal of Personality and Social Psychology, 56,* 586-595.

McKillip, J., and Vierke, M. S. (1980). College smokers: Worried, sick but still puffing. *Journal of the American College Health Association, 28,* 280-282.

Meyer, G. S. and Gibbons, R. V. (1997). House calls to the elderly – a vanishing practice among physicians. *New England Journal of Medicine, 337* (25), 1815-1820.

Moore, E. (1998, March 10). Kicking the habit despite the dangers, twelve million people in the UK smoke. *The Guardian*, 8.

Moreland, R.L. and Zajonc, R.B. (1982) Exposure effects in person perception: Familiarity, similarity, and attraction. *Journal of Experimental Social Psychology, 18*, 395-415.

Morton, P. G. (1989). Health assessment in nursing. Springhouse, Pennsylvania: Springhouse Corporation.

National Bureau of Economic Research Study. (2000). Teen Smoking: Price Matters. *Business Week, 3671*, 32.

National Youth Risk Behavior Survey (2000). Trends in cigarette smoking among high school students- United States, 1991-1999. *Journal of School Health, 70*, 368-375. Office on Smoking and Health, Division of Adolescent and School Health Centers for Disease control and Prevention.

Nelson, Heath, and Kessler, 1998; Temporal progression of alcohol dependence symptoms in the U.S. household population: Results from the National Comorbidity Survey. *Journal of Consulting and Clinical Psychology, 66*, 474-483.

Office of the U.S. Surgeon General. (1988*). Nicotine addiction.* Washington, DC: US Government Printing Office.

Ouellette, J. A., and Wood, W. (1998). Habit and intention in everyday life: The multiple processes by which past behavior predicts future behavior. *Psychological Bulletin, 124* (1), 54-74.

Outten,R., Rowles, P and Chambliss, C.A. Faculty members' attitudes toward students who smoke: The last permitted type of discrimination, Resources in Education, ERIC/CASS, CG032546, 2004.

Page, R. M. (1998). College students' distorted perception of the prevalence of smoking. *Psychological Reports, 82,* 474.

Pechmann, C., and Shih, C. (1999). Smoking scenes in movies and antismoking advertisements before movies: effects on youth. *Journal of Marketing, 63* (3), 1. Retrieved September 22, 1999 from Expanded Academic ASAP (InfoTrac) on the World Wide Web; http://www.infotrac.galegroup.com/itweb

Pechmann, C., Ratneshwar, S. (1994). The effects of anti-smoking and cigarette advertising on young adolescents' perceptions of peers who smoke. *Journal of Consumer Research*, 21, 236-252.

Potkin, S.G. (2004). The association between anger and susceptibility to nicotine. In L. Neergaard, Some predisposed to smoking. *Miami Herald* (p. 3A). February 17, 2004.

Potts, H., Gillies, P., and Herbert, M. (1986). Adolescent smoking and opinion of cigarette advertisements. *Health Education Research: Theory and Practice, 1* (3), 195-201.

Price, J. H., Beach, P., Everett, S., Telljohann, S. K., and Lewis, L. (1998). Evaluation of a three-year urban elementary school tobacco prevention program. *Journal of School Health, 68,1,26-31.*

Reid, D. (1985). Prevention of smoking among school children: Recommendations for policy development. *Health Education Journal, 44* (1), 3-12.

Rigotti, N.A., Lee, J.E., and Wechsler, H. (2000). US college students' use of tobacco products: the results of a national survey. *The Journal of the American Medical Association, 284*, 699.

Rosal, M. C., Ockene, J. K., Hurley, T. G., and Hebert, J. R. (1998). Effectiveness of nicotine-containing gum in the physician delivered smoking intervention study. *Preventive Medicine, 27*, 262-267.

Rosenberg, M. (1965). Society and the adolescent self-image. Princeton, Princeton University.

Rutledge, P.C. and Sher, K.J. (2001). Heavy drinking from the freshman year into early young adulthood: The role of stress, tension-reduction drinking motives, gender, and personality. *Journal of Studies on Alcohol, 62(4),* 457.

Saucier, G. (1992). Mini-Markers: A brief version of Goldberg's unipolar Big-Five markers. *Journal of Personality, 63,* 506-512.

Schooler, C., Feighery, E., and Flora, J.A. (1996). Seventh graders' self-reported exposure to cigarette marketing and its relationship to their smoking behavior. *American Journal of Public Health, 86* (2), 225-230.

Seltzer, C. C. and Oeschsli, F. W. (1985). Psychological characteristics of adolescent smokers before they started smoking: evidence of self-selection. *Journal of Chronic Disorders, 38,* 17-26.

Shogren, E. (1997). Hollywood is urged to act on smoking. *Los Angeles Times,* p.A25.

Special Report: State Tobacco Settlement. (2002, January 15). Report Shows most states falling short in using tobacco settlement funds for prevention. Prepared by the Campaign for Tobacco Free Kids, American Heart Association, American Cancer Society, and American Lung Association. Retrieved July 15,2002 from Campaign for Tobacco Free Kids on the World Wide Web; http://www.tobaccofreekids.org/reports/settlement

Srebro, K., Hodges, J., Authier, and Chambliss, C. (1999). Views of College Student Smoking: A Comparison of Smokers and Nonsmokers. Resources in Education, ERIC/CASS, CG029395.

Stein, J. A., Newcomb, M. D., and Bentler, P. M. (1996). Initiation and maintenance of tobacco smoking: Changing personality correlates in adolescence and young adulthood. *Journal of Applied Social Psychology, 26* (2), 160-187.

Stevens, V. J., and Hollis, J. F. (1989). Preventing smoking relapse, using an individually tailored skills-training technique. *Journal of Consulting and Clinical Psychology, 57,* 420-424.

Stewart, S.H., and Zeithlin, S.B. (1995). Anxiety sensitivity and alcohol use motives. *Journal of Anxiety Disorders, 9,* 229-240.

Stronks, K., van de Mheen, D., Looman, C.W.N., and Mackenbach, J.P. (1997). Cultural, material, and psychosocial correlates of the socioeconomic gradient in smoking behavior among adults. *Preventive Medicine, 26,* 754-766.

Trends in cigarette smoking among high school students—United States, 1991-2001. (2002). *The Journal of the American Medical Association,* 288, 308-310.

U. S. Department of Health and Human Services. (1985) Cancer and chronic lung disease in the workplace: A report of the Surgeon General. Rockville, MD: U. S. Department of Health and Human Services, Office on Smoking and Health.

U.S. Department of Health and Human Services. (1986). The health consequences of involuntary smoking, a report of the Surgeon General (DHHS Publication No. 87-8309). Washington, DC: U. S. Government Printing Office.

U.S. Department of Health and Human Services. (1989). Reducing the Health Consequences of Smoking: 25 Years of Progress: A Report of the Surgeon General 1989. (DHHS Publication No.89-8411) Atlanta, GA: Office on Smoking and Health, Centers for Disease Control and Prevention.

Venuti, J. P., and Chambliss, C. (2000). Effects of Substance Use Education Programs. *Resources in Education,* ERIC/CASS, CG030259.

Venuti, J. P., Conroy, M., Landis, P. and Chambliss, C.A. (2000). Subjective Determinants of Substance Use: Gender Differences in Student Substance Use, *Resources in Education,* ERIC/CASS, CG030260.

Venuti, J., Conroy, M., Bucy, P., Landis, P., and Chambliss, C., (2002). The Relative Stigma Associated with Smoking, Obesity, and Criminality, *Resources in Education,* ERIC/CASS, CG031614.

Venuti, J.P., and Chambliss, C. (2000). Effects of substance use education programs: Cultural Differences in College Substance Use, Resources in Education, ERIC/CASS, CG030259.

Venuti, J.P., Conroy, M., Bucy, P., Landis, P.L., Chambliss, C. (2000). Prejudice against cigarette smokers in higher education, *Resources in Education,* ERIC/CASS, CG030261.

Wagner, M.K. (2001). Behavioral characteristics related to substance abuse and risk-taking, sensation-seeking, anxiety sensitivity, and self-reinforcement. *Addictive Behaviors, 26,* 115-120.

Wechsler, H., Dowdall, G.W., Davenport, A., and Castillo, S. (1995). Correlates of college student binge drinking. *American Journal of Public Health, 85,* 921-926.

Wechsler, H., Rigotii, N.A., Gledhill-Hoyt, J., and Lee, H. (1998). Increased levels of cigarette use among college students: A cause for national concern. *Journal of the American Medical Association, 280* (19), 1673-1678.

Wilson, D. K., Wallston, K. A. and King, J. E. (1990). Effects of contract framing, motivation to quit, and self-efficacy on smoking reduction. *Journal of Applied Social Psychology, 20* (7), 531-547.

Wood, P.B., Cochran, J.K., Pfefferbaum, B., and Arneklev, B.J. (1995). Sensation seeking and delinquent substance use: An extension of learning theory. *The Journal of Drug Issues, 25(1),* 173-193.

Zajonc, R.B. (1965) Social facilitation. *Science, 149,* 269-74.

Zajonc, R.B. (1968) Attitudinal effects of mere exposure. *Journal of Personality and Social Psychology.* Monograph supplement 9: 1-27.

Zinser, O., Kloosterman, R., and Williams, A. (1991). Perceptions of cigarette advertisements by college student smokers, former smokers, and nonsmokers. *Journal of Social Behavior and Personality, 6* (2), 355-366.

Zinser, O., Kloosterman, R., and Williams, A. (1994). Advertisements, volition, and peers among other causes of smoking: Perceptions of college student smokers. *Journal of Alcohol and Drug Education, 39* (3), 13-26.

Zuckerman, M. (1987a). Sensation seeking and the endogenous deficit theory of drug abuse. In: Szara, S.I. (Ed.) Neurobiology of Behavioral Control in Drug Abuse. National Institute on Drug Abuse Research Monograph Series No. 74. Department of Health and Human Services, Publication No. 87-1506, Washington: Government Printing Office, 59-70.

Zuckerman, M. (1987b). Biological connection between sensation seeking and drug abuse. In: Engel, J., Oreland, L., Ingvar, D.H., Pernow, B., Rossner, S., and Pellborn, L.A. (Eds.) *Brain Rewards Systems and Abuse*, New York: Raven Press Publication, 165-176.

Zuckerman, M. (1994). Behavioral Expressions and Biosocial Bases of Sensation Seeking, New York: Cambridge University Press.

Zuckerman, M. (1979). *Sensation Seeking: Beyond the Optimal Level of Arousal,* Hillsdale, NJ: Lawrence Erlbaum Associates, Inc.

In: Smoking Cessation: Theory, Interventions and Prevention   ISBN: 978-1-60021-591-9
Editor: Jerome E. Landow   © 2008 Nova Science Publishers, Inc.

Chapter 3

SMOKING CESSATION AMONG COLLEGE STUDENTS: CHALLENGES AND OUTCOMES

Alexander V. Prokhorov, Kentya H. Ford and Mary Mullin Jones
The University of Texas M. D. Anderson Cancer Center,
Department of Behavioral Science, Houston, Texas, USA

ABSTRACT

Smoking among college students is widespread and represents a significant public health issue. Smoking cessation programs utilizing state-of-the-art theoretical concepts and computer technologies hold considerable promise for this category of young adults. Our research team has conducted a study aimed at designing, evaluating, and testing the impact of a theory-guided intervention utilizing a computer-assisted, counselor-delivered approach. This chapter provides background information on smoking among college students. It also describes our computer-based expert system used for data collection and addressing personal health risks and readiness to change smoking behavior, and the main outcomes from our study. A group-randomized, controlled trial was used to assess the intervention in a sample of 426 students (58.5% females; mean age, 22.8 ± 4.7 years) from 15 pair-matched community colleges located in the Houston, Texas area. The experimental intervention was delivered by a trained counselor who used the computerized expert system, motivational intervention approach, and personalized health feedback. At the 10-month follow-up assessment, the salivary cotinine-validated smoking cessation rates were 16.6% in the experimental condition and 10.1% in the standard care condition ($p=0.068$). Although the statistical significance between the study conditions was not reached, our results indicate that our computer-assisted intervention holds considerable promise in reducing smoking among community college students. Difficulties and solutions in terms of recruitment and retention of our young study participants are discussed. Feasible and effective tobacco control interventions targeting college students, along with adoption of smoke-free campus policies are warranted.

INTRODUCTION

Tobacco use among young adults aged 18-24 years is a growing public health concern (Center for Disease Control, 1997). During the early 1990s, smoking among young adults began to alter after nearly 16 years of sustained decline. Wechsler et al. (Wechsler, Rigotti, Gledhill-Hoyt and Lee, 1998) reported an increase in the prevalence of current use by college students from 22.3% in 1993 to 28.5% in 1997. The highest rates were among freshmen (31.2%) and lowest among college seniors (25.3%). Although 11% of "ever smokers" had their first cigarette before the age of 18 years, 28% of current smokers began to smoke regularly after the age of 18 years (Wechsler, Rigotti, Gledhill-Hoyt and Lee, 1998). Data collected from a nationally representative sample of college students in 1999 showed that over 50% had tried smoking and 28.5% had smoked in the past month (Rigotti, Lee and Wechsler, 2000). The reasons for the increase in smoking among college students is unclear, but Murphy-Hoefer (Murphy-Hoefer et al, 2005) reported that it may reflect a "cohort effect."

More recent data from the Monitoring the Future (MTF) study (2005) and the 2005 National Survey on Drug Use and Health (2006) suggest a decline in past month and past year smoking among college students. While positive results are being seen in this population, the fact remains that more than 25% of the college population are smokers (Johnston, O'Malley, Bachman and Schlunberg, 2005; Substance Abuse and Mental Health Services, 2006). There is still a considerable amount of work to be accomplished.

ADVERSE HEALTH EFFECTS

Cigarette smoking causes more deaths in the United States than AIDS, alcohol abuse, drug abuse, motor vehicle injuries, and suicide combined (Center for Disease Control, 2002). Cigarette smoking is the major risk factor for the development of chronic obstructive pulmonary disease (COPD), coronary heart disease, atherosclerotic peripheral vascular disease, and many cancers (Flay, Ockene and Tager, 1992a; Glynn, 1993; Ockene, 1997; Shopland, Burns, Garfinkel and Samet, 1997; USDHHS, 1984). These and other preventable, smoking related diseases are the underlying cause of more than 430,000 deaths annually in the United States (Center for Disease Control, 2002).

The long-term health problems related to smoking are a function of the duration and amount smoked (USDHHS, 1994). However, youths as young as 10-12 have been shown to have respiratory problems. Moreover, a dose-response relationship seems to exist between respiratory systems and level of smoking (Bland, Bewely, Pollard and Banks, 1978; Higenbottam, Shipley, Clark and G., 1980). Respiratory problems like coughing and phlegm production are found notably more often among teen smokers than nonsmokers (Prokhorov, Emmons, Pallonen and Tsoh, 1996; Prokhorov, Pallonen, Niaura and Prochaska, 1994; Rimpelä and Teperi, 1989; USDHHS, 1994). Other studies have found that the odds of having respiratory symptoms (e.g., shortness of breath, coughing, and wheezing) are at least doubled among high-school smokers compared to nonsmokers (Arday et al, 1995). Similarly, the prevalence of respiratory symptoms is doubled among young smokers who smoked one cigarette or more per week (Bewley and Bland, 1976). It has been hypothesized that initiating smoking at 15 years of age will lead to a reduction in pulmonary functioning – as indicated by tests of forced expiratory volumes and flow rates (FEV_1 and FEF_{25-75}) – to levels that could provide early warning signs of the adverse effects of smoking in otherwise healthy teens (Tager et al, 1985). These early warning signs and symptoms are likely to be even more pronounced among young adult smokers. Our own study of community college students showed that 88% of smokers reported respiratory symptoms, compared to 27% of nonsmokers ($p<0.001$) (Prokhorov et al, 2003). Clinical studies have also demonstrated that smoking cessation is usually associated with a gradual disappearance of respiratory symptoms, and partial cessation is associated with some reduction in symptoms (USDHHS, 1984). The symptoms of cough, phlegm, and wheezing are diminished and/or reversed in former smokers (USDHHS, 1984). Smoking is also associated with premature lipidemic and atherosclerotic plaques, and a relative increased risk of early cardiovascular disease (USDHHS, 1994). A smoker who is less than 65 years old is up to eight times as likely as a nonsmoker to suffer from myocardial infarction, and nearly five times as likely to incur a cerebral vascular incident (Shopland and Burns, 1993). These facts have prompted researchers to study the factors that predict tobacco use in an effort to prevent and treat nicotine dependence.

DIFFICULTY IN QUITTING SMOKING

Evidence indicates that adolescent and young adult smokers experience difficulty in quitting smoking. Although most of the quit attempts that a smoker makes occur early in life (Ershler, Leventhal, Fleming and Glynn, 1989; Fiore et al, 1990; Moss, 1979; Pallonen et al, 1990), an estimated 51% of 15-year-old smokers have tried but failed to quit using tobacco. Importantly, 27% of adolescent smokers think that they will never be able to quit, no matter how hard they try (Revill and Drury, 1980). Among young adult smokers (ages 18 to 24 years), the quitting patterns resemble those of adolescents. Although 57% of young adults report quitting for at least 1 day in the past year, only 14% report having maintained abstinence for a minimum of 1 month. Among young adults who smoke daily for at least 1 year, only 8% maintain abstinence for a minimum of 1 month (CDC, unpublished data). Also, 18% of college smokers have been shown to make five or more quit attempts (Wechsler, Rigotti, Gledhill-Hoyt and Lee, 1998). Both adolescents and young adults routinely fail when they attempt to quit smoking without assistance (Flay, Ockene and Tager, 1992b).

REASONS FOR TOBACCO USE AMONG COLLEGE STUDENTS

Entering college can be an exciting, yet stressful event for young adults. Traditionally, students enter college immediately after high school (age 18 or 19 years) and are faced with adapting to changes in support networks, academic courses, and their new social environment (Von Ah, Ebert, Ngamvitroj and Kang, 2005). Along with these changes and new responsibilities, college students have greater freedom and control over their lifestyles than ever before.Therefore, this transitional period is an opportune time to establish healthy lifestyle behaviors (Dinger and Waigandt, 1997). However, researchers have found that college students engage in tobacco use and other unhealthy behaviors, which may have long-term implications for their health (Johnston, O'Malley, Bachman and Schlunberg, 2005; Substance Abuse and Mental Health Services, 2006). Therefore, identifying factors that influence health-compromising behaviors among college students, such as cigarette smoking, warrant close attention of investigators.

A number of environmental, behavioral, and personal factors have been shown to be associated with smoking initiation and maintenance. For example, considerable volume of research has established a strong link between social influence of families and peers, and the behavior of smoking (Flay et al, 1994; Flay, Phil, Hu and Richardson, 1998; Mayhew, Flay and Mott, 2000; Morrell, Cohen, Bacchi and West, 2005; Stockdale, Dawson-Owens and Sagrestano, 2005). Among youth smoking cessation has been shown to be predicted by fewer friends who smoke, less parental smoking, and fewer household smokers (Chassin, Presson, Sherman and Edwards, 1991). Along with other smoking cessation methods, use of a buddy (spouses, partners, or someone who lived outside the participant's household) who provides social support during the cessation attempt increases the likelihood of successful cessation. Olsen and colleagues (Olsen et al, 1990) found significant improvement in cessation outcomes when there was peer support at the work site. Gruder et al. (Gruder et al, 1993) found that use of the social support system among smokers in an interactive televised smoking cessation program was an effective adjunct to raising smoking abstinence rates. The USDHHS *Clinical Practice Guideline on Treating Tobacco Use and Dependence* indicates that adding social support to pharmacologic treatment seemed to significantly increase long-term quit rates compared to treatment without social support (Fiore et al, 2000).

Smoking among college students also differs by ethnicity (whites smoke at higher rates), education, less religious, members of fraternities or sororities, not participating in athletics, gender (women more likely than men), and among those who consume more alcohol (Emmons, Wechsler, Dowdall and Abraham, 1998; Morrell, Cohen, Bacchi and West, 2005; Ridner, 2005; Wechsler, Rigotti, Gledhill-Hoyt and Lee, 1998). Similarly, cigarette smoking also varies across age groups. In the general population, the current smoking rate tends to peak between 18 and 22 years of age and then falls as experimentation with cigarette smoking decreases (Johnston, O'Malley, Bachman and Schlunberg, 2005). Also, prospective data indicate that alcohol use predicts smoking progression among adolescents and cessation among current smokers (Mayhew, Flay and Mott, 2000). Rigotti and colleagues (Rigotti, Lee and Wechsler, 2000) found that college students, who were binge drinkers, were four times more likely to smoke than those who were not binge drinkers. Those who were marijuana users were nearly five times more likely to be current smokers. Although college students' use of illicit drugs including marijuana is lower than their non-college counterparts (Johnston, O'Malley, Bachman and Schlunberg, 2005), college students have higher rates of alcohol consumption and binge drinking than those in the general population (Schlunberg et al, 2001).

Several studies have examined college students' behavior and attitudes about cigarettes. Hines et al. (Hines, Fretz and Nollen, 1998) found that occasional college smokers felt smoking made them look glamorous, feel daring, and did not make them feel like outcasts. College students have been shown to identify the benefits of smoking as stress reduction, enjoyment, something to do, social acceptance, and weight reduction (DeBernardo et al, 1999; Von Ah, Ebert, Ngamvitroj and Kang, 2005). Recent studies have highlighted the importance of the link between depression (or negative affect) and smoking (Breslau et al, 1998; Kandel and Davies, 1986; Kenford et al, 2002; Windle and Windle, 2001) reported that depressive symptoms among 15- and 16-year-olds were related to their smoking status 9 years later. Choi et al. (Choi et al, 1997) reported that cigarette smoking was related to the onset of depression among 12-18-year-olds. Among 18-19 year old smokers, depression predicted continued smoking 4 years later (Zhu, Sun, Billings and Choi, 1999), and smoking rates are higher among college students who are unhappy (Emmons, Wechsler, Dowdall and Abraham, 1998).

A student's decision to smoke may also be influenced by other environmental factors such as marketing, lack of smoking restrictions in residence halls, and easy accessibility to cigarettes. Marketing targeted at people aged 18 to 24 years may contribute to an increase in college student smoking as young adults are the legal targets of tobacco industry marketing (Ling and Glantz, 2002). A Report of the U.S. Surgeon General (1994) indicated that since the 1960s, smokers aged 25 years or younger have been a major marketing target, and are considered to be critical for the long-term performance and profitability of the tobacco industry (USDHHS, 1994). Marketing to this age group occurs through sponsorship of music and sporting events, parties, and bar promotions (Katz and Lavack, 2002; Ling and Glantz, 2002). Some of the marketing, including tobacco advertisements occurs on many college campuses (Halperin and Rigotti, 2003). Exposure to tobacco promotions at social events has been associated with increased tobacco use by college students (Rigotti, Moran and Wechsler, 2005).

INTERVENTION MEASURES

Recent reports suggest that noticeable progress has been made in adopting tobacco-control policies that affect college students. One study that included 50 large public universities in the United States found that about half of these universities banned smoking in all campus buildings and residence halls (Halperin and Rigotti, 2003).

To discourage tobacco use among college students, tobacco control policies for United States colleges and universities were recommended by the American College Health Association and American Cancer Society (American Cancer Society, 2001; American College Health Association, 2000). Both groups recommend that colleges prohibit smoking in all campus buildings (including student residences and eating areas), prohibit tobacco advertising on campus and in college publications, prohibit tobacco sponsorship of campus events, prohibit the sale of tobacco on campus, and provide ready access to smoking cessation treatment. While there is limited evidence for the efficacy of these recommended policies in the college environment at present, data are beginning to appear. For example, one cross-sectional study found an association between smoke-free policies in student residences and lower smoking prevalence, especially among students who did not enter college as regular smokers (Wechsler et al, 2001).

Nearly one-third of young adults attend a college or university in the United States, making these institutions important channels for influencing young adult behavior (Hingson, Heeren, Zakocs and al, 2002). Colleges and universities offer potential sites for tobacco-reduction interventions and can play a useful role in promoting tobacco prevention and cessation (DeBernardo et al, 1999). However, there is a relatively limited amount of tobacco intervention research targeting college students. Murphy-Hoefer et al. (Murphy-Hoefer et al,

2005) conducted a review to summarize and synthesize college-based interventions since 1980. The authors identified 14 studies, and only five of them received a satisfactory rating based on evaluation criteria. Most of the studies were based on convenience samples and were conducted at 4-year universities. Institutional interventions focused mainly on campus smoking restrictions, smoke-free policies, anti-tobacco messages, and cigarette pricing.

Several lines of evidence suggest that the smoking cessation programs currently available for adults may not be effective for college students. College students are unlikely to be attracted to "traditional" cessation programs, such as lectures, health fairs, and workshops that typically distribute printed literature and educational materials. Although nearly 56% of college health directors report that their college health centers offer some type of smoking cessation program, few students use the programs (Wechsler et al, 2001). Psychosocial cues to smoke, self-perceptions, and low self-efficacy related to cessation are likely to be more prevalent among younger adults than among older adult populations (Budd and Preston, 2001). Researchers suspect that low perceived risk, perceived advantages of smoking, and lack of recognition of the benefits of quitting contribute to smoking behavior among adolescents (Ershler, Leventhal, Fleming and Glynn, 1989; Prokhorov, Emmons, Pallonen and Tsoh, 1996; Stanton, Lowe and Gillespie, 1996; Sussman et al, 1998; van Roosmalen and McDaniel, 1992). Sussman et al (Sussman et al, 1998) reported that the level of baseline smoking, smoking intention, and perceived stress significantly predicted self-initiated quitting among youth. Because these factors are prominent in adolescents, it appears reasonable to expect that they are also prominent in college-aged adults. Young adults in general and college students in particular know that tobacco use damages health (e.g., (Torabi, Yang and Li, 2002), but many students continue to smoke anyway.

Providing innovative programs tailored to the unique preferences and needs of college students might enhance student participation in smoking-cessation programs. However, while substantial effort has been expended in recent years toward developing smoking prevention and cessation programs, very little effort has been made to develop smoking cessation programs specifically for community college students. This might be a contributing factor as to why smoking prevalence among college students has not steadily declined.

WHAT ARE THE GAPS?

Little information exists on the effectiveness tobacco control interventions for college students. Also, few cessation programs are available on college campuses, and the ones that are available have not been evaluated in terms of their effectiveness (Lantz, 2003). College students infrequently visit a health care provider or seek health care advice (Kear, 2002). Fewer than 28% of college students reported receiving information on tobacco use prevention from their college or university (Center for Disease Control, 1997). Therefore, an understanding of factors motivating smoking initiation and continuation in young adults is necessary to develop relevant antismoking messages and effective modes of delivering the message to this group.

PROJECT "LOOK AT YOUR HEALTH"

Overview

Project "Look At Your Health" was a three- year group randomized study, funded by an R01 grant from the NCI (Alexander V. Prokhorov, Principal Investigator). Motivational interviewing (MI) and health status feedback (HF) were used to encourage smokers 18-35 years of age to progress through stages of readiness to quit smoking. The two arms of the intervention included:

1. Look at Your Health (LAYH) experimental intervention group representing the motivational interviewing combined with health status feedback in an individual counseling session, versus
2. A Standard Care (SC) group that received a variety of self-help materials and a brief counseling session specific to these materials.

The project involved a total of 15 community college campuses in the greater Houston area. Our goal was to recruit 38 students from each campus for a total population of 570 students. Each of the campuses was randomized to either the LAYH group or the SC group. The sessions took place at a designated office on each campus. The sessions included a baseline, 2-month follow-up, 4-month follow-up and a 10-month final session.

METHODS

Personalized Intervention

In the intervention group (LAYH), counseling sessions were conducted at on-campus locations by a trained counselor. At the beginning of each session, counselors performed a lung function test (spirometry), assessed expired carbon monoxide (CO), and collected a saliva sample (only at the baseline session and 10-month follow up). At the baseline session, the counselor measured the participant's height without shoes using a medical stadiometer and recorded the participant's personal information (name, address, and unique study identification number) in a computer. The computer was then given to the participant to complete a computerized questionnaire that collected data on sociodemographic characteristics (collected at baseline only), smoking-related beliefs and behaviors, and health status.

Using the Motivational Interviewing technique (Miller and Rollnick, 2002), the counselor then provided an intervention session tailored to the participant's smoking-related characteristics (e.g., nicotine dependence level, decisional balance, and temptations to smoke) and stage of readiness to quit (Prochaska, DiClemente and Norcross, 1992). Motivational interviewing (Miller and Rollnick, 2002; Rollnick, Heather and Bell, 1992) was employed as the intervention style to encourage the students' continuous participation in the study. We hypothesized that this approach based on motivational interviewing and personalized health feedback would be more effective than a self-help manual to quit in helping college student smokers quit and remain abstinent from smoking. An expert system software program provided counselors with real-time, on-screen, tailored feedback and quitting strategies. The system also summarized each participant's data in the form of an individualized newsletter (approximately 10 pages) that the counselor printed out and provided to the participant at the end of each session. To make spirometry results meaningful, the expert system computed a measure of "lung age" for each participant. The counselor discussed the findings during the session and included them in the printed newsletter. A more detailed description of the personalized intervention is presented below.

Expert System

We developed the expert system to facilitate the personalized intervention group participants' receipt of personally tailored counseling. We based the intervention on the transtheoretical model (TTM) of change (Prochaska et al, 1994) and the health belief model (Rosenstock, 1974;, 1990). The TTM of change, conceptualized by Prochaska and colleagues (Prochaska, DiClemente and Norcross, 1992), provides a useful approach to evaluation of the process of change. The model has been studied extensively in the context of self-initiated change of health-related behaviors, especially tobacco use. This model provides a framework for understanding the mechanisms that are hypothesized to mediate change (processes), a temporal ordering of the sequence of events in changing a problem behavior (stages), measures that are sensitive to the earliest signs of change (decisional balance and temptations to smoke), and a means of tailoring education and intervention approaches to an individual's level of readiness for change. According to the model, quitting tobacco use is not a one-step process. Instead, most smokers pass through a series of five *stages of change* in the process of quitting. These stages are precontemplation—not thinking about quitting in the next six months; contemplation—thinking about quitting in the next 6 months but not in the next 30 days; preparation—being ready to quit in the next 30 days and having made a quit attempt in the past 12 months; action—tobacco free for less than 6 months; and maintenance—tobacco free for 6 months or more. Because quitters often return to smoking, the model assumes a cyclical property, in that people who relapse revert to an earlier stage.

In general, the expert system collected data from the computerized questionnaire completed by the study participant near the beginning of the counseling session and then processes the data. This generated (1) a summary screen that helps the counselor structure the counseling session and (2) an individualized printed newsletter that highlights key information and helpful quitting strategies relevant to the participant. Although many expert systems for smoking cessation are based on the transtheoretical model of change and utilize computer-generated reports provided either on-screen (Aveyard et al, 1999) or printed as a personal letter (Velicer and Prochaska, 1999), these systems have produced mixed results. The fundamental difference between the previously designed systems and the system used in our study is that our system combined the advantages of the computer-generated information and stage-matched smoking cessation strategies with the strength of counseling conducted by an individual trained in Motivational Interviewing and delivery of health feedback.

The expert system software for LAYH, was programmed using Microsoft Visual Basic 6.0, and the database used to collect and store data is Microsoft Access. The tailored newsletter component was developed using Seagate Crystal Reports 6. The expert system runs on laptop computers with a Microsoft Windows 95 or higher operating system. Participants entered their responses through a series of pull-down menus, text boxes, and option buttons. The computer program checks each input screen for errors and to ensure that all questions are answered before proceeding to the next screen.

Spirometry and Calculation of Estimated Lung Age

Pulmonary function of personalized intervention group members was calculated by using a computerized spirometer (*SpiroCard*; QRS, Minneapolis, MN) that converts a computer into a spirometer. Spirometers are commonly used to diagnose pulmonary disorders in patient care settings as well as in clinical and epidemiological research. Most information on early signs of obstructive and restrictive pulmonary disorders in young adults can be obtained from separate measurements of forced expiratory volume in 1 second (FEV_1) and forced vital capacity (FVC), as well as by calculation of the FEV_1/FVC ratio.

On the basis of the spirometry data (FEV_1), the computerized expert system computed lung age (the age at which a nonsmoker's lungs would be expected to be in the same condition as the student's lungs) as described by Morris and Temple (Morris and Temple, 1985). Smokers typically have a lung age higher than their chronological age. This indicates aging of the lungs as a result of damage from smoking.

Measurement of Carbon Monoxide in Expired Air

CO levels in expired air were measured using the MicroCO device (Micro Direct, Auburn, ME), which had a portable "traffic light" visual indicators (green for nonsmokers, yellow for light smokers, and red for heavy smokers), and an audible alarm that indicated the end of the required 10-second single breath expiration. The monitor displayed both parts per million CO to air and percentage of carboxyhemoglobin. The monitor also included software and an output connection to a personal computer for data logging. CO levels of eight parts per million or higher are widely used to indicate current smoking e.g., (Berlin, Radzius, Henningfield and Moolchan, 2001).

Counseling Procedures

Throughout the counseling portion of each session, the counselor is guided by the summary screen generated by our expert system in response to the participant's answers to the computerized questionnaire. Graphical icons appear next to text entries that the program designates as most relevant for that participant.

After developing rapport with the student, the counselor discussed the student's smoking behavior (i.e., number of cigarettes smoked per day, number of years smoked, and past attempts to quit). Then, using motivational interviewing strategies, the counselor asks the participant to discuss the pros and cons of smoking, the pros and cons of quitting, and readiness to make behavioral changes that affect smoking. The negative aspects of smoking and the positive aspects of quitting (as identified by the student) are emphasized and discussed in as much detail as the student chooses. If the student quits smoking at any time during the study, slight modifications to the motivational interviewing are required. First, the pros and cons of smoking are discussed in terms of what the student does or does not miss about smoking. Second, the pros and cons of quitting are discussed in terms of obstacles to maintaining abstinence. Finally, behavioral changes are re-assessed to determine their ongoing efficacy.

Baseline Counseling Session

During the baseline counseling session, the counselor first used the baseline summary screen to determine the participant's current stage of change for cessation. The counseling session was then tailored accordingly. The counselor explains the meaning of each component of the screen to participants. As an example, consider an 18-year-old female who entered the project in the preparation stage (considering quitting in the next 30 days). She has smoked for five years and believes that her overall health has been affected by smoking. She reports having no respiratory symptoms caused by smoking. She believes her health is worse than that of a nonsmoker, that her overall health is affected by smoking, that continuing to smoke will result in a decline in her health and that quitting will improve her health. During the session, the counselor would then discuss these beliefs with the participant and discuss the various negative health risks associated with continued smoking. The counselor would also call attention to the section of the summary screen that reports respiratory symptoms and respiratory test results. These are crucial points in explaining how smoking has already affected the student. Also, the counselor would point out how quitting smoking will benefit the student and discusses the student's dependence and the withdrawal symptoms that she has experienced. The counselor asks about specific triggers for smoking and situations in which the student has strong cravings to smoke. The counselor would then outline the stage-appropriate cessation strategies and provides a guideline for the counseling session. The counselor reviews these strategies with the student. Then the counselor would use the system to generate a projection of the student's financial losses due to smoking (e.g., dollars lost as a result of smoking two $2.50 packs of cigarettes a day for 10 years would be $18,250). Finally, the counselor would click the "Print Newsletter" button to cue the printing of a tailored newsletter for the student. The student receives a newsletter at the end of each session. Typically, a baseline counseling session would take up to 30 minutes to complete, not including the time at the beginning of each session dedicated to completion of the computerized questionnaire.

Follow-up Counseling Sessions

Each follow-up session builds on previous sessions. For each participant, data were compared with those of the previous session (baseline or follow-up). At each follow-up session, the student received information reflecting normative (people his/her age, gender, race/ethnicity, etc.) and ipsative (him- or herself during the previous visit) feedback. The counselor reviewed the progress (or absence of progress) for each of the key parameters and communicated these observations to the participant. A follow-up newsletter providing normative and ipsative feedback was printed.

Standard Care Intervention

In the standard care group, individual counseling sessions were also conducted at on-campus locations. At the beginning of each session, the counselor recorded the participant's personal information (name, address, and unique study identification number) in a computer and then gives the computer to the participant. The participant completed a computerized questionnaire that collects data on sociodemographic characteristics (collected at baseline only), smoking-related beliefs and behaviors, and health status. At the baseline assessment, saliva samples were taken for cotinine validation of self-reported smoking status and were analyzed on the spot using an express-diagnostic technology. The saliva tests are repeated at the final assessments.

Following completion of the computerized questionnaire, participants received limited counseling. At the baseline session, the counselor advised the participant to quit smoking and provides the participant with a copy of the National Cancer Institute's *Clearing the Air* self-help manual. At each follow-up session, the counselor gave the participant a different fact sheet extracted from the *Clearing the Air* manual. In addition, the counselor briefly reviewed the participant's progress toward quitting and answers any questions that the participant might have related to smoking cessation (e.g., questions about methods of quitting, coping strategies, and relapse prevention. The initial counseling session lasted approximately 25 minutes, and each follow-up counseling session lasts approximately 15 to 20 minutes. This did not include the time at the beginning of each session dedicated to completion of the computerized questionnaire.

The Computerized Study Questionnaire

At the baseline, both groups completed a computerized questionnaire that assessed sociodemographic characteristics (age, sex, ethnicity, marital status, living conditions, employment, class attendance, and the area of study). Smoking-related beliefs and behaviors, and health status were also assessed. Key constructs assessed via questionnaire are described below. For self-reported nonsmokers, smoking status was validated with salivary cotinine at baseline and at the final (10-month) follow-up. This assessment was done using the NicoMeter™ semi-quantitative dipstick device, which is a convenient, reliable, and cost-effective indicator of tobacco use (Gariti et al, 2002). Self-reported quitters with salivary cotinine values ≤ 5 ng/mL (i.e., level "0" on the NicoMeter™ scale) were considered to be validated quitters.

Stage of Change for Smoking Cessation

The stages of change were identified using the widely used 3-item measure.(Prochaska, DiClemente and Norcross, 1992) Specifically, smokers were classified into the precontemplation stage if they did not intend to quit in the next 6 months; contemplation stage if they intended to quit in the next 6 months; and the preparation stage is they intended to quit in the next 30 days and tried quitting in the past 12 months. Those who reported abstinence for less than 6 months were classified into the action stage of change. The maintenance stage was defined as staying abstinent for more than 6 months.

Decisional Balance

The Decisional Balance scale (Velicer, DiClemente, Prochaska and Brandenburg, 1985) was used to evaluate the "pros and cons" of smoking. The scale score was computed as an unweighted sum of 12 items forming that scale, and scores were standardized to mean = 50 and standard deviation (SD) = 10. The scale is a 5-point Likert scale with responses ranging from "strongly disagree" to "strongly agree." A decisional balance score was computed as pro score (standardized) minus con score (standardized); a score of 0 indicates that the pros and cons are equal; a negative score indicates that the cons outweigh the pros, and a positive score indicates that the pros outweigh the cons.

Temptation to Smoke

Temptations to smoke were measured using a scale developed by Velicer and colleagues (Velicer, DiClemente, Rossi and Prochaska, 1990) Scores were computed as unweighted sums of 13 items describing temptations to smoke. A 5-point Likert scale measured responses ranging from "not at all tempted" to "extremely tempted." Temptations to smoke are based on positive and negative affect, positive social situations, and habitual behavior and cravings. A higher score is indicative of a higher level of temptations.

Withdrawal Symptoms

Withdrawal symptoms were measured using a scale derived from one proposed by Hughes and Hatsukami;(Hughes and Hatsukami, 1986). This scale contains items describing emotional/affective disturbances and physiological disturbances. The score was computed as an unweighted sum of the responses on a 5-point Likert scale ranging from "never" to "always." A higher score indicates greater withdrawal symptoms.

Respiratory Symptoms

We used the American Thoracic Society's inventory to assess the frequency of self-reported respiratory symptoms (Comstock, Tockman, Helsing and Hennesy, 1979). This score was computed as an unweighted sum of the responses on a 5-point Likert scale ranging from "never" to "everyday," with a higher score indicating greater respiratory symptoms.

Other Tobacco Use Variables

Other key variables used to characterize tobacco use status included number of years smoked, number of cigarettes smoked daily, nicotine dependence assessment using the Fagerström Test for Nicotine Dependence,(Heatherton, Kozlowski, Frecker and Fagerström, 1991) and number of quit attempts (a single item assessing the number of 24-hr quit attempts in the past year, ranging from "none" to "six or more" times).

Statistical Analysis

Our primary dependent variable was 7-day point prevalence abstinence. Secondary outcomes included progression through the stages of change, determinants of smoking, and number of quit attempts.

Baseline Comparisons

The study population was characterized using simple descriptive statistics. Scale scores were computed for individuals who provided responses to all of the items underlying a given measure. To detect baseline differences between the treatment groups, we used generalized linear mixed model regression. Because the campus was the unit of randomization, models included the campus as a random effect to adjust for potential correlation of measurements within campuses. All statistical analyses were completed using SAS statistical software version 8.02. (SAS Institute)

Abstinence at 10-Month Follow-up

Generalized linear mixed model regression was used to detect group differences in abstinence at 10-month follow-up. To adjust for potential correlation of measurements within campus, we modeled campus as a random effect nested within treatment condition. The outcome was binary (smoker or nonsmoker at 10-month follow-up), and Proc Glimmix in SAS was used to model the relationships. Both self-reported and biochemically confirmed abstinence rates were analyzed and are presented here.

Progression through the Stages of Change

The percentage distribution across the four stages of change—precontemplation, contemplation, preparation, and action (Prochaska, DiClemente and Norcross, 1992)—was compared between the treatment groups at baseline and at the 10-month follow-up. Contingency tables, Pearson chi-square analysis, and P values were used to summarize the results.

Determinants of Smoking

For determinants of smoking, the primary method of analysis was a pre-post test analysis using mixed-model ANCOVA (PROC MIXED in SAS). In this analysis, primary mediators at the 10-month follow-up were compared between the two groups, while controlling for baseline values of these outcomes. Campus was modeled as a random effect nested within treatment condition, and condition and baseline values were modeled as fixed effects. This approach provided an estimate of the intervention effect in terms of an adjusted difference in the 10-month outcomes. The effect of the intervention at 10 months was evaluated by comparing the mean outcomes between the control and intervention groups adjusted for baseline values and campus effect.

RECRUITMENT OF PARTICIPANTS

Successful participant recruitment is critical to tobacco-cessation research among community college students; therefore, we decided to elaborate on this issue in this chapter. Historically, smoking cessation research programs for this population have garnered limited interest among the students. Reasons for this may include heavy course-load, work commitments, and social activities. There is also the belief that smoking does not appreciably compromise their health and that they will be able to quit at will with no professional help. There also seems to be a misconception among some researchers that "recruitment is recruitment" and that the same methods and techniques that work for older adults will work for this population. All of these reasons present a challenge to any research team hoping to create and implement a smoking-cessation program for college students.Given the growing interest in smoking cessation studies among college students, this information has high research value and practical significance.

We cannot stress the importance of obtaining the appropriate permission to conduct the study on campus, and to have a designated contact on each campus.Visits with these contacts provided information about what recruitment methods might work best with their student populations and some of the possible avenues for recruitment on campus. In Houston, there was great variation from campus to campus, as some were academic and others were technological or trade oriented curriculum.

Based on their experience with a pilot study conducted prior to LAYH, our staff decided to recruit primarily through brief classroom announcements made by faculty members. Fliers asking faculty if they were willing to make classroom announcements were distributed at faculty meetings and workshops, and sent via campus email and faculty mailboxes. Interested faculty members received a packet of recruitment fliers to distribute in class. Attached to each packet was a brief announcement for the faculty member to read aloud in class. Nearly 60 faculty packets on 7 campuses were distributed during two semesters. Several of the campuses would not allow project staff to directly contact staff members and/or use classroom time for project announcements. This recruitment method did not work as well for the actual project as it had for the pilot study.

As a result, the target number of participants was not achieved during the first year of recruitment. Given the potential for inability to conduct statistical analysis in the smaller than planned sample, the research team made subject recruitment a top priority. As a result, the team identified and implemented a series of innovative recruitment and retention strategies.

- Three research assistants whose main responsibility was subject recruitment were hired on an hourly basis. All three individuals were college students and fell into the group of 18-35 year-olds. They operated under the careful supervision of the project director.
- With the start of the second academic year, staff identified and contacted campus activity coordinators and began attending campus activities. "Sign-up" tables with tabletop signage were set up at these activities and the research assistants distributed highlighters and candy with the project name. To recruit study subjects, the project staff attended a variety of campus sponsored activities including: health fairs, blood drives, ice cream socials, concerts, voter registration drive, student organization fairs, campus "game" shows, student appreciation day, class registration, fitness fair, welcome parties, new student orientation, Black History Week celebration, Spanish Heritage celebrations. Volunteer fair, voluntary HIV testing, Great American Smoke-out, and Red Ribbon week celebrations.
- All campuses did not have a designated activities coordinator, and some campuses, had few to no planned student activities. For these campuses, staff set up a table in high-traffic areas such as the student center or cafeteria. Tables were set up on 18 different occasions at nine different campuses. Sign up tables and attendance at planned student activities generated a list of 318 potential participants during a four month time period.
- '"Rolling" recruitment was crucial to the success of the project. Given our limited personnel and budget, this was the only viable option. Our decision to use rolling recruitment was based on practicality and kept the number of project participants at any given time to a manageable number.
- When working within the confines of the academic calendar, the number of students recruited will vary by semester. For example, during the summer months, fewer students were recruited due to smaller pool of students. Campuses schedule fewer classes and activities. It is also important to take into account the following: the time of day, day of week, semester (Fall, Spring, summer), exams, mid terms, etc.

- With a long-term project, personnel will change, space becomes unavailable, and policies are revised. Much of our success can be attributed to maintaining a solid working relationship with campuses. Our staff worked diligently to provide regular updates and to keep their campus contacts apprised of any significant developments using electronic mail, personal visits, and telephone calls. The importance of this cannot be minimized.
- During the course of LAYH, we saw the importance of being flexible in your recruitment approach. We worked to constantly evaluate and revise our approach. What works one semester may not work the next or what works at one campus may not work on another. This is particularly true for large demographically diverse campuses. For the full duration of the recruitment period, we continued to explore a variety of on-campus promotional venues and to identify other on-campus locations for recruitment.

Retention of Participants

As important as participant recruitment is the matter of retention. Perhaps the greatest issue for us was "sign-up versus show-up". While recruiters were able to generate a considerable list of more than enough potential participants over time, this didn't guarantee that participants actually showed up for counseling sessions. Our experience indicates that individuals who register to participate are not always motivated to start and/or complete their actual sessions. There is quite a difference in the number of students that sign up during enrollment, and those that actually show up for first session and sign a consent form.

While participants were given at least three reminders before each appointment, "no shows" continued to be a persistent problem. Numerous participants have been scheduled and rescheduled for their baseline appointment, some up to three times. Our research staff believes that these issues can be attributed to several things. In addition to classes, the majority of these students have jobs and, and many have families. Community college students appear to be a highly transient population making follow-up extremely challenging. On countless occasions, project staff attempted to contact an individual to schedule an appointment only to learn that inadequate or invalid contact information had been provided by the student. Attempts to follow-up by mail only produce returned correspondence. In an attempt to alleviate this problem, recruitment staff collected as much contact information as possible from participants including parent's phone number and address, and a second phone number.

Upon completion of the intervention phase of LAYH, 326 students completed all four sessions (baseline, 2, 4, and 10 month post). Given the transient nature of our population, our research team was pleased to reach 80% of our goal.

RESULTS

Sample Characteristics

The baseline sample consisted of 426 students (80.1% of the targeted *n*, 532). The mean age was 22.8 ± 4.7 years (range, 18 to 35 years). Most participants were female (58.5%) and

Caucasian (55.4%). The majority of students had never been married (82.4%), lived with parents or other family of origin (53.5%), and were employed part-time (42.0%). Most students attended classes on a full-time basis (70.9%), and about one third (30.5%) were enrolled in their first semester of college. The most common area of study cited was "academic" (24.6%). Combined, the "undecided" and "other" areas of study accounted for 36.8% of the sample.

At baseline, there were 207 students in the SC group and 219 in the LAYH group. Although our sample was composed of volunteers, the sample characteristics reflected the overall student populations at the two largest participating community colleges—Houston Community College and San Jacinto College. There were no group differences by age, sex, ethnicity, marital status, number of children, employment, exercise, nicotine dependence, smoking profile (dependence and quit attempts), or the key Transtheoretical Model (Becker, 1974; Miller and Rollnick, 1991; Miller and Rollnick, 2002; USDHHS, 2003), constructs (stages of change, temptations, and decisional balance).

On average, participants smoked 12.5 (standard deviation [SD], 8.5) cigarettes per day, began smoking regularly at 16 years of age (SD, 3.3), and had smoked regularly for 6.6 years (SD, 4.8). At baseline, 10% of students were in the precontemplation stage, 65% were in the contemplation stage, and 25% were in the preparation stage. Nineteen percent had never attempted to quit, 30% had quit once or twice, 24% had quit three to five times, and 27% had quit six or more times. Twenty-seven percent of participants exhibited a substantial degree of nicotine dependence (Fagerström Test for Nicotine Dependence [FTND] score of 5 or more), 38% had a moderate degree of nicotine dependence (FTND score of 2 to 4), and 35% had negligible levels of dependence on nicotine (FTND score of less than 2). The average withdrawal symptom score was 10.16 (SD, 4.60). Salivary cotinine values at baseline confirmed smoking status for 95% of the students; the other 5% of the tests were invalid because of initial methodological deficiencies that were quickly rectified.

A total of 326 students completed all 4 individual sessions with the counselor: 168 (81.1%) in the SC group and 158 (72.1%) in the LAYH group. No group differences on any of the variables were found in the subsample who completed the final 10-month survey. Table 1 summarizes these results.

Table 1. Descriptive characteristics: baseline and 10-month follow-up

	Baseline (n = 426)		10-month follow-up (n = 326)	
Characteristic (p-value)	SC (n = 207)	LAYH (n = 219)	SC (n = 168)	LAYH (n = 158)
Age, years	22.9 (4.6)	22.8 (4.7)	22.9 (4.7)	22.6 (4.4)
Sex (female) (p = .90)	54.0%	63.0%	53.6%	65.8%
Ethnicity				
White	54.6%	56.2%	56.0%	57.6%
African American	15.5%	9.1%	14.3%	7.6%
Hispanic	15.5%	18.3%	14.9%	19.0%
Other	14.5%	16.4%	14.9%	15.8%
Marital status (single) (p = .90)	87.9%	85.3%	88.7%	84.8%
Children = yes (p = .14)	21.7%	26.0%	19.6%	24.7%
Employment				
Full time	21.7%	17.4%	21.4%	18.4%
Part time	44.0%	40.2%	45.8%	42.4%
Not employed	34.3%	42.5%	32.7%	39.2%

Table 1. (Continued)

	Baseline (n = 426)		10-month follow-up (n = 326)	
Exercise				
> 3 times/wk	34.8%	35.6%	32.7%	34.8%
< 3 times/wk	32.9%	34.7%	35.1%	35.4%
Not at all	32.4%	29.7%	32.1%	29.7%
Nicotine dependence score ($p = .60$)	2.9 (2.4)	2.8 (2.3)	2.9 (2.4)	2.8 (2.3)
"Have you ever attempted to quit?" (yes) ($p = .23$)	82.6%	88.6%	83.3%	88.6%
Number of years smoked ($p = .25$)	6.9 (4.7)	6.3 (4.9)	6.9 (4.8)	6.1 (4.7)
Number of cigarettes per day ($p = .14$)	12.9 (9.5)	12.0 (7.5)	12.9 (9.8)	12.0 (7.5)
Stage of Change ($p = .25$)				
Precontemplation	10.6%	9.1%	11.9%	10.8%
Contemplation	65.7%	63.9%	66.1%	62.7%
Preparation	23.7%	26.9%	22.0%	26.6%
Decisional Balance score ($p = .72$)	-0.28 (15.3)	0.27 (15.3)	-.27 (15.2)	-.10 (14.1)
Temptations to Smoke score ($p = .42$)	46.0 (7.8)	46.9 (8.1)	46.2 (7.9)	47.3 (8.0)

*Values in table are mean (standard deviation) or percentages.
Note: SC= Standard Care; LAYH= Look at Your Health.

Quit Rates, by Treatment Condition

Cotinine-validated quit rates (7-day, point-prevalence abstinence) are shown in table 2. At the 10-month follow-up, 86 students (26.4% of total n = 326) self-reported quitting smoking. Self-reported quit rates were 24.4% (n = 41) for the SC group and 28.5% (n = 45) for the LAYH group (p = .21). Upon biochemical verification, of the 326 total cotinine samples (of which 325 underwent validation to verify self-reported quitting status), we observed 43 (13.5%) validated quits—25 (16.6%) in the LAYH group, and 17 (10.1%) in SC (p = .068)

Table 2. Smoking abstinence at 10-month follow-up, by sex and ethnicity

	Quit Rate (%)	
	SC (n = 168)	LAYH (n = 158)
Overall (n = 326)	10.1	16.6
Sex		
Male (n = 132)	2.6	11.1
Female (n = 193)	16.7	19.4
Ethnicity		
White (n = 184)	10.6	14.4
African American (n = 36)	4.2	8.3
Hispanic (n = 55)	20.0	20.0
Other (n = 50)	4.0	24.0

Note: SC= Standard Care; LAYH= Look at Your Health.

Quit Rates, by Sex and Ethnicity

Quit rates by sex and ethnicity are shown in table 2. Higher quit rates were observed among women than among men in both the SC and LAYH groups. For all ethnicities except Hispanics, quit rates were higher in the LAYH group than in the SC group. The results were not statistically significant.

Quit Rates, by Stage of Change

Cotinine-validated quit rates by stage of change at 10-month follow-up are shown in figure 1. For those in the precontemplation and contemplation stages of change, there were no significant differences in quit rates between the SC and LAYH groups. Among students in the preparation stage of change, quit rates were significantly higher for those in the LAYH group than for those in the SC group (31.7% vs. 10.8%, $p < .05$).

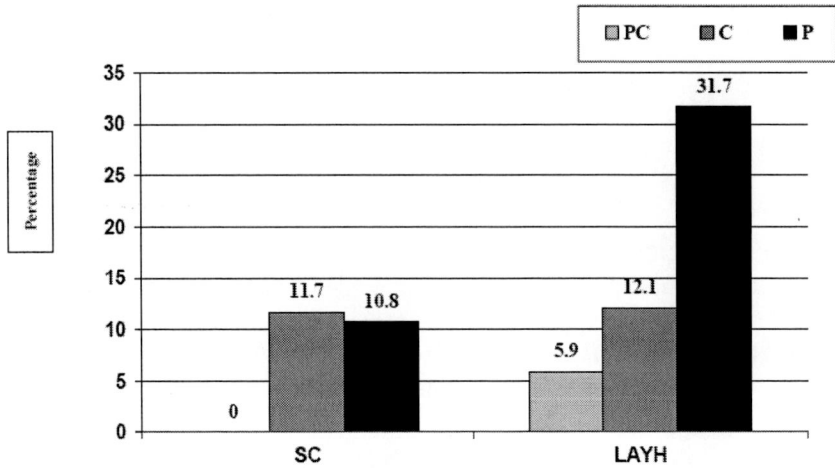

Figure 1. Quitters at 10-Month Follow-up by Stage Change at Baseline.

Movement through the Stages of Change

One hypothesis that we tested was to determine whether LAYH would have a more significant impact than SC on students' progression through the stages of change from the baseline session to the 10-month follow-up (figure 2). As shown, most students were in contemplation or preparation stage at baseline. For students in the precontemplation or contemplation stages at baseline, no significant differences in progression through the stages were observed between the SC and LAYH groups. For students in the preparation stage at baseline, 48% of the LAYH group progressed to action by 10 months, compared to 28% of the SC group, and 14% of the LAYH group regressed to contemplation, compared to 49% of the SC group ($p = .01$). None of the participants reached the maintenance stage.

Panel 1. Precontemplation Stage at Baseline

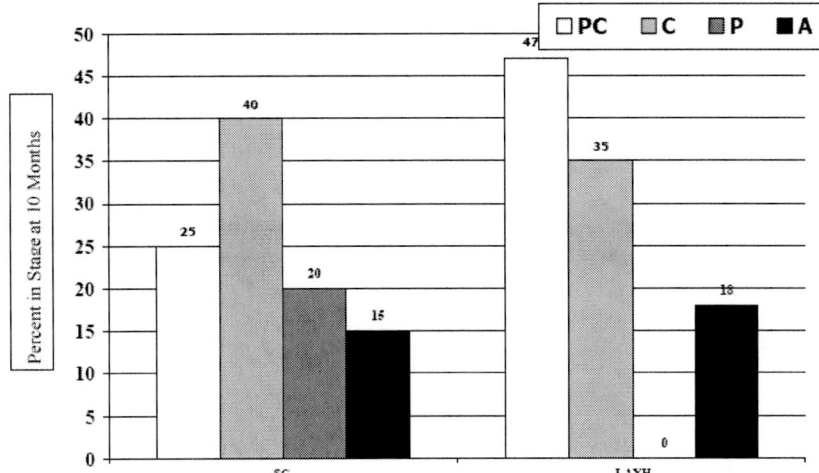

Note: PC=Precontemplation; C= Contemplation; P=Preparation; A=Action; SC= Standard Care; LAYH= Look at Your Health.

Figure 2. Movement through the stages of change from baseline to 10-month follow-up, for patients in the precontemplation (Panel 1), contemplation (Panel 2), and preparation stages (Panel 3) at baseline.

Panel 2. Contemplation Stage at Baseline

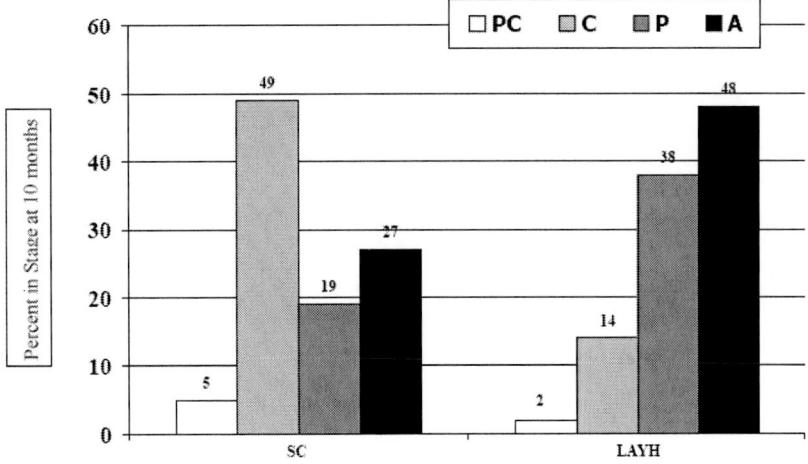

Note: PC=Precontemplation; C= Contemplation; P=Preparation; A=Action; SC= Standard Care; LAYH= Look at Your Health.

Determinants of Smoking

Changes in determinants of smoking between baseline and the 10-month follow-up differed significantly by intervention group. Compared to the SC group, the LAYH group displayed significantly stronger anti-smoking beliefs and perceptions of the benefits of quitting as reflected by changes in the Decisional Balance score[a] (for total sample, changes were 2.1 for SC versus -2.2 for LAYH, adjusted for baseline, $p< .05$; for smokers, changes were 2.57 for SC versus -0.65 for LAYH, adjusted for baseline, $p<.01$). Compared with the SC group, the LAYH group also reported decreased temptations to smoke (for total sample, 42.1 for SC versus 36 for LAYH, adjusted for baseline, $p<.001$; for smokers, 43.1 for SC versus 38.2 for LAYH, adjusted for baseline, $p<.05$); fewer withdrawal symptoms (for total sample, 9.6 for SC versus 7.5 for LAYH, adjusted for baseline, $p<.001$; for smokers, 9.4 for SC versus 7.8 for LAYH, adjusted for baseline, $p<.05$); and milder respiratory symptoms (for total sample, 18.4 for SC versus 16 for LAYH, adjusted for baseline, $p<.001$).

Number of Quit Attempts

Among self-reported non-quitters at 10-month follow-up, there were no significant differences between the LAYH and SC groups in the mean number of quit attempts when adjusted for baseline attempts (3.5 attempts vs. 3.4 attempts). The total number of quit attempts was compared at baseline and at each of the follow-up sessions between intervention and control groups. The results are presented separately for quitters and smokers at 10 months.

At baseline, there were no significant differences between the LAYH and SC groups with respect to the number of quit attempts (3.3 [SD = 1.4] vs. 3.2 [SD=1.5]). The number of quit attempts were compared between LAYH and SC among biochemically validated quitters and smokers at 10 months. At the first follow-up, the mean number of quit attempts was higher for the LAYH group than the SC group (3.6 [SD = 1.2] vs. 2.9 [SD = 1.6]); however, the difference was not statistically significant.

Among students who were smokers at the 10-month follow-up, the mean number of quit attempts was virtually identical for both study conditions (3.4 [SD = 1.3] vs. 3.3 (SD = 1.4]). The mean number of attempts for quitters at 10 months was somewhat higher among the LAYH group compared to SC (3.5 [SD = 1.4) vs. 3.0 (SD = 1.3]), but results were not statistically significant. For smokers, the mean number of quit attempts did not differ significantly (3.3 [SD=1.4] vs. 3.1 [SD = 1.4]). At the final follow-up, the number of quit attempts was recorded for smokers only. The mean number of quit attempts was virtually the same for both conditions and was similar to results seen among smokers at the previous assessment points (3.5 [SD = 1.3] vs. 3.4 [SD=1.4]).

DISCUSSION AND CONCLUSION

Our study evaluated the impact of a novel smoking cessation intervention for community college students. In conjunction with motivational interviewing, counselors used an expert-system software program to provide the participants with individually tailored, highly personalized feedback on respiratory health, presence of alveolar carbon monoxide, quitting strategies, and other smoking-related characteristics.

---

[a] A lower score means the student agrees with reasons to not smoke more than the reasons to smoke.

Our findings suggest that this intervention may reduce the smoking prevalence among community college students. This is particularly important in light of the fact that community college students are a severely understudied population, and few, if any community colleges offer smoking cessation programs to this rapidly growing population of young individuals.

Tailored, personalized, and individualized feedback about the negative consequences of smoking appears to be especially meaningful to this group. Because of their young age, they rarely suffer from chronic diseases, tend to minimize the health effects of smoking, and display limited insight into their personal risks of smoking-attributable illness. To our knowledge, it is the only smoking cessation intervention for this population that brought positive outcomes in terms of increased number of quitters at 10-month follow-up.

Although the differences in biochemically validated quit rates between the intervention and control groups approached but did not achieve statistical significance, we believe that our results show promise. First, our SC condition offered considerably more than students would ordinarily receive. Therefore, cessation rates for this group might be inflated. Second, the impact of our intervention resulted in smoking cessation rates comparable with the state-of-the-science knowledge related to the highest achievable efficacy from individual counseling. Specifically, our results were remarkably similar to efficacy rates described in the corresponding section of the USDHHS *Clinical Practice Guideline for Treating Tobacco Use and Dependence* (Fiore et al, 2000). We found that at the 10-month follow up, 10.1% of SC participants remained abstinent compared with 16.6% in the intervention group (cotinine-validated results). According to the meta-analysis of 58 randomized controlled trials presented in the *Clinical Practice Guideline*, (Fiore et al, 2000) the lowest estimated abstinence rates (10.8%) were among smokers who did not seek treatment with a provider ("no format"), and the highest rates (16.8%; CI=14.7,19.1) were among smokers who received individual cessation counseling. In other words, our intervention appears to exhibit similar efficacy as the current "best practices" reported by the U. S. Department of Health and Human Services in 2000 (USDHHS, 2000). Moreover, when stage of change is taken into account, our intervention yielded abstinence rates that were almost three times greater than of the SC group (31.7% vs. 10.8%) and nearly twice as high as those found in the meta-analysis (16.8%; assuming participants were in the preparation stage upon entering treatment).

A noteworthy finding from this study was the substantial discrepancy between self-reported and biochemically validated abstinence rates at 10 months. Only about half of the self-reported quitters were validated with the cotinine test (16.6% vs. 28.5% in the LAYH group and 10.1% vs. 24.4% in the SC group) suggesting that the rates of misreported quitting among community college students are phenomenally high and a biochemical validation of their self-reports is essential. The rationale for biochemical tests, especially among adult populations, has been debated in the literature; (Luepker, Pallonen, Murray and Pirie, 1989; Velicer, Prochaska, Rossi and Snow, 1992) however, we submit that there might have been a number of possible reasons (e.g., social desirability in general, desire to please the counselor, or embarrassment because of the failure to quit) why students failed to accurately report their current smoking behavior. Another possible contributor to the aforementioned discrepancy could be misreporting of social smoking (captured by the cotinine test) and mistaking it for "quitting." Clearly, this methodological issue requires additional in-depth investigations among community college students.

The intervention group (LAYH) students also made significant progress through the stages of change and through the psychological and physiological determinants of smoking, compared to those in SC. More LAYH participants progressed from preparation to action and fewer regressed from preparation or action to contemplation. The LAYH group espoused significantly higher anti-smoking and pro-quitting beliefs, and fewer temptations to smoke, as well as fewer withdrawal and lower respiratory symptoms. For those not abstinent at 10 months, these outcomes are likely to signify the intervention effect promoting readiness to quit smoking which eventually might move them towards future quit attempts.

Our findings pertinent to the other key Transtheoretical Model constructs (decisional balance and temptations to smoke) indicate that our intervention program resulted in their favorable changes. This was in sharp contrast to the SC that did not exhibit such changes. These findings appear to validate the aforementioned movement of continued smokers through the stages of change in the right direction, as it was shown in previous Transtheoretical-guided studies (Prochaska et al, 1994).

Among the study limitations, the relatively low sample size should be mentioned. Also, at mid-point, one of the targeted LAYH campuses had to be replaced with another one due to unanticipated difficulties with recruitment. Although we continued to treat and follow-up students recruited from both campuses in the same fashion, this glitch might have affected the rigor of the study randomization. Despite these limitations, we believe that this provides us with many important lessons and considerable experience in dealing with the high risk, yet severely understudied population of community college students.

To our knowledge, our investigation was the first attempt to approach community college students with a theory-guided, technology-based, and counselor-delivered smoking cessation program. Although we failed to reach statistical significance between the study conditions, much important information was gathered to continue this line of research in the future. Armed with this knowledge and experience, our investigative team will enhance and refine the intervention approach to achieve better results in helping college students quit tobacco use.

REFERENCES

American Cancer Society. (2001). Mission statement: American Cancer Society's smoke free New England, in advocating for a tobacco free campus: a manual for college and university students.

American College Health Association. (2000). Position statement on tobacco on college and university campuses.

Arday, D. R., Giovino, G. A., Schulman, J., Nelson, D. E., Mowery, P. and Samet, J. M. (1995). Cigarette smoking and self-reported health problems among U.S. high school seniors, 1982-1989. *American Journal of Health Promotion,* 10(2), 111-116.

Aveyard, P., Cheng, K. K., Almond, J., Sherratt, E., Lancashire, R., Lawrence, T., Griffin, C. and Evans, O. (1999). Cluster randomised controlled trial of expert system based on the transtheoretical ("stages of change") model for smoking prevention and cessation in schools. *BMJ,* 319(7215), 948-953.

Becker, M. H. (1974). The Health Belief Model and Personal Health Behavior. *Health Education Mongraphs,* 2(4).

Berlin, I., Radzius, A., Henningfield, J. E. and Moolchan, E. T. (2001). Correlates of expired air carbon monoxide: Effect on ethnicity and relationship with saliva cotinine and nicotine. *Nicotine and Tobacco Research*, 3, 325-331.

Bewley, B. R. Bland, J. M. (1976). Smoking and respiratory symptoms in two groups of school children. *Preventive Medicine*, 5, 63-69.

Bland, M., Bewely, B. R., Pollard, V. and Banks, M. H. (1978). Effect of children's and parents' smoking on respiratory symptoms. *Archives of Disease in Childhood*, 53(2), 100-105.

Breslau, N., Peterson, E. L., Schultz, L. R., Chilcoat, H. D. and Andreski, P. (1998). Major depression and stages of smoking: A longitudinal investigation. *Archives of General Psychiatry*, 55(2), 161-166.

Budd, G. Preston, D. (2001). College students' attitudes and beliefs about the consequences of smoking: development and normative scores of a new scale. *J. of the American Academy of Nurse Practitioners*, 13, 9.

Center for Disease Control. (1997). Youth Risk Behavior Surveillance, National College Health risk behavior survey, United States, 1995. *MMWR-Morbidity and Mortality Weekly Report*, 46(No. SS-6), 1-56.

Center for Disease Control. (2002). Annual smoking-attributable mortality, years of potential life lost, and economic costs - United States, 1995-1999. *MMWR*, 51, 300-303.

Chassin, L., Presson, C., Sherman, S. and Edwards, D. (1991). Four pathways to young adult smoking status: Adolescent social psychological antecedents in a Midwestern community sample. *Health Psychology*, 10, 409-418.

Choi, W. S., Patten, C. A., Gillin, J. C., Kaplan, R. M. and Pierce, J. P. (1997). Cigarette smoking predicts development of depressive symptoms among U.S. adolescents. *Ann. Behav. Med*, 19(1), 42-50.

Comstock, G. W., Tockman, M., Helsing, K. J. and Hennesy, K. M. (1979). Standardized respiratory questionnaires: comparison of the old with the new. . *American Review of Respiratory Disease*, 119, 45-53.

DeBernardo, R. L., Aldinger, C. E., Dawood, O. R., Hanson, R. E., Lee, S. J. and Rinaldi, S. R. (1999). An e-mail assessment of undergraduates' attitudes toward smoking. *Journal of American College Health*, 48(2), 61-66.

Dinger, M. Waigandt, A. (1997). Dietary intake and physical activity behaviors of male and female college students. *American J. of Health Promotion*, 11(5), 360-362.

Emmons, K. M., Wechsler, H., Dowdall, G. and Abraham, M. (1998). Predictors of smoking among US college students. *American Journal of Public Health*, 88(1), 104-107.

Ershler, J., Leventhal, H., Fleming, R. and Glynn, K. (1989). The quitting experience for smokers in sixth through twelfth grades. *Addict. Behav*, 14(4), 365-378.

Fiore, M. C., Bailey, W. C., Cohen, S. J., Dorfman, S. F., Goldstein, M. G., Gritz, E. R., Heyman, R. B., Jaen, C. R., Kottke, T. E., Lando, H. A., Mecklenburg, R. E., Mullen, P. D. et al. (2000). *Treating Tobacco Use and Dependence: Clinical Practice Guideline.* Rockville, MD: U.S. Department of Health and Human Services.

Fiore, M. D., Novotny, T. E., Pierce, J. P., Giovino, G. A., Hatziandreu, E. J., Newcomb, P. A., Surawicz, T. S. and Davis, R. M. (1990). Methods used to quit smoking in the United States: Do cessation programs help? *Journal of The American Medical Association*, 263, 2760-2765.

Flay, B. R., Hu, F. B., Siddiqui, O., Day, L. E., Hedeker, D., Petraitis, J., Richardson, J. and Sussman, S. (1994). Differential influence of parental smoking and friends' smoking on adolescent initiation and escalation of smoking. *Journal of Health and Social Behavior,* 35(September), 248-265.

Flay, B. R., Ockene, J. K. and Tager, I. B. (1992b). Smoking: epidemiology, cessation, and prevention. Task Force on Research and Education for the Prevention and Control of Respiratory Diseases. *Chest,* 102(3 Suppl), 277S-301S.

Flay, B. R., Phil, D., Hu, F. B. and Richardson, J. (1998). Psychosocial predictors of different stages of cigarette smoking among high school students. *Preventive Medicine,* 27(5), A9-A18.

Gariti, P., Rosenthal, D. I., Lindell, K., Hansen-Flaschen, J., Shrager, J., Lipkin, C., Alterman, A. I. and Kaiser, L. R. (2002). Validating a dipstick method for detecting recent smoking. *Canc. Epidemiology Biomarkers and Prevention,* 11, 1123-1125.

Glynn, T. (1993). Improving the health of US children. The need for early interventions in tobacco use. *Preventive Medicine,* 22, 513-519.

Gruder, C. L., Mermelstein, R. J., Kirkendol, S., Hedeker, D., Wong, S. C., Schreckengost, J., Warnecke, R. B., Burzette, R. and Miller, T. Q. (1993). Effects of social support and relapse prevention training as adjuncts to a televised smoking-cessation intervention. *J. Consult. Clin. Psychol,* 61(1), 113-120.

Halperin, A. Rigotti, N. (2003). US public universities' compliance with recommended tobacco-control policies. *J. Am. Coll. Health,* 51, 181-188.

Heatherton, T. F., Kozlowski, L. T., Frecker, R. C. and Fagerström, K. O. (1991). The Fagerström test for nicotine dependence: A revision of the Fagerström tolerance questionnaire. *British Journal of Addiction,* 86(9), 1119-1127.

Higenbottam, T., Shipley, M. J., Clark, T. J. and G., R. (1980). Lung function and symptoms of cigarette smokers related to tar yield and number of cigarettes smoked. *Lancet,* 1(8165), 409-412.

Hines, D., Fretz, A. and Nollen, N. (1998). Regular and occasional smoking by college students: Personality attributions of smokers and nonsmokers. *Psychological Reports,* 83, 1299-1306.

Hingson, R. W., Heeren, T., Zakocs, R. C. and al, e. (2002). Magnitude of alcohol-related mortality and morbidity among U.S. college students ages 18-24. *J. Stud. Alcohol,* 63, 136-144.

Hughes, J. R. Hatsukami, D. (1986). Signs and symptoms of tobacco withdrawal. *Archives of General Psychiatry,* 43(3), 289-294.

Johnston, L., O'Malley, P., Bachman, J. and Schlunberg, J. (2005). Monitoring The Future. National survey results on drug use, 1975-2004: Volume II, College students and adults ages 19-45. National Institute on Drug Abuse. *NIH Publication No.* 05-5728, Bethesda, MD.

Kandel, D. B. Davies, M. (1986). Adult sequlae of adolescent depressive symptoms. *Arch. General Psychiatry,* 43, 255-262.

Katz, S. K. Lavack, A. M. (2002). Tobacco related bar promotions: insights from tobacco industry documents. *Tobacco Control,* 11(suppl I), i92-i101.

Kear, M. (2002). Psychosocial determinants of cigarette smoking among college students. *J. of Community Health Nursing,* 19(4), 245-257.

Kenford, S., Smith, S. S., Wetter, D., Jorenby, D., Fiore, M. and Baker, T. (2002). Predicting relapse back to morning: Contrasting affective and physical models of dependence. *J. of Consulting Clinical Psychology, 70*, 216-227.

Lantz, P. (2003). Smoking on the rise among young adults: implications for research and policy. *Tobacco Control, 12* ((Suppl 1)), i60-i70.

Ling, P. M. Glantz, S. A. (2002). Why and how the tobacco industry sells cigarettes to young adults: evidence from industry documents. *Am. J. Public Health, 92*, 908-916.

Luepker, R. V., Pallonen, U. E., Murray, D. M. and Pirie, P. L. (1989). Validity of telephone surveys in assessing cigarette smoking in young adults. *American Journal of Public Health, 79*(2), 202-204.

Mayhew, K., Flay, B. and Mott, J. (2000). Stages in the development of adolescent smoking. *Drug and Alcohol Dependence, 59*(Suppl 1), S61-S81.

Miller, W. Rollnick, S. (1991). Motivational Interviewing: *Preparing People to Change Addictive Behaviours.* New York, NY: Guilford Press.

Miller, W. R. Rollnick, S. (2002). Motivational interviewing: *Preparing people for change* (2nd editon). New York: Guilford Press.

Morrell, H. E., Cohen, L. M., Bacchi, D. and West, J. (2005). Predictors of smoking and smokeless tobacco use in college students: a preliminary study using web-based survey methodology. *J. Am. Coll. Health, 54*(2), 108-115.

Morris, J. F. Temple, W. (1985). Spirometric "Lung Age" estimation for motivating smoking cessation. *Preventive Medicine, 14*, 655-662.

Moss, J., C.T. (1979). Role of the specialties in family practice teaching: A family practitioner's view. *Journal of the Medical Association of the State of Alabama, 48*, 11-12.

Murphy-Hoefer, R., Griffith, R., Pederson, L. L., Crossett, L., Iyer, S. R. and Hiller, M. D. (2005). A review of interventions to reduce tobacco use in colleges and universities. *Am. J. Prev. Med, 28*(2), 188-200.

Ockene, I. M., N. (1997). Cigarette smoking, cardiovascular disease, and stroke. *Circulation, 96*, 3243-3247.

Olsen, G. W., Shellenberger, R. J., Lacy, S. E., Fishbeck, W. A. and Bond, G. G. (1990). A smoking cessation incentive program for chemical employees: design and evaluation. *Am. J. Prev. Med, 6*(4), 200-207.

Pallonen, U., Murray, D. M., Schmid, L., Pirie, P. and Luepker, R. (1990). Patterns of self-initiated smoking cessation among young adults. *Health Psychology, 9*(4), 418-426.

Prochaska, J. O., DiClemente, C. C. and Norcross, J. C. (1992). In search of how people change: Applications to addictive behaviors. *American Psychologist, 47*(9), 1102-1114.

Prochaska, J. O., Velicer, W. F., Rossi, J. S., Goldstein, M. G., Marcus, B. H., Rakowski, W., Fiore, C., Harlow, L. L., Redding, C. A., Rosenbloom, D. and Rossi, S. R. (1994). Stages of change and decisional balance for 12 problem behaviors. *Health Psychol, 13*(1), 39-46.

Prokhorov, A. V., Emmons, K. M., Pallonen, U. E. and Tsoh, J. Y. (1996). Respiratory response to cigarette smoking among adolescent smokers: a pilot study. *Prev. Med, 25*(5), 633-640.

Prokhorov, A. V., Pallonen, U. E., Niaura, R. and Prochaska, J. O. (1994). Nicotine dependence in vocational school students and adults. *Annals of Behavioral Medicine, 16*, 115S.

Prokhorov, A. V., Warneke, C., de Moor, C., Emmons, K. M., Mullin Jones, M., Rosenblum, C., Hudmon, K. S. and Gritz, E. R. (2003). Self-reported health status, health vulnerability, and smoking behavior in college students: implications for intervention. *Nicotine Tob. Res,* 5(4), 545-552.

Revill, J. Drury, C. G. (1980). An assessment of the incidence of cigarette smoking in fourth year school children and the factors leading to its establishment. *Public Health,* 94(4), 243-260.

Ridner, S. L. (2005). Predicting smoking status in a college-age population. *Public Health Nursing,* 22(6), 494-505.

Rigotti, N., Moran, S. and Wechsler, H. (2005). US College Students' exposure to tobacco promotions: prevalence and association with tobacco use. *Am. J. of Public Health,* 95(1), 138-144.

Rigotti, N. A., Lee, J. E. and Wechsler, H. (2000). US college students' use of tobacco products: results of a national survey. *Journal of the American Medical Association,* 284(6), 699-705.

Rimpelä, A. Teperi, J. (1989). Respiratory symptoms and low tar cigarette smoking: A longitudinal study on young people. *Scandinavian Journal of Social Medicine,* 17(2), 151-156.

Rollnick, S., Heather, N. and Bell, A. (1992). Negotiating behaviour change in medical settings: the development of brief motivational interviewing. *Journal of Mental Health,* 1, 25-37.

Rosenstock, I. M. (1974). The health belief model and preventative health behavior. *Health Education Quarterly,* 11, 1-47.

Rosenstock, I. M. (1990). The health belief model: explaining health behavior through expectancies. San Francisco: Jossey-Bass. SAS Institute, I. Carey, NC.

Schlunberg, J., Maggs, J., Long, S., Sher, K., Gotham, H., Kivlahan, D., Marlatt, G. and Zucker, R. (2001). The problem of college drinking: insights from a developmental perspective. *Alcoholism: Clinical and Experimental Research,* 25(3), 473-477.

Shopland, D. Burns, D. (1993). *Nicotine addiction: Principles and management.* New York: Oxford University Press.

Shopland, D., Burns, D., Garfinkel, L. and Samet, J. (1997). Changes in cigarette-related disease risks and their implications for prevention and control. Retrieved. from.

Stanton, W. R., Lowe, J. B. and Gillespie, A. M. (1996). Adolescents' experiences of smoking cessation. *Drug Alcohol Depend,* 43(1-2), 63-70.

Stockdale, M. S., Dawson-Owens, H. L. and Sagrestano, L. M. (2005). Social, attitudinal, and demographic correlates of adolescent vs college-age tobacco use initiation. *Am. J. Health Behav,* 29(4), 311-323.

Substance Abuse and Mental Health Services. (2006). Results from the 2005 national survey on drug use and health: National Findings. Office of Applied Studies, NSDUH Series H-30, DHHS Publication No. SMA 06-4194. Rockville, MD.

Sussman, S., Dent, C. W., Severson, H., Burton, D. and Flay, B. R. (1998). Self-initiated quitting among adolescent smokers. *Prev. Med,* 27(5 Pt 3), A19-28.

Tager, I. B., Minnoz, A., Rosner, B., Weiss, S. T., Carey, V. and Speizer, F. E. (1985). Effect of cigarette smoking on the pulmonary function of children and adolescents. *American Review of Respiratory Disease,* 131, 752-759.

Torabi, M. R., Yang, J. and Li, J. (2002). Comparison of tobacco use knowledge, attitude and practice among college students in China and the United States. *Health Promotion International,* 17, 247-254.

USDHHS. (1984). The health consequences of smoking, chronic obstructive lung disease: A Report of The Surgeon General. Rockville, MD: United States Department of Health and Human Services, Public Health Service, Centers for Disease Control, Center for Chronic Disease Prevention and Health Promotion. Office on Smoking and Health, United States Government Printing Office, DHHS Publication No. CDC 84-50205.

USDHHS. (1994). Preventing tobacco use among young people: A Report of The Surgeon General. Atlanta, GA: United States Department of Health and Human Service, Public Health Service, Centers for Disease Control and Prevention, National Center for Chronic Disease Prevention and Health Promotion, Office on Smoking and Health.

USDHHS. (2000). Reducing Tobacco Use: A Report of the Surgeon General. Atlanta, GA: US Department of Health and Human Services, Centers for Disease Control and Prevention, National Center for Chronic Disease Prevention and Health Promotion, Office on Smoking and Health.

USDHHS. (2003). Clearing the air: quit smoking today. NIH Publication No. 03-1647. Bethesda, MD: National Institutes of Health.

van Roosmalen, E. McDaniel, S. (1992). Adolescent smoking intentions: gender differences in peer context. *Adolescence,* 27(105), 87-105.

Velicer, W. F., DiClemente, C. C., Prochaska, J. O. and Brandenburg, N. (1985). Decisional balance measure for assessing and predicting smoking status. *Journal of Personality and Social Psychology,* 48(5), 1279-1289.

Velicer, W. F., DiClemente, C. C., Rossi, J. S. and Prochaska, J. O. (1990). Relapse situations and self-efficacy: An integrative model. *Journal of Addictive Behaviors,* 15(3), 271-283.

Velicer, W. F. Prochaska, J. O. (1999). An expert system intervention for smoking cessation. *Patient Education Couns,* 36(2), 119-129.

Velicer, W. F., Prochaska, J. O., Rossi, J. S. and Snow, M. G. (1992). Assessing outcome in smoking cessation studies. *Psychol. Bull,* 111(1), 23-41.

Von Ah, D., Ebert, S., Ngamvitroj, A. and Kang, D. (2005). Issues and innovators in nursing practices. Predictors of health behaviors in college students. *J. of Advanced Nursing,* 48(5), 463-474.

Wechsler, H., Kelley, K., Seibring, M., Kuo, M. and Rigotti, N. A. (2001). College smoking polilcies and smoking cessation programs: Results of a survey of college health center directors. *Journal of American College Health,* 49, 205-212.

Wechsler, H., Rigotti, N. A., Gledhill-Hoyt, J. and Lee, H. (1998). Increased levels of cigarette use among college students: a cause for national concern. *Journal of the American Medical Association,* 280(19), 1673-1678.

Windle, M. Windle, R. C. (2001). Depressive symptoms and cigarette smoking among middle adolescents: Prospective associations and intrapersonal and interpersonal influences. *Journal of Consulting and Clinical Psychology,* 69(2), 215-226.

Zhu, S., Sun, J., Billings, S. and Choi, W. (1999). Predictors of smoking cessation in U.S. adolescents. *American Journal of Preventive Medicine,* 16, 202-207.

In: Smoking Cessation: Theory, Interventions and Prevention   ISBN: 978-1-60021-591-9
Editor: Jerome E. Landow   © 2008 Nova Science Publishers, Inc.

Chapter 4

PHYSICIAN INTERVENTION FOR SMOKING CESSATION

Norman Hymowitz[*]

University of Medicine and Dentistry of New Jersey;
New Jersey Medical School, Newark, New Jersey, USA

I. INTRODUCTION

Since the first Surgeon General's report on smoking and health was published in 1964, there have been more than 12 million premature deaths attributable to smoking in the United States (American Cancer Society [ACS], 2006). In the United States, tobacco use is responsible for nearly one in five deaths, an estimated 438,000 premature deaths each year between 1997-2001 (ACS, 2006). In addition, it is estimated that another 8.6 million persons suffer from smoking-caused chronic conditions, including chronic bronchitis, emphysema, and cardiovascular disease. Moreover, smoking accounts for 30% of all cancer deaths and 87% of lung cancer deaths (ACS, 2006).

In 2003, the number of smokers in the world was estimated at about 1.3 billion people. This figure is expected to increase to at least 1.7 billion by 2025, with the doubling in the number of female smokers making the greatest contribution to the increase (ACS, 2006). In 2000, there were about 4.8 million smoking-related premature deaths worldwide, nearly evenly divided between developed and developing nations. Based on current patterns, smoking-attributable diseases will kill about 650 million of the world's 1.3 billion smokers alive today (ACS, 2003).

The *Healthy People 2010* objectives regarding adult tobacco use in the United States (U.S. Department of Health and Human Services [U.S. DHHS], 2000) are to reduce the prevalence of cigarette smoking to 12%, cigar smoking to 1.2%, use of smokeless tobacco to 0.4%, and to increase cessation attempts among adults to 75.0%. A Centers for Disease Control (CDC) report indicated lagging progress on all four objectives (Mariolis, Rock,

---

[*] Address for correspondence; University of Medicine and Dentistry of New Jersey, New Jersey Medical School; 183 South Orange Avenue; Newark, New Jersey 07103; (973) 972-54245; Hymowitz@umdnj.edu

Asman, et al., 2006). In 2005, approximately 20.9% of U.S. adults were current cigarette smokers, the same percentage as in 2004, suggesting that the 8-year decline in smoking prevalence among adults in the United States might be stalling, mirroring a similar lack of decline in smoking among adolescents since 2002 (Mochizuki-Kobayashi, Fishburn, Baptiste, et al., 2006). In addition, in 2005, an estimated 2.2% of U.S. adults were current cigar smokers, 2.3% used smokeless tobacco, and 42.5% of current cigarette smokers had stopped smoking for at least 1 day in the preceding 12 months because they were trying to quit. (Mariolis, et al., 2006).

These figures demand the attention of the medical and public health communities, and physicians, in particular, have a unique and important role to play in the anti-smoking arena. In the United States, they literally see about 70% of smokers each year (Burns, 1994), and some, such as pregnant women and parents of newborn babies, on numerous occasions. Obstetricians are uniquely positioned to encourage expectant mothers to quit smoking, and pediatricians may utilize well baby visits to counsel parents about the harmful effects of environmental tobacco smoke (ETS), to encourage mothers who quit smoking during their pregnancy to remain abstinent, and to help parents who smoke to quit. On other occasions, pediatricians may play a role in the prevention of smoking onset in children and adolescents and help young people who smoke to quit (cf. Stein, Haddock, O'Byrne, et al., 2000).

Other primary care physicians, as well as specialists, may take advantage of their position in society to influence the health behavior of patients of all ages, not only by encouraging cessation of all tobacco use, but by offering effective assistance. As health care providers, physicians have a solemn obligation to help patients avoid illness and promote good health as well as treating the infirmed. With respect to tobacco prevention and control, physicians have played a leadership role in identifying the harm caused by tobacco products, formulating policy and legislation to protect the public, and the management of tobacco addiction in office, clinic, and hospital settings. However, more must and can be done.

The purpose of the present chapter is to provide an overview of what can be accomplished by practicing physicians who address tobacco in clinical settings. The chapter is less of a critical review and critique of the existing literature on the efficacy and effectiveness of physician intervention (cf. Lancaster and Stead, 2004) and more of a commentary on how contemporary physicians' may use their growing armamentarium and state-of-the-art interventions to help patients quit smoking. In so doing, I present a historical perspective to highlight the foundations on which contemporary approaches to physician office-based intervention on tobacco stand.

II. HISTORICAL PERSPECTIVE

Medicinal Value of Tobacco

"...The leaves thereof being dried and brought into powder; they used to take the fume or smoke thereof by sucking it through pipes made of clay into their stomach and head: from whence it purgeth superfluous flame and other gross humors, openeth all the pores and passages of the body: by which means the use thereof, not only preserveth the body from obstructions: but also if any may be, so that they have not been too long continuance, in short time breaketh them: whereby their bodies are notably preserved in health, and know not many grievous diseases where withal we in England are often times afflicted..."

(Hariot, 1588; in Koskowski, 1955)

Tobacco has been used in primitive medicine since ancient times. The Cohuilla Indians of California used tobacco to ward off evil spirits named *Sespes*, which caused insomnia. Indians of other tribes chewed small pills of fresh tobacco leaves or the leaves themselves, enabling them to go without food and drink for several days. They believed that tobacco reinforced the heart and stomach, opened the bosom, removed mucous, killed worms, and calmed pain in bile colic. Tobacco was also administered against lice, and it was used to cure frostbite, burns, rashes, venereal ulcerations and malignant tumors. It was used to protect against poisoned arrows, as an analgesic, to neutralize the venom in wounds after the bite of a mad dog, and against fainting, gout, and oedema (Koskowski, 1955).

In 1597, John Gerard published *Herball*, a volume which was long considered a text-book of therapeutics (Koskowski, 1955). Gerard described the medicinal qualities of tobacco for the treatment of headache, rheumatism, "pain of the lungs", catarrh, and in removing humors. The English invented the tobacco enema, whereby tobacco smoke was puffed into the rectum. Boyle recommended the tobacco enema in the treatment of intestinal colic, and Dr. Hartman used tobacco water in the treatment of fever (Koskowski, 1955).

Among others who claimed medicinal properties for the tobacco plant were the 16th Century physicians Leibault and Gohury of Paris and Nicholas Nomartes from Sevilla (Van Lancker, 1977). The publications of these physicians contained tobacco-based recipes for external and internal use. Tobacco ointments, pastes and poultices were credited to cure ulcers, wounds, contusions, nolimetangere, scrofula, and scabies. Nomartes claimed to have cured headaches, coughs, asthma, gout, stomach pains, constipation, renal stones, flatulence, rheumatism, toothache and hemoptysis with either tobacco syrups, tobacco enemas or, in practically all cases, by inhalation of tobacco smoke (Van Lanker, 1977).

During the plague of London in 1665, tobacco chewing was considered the most effective prophylactic measure against infection. Physicians visiting their patients and gravediggers burying plague victims always smoked pipes during their work (Koskowski, 1955). In an effort to gain protection against plague, all Eton boys were asked to smoke tobacco before entering their classrooms. Many years later, one Eton alumnus reported that he was never whipped so much in his life as he was one morning for not smoking (Apperson, 1914).

It was believed that not one London tobacconist died from that disease during the cholera epidemics of 1831, 1849, and 1866 (Apperson, 1914). Across the sea, 10 per cent of the population of Philadelphia died of yellow fever in the summer of 1793. Men, women, and children smoked strong cigars and drank beer as protection against the "American plague", and houses were fumigated with smoke produced from a mixture of gunpowder and tobacco (Koskowski, 1955).

Scientific and Medical Concerns

Early use of tobacco was not without its detractors. James I of England not only believed that tobacco did not have any medicinal properties; he compared its black smelly smoke to horrible vapors that exhale from hell (Van Lancker, 1977). In 1605, the king organized the first public debate on the effects of tobacco. Black brains and black viscera, allegedly obtained from the dead bodies of inveterate smokers, were produced for everyone to examine with horror (Van Lancker, 1977).

In 1642, the famous bull of Pope Urban VIII was published, condemning the use of tobacco, especially in churches (Koskowski, 1955). In Russia, by a decree of 1634, those who traded in tobacco were threatened with slitting the nose, castration, flogging, and banishment. In Turkey, the Emperor Ibrahim imposed heavy punishments in 1640, believing that use of tobacco might produce sterility and reduce a man's fighting quality. Comparable edicts were passed in Persia, Ethiopia, China, and Germany (Koskowski, 1955).

Scientific evidence against tobacco started to accumulate very early on (Adda and Lechene, 2004). In 1670, the Dutch anatomist Kerckring described the results of his autopsies of heavy smokers as follows: "The tongue of the cadaver is black and gives off an odor of poison; the trachea is coated with soot, like a cooking pot; the lungs are dried-out and almost friable. The corpse gives the overall impression that someone had lit a fire among the organs" (Adda and Lechene, 2004). In 1689, the Medical School of Paris examined the problem of tobacco smoking and its influence on the length of life. They concluded that smoking shortens life (Koskowski, 1955). A century later, the English physician, Jon Hill, published *Cautions Against the Immoderate Use of Snuff* (Hill, 1761). Hill observed that the consumption of snuff appeared to be associated with cancer of the nose. In 1795, an article appeared in a medical journal that linked pipe smoking with cancer of the lip (Terry, 1970). As noted by Adda and Lechene (2004), similar studies were conducted throughout the 18th and 19th centuries, but without causing any major stir. However, from the 1920s onwards, attitudes in the scientific and medical communities started to change.

Broders (1920) published an article in the *Journal of the American Medical Association* linking tobacco use and lip cancer, and Lombard and Doering (1928) reported in the *New England Journal of Medicine* that cancer was more common among smoking patients than among control groups. In a paper published in *Science*, Pearl (1938) showed that smokers do not live as long as non-smokers. In 1940, Muller reported a case-control study implicating a link between tobacco smoking and lung cancer in Germany, but the message was largely lost as the medical community was distracted by the disaster of World War II (Miller, 2005). Wynder and Graham (1950) published the results of a major epidemiological study definitively linking smoking to lung cancer, and Doll and Hill (1950) published a paper in the *British Medical Journal* reporting that heavy smokers are fifty times as likely as nonsmokers to develop cancer of the lung. In 1952, a *Reader's Digest* article entitled *Cancer by the Carton* was influential in informing the public of the connection between smoking and lung cancer (Norr, 1952).

Ten years later the Royal College of Physicians (1962) issued a landmark document that concluded, "Cigarette smoking is the most likely cause of the recent world-wide increase in deaths from lung cancer …is an important predisposing cause of the development of chronic bronchitis…probably increases the risk of dying from coronary heart disease…has an adverse effect on healing of [gastric and duodenal] ulcers…[and] may be a contributing factor in cancer of the mouth, pharynx, oesophagus, and bladder".

From November 1962 through December 1963, the United States Surgeon General's *Advisory Committee on Smoking and Health* held meetings in which they reviewed more than 7000 publications pertaining to smoking and health, including more than 3000 articles published after 1950 (U.S. DHHS, 1989). The final *Report of the Advisory Committee* was released on January 11, 1964 (United States Public Health Service [U.S. PHS], 1964). The *Report* concluded that "Cigarette smoking is causally related to lung cancer in men; the magnitude of the effect of cigarette smoking far outweigh all other factors. The data for women, though less extensive, point in the same direction.... The risk of developing lung cancer increases with duration of smoking and the number of cigarettes smoked per day, and is diminished by discontinuing smoking."

The *Report* also concluded that pipe smoking is causally related to lip cancer, cigarette smoking is causally linked to laryngeal cancer in men, and cigarette smoking is the most common cause of chronic bronchitis. The *Advisory Committee* identified significant associations between smoking and cancer of the esophagus, cancer of the urinary bladder, coronary artery disease, emphysema, peptic ulcer disease, and low- birth weight babies. However, the *Committee* did not consider the available data to be sufficient to label these associations causal (U.S. DHHS, 1989).

The *1964 Report of the Advisory Committee* heralded an anti-smoking movement in the United States that is still very much alive today. The *1964 Report* was followed by a series of *Reports* that further elucidated the relationship between smoking and health, the addictive nature of nicotine, specific effects on the young, women, and minorities, as well as the adverse consequences of environmental tobacco smoke (ETS). Governmental and voluntary agencies, as well as private citizens and other entities, embarked on campaigns to inform and educate the public about the harm of tobacco use and exposure to tobacco smoke to help smokers and users of other forms of tobacco to quit, to prevent the onset of tobacco use in the young, and to create an environment in which non-smokers are protected from the harmful effects of involuntary tobacco smoke. Physicians and others in the medical community played a leadership role in these endeavors, with former Surgeon General, C. Everett Koop, M.D., declaring that cigarette smoking was the single most important preventable cause of morbidity and mortality in our society and the most important public health problem of our time (U.S. DHHS, 1989).

III. PHYSICIAN INTERVENTION

The Physician's Role

In 1968, Donald Fredrickson, MD, Director, Smoking Control Program, New York City Department of Health, stated, "The overwhelming weight of scientific evidence clearly establishes cigarette smoking as a grave threat to personal health. This unpleasant fact can no longer be ignored. Nor can we deny that as physicians we forfeit an unparalleled opportunity to practice highly effective preventive medicine when we fail to counsel all patients and, in particular, younger patients, on the dangers of smoking" (Fredrickson, 1968). Mausner and Mausner (1967), Russell (1971), and Steinfeld (1972) were among the early leaders in the field who similarly stressed the important role that physicians may play, a call echoed more recently by former Surgeon General Koop (1985) and former Secretary of Health and Human Services Sullivan (1990).

Fredrickson (1968) encouraged physicians to serve as nonsmoking role models, to be informed about the adverse health effects of smoking, to take advantage of clinical opportunities or teachable moments to deliver personalized health messages, to utilize pamphlets and other resources to support educational and behavior change interventions, and to utilize nurses and other office personnel in the anti-smoking effort. These recommendations still hold true today, as witnessed by the fact that the medical profession has led all others in quitting smoking (Glynn, Manley, and Mecklenburg, 1994); efforts to inform physicians about tobacco now take place in Medical School (Kristeller and Ockene, 1996; Ferry, Grissino, and Runfola, 1999), residency training (Ockene, Quirk, Goldberg, et al., 1988; Humair and Cornuz, 2003; Hymowitz, Schwab, Haddock, et al, 2004) and continuing medical education (Lindsay, Ockene, Hymowitz, et al., 1994; Borrelli, 2006). The concept of clinical opportunities or teachable moments for addressing tobacco is now well entrenched (U.S. DHHS, 1992; McBride, Emmons, and Lipkus, 2003), as is the treatment of tobacco use as a vital sign (Fiore, 1991). Implementation of office *systems* to enhance and coordinate smoking cessation efforts (cf., Duncan, Stein, and Cummings, 1991; Fiore, Bailey, Cohen, et al., 2000), use of nurses and office staff to enhance intervention and follow-up (Hurt, Dale, Fredrickson, et al., 1994), and the use of educational and quit smoking material available in print (e.g., Glynn and Manley, 1995) and electronic media (e.g., Gerbert, Berg-Smith, Mancuso, et al., 2003) to support physician smoking cessation efforts is now common practice.

Recognizing the unique nature of the physician-patient relationship, Fredrickson (1968) advocated genuine empathy and understanding to motivate and win over patients, and he emphasized the need to take advantage of subsequent office visits for follow-up and reinforcement. Frederickson (1968), Russell (1971), and Mausner and Mausner (1967) viewed the smoking cessation process as one of relearning; involving three basic steps (motivation, implementing systematic behavior change strategies, and reinforcement). Based on the available scientific literature of the time (cf. Bernstein, 1969), they recommended behavior modification strategies to help patients quit smoking (e.g., self monitoring of smoking behavior, identifying and coping with smoking "triggers", developing alternative/substitute behaviors, preparing for a quit date, and obtaining support for remaining abstinent). These and other behavioral strategies for helping patients stop smoking can readily be accommodated in busy office/clinic settings, and are very much in vogue today (Hymowitz, 1999; 2005).

Early Studies

In the 1960s and early 70s, the theoretical and empirical basis for how best to help people quit smoking was in its infancy, the concept of nicotine replacement therapy (NRT) had yet to fully emerge, and the application of patient-centered and motivational interviewing techniques to tobacco prevention and control was virtually unknown. However, concerns about the adverse health effects of cigarette smoking and other forms of tobacco use were mounting, and more than 50% of America's adults smoked cigarettes. While the early studies of physician intervention on tobacco lacked the methodological and scientific rigor that we have come to expect today (Lichtenstein and Danaher, 1976; Pederson, 1982), they are important from a historical point of view. They formed the foundation for research activities that continue today, and they planted the seeds that underlie current approaches to tobacco prevention and control in office, clinic, and hospital settings.

Mausner, Mausner, and Rial (1968) were among the first to study the influence of physician advice on the smoking behavior of patients. Previous work (Bass and Wilson, 1964) showed that telephone messages from a "safety organization" and letters from a pediatrician were relatively ineffective in influencing people to purchase seat belts for their automobiles. However, a brief recommendation about seat belts by a pediatrician during a routine office visit proved quite successful. Mausner, et al. (1968) sought to determine if the physician's influence similarly extended to smoking behavior.

Two general practice (GP) physicians who shared office facilities delivered the intervention. One, the "control physician," did not specifically address tobacco. The other, the "study physician", asked whether the patient smoked and indicated that smoking is harmful to health. He also distributed a pamphlet with instruction on how to stop smoking and a supply of Nicoban, a lobeline preparation (Mausner, et al., 1968). The two groups were similar with respect to demographics, although the "study group" contained a greater proportion of heavy smokers than the comparison group. Despite this, telephone interviews 1 week and 3 months later showed that a greater proportion of smokers in the study group (33% at 3 months; 31/93) reduced their smoking (either quit or reduced smoking by one-half pack of cigarettes or more per day) than in the control group (9% at 3 months; 3/32).

A study by Williams (1969) involving a series of patients in a chest clinic at Whittington Hospital, London, also underscored the importance of physician advice. Only patients who smoked 10 or more cigarettes per day were included in the study. The participants were either new patients or patients who had never been advised to give up smoking previously by clinic staff. The study extended over 9 months, with a follow-up of 6 months. Patients were advised by their physician to quit smoking. While the physician saw them again at subsequent visits, no further discussion of smoking ensued.

Of the 160 participants for whom information was available for 6 months, 59 (37%) reported that they quit smoking, 39 (24%) reduced their intake by half, 41 (26%) relapsed after either quitting or cutting down, and 21 (13%) made little or no change in smoking (Williams, 1969). Of the 59 patients who were not smoking at the 6-month follow-up, 37 (23%) quit immediately following the initial interview. These results, like those of Mausner, et al. (1968), support the value of physician intervention on smoking, although failure to employ a no-treatment control group, to use an objective measure of smoking, and to adequately deal with follow-up issues compromises the confidence one may place in the study outcome.

Pincherle and Wright (1970) compared the success rate of individual doctors who provided annual physical examinations for business executives at the Institute of Directors' Medical Centre in England. All doctors were encouraged to be "evangelistic in this matter and a fierce and factual anti-smoking booklet was available for distribution." After the initial examination and advice from the physician to quit smoking, 24% of the 1,493 smokers who had returned at least once for a repeat visit a year or more afterwards reported that they stopped or reduced smoking by 30% or more. The success rate in helping smokers quit or "cut down" by the 10 doctors who saw the group varied from 17% to 35%. The authors concluded, "This variation is statistically significant and indicates that individual doctors might benefit by studying the effectiveness of the way in which they advise their patients," an issue that continues to receive considerable attention today.

Burt, Illingworth, Shaw, et al. (1974) studied smoking cessation after myocardial infarction. One hundred and twenty-five survivors of acute myocardial infarction were given detailed explanation followed by firm advice to stop smoking. This was reinforced by written advice and follow-up. Sixty-two percent of the patients reported that they stopped smoking and were still abstinent 1-3 years later. In a similar group of 85 patients who were treated in the same coronary care unit but thereafter given conventional advice and not followed-up, 27.5% were non-smokers 1-3 years later. The authors attributed their impressive results to "a forceful approach by the physician after he had established a personal relationship with the patient, support by the junior medical and the nursing staff, reinforcement of the advice at intervals in a follow-up clinic together, in many cases, with a visit to the home by a health visitor".

Lichtenstein and Danaher (1976), Pederson (1982), and Schwartz (1987) provide excellent reviews and critiques of these and other early studies. In addition to noting the need for more methodological rigor, they observed that smoking intervention was more effective in patients with frank disease and symptoms than in patients that were disease and symptom-free. This observation is still true today and is consistent with the Health Belief Model (Becker, 1974) that holds that certain beliefs must be present before patients will make lasting changes in health behavior. Patients must (1) be aware of the harm that cigarettes and other forms of tobacco cause; (2) believe that they are vulnerable to these harms; (3) believe that there is something that can be done to prevent or reduce the harm; (4) believe that the treatment recommended by the physician is effective; and (5) believe that the perceived costs of making the changes do not outweigh the perceived benefits.

Most smokers cite health improvement as a reason for stopping (Duncan, Cummings, Hudes, et al., 1992), and a recent survey of primary care patients showed that those who believed their symptoms were related to smoking were significantly more motivated to try to quit than those who did not (Coleman, Barrett, Wynn, et al., 2003). As such, visits to physician offices are ripe with opportunities to take advantage of teachable moments (McBride, et al., 2003). Quit rates and desire to quit smoking for patients diagnosed with heart disease (Freund, D'Agustino, Belanger, 1992) and head and neck cancer (Gritz, Carr, Rapkin, et al., 1991) may exceed 50%, as may quit smoking rates for pregnant women (McBride, Pirie, and Curry, 1992). However, the presence of a serious health event is no guarantee that a smoker will quit or remain abstinent. Most women who quit smoking during pregnancy return to smoking soon after their baby is born (McBride, Curry, and Lando, 1999), and when patients with frank disease begin to feel better, it is all too easy for them to believe that *this* particular cigarette will not tip the balance. By the same token, preventive efforts aimed at helping patients stop smoking before they develop frank disease are not as successful as one would like. Denial is a common defense mechanism, and smokers who quit and relapse many times may be reluctant to try again. Physicians would do well to ascertain whether the appropriate health beliefs are in place before concluding that their recommendations for quitting smoking, even with high risk and ill patients, will be followed.

Recent Studies

Interest in the role of physicians in tobacco prevention and control increased dramatically from the 1960s to the present, as did the methodological rigor of the research studies (e.g., random assignment of subjects to experimental conditions, more attention to sample size and follow-up issues, use of objective measures of smoking status, etc.). Physician intervention moved beyond *advice* to include *assistance* for stopping smoking in the form of brief behavioral interventions, self-help quit smoking materials, and/or the use of pharmacological therapy, such as NRT and Bupropion (cf. Frishman, Mitta, Kupersmith, et al., 2006).

Russell, Wilson, Taylor, et al. (1979) carried out an important and influential study in which they assessed the effects of GPs' advice against smoking. Twenty-eight doctors in five group practices in London took part. The sample comprised all cigarette smokers aged 16 or more who attended the surgeries to see a doctor during a specific 4-week period. A total of 2138 eligible cigarette smokers participated, of whom 88% provided data at 1-month follow-up and 73% provided data at one year.

Patients were assigned to one of four groups based on the day they attended the practice (Russell, et al., 1979). Group 1 comprised non-intervention controls; group 2, questionnaire-only controls; group 3, advice by the GP to stop smoking; and group 4, advice to stop smoking, a leaflet on how to stop smoking, and follow-up. The advice to stop smoking was simple and firm. It was given in the doctors' own style over one or two minutes during the routine consultation. Validation of self-reported outcome was obtained in a small sample of patients (n = 23) by measuring nicotine concentrations in saliva. Of the 14 patients who reported that they stopped smoking, the salivary nicotine level was consistent with no smoking in all but one patient, yielding a deception rate of 7% (Russell, et al., 1979).

The quit rates for the four groups at 1-month follow-up were: Group 1, 3.0%; Group 2, 3.0%; Group 3, 4.6%; and Group 4, 7.5%. Compared to the controls (Groups 1 and 2), participants in Group 4 were significantly more likely to stop smoking at one month. Data for Year 1 were as follows: Group 1, 10.3%; Group 2, 14.0%; Group 3: 16.7%; and Group 4, 19.1%. It is noteworthy that 5.1% of the patients in Group 4 stopped smoking at 1 month and remained abstinent through 1 year (Russell, et al., 1979).

Russell, et al. (1979) noted that GPs in Great Britain see over 18 million of the 20 million smokers in Britain at least once every five years, and most of them much more often. The potential of GPs working collectively to address smoking in their practices is so immense that a modest annual smoking cessation success rate of 5% nationally would have a dramatic effect on the health of the nation. The public health implications of this study were not lost on those in the United States (cf. Glynn, et al., 1994), Australia (cf., Wilson, Wakefield, Steven, et al., 1990; Richmond, 1994), and elsewhere around the globe.

When one adds pharmacotherapy, self-help quit smoking aids, such as books, CDs, computer programs, telephone counseling, telephone "hot lines", personalized computer-generated reports, and serialized quit materials or modules mailed in installments, to the physician's armamentarium, the success rates achieved by GPs and others in office, clinic, or hospital settings may be significantly enhanced (cf. Orleans, 1993). For physicians who are able to devote more time to smoking cessation efforts, quit rates may approach, if not exceed, the levels of success that are typically achieved in formal intensive quit smoking programs.

Rose and Hamilton (1978) carried out a randomized control trial of the effect on middle-aged men of advice to stop smoking. The participants were drawn from men who had undergone a cardio respiratory screening examination in the Whitehall study of male civil servants in London. Fourteen hundred and forty-five high-risk men entered the trial, and they were allocated randomly to the intervention group (714 men) or "normal care" control group (731 men).

For men in the "normal care" group, a full report of the screening results was sent to their general physician. The men were not aware that they were participating in a trial. At 1- and 3-year points in the study, they were asked to return for an examination to help the research. Men in the intervention group received a letter inviting them to a 15-minute visit with one of the study doctors. There were no defaulters. At the visit, the doctor talked with them about the risks that smoking posed and the benefits that would accrue if they quit. The doctor briefly reviewed some of the "practicalities" of stopping, urged the men to consider quitting smoking, gave them two booklets, and invited them to return in one week.

By the second visit, about half of the men reported quitting smoking. Of all the men who stopped within the first year, 80% did so immediately after the first interview (Rose and Hamilton, 1978). Unfortunately, the study did not include an objective measure of smoking status. For those that did not quit, the doctors answered questions, discussed techniques for stopping, and distributed smoking "report cards" to be completed daily and returned after three weeks. On receiving it, the doctors sent a personal reply. Further 15-minute interviews took place at the 10-week and 6-month points, with intervening use of record cards and replies where appropriate.

Examinations of men in both groups were carried out at 1 and 3 years. The follow-up rates were 81% and 64% at years 1 and 3, respectively, for the Intervention Group and 86% and 70% at years 1 and 3, respectively, for the Normal Care Group. Quit rates, whether conservatively based on intent to treat (include all subjects enrolled in the study) or on responders only, were superior for men assigned to the Intervention Group (intent to treat, 51% and 36% at years 1 and 3; responders only, 63% and 58% at years 1 and 3). For the Normal Care Group, the quit rates were about 10% and 14%, at years 1 and 3, respectively, for the analyses based on intent to treat as well as on those who responded.

In a study conducted in Sydney, Australia, Richmond and Webster (1985), 200 smoking patients were randomly assigned to one of two conditions. One group (n=100) received a brief but structured multi-component behavioral change intervention consisting of six visits to a GP over a 6-month period: one assessment, one patient education, and four follow-up visits. The control group received no intervention.

At the first visit, the patient's weight, height, and lung function were measured, a sample of blood was taken for measurement of tobacco products (cotinine, carboxyhemoglobin, and thiocyanate), and a detailed smoking history was taken by a research assistant. The patient was asked by the doctor to use a daily diary to monitor smoking behavior over the following week. At the second visit, one week later, the doctor delivered a personalized health message using the patient's blood and lung function test results, and he/she gave the patients a self-help quit smoking booklet. The latter contained suggestions for modifying cigarette smoking and preparing for a quit date, managing weight gain and stress, and remaining cigarette-free. The doctor also offered advice on how to cope with withdrawal symptoms and encouraged patients to attend follow-ups at 1 and 3 weeks and 3 and 6 months.

The point prevalence biochemical validated abstinence rates at 6 months were 33% for the treatment group and 3% for the control group, a highly significant difference. Follow-up at 3 years yielded a point prevalence abstinent rate for the treatment group of 36%, while the continuous abstinence rate at 3 years was 23%. The point prevalence and continuous abstinence rates at 3 years for a second control group were 3% and 2%, respectively. Among the 37% who self-selected to complete the treatment program by attending all of the sessions,

57% were abstinent at 3 years compared to 23% for those who did not attend all of the follow-up sessions (Richmond and Webster, 1985).

The quit rates for the treatment groups obtained in the studies by Rose and Hamilton (1978) and Richmond and Webster (1985) far exceed those of the typical physician-office interventions which feature advice and/or brief interventions for smoking cessation in patients without frank disease or symptoms. The reason for this probably lies in the intensity of the physician intervention effort. Patients were seen on multiple occasions, and Treatment Group physicians used lung function and other health data to support a personalized approach to patient education and advice. They also provided instruction and material on how to quit smoking and a series of follow-up sessions to help patients cope with withdrawal symptoms and lapses.

While more may be better, there is a general recognition that physicians rarely have time for intensive intervention on tobacco in busy office, clinic, and hospital settings. In 1984, the United States National Cancer Institute (NCI) supported five randomized controlled trials aimed at the development of brief intervention protocols for physicians and dentists to use in treating patients who smoke (Glynn, et al., 1994). The trials involved more than 30,000 patients and 1000 physicians and dentists, and they were conducted in a variety of outpatient medical and dental settings (private offices, public clinics, health maintenance organizations, and residency training programs).

In all but one trial, entire practices were randomized, not individual patients. In the experimental practices, clinicians and other clinical staff were trained in smoking cessation techniques. In the control practices, no training was provided. All the trials examined long-term (12 months) cessation rates, and patients who claimed to have stopped smoking were treated as smokers unless cessation was biochemically validated. The interventions used by the clinicians were brief, and best described as "clinician-guided self-help programs". Brief counseling, use of self-help stop smoking booklets, and some use of nicotine gum were the common intervention techniques. Two studies incorporated office reminder systems to increase the compliance of clinicians and other staff in the use of smoking cessation protocols (Glynn, et al., 1994).

In all the trials, the clinicians who were trained in smoking cessation techniques used them. In comparison with untrained clinicians, trained clinicians were more likely to advise patients to quit smoking and to ask their patients to select a specific quit date. Trained clinicians prescribed nicotine gum more appropriately, and their patients were more likely to use the gum correctly (Glynn, et al., 1994).

Smoking cessation rates were calculated for entire practices, not for individual patients (i.e., all smokers seen in a practice, not just those who received advice and intervention from the clinician). While there was considerable variability among the studies, cessation rates of up to 15% were obtained. Training in brief intervention techniques alone did not significantly alter smoking cessation rates among patients. Only when trained clinicians were routinely reminded to intervene with all smoking patients through chart stickers or other mechanisms did smoking cessation rates among patients increase significantly (Glynn, et al., 1994).

Based on these results, the National Cancer Institute (NCI) recommended the following clinical interventions: Ask all patients about smoking; Advise smokers to stop; Assist their efforts with self-help materials, and possible nicotine replacement; and Arrange follow-up (Glynn and Manley, 1995). The NCI also recommended changes in office procedures that will increase significantly the clinician's effectiveness in treating patients who smoke. These include selecting an office coordinator, making the office smoke-free, systematically identifying and monitoring smokers, and involving staff members with follow-up support.

Russell, Merriman, Stapleton, et al. (1983) carried out a study to determine whether the offer and prescription of nicotine chewing gum would enhance the efficacy of GP's advice to stop smoking. A sample of 1938 cigarette smokers who attended the surgeries of 34 GPs in 6 group practices were assigned by week of attendance (in a balanced design) to one of three conditions: nonintervention control, advice plus booklet, and advice, plus booklet, plus nicotine chewing gum (Nicorette 2 mg). Follow-up visits were scheduled at 4 months and 1 year, and smoking status was verified by measurement of expired air carbon monoxide (Russell, et al., 1983).

The proportion of subjects who were abstinent at 4 months and were still abstinent at 1 year was 3.9%, 4.1%, and 8.8% for advice only, advice plus booklet, and advice plus booklet plus nicotine gum, respectively. The percentages were based on all cigarette smokers enrolled in the study, including those who did not wish to stop and those in the nicotine gum group who did not try the gum (47%). The selected subgroup of 8% who used more than one box of 105 pieces of gum achieved a success rate of 24% (Russell, et al., 1983).

The literature on various forms of NRT (gum, transdermal patch, inhaler, nasal spray, lozenge) has since grown quite vast (Maseeh and Kwatra, 2005; Frishman, et al., 2006), and these medications have literally transformed physician office-based approaches to smoking cessation. The general consensus is that NRT and Bupropion lead to a doubling of quit rates obtained without the use of medication (Rennard and Daughton, 1998), and the impact is greatest when medication is combined with behavioral interventions and follow-up (Orleans, 1993).

Clinical Practice Guidelines

The Clinical Practice Guideline, entitled *Treating Tobacco Use and Dependence* (Fiore, et al., 2000), was based on the review and analysis of 6000 articles published between 1975 and 1999, and it recommended that physicians should offer an approved form of pharmacotherapy to all of their patients who want to stop smoking, except in the presence of special circumstances (e.g., patients with medical contraindications, those smoking fewer than 10 cigarettes per day, pregnant/breastfeeding women, and adolescent smokers). If pharmacotherapy is used with lighter smokers, clinicians should consider reducing the dose of first-line NRT pharmacotherapies. No adjustments are necessary when using Bupropion (Fiore, at al., 2000).

Five *first-line* pharmacotherapies were identified that reliably increase long-term smoking abstinences:

- Buproprion SR (Zyban)
- Nicotine gum
- Nicotine inhaler
- Nicotine nasal spray
- Nicotine patch.

Since the *Guidelines* were published, a nicotine lozenge was introduced and shown to be as effective as other nicotine products (Shiffman, Dresler, Hajek, et al., 2002; Maseeh and Kwatra, 2005). It is now FDA-approved as a smoking cessation aid. In addition, a new non-nicotine containing drug, Verinicline, a selective alpha-4-beta 2 nicotinic receptor partial agonist marketed by Pfizer as Chantix, has been shown to be as or more effective than Bupropion (Frishman, et al., 2006). It is also FDA-approved for use in smoking cessation.

Two *second-line* pharmacotherapies were identified as efficacious and may be considered by clinicians if first-line pharmacotherapies are not effective. They are Clonidine and Nortriptyline (Fiore, et al., 2000). In the near future, it is likely that many new pharmaceuticals, including vaccines and a variety of non-nicotine smoking cessation pharmacotherapies (Maseeh and Kwatra, 2005; Frishman, et al., 2006), will be added to physicians' armamentarium.

The *Guidelines* also suggest that physicians implement an office-wide system that ensures that, for every patient at every clinic visit, tobacco use status is queried and documented. To do this, physicians may have to call upon nurses and other office staff to assist with screening, intervention, and follow-up activities. Key steps for helping patients who are willing to try to quit smoking include:

- Help the patient with a quit plan (set a quit date, tell family, friends and coworkers about quitting, anticipate challenges to planned quit attempt, remove tobacco products from environment)
- Provide practical counseling (problem solving and skill acquisition)
- Provide intra-treatment social support
- Help patient obtain extra-treatment social support
- Recommend the use of approved pharmacotherapy, except in special circumstances
- Provide supplementary materials
- Schedule follow-up

The Clinical Practice Guideline also emphasized the use of the "5 A's" for brief intervention. They are:

- Ask about tobacco use (Identify and document tobacco use status for every patient at every visit)
- Advise to quit (In a clear, strong, and personalized manner, urge every tobacco user to quit)
- Assess willingness to make a quit attempt (Is the tobacco user willing to make a quit attempt at this time?)
- Assist in quit attempt (For the patient willing to make a quit attempt, use counseling and pharmacotherapy to help him or her quit)
- Arrange follow-up (Schedule follow-up contact, preferably within the first week after the quit date)

The addition of the *assess* step is important, because it encourages the physician to take into account the patient's willingness to try to quit smoking. This enables physicians to use their time more efficiently and to avoid the frustration that often results from trying to help patients stop smoking when they are not ready or willing. If the patient is not willing to try to stop smoking, physicians should not devote precious time and energy in the busy office environment encouraging the patient to select a quit date or teaching the smoker how to use NRT. Similarly, if the patient is willing to try to quit, it may not be necessary to devote time to educating the patient about the harm of smoking and benefits of quitting. Instead, physicians may address motivation and barriers to quitting in the former case and how best to quit in the latter. In addition, it is no longer necessary to evaluate the success of every encounter with a smoker on the basis of whether or not the patient quit smoking. Rather, a successful encounter may be viewed as one in which the doctor-patient interchange leads to an increase in the patient's *willingness* or *readiness* for quitting smoking, even if, at first, the doctor simply plants the seed that causes the patient to think differently about continuing to smoke or quitting.

For the patient unwilling to quit, the *Guidelines* recommend use of a brief motivational intervention ("5 R's") (Fiore, et al., 2000). These include:

- Relevance (why quitting is personally relevant to this particular patient)
- Risks (ask patient to identify negative consequences of smoking)
- Rewards (ask patient to identify potential benefits of stopping smoking)
- Roadblocks (ask the patient to identify barriers or impediments to quitting and note elements of treatment [problem solving, weight management, pharmacotherapy] that could address barriers
- Repetition (repeat motivational intervention every time the unmotivated patient visits the clinic/office)

For patients who recently quit smoking, the physician should take a few minutes to encourage and support continued abstinence (Fiore, et al., 2000). The *Guidelines* suggest using open-ended questions to facilitate discussion of the benefits of quitting and ways in which the patient can continue his/her success (e.g., *"How has stopping helped you"*, *"How are you dealing with weight gain"*, *"What problems do you anticipate"* *"How might you cope with them"*). The physician may encourage the patient to engage in brainstorming or problem-solving exercises to cope with potential obstacles to remaining abstinent.

The theoretical underpinnings for this approach derive from the seminal work of Prochaska and his colleagues (Prochaska and DiClemente, 1983; DiClemente, Prochaska, Fairhurst, et al., 1991; Prochaska, Velicer, Rossi, 1994) who view smoking cessation as a process in which smokers cycle through a series of stages, often many times in their lifetime, before finally quitting smoking for good. Depending on the patient's stage of change, he/she will be more or less ready (or willing) to try to stop smoking. The physician's task is to assess stage of change, utilize an intervention that is appropriate for that particular stage (stage-dependent intervention), and attempt to move the patient along the continuum of change (i.e., from a stage in which a patient may not even be thinking about stopping smoking [*pre-contemplation*], to one in which they are considering stopping but may be quite ambivalent about it [*contemplation*], and, ultimately, to one where they actually take steps to modify their behavior [*preparation, action*] or remain cigarette-free [*maintenance*]).

Motivational Interviewing

Assessing stage of change and utilizing stage-dependent interventions within the context of a busy office setting may appear a bit daunting to physicians who are not familiar with state-of-the-art interviewing techniques, behavioral interventions for smoking modification, and factors that increase the likelihood of quitting (i.e., degree of nicotine addiction, level of education, support from spouse or others, etc.) or the return to smoking once the smoker quits (i.e., withdrawal symptoms, stress, weight gain, lack of support, etc.). Motivational Interviewing (Botelho and Skinner, 1995; Miller and Rollnick, 1991; Lockyear, 2004) enables the doctor to build upon his/her relationship with the patient and to create an atmosphere that will enhance prospects for successful interaction and behavior change. It is based upon a person-centered approach to doctor-patient communication (cf. Levenstein, McCracken, McWhinney, et al., 1986) and a *partnership model* (Denmark, 2004) in which the patient accepts responsibility for change and becomes a full participant in treatment planning. Important goals of motivational-interviewing are to help patients resolve ambivalence in a way that increases their willingness to try to quit smoking and to create an environment in which patients feel free to share their concerns about changing or not changing behavior (cf. Borelli, 2006). The doctor must be prepared to *roll* with resistance and to encourage patients who are not yet ready for change to carefully weigh the costs and benefits of changing and not changing their behavior (Decision Balance) (Miller and Rollnick, 1991).

While each patient has a different *story* to tell, open-ended questions, careful listening, empathy, genuine concern, a non-judgmental attitude and the ability to reframe and summarize what the patient is saying enable doctors who are neither experts in smoking cessation nor totally familiar with the patient to encourage discussion and to take advantage of the resources that patient's bring to bear. Seventy to eighty percent of smokers, young and old, have tried to quit smoking in the past (Hymowitz, 2005). They have a good sense of factors that influence their behavior, what works for them and what does not, what went wrong in the past, and what they must do differently in the future. Open-ended questions, such as *"What are your thoughts about stopping smoking", "What was it like for you when you quit smoking in the past", "What caused you to return to smoking", "What will it take for you to give stopping smoking another try", "What obstacles do you foresee"*, and *"How might you deal with them"*, foster patient participation and enable the doctor to gain insight into the issues at hand, assess willingness to change, learn about patients' health beliefs, and work with the patient to develop a treatment plan. While motivational-interviewing may add a few minutes to the doctor-patient encounter, the benefits, in terms of physician and patient satisfaction and enhanced likelihood of success, far outweigh the costs.

Patients that never quit smoking in the past also have interesting stories to tell, and it is not difficult to draw them into a discussion concerning their views on smoking and quitting, perceived barriers and issues, and possible resources that may help them when they decide to try quitting smoking. Scaling questions, such as *"On a scale of "1" to "10", where "1" means not very motivated and "10" means very motivated, how motivated are you to quit smoking"*, often are effective ways to encourage patient participation and to gain insight into motivation for change. As the reader might imagine, a good follow-up question might be *"What will it take to increase your motivation"*. By drawing patients into a discussion, using the patient as a resource, and allowing them to participate in the development of a stage-dependent treatment plan, the doctor need not be an *expert* in smoking cessation to facilitate patients' quit attempts. Yet, he/she can become a very effective agent of change and *facilitator* of smoking cessation.

A similar approach also may be effective in helping parents create a smoke-free environment for their children, preventing the onset of smoking in young people, and preventing the return to smoking in postpartum women who quit smoking during pregnancy. In each case, the physician may utilize the "5As" algorithm, assess stage of change, and employ open-ended questions to encourage the patient (or parent of the patient) to identify factors that facilitate or hinder change and join with the physician in developing a stage-dependent treatment plan.

The *partnership model* fosters a sense of self-efficacy in the patient, and patients who participate in the development of a treatment plan are more likely to "buy into" and adhere to the plan of action. They also are more likely to be satisfied with the office visit, whether the visit focused on smoking cessation, diet, or other health behaviors (Simpson, Buckman, Stewart, et al., 1991).

While many physicians may not feel comfortable about addressing tobacco (Cantor, Baker, and Hughes, 1993), formal training programs have been shown to enhance physicians' confidence and increase their likelihood of addressing tobacco in clinical practice (Cabana, Rand, Slish, et al., 2004). The basic tenets of person-centered and motivational interviewing, as well as an emphasis on *active* learning (e.g., role playing, modeling, behavioral rehearsal), now form an important component of training for medical students and residents (Ockene, Quirk, Goldberg, et al., 1988; Cornuz, Humair, Seematter, et al., 2002; Humair and Cornuz, 2003; Lee, Hishinuma, Derauf, et al., 2004; Hymowitz, 2006), as well as for physicians in clinical practice (Ockene and Zapka, 2000; Borelli, 2006). It is anticipated that future physicians who undergo formal training in person-centered or motivational interviewing will be better prepared to address tobacco and other health behaviors in clinical settings.

IV. CONCLUSION

Physicians have a unique and important role to play in the anti-smoking arena, and the need for future physicians to join the fray will not decrease any time soon. Worldwide tobacco-related deaths are expected to increase from about 4 million per year in 1999 to about 10 million per year by the 2030s. This is a higher death toll than is expected from malaria, maternal and major childhood conditions, and tuberculosis combined (American Cancer Society, 2003).

While rates of smoking in the United States have declined since the 1950s and 60s, the population has increased, surpassing 300 million people in recent months. The net result is that millions of Americans continue to smoke, young people start smoking every day, and the toll of tobacco-related morbidity and mortality remains at epidemic proportions. The tobacco industry spends in excess of 15 billion dollars per year in the United States alone on advertising and promotion efforts (Mariolis, Rock, Asman, et al., 2006), and it is unlikely that they will soon curtail their efforts to attract new smokers and maintain the old ones.

In 2002, Tommy G. Thompson, Secretary of the United States Department of Health and Human Services, requested that the United States Interagency Committee on Smoking and Health (ICSH) establish a subcommittee to develop recommendations for promoting smoking cessation in the United States (Fiore, Croyle, Curry, et al., 2004). The resulting *National Action Plan for Tobacco Cessation* comprises 10 recommendations, 6 federal initiatives and four public-private partnership initiatives. The federal initiatives are as follows:

- Establish a federally funded National Tobacco Quitline network that will provide universal access to evidence-based counseling and medications for tobacco cessation.
- Launch an ongoing, extensive, paid media campaign to help Americans quit using tobacco.
- Include evidence-based counseling and medications for tobacco cessation in benefits provided to all federal beneficiaries and in all federally funded healthcare programs.
- Invest in a new, broad and balanced research agenda (basic, clinical, public health, translational, and dissemination to achieve future improvements in the reach, effectiveness, and adoption of tobacco dependence interventions across both individuals and populations.
- Invest in training and education to ensure that all clinicians in the United States have the knowledge, skills, and support systems necessary to help their patients quit tobacco use.
- Establish a Smoker's Health Fund by increasing federal excise tax on cigarettes and other Tobacco products.

The public-private partnership initiatives are:

- Mobilize health insurers, employers and others to foster evidence-based tobacco dependence coverage for all covered lives.
- Mobilize health systems to implement system-level changes to foster effective utilization of tobacco dependence treatments.
- Mobilize national quality assurance and accreditation organizations, clinicians, health systems, and others to establish and measure the treatment of tobacco dependence as part of the standard of care.
- Mobilize communities to ensure that policies and programs are in place to increase demand for services and to ensure access to such services, especially for underserved populations.

The impact of these recommendations for practicing physicians, both in primary care and specialty areas, will be substantial. There will be greater emphasis on training physicians to address tobacco. More specifically, the subcommittee recommended that the U.S. DHHS (1) provide grants to medical and other health care professional schools to develop, implement, and evaluate curricula for treatment of tobacco dependence; (2) establish partnerships with health care professional organizations and licensing bodies to ensure that licensure and certification examinations assess knowledge of tobacco dependence and its treatment; and (3) convene a diverse group of experts to ensure that competency in tobacco dependence interventions is a core graduation requirement for all new physicians and other key health care professionals.

It is anticipated that the result of these initiatives will be generations of physicians skilled in communication and intervention skills, knowledgeable in tobacco prevention and control, as well as in the management of health behavior in general, who will be able to intervene successfully on tobacco and other health behaviors within the context of busy practice settings. They will understand how to capitalize on teachable moments, conduct a comprehensive tobacco history, assess health beliefs and stage of change, and utilize a partnership model to develop effective patient-centered treatment plans. In so doing, the physicians will be knowledgeable about behavioral and pharmacological aspects of treatment and utilize diverse supplementary material to facilitate behavior change. The skilled physician also will understand the value of office management systems, utilizing office staff and nurses to support and follow-up intervention efforts.

Support for insurance coverage of tobacco treatment will remove a powerful barrier to physician intervention on tobacco and the time spent doing it, system level changes in health care settings will enable physicians and their staffs to accommodate and follow more smokers, while the tobacco quitlines and media campaigns will increase the demand for physician support for smoking cessation. Additional money for research will lead to new and more powerful tools for smoking cessation interventions (i.e., new medications, computer-assisted technologies, and behavioral treatments).

There is little doubt that physicians and the medical community are up to the task, as witnessed by recent advances in the area of pediatric interventions for smoking prevention and cessation and the management of environmental tobacco smoke (ETS) (Sargent and DiFranza, 2003). Current efforts to take advantage of teachable moments to address tobacco in emergency rooms (Bernstein and Becker, 2002; Sockrider, Abramson, Brooks, et al., 2006) as well as in oncology (Gritz, Fingeret, Vidrine, et al., 2006), pulmonary (Wagena, van der Meer, Ostelo, et al., 2004), cardiology (Wilkes, Evans, Henderson, et al., 2005), diabetes management (Persson and Hjarlmarson, 2006), surgical (Warner, Sarr, Offord, et al., 2004), kidney transplant (Ehlers, Rodrigue, Patton, et al., 2006), and psychiatric (American Psychiatric Association, 1996; Lawn and Pols, 2005) settings have expanded the venues in which physician tobacco interventions occur. Future advances in pharmacotherapy, behavioral intervention, and the quality of doctor-patient communication will continue to enhance the physicians' armamentarium and effectiveness, and, ultimately, the medical community's continued dedication to the health and well being of patients and the general public will win the day.

REFERENCES

Adda, J., and Lechene, V. (2004). On the identification of the effect of smoking on mortality. CeMMap working paper cwp13/04, Centre for Microdata Methods and Practice, Institute for Fiscal Studies.

American Cancer Society. (2003). *Cancer Facts and Figures 2003.* Atlanta: Author.

American Cancer Society. (2006). *Cancer Facts and Figures 2006.* Atlanta: Author.

American Psychiatric Association. (1996). Practice guideline for the treatment of patients with nicotine dependence. *American Journal of Psychiatry*, 153, S1-S31.

Apperson, G. L. (1914). *The Social History of Smoking.* London: Martin Secher.

Bass, L.W., and Wilson, T.R. (1964). The pediatrician's influence in private practice measured by controlled seat belt study. *Pediatrics*, 33, 700-704.

Becker, M.H. (1974). The health belief model and personal health behavior. *Health Education Monographs*, 2, 409-419.

Bernstein, D. A. (1969). Modification of smoking behavior: An evaluative review. *Psychological Bulletin*, 71, 418-440.

Bernstein, S.L., and Becker, B.M. (2002). Preventive care in the emergency department: Diagnosis and management of smoking and smoking-related illness in the emergency department: a systematic review. *Academic Emergency Medicine*, 9, 720-729.

Borrelli, B. (2006). Using motivational interviewing to promote patient behavior change and enhance health. http://www.medscape.com/viewprogram/5757_pnt.

Botelho, R.J., and Skinner, H. (1995). Motivating change in health behavior. *Primary Care*, 22, 565-589.

Broders, A.C. (1920). Squamous-cell epithelium of the lip. *Journal of the American Medical Association*, 74, 656-664.

Burns, D. (1994). Overview of office-based smoking cessation assistance. In D.R. Shopland, D.M. Burns, S.J. Cohen, T.E. Kottke, and E.R. Gritz (Eds.), *Tobacco and the Clinician* (3-11). U.S. Department of Health and Human Services. (NIH Publication No. 94-3693). Washington, D.C.: Government Printing Office.

Burt, A., Illingworth, D., and Shaw, T.R.D., et al. (1974). Stopping smoking after myocardial infarction. *The Lancet*, 304-306.

Cabana, M.D., Rand, C., and Slish, K., et al. (2004). Pediatrician self-efficacy for counseling parents of asthmatic children to quit smoking. *Pediatrics*, 113, 78-81.

Cantor, J.C., Baker, L.C., and Hughes, R.G. (1993). Prepared for practice. Young physicians' views of their professional education. *Journal of the American Medical Association*, 270, 1035-1040.

Colman, T., Barrett, S., and Wynn, A., et al. (2003). Comparison of the smoking behavior and attitudes of smokers who believe they have smoking-related problems with those who do not. *Family Practice*, 20, 520-523.

Cornuz, J., Humair, J.P., and Seematter, L., et al. (2002). Efficacy of resident training in smoking cessation: A randomized, controlled trial of a program on application of behavioral theory and practice with standardized patients. *Annals of Internal Medicine*, 136, 429-437.

Denmark, D. (2004). Patient-physician partnering to improve chronic disease care. *Family Practice Management*, 11, 55.

DiClemente, C.C., Prochaska, J.O., and Fairhurst, S.K., et al. (1991). The process of smoking cessation: an analysis of precontemplation, contemplation, and preparation stages of change. *Journal of Consulting and Clinical Psychology*, 59, 295-304.

Doll, R., and Hill, A. B. (1950). Smoking and carcinoma of the lung. Preliminary report. *British Medical Journal, ii,* 739-748.

Duncan, C.L., Cummings, S.R., and Hudes, E. S., et al. (1992). Quitting smoking: reasons for quitting and predictors of cessation among medical patients. *Journal of General Internal Medicine*, 7, 398-404.

Duncan, C., Stein, M.J., and Cummings, S.R. (1991). Staff involvement and special follow-up time increase physicians' counseling about smoking cessation: A controlled trial. *American Journal of Public Health*, 81, 899-901.

Ehlers, S.L., Rodrigue, J.R., and Patton, P.R., et al. (2006). Treating tobacco use and dependence in kidney transplant recipients: Development and implementation of a program. *Progress in Transplantation*, 16, 33-37.

Ferry, L.H., Grissino, L.M., and Runfola, P.S. (1999). Tobacco dependence curricula in US undergraduate medical education. *Journal of the American Medical Association*, 282, 825-829.

Fiore, M.C. (1991). The new vital sign. *Journal of the American Medical Association*, 266, 3183-3184.

Fiore, M.C., Bailey, W.C., and Cohen, S.J., et al. (2000). *Treating Tobacco Use and Dependence*. Clinical Practice Guideline. Rockville, MD: U.S. Department of Health and Human Services. Public Health Service.

Fiore, M.C., Croyle, R.T., and Curry, S.J., et al. (2004). Preventing 3 million premature deaths and helping 5 million smokers quit: A national action plan for tobacco cessation. *American Journal of Public Health*, 94, 205-210.

Fredrickson, D.T. (1968). How to help your patient stop smoking-Guidelines for the office physician. *Diseases of the Chest*, 54, 28-34.

Freund, KM, D'Agostino, R.B., and Balanger, A.J., et al. (1992). Predictors of smoking cessation: The Framingham Study. *American Journal of Epidemiology*, 135, 957-964.

Frishman, W.H., Mitta, W., and Kupersmith, A., et al. (2006). Nicotine and non-nicotine smoking cessation pharmacotherapies. *Cardiology in Review*, 14, 57-73.

Gerbert, B., Berg-Smith, S., and Mancuso, M., et al. (2003). Using innovative video doctor technology in primary care to deliver brief smoking and alcohol intervention. *Health Promotion Practice*, 4, 249-261.

Glynn, T.J., and Manley, M.W. (1995). *How to Help Your Patients Stop Smoking*: *A National Cancer Institute Manual for Physicians.* (NIH Publication No.95-3064). Bethesda: National Cancer Institute.

Glynn, T.J., Manley, M.W., and Mecklenburg, R. (1994). Involvement of physicians and dentists in smoking cessation: A public health perspective. In R. Richmond (ed.), *Interventions for Smokers: An International Perspective* (pp. 195-216). Baltimore: Williams and Wilkens.

Gritz, E.R., Carr, C.R., and Rapkin, D., et al. (1991). A smoking cessation intervention for head and neck cancer patients: trial design, patient accrual, and characteristics. *Cancer Epidemiology, Biomarkers, and Prevention*, 1, 67-73.

Gritz, E.R., Fingeret, M.C., and Vidrine, D.J., et al. (2006). Successes and failures of the teachable moment. *Cancer*, 106, 17-27.

Hariot, T. (1588). Briefe and True Report of the New Found Land of Virginia. London: (no publisher listed).

Hill, J. (1761). Cautions Against the Immoderate Use of Snuff and the Effects It Must Produce When This Way Taken into the Body. London: Baldwin and Jackson.

Humair, J.P., and Cornuz, J. (2003). A new curriculum using active learning methods and standardized patients to train residents in smoking cessation. *Journal of General Internal Medicine*, 18, 1023-1027.

Hurt, R.D., Dale, C., and Fredrickson, P.A., et al. (1994). Nicotine patch therapy for smoking cessation combined with physician advice and nurse follow-up. *Journal of the American Medical Association*, 271, 595-600.

Hymowitz, N. (1999). Smoking cessation. In N.S. Cherniack, M.D. Altose, and I. Homma (Eds.), *Rehabilitation of the Patient with Respiratory Disease* (pp. 319-353). New York: McGraw-Hill.

Hymowitz, N. (2005). Tobacco. In R.F. Frances, S.I. Miller, and A.H. Mack (Eds.), *Clinical Textbook of Addictive Disorders, 3rd Edition* (pp. 105-137). New York: The Guilford Press.

Hymowitz, N. (2006). Pediatric residency training on tobacco: Review and critique of the literature. *Journal of the National Medical Association*, 98, 1489-1497.

Hymowitz, N., Schwab, J., and Haddock, C.K., et al. (2004). The Pediatric Residency Training on Tobacco Project: baseline findings from the resident tobacco survey and observed structured clinical examinations. *Preventive Medicine*, 39, 507-516.

Koop, C.E. (1985). The pediatrician's obligation in smoking education. *American Journal of Diseases of Children*, 139, 973.

Koskowski, W. (1955). *The Habit of Tobacco Smoking*. London: Staples Press Limited.

Kristeller, J.L., and Ockene, J.K. (1996). Tobacco curriculum for medical students, residents and practicing physicians. *Indiana Medicine*, 89, 199-204.

Lancaster, T., and Stead, L. (2004). Physician advice for smoking cessation. *Cochrane Database of Systematic Reviews*, 4, CD000165.

Lawn, S., and Pols, R. (2005). Smoking bans in psychiatric settings? A review of the research. *Australian and New Zealand Journal of Psychiatry*, 39, 866-885.

Lee, M.T., Hishinuma, E.S., and Derauf, C., et al. (2004). Smoking cessation counseling training for pediatric residents in the continuity clinic setting. *Ambulatory Pediatrics*, 4, 289-294.

Levenstein, J.H., McCracken, E.C., and McWhinney, I.R., et al. (1986). Patient-centred clinical method. I. A model for doctor-patient interaction in family medicine. *Family Practice*, 3, 24-30.

Lichtenstein, E., and Danaher, B.G. (1976). The modification of smoking behavior: A critical analysis of theory, research, and practice. *Progress in Behavior Modification*, 3, 79-132.

Lindsay, E. A., Ockene, J.K., and Hymowitz, N., et al. (1994). Physicians and smoking cessation: A survey of office procedures and practices in the Community Intervention Trial for Smoking Cessation. *Archives of Family Medicine*, 3, 341-348.

Lockyear, P.L.B. (2004). Physician-patient communication: Enhancing skills to improve patient satisfaction. http://www.medscape.com/view program/3679_pnt.

Lombard, H.L., and Doering, C.R. (1928). Classics in oncology. Cancer studies in Massachusetts habits, characteristics and environment of individuals with and without cancer. *New England Journal of Medicine*, 198, 481-487.

Mariolos, P., Rock, V.J., and Asman, K., et al. (2006). Tobacco use among adults-United States, 2005. *Morbidity and Mortality Weekly Report*, 55, 1145-1151.

Maseeh, A., and Kwatra, G. (2005). A review of smoking cessation interventions. *Medscape General Medicine, 7.* http://www.medscape.com/viewarticle/504516_print.

Mausner, J.S., and Mausner, B. (1967). The role of the physician in the control of smoking. *World Conference on Smoking and Health: A Summary of the Proceedings* (pp. 211-216). New York: American Cancer Society.

Mausner, J.S., Mausner, B., and Rial, W.J. (1968). The influence of a physician on the smoking of his patients. *American Journal of Public Health*, 58, 46-53.

McBride, C.M., Curry, S.J., and Lando, H.A., et al. (1999). Prevention of relapse in women who quit during pregnancy. *American Journal of Public Health*, 89, 706-711.

McBride, C.M., Pirie, P.L., and Curry, S.J. (1992). Postpartum relapse to smoking: a prospective study. *Health Education Research*, 7, 381-390.

McBride, C.M., Emmons, K.M., and Lipkus, I.M. (2003). Understanding the potential of teachable moments: the case of smoking cessation. *Health Education Research*, 18,156-170.

Miller, W.R., and Rollnick, S. (1991). *Motivational Interviewing*. Preparing People to Change. New York: The Guilford Press.

Miller, Y.E. (2005). Pathogenesis of lung cancer. *American Journal of Respiratory Cell and Molecular Biology*, 33, 216-223.

Mochizuki-Kobayashi, Y., Fishburn, B., and Baptiste, J., et al. (2006). Cigarette use among high school students-United States, 1991-2005. *Morbidity and Mortality Weekly Report*, 55, 724-726.

Norr, R. (1952). Cancer by the carton. *The Reader's Digest*, 61, 7-8.

Ockene, J., Quirk, M., and Goldberg, R., et al. (1988). A resident's training program for the development of smoking intervention skills. *Archives of Internal Medicine*, 148, 1039-1045.

Ockene, J., and Zapka, J.G. (2000). Provider education to promote clinical practice guidelines. *Chest*, 118, 33S-39S.

Orleans, C.T. (1993). Treating nicotine dependence in medical settings: A stepped care model. In C.T. Orleans and J. Slade (Eds.), *Nicotine Addiction Principles and Management* (pp. 145-161). New York: Oxford University Press.

Pearl, R. (1938). Tobacco smoking and longevity. *Science*, 87, 2253-2254.

Pederson, L.L. (1982). Compliance with physician advice to quit smoking: A review of the literature. *Preventive Medicine*, 11, 71-84.

Persson, L.G., and Hjarlmarson, A. (2006). Smoking cessation in patients with diabetes mellitus: results from a controlled study of an intervention programme in primary healthcare in Sweden. *Scandinavian Journal of Primary Health Care*, 24, 75-80.

Pincherle. G., and Wright, H.B. (1970). Smoking habits of business executives: Doctor variation in reducing cigarette consumption. *Practitioner*, 205, 209-212.

Prochaska, J.O., and DiClemente, C.C. (1983). Stages and processes of self-change of smoking: Toward an integrative model of change. *Journal of Consulting and Clinical Psychology*, 51, 390-395.

Prochaska, J.O., Velcier, W.F., and Rossi, J.S., et al. (1994). Stages of change and decision balance for 12 problem behaviors. *Health Psychology*, 13, 39-46.

Rennard, S.I., and Daughton, D.M. (1998). Nicotine replacement therapy: What are the options today? *The Journal of Respiratory Diseases*, 19, S20-S25.

Richmond, R. (1994). General practitioner interventions for smoking cessation: Past and future initiatives. In R. Richmond (Ed.), *Interventions for Smokers: An International Perspective* (pp. 217-256). Baltimore: Williams and Wilkins.

Richmond, R., and Webster, I. (1985). Evaluation of general practitioners' use of a smoking intervention programme. *International Journal of Epidemiology*, 14, 396-401.

Rose, G., and Hamilton, P.J.S. (1978). A randomized controlled trial of the effect on middle-aged men of advice to stop smoking. *Journal of Epidemiology and Community Health*, 32, 275-281.

Royal College of Physicians of London. (1962). *Smoking and Health Now*. London: Pitman Medical Publishing Co. Ltd.

Russell, M.A.H. (1971). Cigarette dependence: II-Doctor's role in management. *British Medical Journal*, 2, 393-395.

Russell, M.A.H., Merriman, R., and Stapleton, J., et al. (1983). Effect of nicotine chewing gum as an adjunct to general practitioner advice against smoking. *British Medical Journal*, 287, 1782-1785.

Russell, M.A.H., Wilson, C., and Taylor, C., et al. (1979). Effect of general practitioners' advice against smoking. *British Medical Journal*, 2, 231-235.

Sargent, J.D., and DiFranza, J.R. (2003). Tobacco control for clinicians who treat adolescents. *CA Cancer Journal for Clinicians*, 53, 102-123.

Schwartz, J.J. (1987). *Review and Evaluation of Smoking Cessation Methods: The United States and Canada, 1978-1985*. U.S. Department of Health and Human Services. (NIH Publication No. 87-2940). Washington, D.C. U.S.: Government Printing Office.

Shiffman, S., Dresler, C.M., and Hajek, P., et al. (2002). Efficacy of a nicotine lozenge for smoking cessation. *Archives of Internal Medicine*, 162, 1267-1276.

Simpson, M., Buckman, R., and Stewart, M., et al. (1991). Doctor-patient communication: the Toronto consensus statement. *British Medical Journal*, 303, 1385-1387.

Sockrider, M.M., Abramson, S., and Brooks, E., et al. (2006). Delivering tailored asthma family education in a pediatric emergency department setting: A pilot study. *Pediatrics*, 117, S135-S144.

Stein, R.J., Haddock, C.K., and O' Byrne, K.K., et al. (2000). The pediatrician's role in reducing tobacco exposure in children. *Pediatrics*, 106, (http://www.pediatrics.org/cgi/content/full/106/5/e66).

Steinfeld, J.L. (1972). I. The physician's role: The physician's responsibility to his smoking patient. *Rhode Island Medical Journal*, 55, 119-123. (a)

Sullivan, L. (1990). An opportunity to oppose: Physicians' role in the campaign against tobacco. *Journal of the American Medical Association*, 264, 1581-1582.

Terry, L.I. (1970). Today's campaign. *Today's Health*, February, 21-76.

U.S. Department of Health and Human Services. (1989). *Reducing the Health Consequences of Smoking: 25 Years of Progress*. (DHHS Publication No. CDC 89-8411). Washington, DC: U.S. Government Printing Office.

U.S. Department of Health and Human Services. (1992). *Clinical Opportunities for Smoking Intervention*. (NIH Publication No. 92-2178). Washington, D.C.: U.S. Government Printing Office.

U.S. Department of Health and Human Services. (2000). *Healthy People 2010. 2nd ed.* With Understanding and Improving Health and Objectives for Improving Health. 2 vols. Washington, DC: U.S. Government Printing Office.

U.S. Public Health Service. (1964). *Smoking and Health. Report of the Advisory Committee to the Surgeon General of the Public Health Service*. U.S. Department of Health, Education, and Welfare. (Public Health Service Publication No. 1103). Washington, D.C.: U.S. Government Printing Office.

Van Lancker, J.L. (1977) Smoking and Disease. In M.E. Jarvik, J.W. Cullen, and E.R. Gritz, et al. (Eds.), *Research on Smoking Behavior* (pp.230-280). National Institute on Drug Abuse Research Monograph Series 17. (DHEW Publication No. (ADM) 78-581). Washington, D.C.: U.S. Government Printing Office.

Wagena, E.J., van der Meer, R.M., and Ostelo, R.J.W.G., et al. (2004). The efficacy of smoking cessation strategies in people with chronic obstructive pulmonary disease: results from a systematic review. *Respiratory Medicine*, 98, 805-815.

Warner, D.O., Sarr, M.G., and Offord, K.P., et al. (2004). Anesthesiologists, general surgeons, and tobacco interventions in the perioperative period. *Anesthesia and Analgesia*, 99, 1766-1773.

Wilkes, S., Evans, A., and Henderson, M., et al. (2005). Pragmatic, observational study of bupropion treatment for smoking cessation in general practice. *Postgraduate Medical Journal*, 81, 719-722.

Williams, H.O. (1969). Routine advice against smoking. *The Practitioner*, 202, 672-676.

Wilson, D.H., Wakefield, M.A., and Steven, I.D., et al. (1990). "Sick of Smoking": Evaluation of a targeted minimal smoking cessation intervention in general practice. *Medical Journal of Australia*, 152, 518-521.

Wynder, E., and Graham, E. (1950). Tobacco smoking as a possible etiologic factor in bronchogenic carcinoma. *Journal of the American Medical Association*, 143, 329-336.

In: Smoking Cessation: Theory, Interventions and Prevention   ISBN: 978-1-60021-591-9
Editor: Jerome E. Landow   © 2008 Nova Science Publishers, Inc.

Chapter 5

GROUNDING RESEARCH FOR TESTING MODELS OF SMOKING CESSATION BEHAVIOR: THEORY OF REASONED ACTION AND THEORY OF PLANNED BEHAVIOR

*Linda K. Bledsoe**

University of Louisville, Louisville, Kentucky, USA

ABSTRACT

Even though a large body of research elucidating the negative health impact of cigarette smoking has become more widely known by the public in recent years, smoking remains as the single most preventable cause of morbidity and mortality in the U. S. In fact, according to the most recently available prevalence estimates, 20.9% of the American population over 18 years of age were smokers in 2005, which is unchanged from 2004 estimates (Schiller, Martinez, and Barnes, 2006, June). Continuing high levels of smoking among adults emphasize the need for additional research in areas that can inform our understanding and knowledge of smoking cessation behavior. Both the Theory of Reasoned Action (Fishbein and Ajzen, 1975) and the Theory of Planned Behavior (Ajzen, 1985) have been applied to modeling smoking behavior. Although the importance of elicitation or grounding research to subsequent model testing has been emphasized by Ajzen and Fishbein (1980) and others (e.g., Montaño, Kasprzyk, and Taplin, 1997), a search of the literature revealed that very few studies provided details of beliefs used to assess attitudes and social norms or how these beliefs were chosen for the measures developed. This study addressed that gap by conducting elicitation research with adult smokers recruited from an urban Midwestern university (n = 30) and from the community in which the university is located (n = 38). The purpose of the research reported in this chapter was to identify salient behavioral outcomes, social referents, and control beliefs for smoking cessation among adult men and women smokers. Content analysis was conducted on the responses to the elicitation questionnaire in order to determine

---

* Email: linda.bledsoe@louisville.edu; Telephone: 502-852-0421; Fax: 502-852-5887

salient modal beliefs related to quitting smoking. A discussion of the findings and implications is provided.

INTRODUCTION

The purpose of the research reported in this chapter was to identify salient behavioral outcomes, social referents, and control beliefs for smoking cessation in the population under consideration; adult men and women smokers. Although Ajzen and Fishbein (1980) and others who have developed and applied the Theory of Reasoned Action and the Theory of Planned Behavior (e.g., Montaño, Kasprzyk and Taplin, 1997) emphasize the importance of the elicitation phase in testing and applying these models, the process or results the elicitation phase in model testing are rarely reported in the literature.

In a search of the literature related to TRA, TPB, and smoking, it was found that most studies did not list the beliefs that were used to assess attitude and social norm, but gave one or two examples instead (e.g., Chassin et al., 1981; Braithwaite, Sutton, and Steggles, 2002). Generally, the completed research with any population or behavior using TRA or TPB has not included the elicitation phase (e.g., Conner, Sandberg, McMillan, and Higgins, 2006; Hanson, 2005). An example of this approach is Bursey and Craig's (2000) study that applied TPB to smoking cessation in adults after coronary artery bypass surgery in which the authors based salient beliefs for the study on empirical literature. Many of the reported studies described using four or five semantic differential items to measure attitude (e.g., Grube, Morgan, and McGree, 1986; McMillan, Higgins, and Conner, 2005; Sherman et al., 1982). However, three studies were located that used the methods suggested by Ajzen and Fishbein and also provided a list of the beliefs that were elicited (Chung and Fishbein, as cited in Fishbein, 1982; Budd, 1986; De Vries and Kok, 1986). Chung and Fishbein's sample consisted of 63 young college women; Budd's sample consisted of 50 college undergraduate students; and De Vries and Kok's sample consisted of 85 Dutch third graders. The dates when these data were collected and the mostly younger ages of the participants underscore the importance for conducting an elicitation study, particularly with adults smokers recruited from the community.

In discussing TRA as applied to smoking behavior, Fishbein (1982) stressed that a person's attitude toward a behavior is based on *salient* beliefs about that behavior. Fishbein also makes the distinction between general and personal beliefs and attitudes. In TRA (and TPB), it is the personal beliefs and attitudes toward the individual's own performance of a particular behavior that are involved in the formation of intention. The concept of modal salient beliefs as those beliefs elicited most frequently within a given population was developed in order to apply TRA cross-sectionally (Fishbein, 1993). Likewise, salience of each referent (i.e., important other) is also required in assessment of social norms.

No doubt the extensive support for and the application of TRA and TPB to a wide range of behaviors has influenced many researchers to undervalue the integral role of the elicitation phase to these theories. Other writers in the field have commented on the importance of elicitation research. In reviewing various theories applied to health related behaviors, Rimer (1997) considers the grounding of TRA and TPB through elicitation of salient beliefs and referents relevant to the behavior and population under study to be one of the most important characteristics of these theories. Montaño, et al. (1997) conclude that a poorly conducted elicitation phase will likely result in inadequately constructed TRA measures and less than adequate behavioral prediction. After reviewing the available relevant literature, a review of the Theories of Reasoned Action and Planned Behavior is provided followed by the details of the completed elicitation research. A discussion of the findings and implications is provided.

BACKGROUND: THEORETICAL FRAMEWORK

Theory of Reasoned Action

Fishbein and Ajzen's (1975) theoretical approach views people as rational beings, who use available information to make judgments, form evaluations, and make decisions. The Theory of Reasoned Action (TRA) uses an information processing approach with the aggregate of a person's beliefs serving as the informational base that ultimately determines attitudes, intentions, and behavior. This theory is concerned with attitude toward behavior, not attitude toward targets, and attempts to account for proximal causation of volitional behavior. All distal variables, such as attitudes toward targets, are seen as external to the model and are assumed to affect behavior only through their influence on the model's variables (Eagly and Chaiken, 1993). Viewing social behavior as volitional, it is expected that a person will perform those behaviors intended (Fishbein and Ajzen, 1975). Although this assumption of TRA may be problematic for application to smoking behavior which includes an addictive component, TRA has been often used to predict smoking behavior and intentions with a fair degree of success as will be discussed later.

Behavioral intention is determined by attitude toward the behavior in question and the subjective norm concerning this behavior. Attitude toward the behavior is the result of salient beliefs about consequences of the behavior and the evaluation of these consequences. Subjective norm is the result of beliefs about what referents think the person should or should not do and the person's motivation to comply with these wishes. Finally, behavioral intention is viewed as the immediate determinant of the corresponding behavior. The model put forth by this theory has been algebraically represented by Ajzen and Fishbein as follows:

$$B \approx BI = w_1A_b + w_2SN$$

where B is behavior, BI is behavioral intention, A_b is attitude toward the behavior, SN is the subjective norm, and w_1 and w_2 are empirical weights. These weights may vary based on the particular behavior under consideration and also based on such factors as gender or age (Ajzen and Fishbein, 1980).

TRA posits that a strong relationship between intention and behavior depends upon three boundary conditions (Fishbein and Ajzen, 1975). First, the measure of intention must correspond in its level of generality or specificity to that of the behavioral criterion with respect to action, target, context, and time (Ajzen and Fishbein, 1977; Ajzen and Madden, 1986). For example, to predict a specific behavior, such as, signing an organ donor card, we must assess the specific intentions to sign such a card. Second, the intention must be stable in the interval between measurement of intention and the time at which behavior is observed.

Generally, the accuracy of prediction will vary inversely with the length of time between measurement of intention and observation of behavior. The third requirement is that the behavior be under volitional control. The first of these boundary conditions, sometimes referred to as the principle of correspondence, also points to the importance of grounding TRA variables in the population under study before applying the TRA model.

Support for Theory of Reasoned Action

Early tests of TRA demonstrated consistent predictive ability of this theoretical approach (e.g., Ajzen and Fishbein, 1977; 1980). Sutton (1998) reviewed the literature related to TRA and TPB and his evaluation of these models was supportive of their ability to predict and explain intention and behavior. TRA has been applied to a wide range of behaviors and for various purposes, such as, predicting organization misbehavior (Vardi and Weitz, 2002), understanding intention to participate in genetic testing for hereditary cancer (Braithwaite, Sutton, and Steggles, 2002), and using TRA constructs as part of a scale to measure attitudes toward reproductive health and related behavior among female adolescents (Charron-Prochownik, Wang, Sereika, Kim, and Janz, 2006).

More recent research has continued to explore relationships between the TRA variables. Interestingly, Braithwaite, et al. (2002) found that TRA outperformed Theory of Planned Behavior (TPB) in predicting intention to participate in genetic testing for hereditary cancer (breast cancer or colon cancer) in two samples. The authors concluded this finding might have been the result of participants' lack of awareness of possible barriers to having the test. Park (2000) investigated the previously reported moderate to high correlation between attitude and subjective norm by parsing attitude toward behavior into social and personal aspects. Park found that attitudes that are social in nature display more correlation to subjective norm. In the same study, comparisons across cultures (Korean versus U.S.) indicated that respondents from the collectivistic culture tended to endorse subjective norms and social attitudes more, but this did not necessarily contribute to the prediction of behavioral intention.

Theory of Reasoned Action Applied to Smoking Behavior

Much of the research applying TRA to smoking behavior has investigated extensions of the original TRA by the addition of other variables. For example, Chassin and colleagues (Chassin et al., 1981; Chassin, Presson, Sherman, Corty, and Olshavsky, 1984) added 17 distal variables from Jessor and Jessor's problem-behavior theory (1977; as cited in Chassin et al., 1981) and found that these variables increased explained variance in intentions by less than 5% among experimental smokers and by 12-15% among regular smokers. It is also interesting that Chassin et al. (1981) predicted transition in smoking status even though there was imperfect correspondence between the measures, and there was a one year follow-up period.

Along similar lines, Budd (1986) attempted to extend TRA by adding measures of attitudinal, normative, and belief salience. In support of TRA, Budd found that attitude and subjective norms in this sample of smokers and nonsmokers predicted intention to smoke and that intention predicted smoking behavior. The addition of salience of evaluative beliefs produced only a small effect, suggesting such measures do not add to the predictive ability of the TRA model. This finding is consistent with the idea that salience has already been accounted for in the elicitation phase of the research.

Flay et al. (1994) used structural equation modeling to test models for smoking initiation and for smoking escalation that included behavioral intention but were not strictly tests of TRA alone. Both of the models tested included smoking intentions, but not social norms. The relationships between smoking intentions and smoking initiation and between intentions and smoking escalation were found to be significant ($p < .001$). These results provide additional support for the relationship between intention and behavior as predicted by TRA.

Sherman et al. (1982) examined the role of level of direct smoking experience in TRA and found that the weight of attitude in predicting behavioral intentions increased with greater direct experience. This finding runs counter to Fishbein and Ajzen's (1980) assertion that direct experience only affects the attitude-behavior relation through its effect on the stability of the attitude and would not be useful to in the prediction of behavioral intention from current attitude. Sherman et al. (1982) concluded that attitudes resulting from direct experience are more predictive of behavioral intentions because they are more accessible and are therefore more influential in judgments of behavioral intentions and actual behavioral decisions.

In a study that tested a model for motivation and prediction of progress through the stages of change (Prochaska and DiClemente, 1983) for quitting smoking, Bledsoe (2006) found that TRA predicted change but TPB did not. It was expected that TPB would be superior to TRA for smoking behavior due to the addiction factor involved which reduces the volitional nature of the target behavior. This finding may have been in part due to measurement problems encountered for perceived behavioral control. Although measures were developed based on elicitation research described in this chapter and were constructed as guided by theory (see below), the resulting measure for perceived behavioral control had low reliability.

Theory of Planned Behavior

The Theory of Planned Behavior (TPB; Ajzen, 1985; Schifter and Ajzen, 1985) is a revision and extension of the earlier Theory of Reasoned Action and addresses the volitional behavior boundary problem in TRA by adding the concept of behavioral control to attitude and social norm as determinants of behavioral intention. Like its predecessor, the Theory of Planned Behavior is concerned with attitude toward behavior, not attitude toward targets, and claims to account for proximal causation of behavior. All distal variables, such as attitudes toward targets, are seen as external to the model and are assumed to affect behavior only through their influence on the model's variables.

Perceived behavioral control (PBC) is a person's belief about how easy or difficult performance of a particular behavior is likely to be. PBC has been operationalized as the sum of the products for each control belief (c_i) multiplied by the perceived power (p_i) of that particular control factor to facilitate or hinder the target behavior ($\Sigma c_i p_i$, Ajzen,1991).

Ajzen and Madden (1986) suggested two versions of TPB. The first version assumed that perceived behavioral control has a direct causal effect on intention which is not mediated by attitude or subjective norm and that the effect of perceived behavioral control on behavior is completely mediated by intention. The second version of TPB added a direct effect of perceived behavioral control on behavior. However, a strong direct effect of perceived behavioral control is expected only under two conditions. First, the behavior must not be under complete volitional control; and secondly, the perceptions of perceived behavioral control must have some accuracy in reflecting actual control.

Support for the Theory of Planned Behavior

Ajzen and Madden (1986) reported the results of two studies designed to test each of the two versions of the TPB model. The target behavior in the first study was class attendance with 169 undergraduate college students as participants. TRA variables (attitude toward class attendance, subjective norms, and intentions) were measured using standard methods. Perceived behavioral control was measured by asking participants to estimate the frequency of occurrence of ten factors (developed in a pilot study with other college students) that could prevent class attendance. A second measure of perceived behavioral control asked the participants to estimate the degree to which they felt in control of attending all class sessions. Results of hierarchical regression analysis indicated that perceived behavioral control resulted in a significant increment in the explained variance ($p < .01$), indicating that perceived behavioral control had a direct effect on intention. Since this was a situation in which actual control was high, as expected perceived behavioral control did not have a direct effect on the prediction of behavior.

In the second study, Ajzen and Madden tested TPB under conditions in which volitional control of behavior was expected to be lower. Ninety undergraduates participated in this study which assessed their expectations of getting an "A" in a particular course. Attitudes, social norms, and intention were again measured as in the first study. Perceived behavioral control was measured by agreement with beliefs related to eight facilitating or inhibiting factors and by asking participants to indicate the level of control they believed they had in getting an "A" in the course. The results of hierarchical regression found that perceived behavioral control significantly added to the prediction of intentions and also to the prediction of actual grades obtained, thus supporting the effects of perceived behavioral control as described in the second version of TPB.

Madden, Ellen, and Ajzen (1992) extended the above research by comparing TPB to TRA in predicting ten behaviors that varied on degree of volitional control. After developing the list of ten behaviors in a series of pretests, a group of 82 undergraduates were asked to provide information about their attitudes, subjective norms, perceived behavioral control, and intentions for performing each of these ten behaviors during a two week period. At the end of this time, the same participants were asked to report the number of times they had performed each of these ten behaviors in the specified time period.

A within-subjects regression analysis was conducted in which explained variance in intentions and behaviors using both TRA and TPB was estimated for each participant. Including perceived behavioral control resulted in an average increase of 0.21 in the multiple correlation for behavioral intentions. The authors concluded that TPB significantly increased the prediction of behavioral intentions and also resulted in a significant increase in prediction of the target behavior. In order to further compare the ability of TRA and TPB to predict behaviors which varied in degree of perceived behavioral control, a between-subjects regression model was fit to each the ten behaviors and behavioral intentions. The addition of perceived behavioral control increased the prediction of behavioral intention for each of the ten behaviors, with the increase in R^2 ranging from 0.01 to 0.20. However, the addition of perceived behavior control contributed only to the prediction of behaviors that were rated as low in control. Thus, Madden et al. found support for perceived behavioral control acting as an exogenous variable increasing the prediction of intention in comparison with TRA when the behavior was perceived not to be volitional.

These early tests of TPB by Ajzen and others (Ajzen and Madden,1986; Madden, Ellen, and Ajzen, 1992) found that perceived behavior control added to the prediction of behavioral intention and behavior and that the performance of TPB and PBC varied as expected with the level of volitional control of target behavior under study.

More recently, Armitage and Conner's (2001) extensive review and meta-analysis of 185 published studies implementing TPB found that TPB accounted for 27% of the variance in behavior and 39% of the variance in intention. Overall, PBC was found to add 6% to the prediction of intention over and above the original TRA variables. Hausenblas, Carron, and Mack (1997) completed a meta-analysis comparing the efficacy of TRA to TPB for exercise behavior and found that generally TPB was superior to TRA. Albarracín, Johnson, Fishbein, and Muellerleile (2001) found support for both TRA and TPB in their meta-analysis of condom use. However, perceived behavioral control did not contribute significantly to prediction of condom use. Much research has been reported that provides support for the applicability of TPB to different content areas (e.g., condom use, De Wit, Stroebe, De Broome, Sandfort, and Van Griensven, 2000; alcohol use, Trafimow, 1996; use of illegal substances, Conner and McMillan, 1999; physical activity, Courneya, Friedenreich, Arthur, and Bobick, 1999). So much so, that Ajzen (2001) concluded that additional research testing TPB's applicability to specific domains was not warranted.

The Theory of Planned Behavior Applied to Smoking Behavior

Godin and Lepage (1988) used attitude, subjective norm, habit (which was a measure of past smoking behavior), and perceived self-efficacy to predict intention to smoke after pregnancy for a group of 63 pregnant women. This study found support for TPB; however, instead of measuring perceived behavioral control as described by Ajzen and Madden (1986), perceived self-efficacy was measured by asking subjects to indicate to what extent they expected to be capable of not smoking cigarettes in the nine months following delivery.

Babrow, Black, and Tiffany (1990) found that smokers' intentions to participate in a stepped smoking cessation program were significantly associated with attitude, subjective norms, and perceived behavioral control as specified by TPB. In a related study, Black and Babrow (1991) found that smokers' attitude toward participation was the strongest predictor of interest in each of the five steps of program participation, followed by perceived behavioral control, and then normative beliefs. Although interest in each of the five steps of the intervention program was used as a dependent variable, the authors reported a high correlation between interest and intention $r_{(191)} = .69, p < .001$).

Godin, Valois, Lepage, and Desharnais (1992) conducted longitudinal research on TPB's ability to predict cigarette smoking intentions and behavior among a group of 346 adults and also for group of 136 pregnant women. TPB variables were measured using methodology suggested by Ajzen and Madden (1986). For smokers in the general population group, perceived behavior control, attitudes, and subjective norms explained intention, with perceived behavioral control contributing the most ($\beta = 0.50$, $p < .001$). Habit, which was a measure of past smoking behavior, did not add to the prediction of intentions. For smokers among the pregnant women, intention was predicted by perceived behavioral control and attitude. Perceived behavioral control ($\beta = 0.66$, $p < .001$) was the only significant predictor of smoking behavior in this group when intention, perceived behavioral control, and habit were all entered into the equation. In general, Godin et al. (1992) provided a strong test of TPB and the results were supportive of TPB. However, intention was not a predictor of smoking behavior in either group, which is a serious problem for both TPB and TRA. The authors suggested that this may be because of low self-efficacy for quitting among these smokers. Contrary to other studies (e.g., Bentler and Speckart, 1979; Bagozzi, 1981), these results do not support the influence of habit on intention and tend to support Ajzen's (1988) opinion that perceived behavioral control mediates the effect of habit on intention.

Hanson (2005) examined ethnic differences among African American, Puerto Rican, and non-Hispanic white female adolescents in intention to smoke using TPB. White teenagers had stronger intention to smoke than the other groups, and the relative strength of TPB variables as predictors also differed between groups. Perceived behavioral control contributed more to prediction for African Americans in this sample, while attitude was the most predictive of intention for Puerto Rican and white teenagers.

Moan and colleagues (Moan and Rise, 2005; Moan, Rise, and Andersen, 2005) have tested TPB with the addition of variables designed to measure moral norms, identity, and positive and negative affect in a sample of students and also in a sample of parents in Norway. In the student sample, TPB variables accounted for 36% of the intention to smoke and the additional variables increased explained variance by 9%. In the parent sample, TPB variables accounted for 56% of the variance in intention not to smoke indoors around their children, and the additional variables contributed another 19%.

In another study on adolescent smoking by Higgins and Conner (2003), TPB was found to account for a significant proportion of the variance in intention to smoke both cross-sectionally and prospectively. Past smoking behavior was significant only in the prospective analyses and implementation intentions did not add to prediction. McMillan and Conner (2003) explored TPB and the additional variables of descriptive and moral norms applied to alcohol and tobacco use in a group of university students. Their results again support TPB for prediction of smoking intentions and behavior. Although descriptive norms added to the prediction of intention for smoking beyond TPB variables, moral norms did not. McMillan, Higgins, and Conner (2005) extended this work by examining the effectiveness of TPB to predict smoking intentions and behavior in a group of school children aged 12 and 13 years old. The results for TPB variables were similarly significant. However, in this case only moral norm explained additional variance in intention but not smoking.

In summary, tests of TPB have generally been supportive of the addition of perceived behavior control to the original TRA. However, measurement issues and modifications of the original model by addition of variables continue to be investigated with varying results. It is my contention that in order to test TRA or TPB and to apply either of these theories to the best advantage for prediction of smoking behavior, it is necessary to first complete the elicitation phase to identify salient behavioral outcomes, social referents, and control beliefs for smoking cessation in the population under consideration. The remainder of this chapter reports on the results of an elicitation study as applied to smoking behavior.

METHOD

Participants

Participants were 68 adult smokers who were recruited from undergraduate psychology students at an urban Midwestern university ($n = 30$) and also from the community ($n = 38$). The study protocol and informed consent form were reviewed by the Human Studies Protection Program at the university prior to implementation. The students selected from several available studies and received course credit for their participation.

Community participants were recruited using flyers posted in the community at various locations, including several coffee shops, bookstores, and a state office building. All flyers included brief information about the study, stated that a drawing would be held at the end of the study with the winner receiving $75, and included a telephone number for potential volunteers to contact the experimenter. The author met individually with participants at the various locations where they had learned of the study from the flyers; and administered the questionnaire after obtaining signed consent. Demographics, descriptors of smoking behavior, and stage of change are provided in Table 1.

Table 1. Demographics, Descriptors of Smoking Behavior,
and Stage of Change
(N = 68)

	Student sample (n = 30)	Community sample (n = 38)
Sex (%)		
Male	50	55.3
Female	50	44.7
Ethnicity (%)		
African American	13.3	7.9
White	83.3	86.8
Age		
Mean	19.3	39.6
SD	1.7	11.4
Cigarettes / day		
Mean	13.7	23.5
SD	11.8	14.9
Years as smoker		
Mean	3.8	21.9
SD	2.3	11.3
N (%) with 24-hr quit		
attempt in past year	27 (90%)	18 (47.4%)
N / stage of change		
Precontemplation	10	14
Contemplation	10	19
Preparation	10	5

Measures

Demographics and Smoking History

Participants were asked to provide information about how long they had been a smoker (in years), usual number of cigarettes smoked each day, if they had quit smoking for at least 24 hours during the past 12 months, their age, sex, and ethnic background.

Correspondence: Stage of change assessment

Correspondence on all the elements of behavior (action, target, context, time) and other measures in the TPB model is considered to be very important to the model's predictive ability (Ajzen and Fishbein, 1980). The Stage of Change (SOC, Prochaska and DiClemente, 1983) was assessed as one method of exploring correspondence between intention and behavior on the time element. No a priori assumptions were made concerning possible differences in response to elicitation questions among smokers based on stage of change; this issue was explored as part of the content analysis.

A revision of Prochaska and DiClemente's dichotomous staging algorithm (e.g., DiClemente, et al., 1991, Velicer, DiClemente, Prochaska, and Brandenburg, 1985) was used to determine stage of change. The continuous response staging algorithm (Bledsoe and Birkimer, 2004) has demonstrated expected relationships to the Decisional Balance Scale for smoking (Velicer, et al.,1985) and to Processes of Change for smoking (Prochaska, Velicer, DiClemente, and Fava, 1988), while facilitating more precise classification of smokers in the early stages of change. The continuous response staging algorithm allows smokers to indicate degree of agreement with the following statements: a) "I intend to quit smoking sometime", b) "I intend to quit smoking sometime in the next 6 months", c) "I intend to quit smoking sometime in the next 30 days". Participants responded on a scale from 0 (*Don't Agree at All*) to 6 (*Agree Completely*), and responses to all 3 items were summed. Participants who scored between zero and six were classified as precontemplators; those who scored between seven and 12 were contemplators, and those participants who scored over 12 and who had a 24 hour quit attempt during the last 12 months were considered to be in the preparation stage of change.

Elicitation Questions

After determining the participant's stage of change, the experimenter provided the appropriate version of the questions as described below. The only difference in these questions was the time frame referenced. No time reference was included in the version given to those smokers in the precontemplation stage; reference to quitting smoking in the next six months was included in the version given to smokers in the contemplation stage; and reference to quitting smoking in the next 30 days was made in the version given smokers in the preparation stage. All of these questions used an open-ended response format. (See Appendix A for questions.)

Based on Ajzen and Fishbein's (1980) recommendations, the following method was used to structure the items for determining modal salient beliefs for the population under consideration. To assess attitude, participants were asked about advantages and disadvantages of quitting smoking separately in order to encourage both types of responses. Then, the respondent was asked if there is anything else he or she associated with quitting smoking.

In order to elicit information concerning salient social referents, the participants were asked about any persons or groups who would approve or disapprove of their quitting smoking. Again, information about approval or disapproval of salient referents was requested in separate questions. Also, participants were asked if any other groups or people come to mind when thinking about quitting smoking.

Relevant to perceived behavioral control, participants were asked to separately list conditions or circumstances that might facilitate or hinder their efforts to quit smoking.

Procedure

Participants in the student sample met with either the author or a trained assistant in small groups and were first given an informed consent form to read and sign. In order to avoid any possible effects of state dependency on responding due to nicotine craving, students were told that they could take a break at any time to go to a nearby area where smoking was permitted. None of the students opted for a "smoke break" perhaps because they are accustomed to being without cigarettes during classes and the time necessary to complete the questionnaire was 30 minutes or less. Participants were asked to complete the first page of the survey which contained general demographic questions and questions used to determine stage of change. After determining stage of change for each participant, the experimenter provided the appropriate version of the elicitation questions with the time frame referenced matched to stage of change as described above. In order to avoid the need for any identifying information on the questionnaires, participants were asked to provide the last four digits of their social security number to be used later in matching the two parts of the questionnaire. After completing the questionnaire, respondents were debriefed and thanked for their participation in this study. Information about local resources for quitting smoking and a brief summary of research findings about quitting were available for all participants during debriefing.

The same procedures described above were followed in the community sample with two exceptions. Participants met individually with the experimenter and usually smoked during completion of the questionnaire.

RESULTS

After preliminary analyses that explored possible differences by sample and by stage, content analysis was conducted on the full sample of responses to the elicitation questions in order to determine modal salient beliefs related to quitting smoking.

Preliminary Analyses

The following preliminary analyses were conducted for the purpose of exploring possible differences in the number and content of responses by stage to check the relevance of including stage-matched time references in the questions (e.g., the next 30 days for those in the preparation stage) and to make a decision as to whether the responses from both subsamples (student and community) could be combined for further analyses.

Differences by Stage of Change

As a gross measurement, a count was made of the total number of words produced by participants in each of the three stages for all elicitation questions. The results were not as might be predicted by the Transtheoretical Model of Change (TTM). Based on this theory, it would be reasonable to expect those participants in the contemplation stage to produce the largest volume of responses. The contemplation stage has been characterized by awareness of the problem and active weighing the pros and cons of changing the problem behavior (e.g., DiClemente et al., 1991; Prochaska, 1995). It is in this stage that the pros start to outweigh the cons of changing. In this study however, smokers in the preparation stage produced the largest average number of words in their responses (107.07), which could be seen as consistent with TTM theory in that these smokers are to be expected to be very involved in beginning the process of quitting. Contrary to expectation, the next largest average number of words produced was from for smokers in the precontemplation stage (32.25), and the least average number of words produced in response to the survey was made by smokers in the contemplation stage (28.69), ($\chi^2_{(2)} = 70.35$, $p < .01$).

In all three stages, the largest number of responses were made to "What do you see as the advantages of your quitting smoking?," followed by the number of responses made to "What do you see as the disadvantages of your quitting smoking?"

Differences in Content of Responses by Sample and Stage

In order to obtain some indication of possible differences in content of the responses by stage and by sample, two independent coders were given copies of the responses to the survey questions that had been grouped by stage and sample and were asked to attempt to identify the sets of questions by stage (precontemplation, contemplation, or preparation) and sample (student or community).

The first coder was able to correctly distinguish the community sample from the student sample responses by noticing references to jobs, professions, spouses, and children in the community responses. This coder also correctly identified the responses by stage in the community sample. However, she was unable to correctly identify any of the three stages in the student sample. The second coder did not correctly identify the community or student sample or any of the stages within each sample. From these results, it was decided to combine all the responses for each question across stage and sample for determination of modal salient beliefs.

Determination of Modal Salient Beliefs

Responses to one question ("Are there any other groups or people who come to mind when you think about quitting smoking?") had to be dropped from analysis. This question was included as the third item to elicit information concerning salient social referents after first asking participants about any persons or groups who would approve or who would disapprove of their quitting smoking. Although this approach was effective with attitude toward quitting, the responses here were ambiguous. In general, there were fewer responses to this item and participants did not provide enough information to determine if these others were important in their decision about quitting smoking and if so, in what way important. Examples of some of the uninterpretable responses are "Phillip Morris," "farmers who farm tobacco," and " I think of people who smoke weed, I wish they would try to stop."

The responses to the remaining seven questions were coded independently by the author and one other coder. For each question, similar responses were grouped together, and the frequency of each recorded. It should be noted that responses to "Is there anything else you associate with your quitting smoking [or in the next 30 days or 6 months] ?" were classified as advantages or disadvantages to quitting smoking. Second, a decision was made as to whether outcomes in any given group should be considered as a single belief or separate beliefs. If this is not immediately clear, Ajzen and Fishbein (1980) recommended asking whether the two responses could have been reasonably made by the same person. If this was the case, these responses were retained as separate beliefs. Third, small numbers of related beliefs that were low in frequency were combined. Throughout the process, the final wording was kept as close as possible to the most frequent wording used by respondents.

Next, a decision was made as to how many of the beliefs to retain as salient. Ajzen and Fishbein (1980) acknowledged that although it is generally thought that a person may hold a large number of beliefs about any given object, that person can attend to only a small number of beliefs at one time; perhaps five to nine. However, there is no way to determine at what point in an individual's list of beliefs they cease to be salient. One rule suggested, and the rule that was used here, is to rank order responses by frequency and include as many beliefs as necessary to account for seventy-five percent of all beliefs provided by the participants. As a final step, the experimenter and coder consulted on the resulting lists of beliefs and resolved any differences by discussion.

Reliability

As a measure of interrater reliability, Cohen's Kappa (Siegal and Castellan, 1988) was calculated for the lists of beliefs compiled by two independent coders based on the responses to the elicitation questions before the lists were combined (see Table 2). Kappa was calculated based on the most frequent seventy-five percent of responses from each list as this rule used to decide how many beliefs to retain.

Bakeman and Gottman (1986) state that any value of .70 or greater for Kappa indicates acceptable reliability. The reported Kappa for referents who approve of quitting and the Kappa for hindrances to quitting smoking are lower than this suggested standard (.60 and .57). Although these low Kappas raise concerns about the reliability of these items, it should be noted that categories were not created previous to coders assigning the statements of respondents to categories. In other words, raters were not given a set of statements and a set of categories to which these statements were to be assigned. Coders, in effect, created the categories as they classified and combined similar responses, as based on the method as suggested by Ajzen and Fishbein (1980). However, a difference in the level of data reduction applied had a significant impact on Kappa for any set of responses to a given question. For example, on the responses about advantages of quitting, one coder combined references to improved health and reduction in health risks, while the other did not. Concerns about breathing and improved health were placed in the same category by one rater, but not by the second rater.

In general, the most frequent categories that accounted for seventy-five percent of all responses were very similar, if not the same, for each rater on each set of responses. Although Cohen's Kappa may not be an accurate measure of reliability for these results, another more appropriate reliability estimate is unavailable. Cohen's Kappa includes a correction for agreement by chance and here it may be over correcting. For that reason, percentage of agreement is also given for each category in Table 2. If these reported Kappas are reflecting the actual reliabilities of these items, then subsequent measurement of social norm and perceived behavioral control for model estimations could be adversely affected.

**Table 2. Cohen's Kappa Interrater Reliabilities and
Percent Agreement for Elicitation Questions (N = 68)**

Question	Kappa	% agreement
Advantages of quitting	.77	77
Disadvantages of quitting	.83	85
Referents – approve of quitting	.60	68
Referents – disapprove of quitting	.79	89
Facilitating factors for quitting	.81	84
Hindering factors for quitting	.57	61

Modal Salient Beliefs

The following beliefs about advantages of quitting smoking were retained based on the procedure described above (all lists are in order of decreasing frequency): improved health, reduction of health risks (for example, cancer and heart disease), saving money, improved smell of self and clothing, better breathing and increased lung capacity, and improved ability for physical activity. The following beliefs about disadvantages of quitting smoking were retained: increased stress, increased nervous energy, weight gain, loss of enjoyment of smoking, and withdrawal symptoms. This list of advantages and disadvantages differed from previously reported lists in that it did not include nausea, irritated eyes, or getting wrinkles.

The following social referents who supported quitting smoking were retained: most family members, friends who don't smoke, coworkers, and relationship partner (spouse, boyfriend, girlfriend). The following social referents who supported continuing to smoking were retained: cigarette companies and friends who smoke. This list of referents differed from previously reported lists in that physician was not included, but coworker was.

The following facilitating factors related to control beliefs were retained: members of family quitting or trying to quit and being able to afford nicotine replacement, such as, nicorette gum or the "patch" to help with quitting. The following hindering factors related to control beliefs were retained: being in stressful situations or increased stress in general, spending time with people who are smoking, living with people who smoke, being in places and situations where cigarettes are easily available, and people nagging about the need to quit smoking.

CONCLUSION

The results of the exploratory analyses regarding possible differences in the number and content of responses by stage of change in order check the relevance of including stage-matched time references in the elicitation questions (e.g., the next 30 days for those in the preparation stage) were not as expected. Based on both the Transtheoretical Model of Change and the Theories of Reasoned Action and Planned Behavior, it might be expected that those persons in the contemplation stage would produce the largest number of salient beliefs, referents, and control factors. On the contrary, the least number of responses were produced by those smokers in the contemplation stage of change, with responses by smokers in the precontemplation stage outnumbering those in the contemplation stage. No differences in content of the responses to elicitation questions by stage or sample could be reliably detected by two independent coders.

Lower than desirable Cohen's Kappa for referents who approve of quitting and for hindrances to quitting smoking (.60 and .57) raised concerns about the reliability of these items. Upon closer inspection of coding, a clear difference was found in the level of data reduction applied by each of the two coders. Although this result might be expected since categories were not created previous to coders assigning the statements of respondents to categories, it had a significant impact on Kappa for any set of responses to a given question. This difficulty is one example of why elicitation research, with its primarily qualitative approach is at times quite challenging.

The resultant salient modal beliefs and social referents for quitting smoking differed somewhat from those previously reported in the literature. Advantages and disadvantages of quitting smoking differed from those previously reported in that nausea, irritated eyes, or getting wrinkles were not included. Social referents differed from those previously reported in that physician was not included, but coworker was.

Implications

In part due to the success of the Theories of Reasoned Action and Planned Behavior, elicitation research is rarely conducted in current research. However, the findings from elicitation research remain important to the testing and application of both of these models and have important practical implications for helping smokers quit. A great deal of research has been completed on attitude and behavior change that could be brought more effectively to bear on the problem of cigarette smoking both on a societal and individual level, and elicitation research in particular has been underutilized.

For example, persuasion techniques using the public media have been shown to be successful in increasing smoking cessation rates and could be made more so by using elicitation research to inform content directed at particular groups of smokers. Certainly, the effects of advertising in many areas have been repeatedly demonstrated (e.g., effects of cigarette advertising on smoking initiation among children and adolescents, Pierce and Gilpin, 1995). Elicitation research has the potential to add to the understanding of relevant cultural differences in smoking and smoking cessation. In one such study by Marin, Marin, Perez-Stable, Otero-Sabogal, and Sabogal (1990), the authors used the elicitation phase of

TRA to explore specific consequences of smoking versus quitting that are salient to Hispanics. They identified significantly different normative beliefs that would be important to the development of an anti-smoking campaign for Hispanics.

Although it is difficult to be certain of the exact effect of counter advertising and public service announcements due to the inability to isolate all other operating factors (McAuliffe, 1988), these strategies to have played an important role in facilitating a reduction in total and per capita cigarette consumption (Schuster and Powell, 1987; Warner, 1977). However, warnings of health risks on cigarette packages and advertising warnings have been relatively less successful (Andrews, 1995). Specifically, it seems that a public service campaign similar to that used to encourage seat belt use when they first became widely available would be well advised with smoking cessation. Based on the responses supplied by smokers in the elicitation phase, the content of these ads could encourage important others to let the smoker know that it is important to them that he or she quit. However, nagging would be discouraged as counterproductive. Equivalent exposure to health messages and availability of resources become issues here (Andrews, 1995). At one time, the Federal Trade Commission estimated that there was one anti-smoking public service announcement for every 4.4 cigarette advertisements (Schuster and Powell, 1987). A larger commitment of resources is required if public service announcements are to have a larger impact on smoking cessation rates.

Such a public service campaign could also address specific concerns about health effects of smoking. With cigarette warning labels, it has been found that labels listing specific risk outcomes are significantly more believable than labels suggesting quitting or listing harmful contents (Beltramini, 1988). Public service announcements and other media campaign elements could benefit from more specific messages based on what we learn from elicitation research about smokers' specific concerns.

On an individual level, TRA offers methodology for measuring smokers' attitudes which could then be used to help the individual make progress through the stages of change in part through the application of attitude change theories. For example, cognitive dissonance theory (Festinger, 1957) provides guidance as to some of the resistance to change in smokers. Cognitive dissonance theory has shown that people will attempt to reduce dissonance by changing cognitions or adding consonant, even if inaccurate cognitions, such as, "more people die from car accidents than smoking". Most smokers today are generally aware of the serious health risks associated with continuing to smoke. This awareness of risks coupled with continuing to smoke can lead to a great deal of dissonance which in turn may lead to denial of the problem and keep a smoker from attempting change. However, by having access to better information about a smoker's attitude and the specific beliefs that form the basis for that attitude, it is possible that the clinician could reduce resistance by first attempting to change any relevant cognitions.

Limitations

Lower than desirable Cohen's Kappa for referents who approve of quitting and for hindrances to quitting smoking raised concerns about the reliability of these items. The difference in the level of data reduction applied by each of the two coders that emerged could perhaps have been addressed by adding a third coder had resources permitted. Also, Cohen's Kappa may have given a better estimate of the reliabilities, and the reliabilities may in fact have been higher, if separate coders had first created categories and a second group coders had then classified each response into one of these categories.

Generalizability of the results to the population of adult smokers may be adversely affected by self-selection among the volunteer participants for this research. It is not clear how they might be different from randomly selected smokers from the general population of smokers in the U. S. Even so, the inclusion of a community sample provided data from a wider spectrum of smokers and should result in information that is more representative of smokers in general.

Future Directions

In addition to the need for more direct application of elicitation research to smoking interventions and public health efforts as discussed above, continued research on the methods used in elicitation of salient beliefs is needed. The following are two examples of highly informative research using elicitation methodology. Sutton et al. (2003) examined the effects of question wording on resulting responses in elicitation research related to increasing physical activity by comparing questions that had an instrumental focus to questions with an affective focus. They also completed an extensive analysis of the impact of choice of decision rule for retaining beliefs in the final modal set (i.e., include ten or twelve most frequent responses, include all responses that are mentioned by 10 or 20 percent of the sample, or include as many responses as needed to account for 75 percent of all responses, Ajzen and Fishbein, 1980). They found systematic differences in responses based on the type of focus in the question. The "advantages" question resulted in more responses that would be considered instrumental, e.g., better appearance, improved health, and increased fitness. Whereas, the "like/enjoy" questions resulted in responses related to intrinsically enjoyable activities. Sutton et al. concluded that employing different decision rules resulted in very different sets of modal beliefs, underscoring the need for additional research in this area.

Dean et al. (2006) compared three methods of eliciting emotions, morals, and cognitions about organic foods. Dean et al. were particularly interested in how best to capture non-cognitive factors since people generally have emotional associations with food. The usual type of questions (advantages/disadvantages) used in TRA/TPB elicitation research were compared to a word association task and a open-ended method in which participants were asked to list beliefs, emotions, and behaviors in response to a food item. The traditional method elicited the most responses for all food items and was found to be the most successful in eliciting cognitive responses. Dean et al. found that only the open-ended task that specifically asked about emotions elicited any emotional words in responses. They found the word association task not to be as effective, but recommended further testing of the addition of the open-ended method to the traditional approach particularly when affective responses need to be included. In this same study, cultural differences in response patterns were found across three countries – the U. K., Italy, and Finland.

In summary, while much has been learned from the application of the Theories of Reasoned Action and Planned Behavior, the elicitation component of this approach has been underutilized in most current work. Elicitation research has much to offer in terms of theoretical and practical applications. Lastly, future research should include examination of the possible impact of completing elicitation research prior to model application versus not implementing this phase, optimal wording in questions used, and increasing our understanding of the best possible decision rule for inclusion of responses in the final modal set.

REFERENCES

Ajzen, I. (1985). From intentions to actions: A theory of planned behavior. In J. Kuhl and J. Beckman (Eds). *Action-control: From cognition to behavior* (pp.11-39). Heidelberg: Springer.

Ajzen, I. (1988). *Attitudes, personality, and behavior*. Chicago: The Dorsey Press.

Ajzen, I. (1991). The Theory of Planned Behavior. Organizational Behavior and Human Decision Processes, 50, 179-211.

Ajzen, I. (2001). Nature and operation of attitudes. *Annual Reviews: Psychology, 52*, 27-58.

Ajzen, I., and Fishbein, M. (1977). Attitude-behavior relations: A theoretical analysis and review of empirical research. *Psychological Bulletin, 84*, 888-918.

Ajzen, I., and Fishbein, M. (1980). *Understanding attitudes and predicting social behavior*, Englewood Cliffs, NJ: Prentice-Hall.

Ajzen, I., and Madden, T. J. (1986). Prediction of goal-directed behavior: Attitudes, intentions, and perceived behavioral control. *Journal of Experimental Social Psychology, 22*, 453-474.

Albarracín, D., Johnson, B. T., Fishbein, M., and Muellerleile, P. A. (2001). Theories of reasoned action and planned behavior as models of condom use: A meta-analysis. *Psychological Bulletin, 127*(1), 142-161.

Andrews, J. C. (1995). The effectiveness of alcohol warning labels: A review and extension. *American Behavioral Scientist, 38*(4), 622-632.

Armitage, C. J., and Conner, M. (2001). Efficacy of the theory of planned behaviour: A meta-analytic review. *British Journal of Social Psychology, 40*, 471-499.

Babrow, A. S., Black, D. R., and Tiffany, S. T. (1990). Beliefs, attitudes, intentions, and a smoking cessation program: A planned behavior analysis of campaign development. *Health Communication, 2,* 145-163.

Bagozzi, R. P. (1981). Attitudes, intentions, and behavior: A test of some key hypotheses. *Journal of Personality and Social Psychology, 41,* 607-627.

Bakeman, R., and Gottman, J. M. (1986). *Observing interaction: An introduction to sequential analysis*. New York: Cambridge University Press.

Beltramini, R. F. (1988). Perceived believability of warning label information presented in cigarette advertising. *Journal of Advertising, 17(1),* 26-32.

Bentler, P. M., and Speckart, G. (1979). Models of attitude-behavior relations. *Psychological Review, 86,* 452-464.

Black, D. R., and Babrow, A. S. (1991). Identification of campaign recruitment strategies for a stepped smoking cessation intervention for a college campus. *Health Education Quarterly, 18*(2), 235-247.

Bledsoe, L. K. (2006). Smoking cessation: An application of Theory of Planned Behavior to understanding progress through Stages of Change. *Addictive Behaviors, 31, 1271-1276.*

Bledsoe, L. K., and Birkimer, J. C. (2004). Smoking cessation: Two pilot studies exploring the use of continuous response format algorithm to identify subgroups within stage. *Substance Use and Misuse, 39*, 527-548.

Braithwaite, D., Sutton, S., and Steggles, N. (2002). Intention to participate in predictive genetic testing for hereditary cancer: The role of attitude toward uncertainty. *Psychology and Health, 17*(6), 761-772.

Budd, R. J. (1986). Predicting cigarette use: The need to incorporate measure of salience in the Theory of Reasoned Action. *Journal of Applied Social Psychology, 16*(8), 663-685.

Bursey, M. , and Craig, D. (2000). Attitudes, subjective norm, perceived behavioral control, and intentions related to adult smoking cessation after coronary artery bypass graft surgery. *Public Health Nursing, 17*(6), 460-467.

Charron-Prochownik, D., Wang, S., Sereika, S. M., Kim, Y., and Janz, N. K. (2006). A theory-based reproductive health and diabetes instrument. *American Journal of Health Behavior, 30*(2), 208-220.

Chassin, L., Corty, E., Presson, C. C., Olshavsky, R. W., Bensenberg, M., and Sherman, S. J. (1981). Predicting adolescents' intentions to smoke cigarettes. *Journal of Health and Social Behavior, 22*, 445-455.

Chassin, L., Presson, C. C., Sherman, S. J., Corty, E., and Olshavsky, R. W. (1984). Predicting the onset of cigarette smoking in adolescents: A longitudinal study. *Journal of Applied Social Psychology, 14*(3), 224-243.

Conner, M., and McMillan, B. (1999). Interaction effects in the theory of planned behavior: Studying cannabis use. *British Journal of Social Psychology, 38*, 295-317.

Conner, M., Sandberg, T., McMillan, B., and Higgins, A. (2006). Role of anticipated regret, intentions and intention stability in adolescent smoking initiation. *British Journal of Health Psychology, 11*, 85-101.

Courneya, K. S., Friedenreich, C. M. , Arthur, K., and Bobick, T. M. (1999). Understanding exercise in colorectal cancer patients: A prospective study using the theory of planned behavior. *Rehabilitation Psychology, 44*, 68-84.

Dean, M., Arvola, A., Vassallo, M., Lähteenmäki, L., Raats, M. M., Saba, A., and Shepard, R. (2006). Comparison of elicitation methods for moral and affective beliefs in the theory of planned behavior. *Appetite, 47*, 244-252.

De Vries, H., and Kok, G. J. (1986). From determinants of smoking behavior to implications for a preventative program. *Health Education Research, 1*, 85-94.

De Wit, J. B. F., Stroebe, W., De Vroome, E. M. M., Sandfort, T. G. M., and Van Griensven, G. J. P. (2000). Understanding AIDS preventive behavior with casual and primary partners in homosexual men: The theory of planned behavior and the information-motivation-behavior-skills model. *Psychology and Health, 15*, 325-340.

DiClemente, C. C., Prochaska, J. O., Fairhurst, S. K., Velicer, W. F., Velasquez, M. M., and Rossi, J. S. (1991). The process of smoking cessation: An analysis of precontemplation, contemplation, and preparation stages of change. *Journal of Consulting and Clinical Psychology, 59*, 295-304.

Eagly, A. H., and Chaiken, S. (1993). *The psychology of attitudes.* New York: Harcourt Brace Jovanovich Publishers.

Festinger, L. (1957). *A theory of cognitive dissonance.* Evanston, IL: Row, Peterson.

Fishbein, M. (1982). Social psychological analysis of smoking behavior. In J. R. Eiser (Ed.), *Social psychology and behavioral medicine* (pp. 179-197). New York: John Wiley and Sons.

Fishbein, M. (1993). Introduction. In D. J. Terry, C. Gallois, and M. McCamish (Eds.). *The Theory of Reasoned Action: Its application to AIDS-Preventive Behaviour* (pp. xv – xxv). Oxford, England: Pergamon Press Ltd.

Fishbein, M. and Ajzen, I. (1975). Belief, attitude, intention, and behavior: An introduction to theory and research. Reading, MA: Addison-Wesley Publishing.

Flay, B. R., Hu, F. B., Siddiqui, O., Day L. E., Hedeker, D., Petraitis, J., Richardson, J., and Sussman, S. (1994). Differential influence of parental smoking and friends' smoking on adolescent initiation and escalation of smoking. *Journal of Health and Social Behavior, 35,* 248-265.

Godin, G., and Lepage, l. (1988). Understanding the intentions of pregnant nullipara to not smoke cigarettes after childbirth. *Journal of Drug Education, 18*(2), 115-124.

Godin, G., Valois, P., Lepage, L., and Desharnais, R. (1992). Predictors of smoking behaviour: An application of Ajzen's Theory of Planned Behaviour. *British Journal of Addiction, 87,* 1335-1343.

Grube, J. W., Morgan, M., and McGree, S. T. (1986). Attitudes and normative beliefs as predictors of smoking intentions and behaviors: A test of three models. *British Journal of Social Psychology, 25*(2), 81-93.

Hanson, M. J. S. (2005). An examination of ethnic differences in cigarette smoking intention among female teenagers. *Journal of the American Academy of Nurse Practitioners, 17*(4), 149-155.

Hausenblas, H. A., Carron, A. V., and Mack, D. E. (1997). Application of the theories of reasoned action and planned behavior to exercise behavior: A meta-analysis. *Journal of Sport & Exercise Psychology, 19*(1), 36-51.

Higgins, A., and Conner, M. (2003). Understanding adolescent smoking: The role of the Theory of Planned Behavior and implementation intentions. *Psychology, Health, and Medicine, 8*(2), 173-186.

Madden, T. J., Ellen, P. S., and Ajzen, I. (1992). A comparison of the Theory of Planned Behavior and the Theory of Reasoned Action. *Personality and Social Psychology Bulletin, 18*(1), 3-9.

Marin, B. V., Marin, G., Perez-Stable, E. J., Otero-Sabogal, R., and Sabogal, F. (1990). Cultural differences in attitudes toward smoking: Developing messages using the Theory of Reasoned Action, *Journal of Applied Social Psychology, 20*(6), 478-493.

McAuliffe, T. (1988). The FTC and the effectiveness of cigarette advertising regulation. *Journal of Public Policy and Marketing, 7,* 49-64.

McMillan, B., and Conner, M. (2003). Using the theory of planned behaviour to understand alcohol and tobacco use in students. *Psychology, Health and Medicine, 8,* 317-328.

McMillan, B., Higgins, A. R., and Conner, M. (2005). Using an extended theory of planned behavior to understand smoking amongst schoolchildren. *Addiction Research and Theory, 13* (3), 293-306.

Montaño, D. E., Kasprzyk, D., and Taplin, S. H. (1997). The theory of reasoned action and the theory of planned behavior. In K. Glanz, F. M. Lewis, and B. K. Rimer (Eds.), *Health behavior and health education: Theory, research, and practice* (2nd ed., pp. 85-112). San Francisco: Jossey-Bass Inc.

Moan, I. S., and Rise, J. (2005). Quitting smoking: Applying an extended version of the Theory of Planned Behavior to predict intention and behavior. *Journal of Applied Biobehavioral Research, 10*(1), 39-68.

Moan, I. S., Rise, J., and Andersen, M. (2005). Predicting parents' intentions not to smoke indoors in the presence of their children using an extended version of the theory of planned behavior. *Psychology and Health, 20*(3), 353-371.

Park, H. S. (2000). Relationships among attitudes and subjective norms: Testing the theory of reasoned action across cultures. *Communication Studies, 51*(2), 162-176.

Pierce, J. P., and Gilpin, E. A. (1995). A historical analysis of tobacco marketing and the uptake of smoking by youth in the United States: 1890-1977. *Health Psychology, 14(*6), 500-508.

Prochaska, J. O. (1995). An eclectic and integrative approach: Transtheoretical therapy. In A. S. Gurman and S. B. Messer (Eds.), *Essential psychotherapies: Theory and practice (pp. 430-440).* New York: Guilford Press.

Prochaska, J. O., and DiClemente, C. C. (1983). Stages and processes of self-change in smoking: Toward an integrative model of change. *Journal of Consulting and Clinical Psychology, 51,* 390-395.

Prochaska, J. O., Velicer, W. F., DiClemente, C. C., and Fava, J. (1988). Measuring processes of change: Application to the cessation of smoking. *Journal of Consulting and Clinical Psychology, 56*(4), 520-528.

B. K. Rimer. (1997). Perspectives on intrapersonal theories of health behavior. In K. Glanz, F. M. Lewis, and B. K. Rimer (Eds.), *Health behavior and health education: Theory, research, and practice* (2nd ed., pp. 139-147). San Francisco: Jossey-Bass Inc.

Schifter, D. B., and Ajzen, I. (1985). Intention, perceived control, and weight loss: An application of the theory of planned behavior. *Journal of Personality and Social Psychology, 49,* 843-851.

Schiller J.S., Martinez M., and Barnes P. (2006, June). *Early release of selected estimates based on data from the 2005 National Health Interview Survey.* National Center for Health Statistics. http://www.cdc.gov/nchs/nhis.htm.

Schuster, C. P., and Powell, C. (1987). Comparison of cigarette and alcohol controversies. *Journal of Advertising, 16*(2), 26-33.

Sherman, S. J., Presson, C. C., Chassin, L., Bensenberg, M., Corty, E., and Olshavsky, R. W. (1982). Smoking intentions in adolescents: Direct experience and predictability. *Personality and Social Psychology Bulletin, 8*(2), 376-383.

Siegal, S., and Castellan, Jr., N. J. (1988). *Nonparametric statistics for the behavioral sciences.* New York: McGraw-Hill.

Sutton, S. (1998). Predicting and explaining intentions and behaviors: How well are we doing? *Journal of Applied Social Psychology, 28*(15), 1317-1338.

Sutton, S., French, D. P., Hennings, S. J., Mitchell, J., Wareham, N. J. , Griffin, S., Hardeman, W., and Kinmonth, A. L. (2003). Eliciting salient beliefs in research on the Theory of Planned Behavior: The effect of question wording. *Current Psychology: Developmental, Learning, Personality, Social, 22* (3), 234-251.

Trafimow, D. (1996). The importance of attitudes in the prediction of college students' intentions to drink. *Journal of Applied Social Psychology, 26,* 2167-2188.

Vardi, Y., and Weitz, E. (2002) Using the theory of Reasoned Action to predict organizational misbehavior. *Psychological Reports, 91,* 1027-1040.

Velicer, W. F., DiClemente, C. C., Prochaska, J. O., and Brandenburg, N. (1985). A decisional balance measure for predicting smoking cessation. *Journal of Personality and Social Psychology, 48,* 1279-1289.

Warner, K. E. (1977). The effects of the anti-smoking campaign on cigarette consumption. *American Journal of Public Health, 67,* 645-650.

APPENDIX A

For each of the following statements, please circle the number that best describes your agreement with that statement.

Q-1. I intend to quit smoking sometime						
Don't agree at all			Don't Agree Or Disagree			Agree Completely
0	1	2	3	4	5	6
Q-2. I intend to quit smoking sometime in the next 6 months.						
Don't agree at all			Don't Agree Or Disagree			Agree Completely
0	1	2	3	4	5	6
Q-3. I intend to quit smoking sometime in the next 30 days.						
Don't agree at all			Don't Agree Or Disagree			Agree Completely
0	1	2	3	4	5	6

Q-4.   How long have you been a smoker? _____ YEARS

Q-5.   How many cigarettes do you usually smoke during a day? _____

Q-6.   Did you quit smoking for at least 24 hours any time during the last 12 months?

                            (Circle the number of your answer.)
                            1 Yes
                            2 No

Q-7.   Your present age: _____ YEARS

Q-8.   Your gender: (Circle number of your answer.)
                            1 MALE
                            2 FEMALE

Q-9.   What is your ethnic background?

1 AFRICAN AMERICAN
2 ASIAN AMERICAN
3 AMERICAN INDIAN
4 CAUCASIAN (WHITE)
5 HISPANIC
6 OTHER (Please specify.) _____

Please list as many answers to the following questions as possible. There are no right or wrong answers. Your responses will be held in strictest confidence. Your participation today contributes a great deal to our work.

1. What do you see as the advantages of your quitting smoking [or in the next 30 days or 6 months] ?
2. What do you see as the disadvantages of your quitting smoking [or in the next 30 days or 6 months] ?
3. Is there anything else you associate with your quitting smoking [or in the next 30 days or 6 months] ?
4. Are there any groups or people who would approve of your quitting smoking [or in the next 30 days or 6 months] ?
5. Are there any groups or people who would disapprove of your quitting smoking [or in the next 30 days or 6 months] ?
6. Are there any other groups or people who come to mind when you think about quitting smoking [or in the next 30 days or 6 months] ?
7. What would make it easier for you to quit smoking [or in the next 30 days or 6 months] ?
8. What would make it difficult or impossible for you to quit smoking [or in the next 30 days or 6 months] ?

Chapter 6

NEW RESEARCH ON SMOKING CESSATION WITH ALCOHOL AND/OR DRUG USERS

Eve J. Wiseman

Special Treatment Section, Central Arkansas, USA
Veterans Healthcare System, Little Rock, Arkansas, USA
Departments of Psychiatry and Pharmacology,
University of Arkansas for Medical Sciences, Little Rock, Arkansas, USA

ABSTRACT

Although the smoking rate is declining in the general population, smoking remains highly prevalent among substance abusers. Very little is known about optimal treatments for the reduction of cigarette use in persons dually-dependent on nicotine and other substances, and investigators frequently exclude alcohol and drug abusers from anti-smoking research projects. Researchers are beginning to study the effectiveness of anti-smoking interventions, previously tested only in the general population, in people with other chemical dependencies. Issues impacting effectiveness of standard anti-smoking interventions in people with non-nicotine chemical dependencies include: timing of smoking cessation attempts relative to other substance use and relative to treatment for non-nicotine addictions, interrelated patterns of cigarette smoking with other substance use, and unique barriers to quitting or reasons for continued smoking among substance abusers. Novel anti-smoking strategies, which may be particularly effective for this dually-dependent population, are under development. Data indicate that substance-abusing populations, responsive to the systematic application of behavioral contingencies to reduce drug use, also benefit from behavioral strategies to reduce cigarette smoking.

INTRODUCTION

Although the smoking rate is declining in the general population, 80 to 90% of substance abusers still smoke cigarettes (Miller and Gold, 1998; Sees and Clark, 1993), and, despite the likelihood of their continuing to smoke, are frequently excluded from studies of anti-smoking treatments (Hall et al., 1985; Sirota et al., 1985; Stitzer and Bigelow, 1985; Stitzer et al., 1986; Bowers et al., 1987; Risser and Belcher, 1990; Kenford et al., 1994; Cinciripini et al., 1995; Crowley et al., 1991 and 1995). "Carving out" this population from smoking cessation research and from treatment efforts has important public health implications, since the higher rate of continued smoking puts substance abusers at higher risk for subsequent smoking-related problems. In addition to the problems attributed to cigarettes by themselves, combining smoking with alcohol and/or illegal drugs can increase risk of specific smoking-related problems (Brown, 2005; Tashkin et al., 1992; Visscher et al., 2003). In combination with smoking, alcohol increases risk for cancers of the oral cavity, pharynx, esophagus, and larynx (Brown, 2005). The impact of combined smoking and illegal drug use is less clear. However, substance abusers who smoke illegal drugs, such as cocaine, may prefer to smoke the drug mixed in a tobacco cigarette (Gorelick et al., 1997), and habitual smoking of illegal drugs can be associated with acute respiratory symptoms, obstructive ventilatory abnormalities, and impaired diffusing capacity of the lung (Tashkin et al., 1992). Visscher et al. (2003), in a study of the impact of substance use during pregnancy, determined that use of cigarettes, marijuana, and heroin predicted lower birth-weight infants at risk for adverse health consequences. Habitual smoking of cigarettes, in addition to habitual use of alcohol and/or illegal drugs, may have additive or synergistic effects with considerable associated morbidity and mortality.

Smoking many cigarettes per day and/or a higher degree of nicotine dependence may be markers of more severe substance use disorders or of particular types of substance use disorders in dually-dependent individuals (Frosch et al., 2000; Hershberger et al., 2004; Hertling et al., 2005; Hurt, 1995). Frosch et al. (2000) observed that, among methadone-maintained opiate-dependent subjects, illicit substance use increased in a stepwise fashion with number of cigarettes smoked per day, and smoking status was a better predictor of cocaine and opiate use than daily methadone dose. Illicit drug users in another study were found to have a higher degree of nicotine dependence if they smoked "crack" cocaine as well as injecting drugs, and significant relationships were found between nicotine dependence and risk behaviors for transmission of Human Immunodeficiency Virus (Hershberger et al., 2004). In a study of subjects with both alcohol and nicotine dependence (Hertling et al., 2005), alcohol-dependent smokers had more severe nicotine dependence than non-alcohol-dependent smokers, experienced significantly increased craving to smoke, and were likely to report depressive symptoms and sleep disturbances. Data linking nicotine dependence to problems with alcohol (DiFranza and Guerrera, 1990; Hertling et al., 2005) support Hurt's hypothesis (1995) that heavy smoking might be a marker for alcohol abuse. Genetic factors, such as a particular monoamine oxidase A genotype (Wiesbeck et al., 2006), may contribute to the frequent association of heavy smoking with alcohol dependence.

Substance abusers who smoke cigarettes, unlike other cigarette smokers, may have alcohol-specific and/or drug-specific reasons for continuing to smoke, especially in combination with alcohol and/or illegal drugs (Wiseman and McMillan, 1996 and 1998a; Okuyemi et al., 2006). In a study of the combined use of cigarettes with alcohol and/or cocaine, subjects were likely to report concurrent use (within the same month), simultaneous use (at the same time or within a couple of hours of the non-nicotine substance), and increased or improved alcohol and/or cocaine effect attributed to smoking cigarettes (Wiseman and McMillan, 1996). In another study of reasons for combining cocaine and cigarette use and for preferring either mentholated or non-mentholated cigarettes, subjects frequently reported sedating, stimulating, or addictive effects as reasons for the combined use of cigarettes with cocaine (Wiseman and McMillan, 1998a). Sedating or calming effects of cigarette smoking included reduction of cocaine-induced paranoia, and cocaine-substituting and cocaine-enhancing effects of cigarette smoking, especially from mentholated cigarettes, were categorized as stimulating effects. Addictive effects included craving for cigarette smoking that was triggered by cocaine use. Focus groups of persons in homeless settings also reported frequent cigarette smoking in combination with alcohol or illegal drugs or to achieve a substitute "high" (Okuyemi et al., 2006). Similar patterns of brain metabolic changes may explain some of the connections between smoking and alcohol/drug use: Brody et al. (2002) observed activation of brain regions associated with arousal, compulsive repetitive behaviors, sensory integration, and episodic memory when heavy smokers were exposed to cigarette-related cues and cigarette craving, resembling findings with other addictive substances.

Despite the strong link between non-nicotine substance use and cigarette smoking, substance abuse treatment focused on decreasing subsequent use of alcohol and illegal drugs may not impact cigarette smoking or craving to smoke cigarettes (Wiseman and McMillan, 1995, 1996, and 1998b). When followed over the course of intensive treatment for alcohol and illegal drugs, craving for cigarettes remained essentially unchanged while craving for non-nicotine substances declined precipitously (Wiseman and McMillan, 1995 and 1996). Other data showed that over 80% of subjects sampled from an outpatient or aftercare treatment setting still met Fagerstrom Tolerance Questionnaire criteria for medium to high nicotine dependence, despite long-standing abstinence from alcohol and illegal drugs in some cases (Wiseman and McMillan, 1998b). Light or moderate smokers (16-24 cigarettes per day) in this study sometimes reported smoking a larger number of cigarettes per day after cessation of non-nicotine substance use. These data suggest that the target behavior of abstinence from alcohol and illegal drugs may be independent of the target behavior of smoking cessation, in that abstinence from alcohol and illegal drugs achieved during substance abuse rehabilitation infrequently correlated with successful smoking cessation.

However, dually-dependent subjects reporting reduced cigarette smoking over long-term follow-up or participating in anti-smoking treatment concurrent with other substance abuse treatment may have better outcomes for alcohol and/or drug use (Shoptaw et al., 2002; Prochaska et al., 2004; Friend and Pagano, 2005). Friend and Pagano (2005) noted that smokers whose cigarette consumption decreased during Project MATCH, which followed alcohol-dependent subjects for 15 months, were less likely to relapse to alcohol use than subjects whose cigarette consumption increased or remained unchanged. During a 28-day intervention for methadone-maintained tobacco smokers, data supported a link between decreased cigarette use and decreased use of cocaine (Shoptaw et al., 1996). This finding was replicated during a 12-week smoking cessation intervention, also in methadone maintenance settings, with subjects providing more opiate-free and cocaine-free urines during weeks when they met criteria for smoking abstinence than during weeks when they did not meet these criteria (Shoptaw et al., 2002). In a meta-analysis of smoking cessation interventions with individuals in substance abuse treatment or recovery, Prochaska et al. (2004) concluded that smoking cessation interventions provided during addictions treatment were associated with a 25% increased likelihood of long-term abstinence from alcohol and illicit drugs, although the long-term intervention effects for smoking cessation were usually nonsignificant. Thus, reductions in tobacco use, including short-term reductions during concurrent treatments for nicotine and non-nicotine substances, may be associated with better long-term drinking and drug use outcomes in substance abuse treatment.

All of the above factors support the critical need for researchers to develop and for clinicians to implement effective anti-smoking interventions for dually-dependent persons. Based on the high prevalence of continued smoking among substance abusers and the tendency to be "carved out" of smoking cessation research (described above), this population is at risk to be among the last to quit smoking, possibly resulting in tremendous personal and societal costs. The above data also support that cigarette smoking may have multiple connections to alcohol and illegal drug use, ranging from being a possible marker for severity and/or specific types of alcohol/drug use to being a means to modify or substitute for effects of other substances. Additional data, cited above, suggest that patients reporting reduction of cigarette smoking may have a better prognosis for recovery from non-nicotine substances. Therefore, treatment providers who focus on smoking cessation, in addition to focusing on abstinence from alcohol and illegal drugs, may achieve better long-term drinking and drug use outcomes for their patients. However, interventions have yet to be developed that achieve long-term reductions in tobacco use in the dually-dependent population.

ANTI-SMOKING INTERVENTIONS TARGETING SUBSTANCE ABUSERS

Cigarette smoking has not been a treatment focus for substance-abusing patients, yet some substance-abusing patients have participated in anti-smoking interventions with favorable results (Joseph, 1993; Hurt et al., 1994 and 2005; Shoptaw et al., 1996 and 2002; Johnson et al., 2005; Richter et al., 2005; Wiseman et al., 2005). Single component interventions have included anti-smoking medications for alcohol-dependent subjects (Hurt et al., 2005; Johnson et al., 2005) and a contingency management intervention for methadone-maintained tobacco smokers (Shoptaw et al., 1996). Multi-component interventions have incorporated a combination of non-pharmacological and pharmacological techniques, with non-pharmacological techniques ranging from educational approaches (Joseph, 1993) to group therapy (Hurt et al., 1994) to behavioral techniques, such as motivational interviewing (Richter et al., 2005) and contingency management (Shoptaw et al., 2002; Wiseman et al., 2005). Pharmacotherapy in multi-component interventions has ranged from clonidine (Joseph, 1993) to nicotine replacement (Hurt et al., 1994; Shoptaw et al., 2002; Wiseman et al., 2005) to bupropion combined with nicotine replacement (Richter et al., 2005). Some studies incorporating multi-component interventions have explored the separate effects of the pharmacological and non-pharmacological components of the interventions (Shoptaw et al., 2002; Wiseman et al., 2005).

Single component studies of anti-smoking medications among alcohol-dependent subjects indicate that higher than usual doses of nicotine replacement may be needed (Hurt et al., 2005) and that off-label use of medications may assist in promoting smoking abstinence (Johnson et al., 2005). Hurt et al. (2005) tailored nicotine patch therapy to baseline serum cotinine in their treatment of 195 nondepressed smokers with alcohol dependence in sustained full remission. Based on their baseline serum cotinine levels, subjects' nicotine patch doses ranged from 22 milligrams to 44 milligrams per day, yet there was no evidence of severe nicotine toxicity. These higher than usual doses of nicotine replacement resulted in over half of the subjects achieving smoking abstinence at the end of the 8 weeks of nicotine patch treatment. In a study of off-label medication, Johnson et al. (2005) used up to 300 milligrams per day of oral topiramate, an anticonvulsant possibly associated with reduction of alcohol and/or cocaine use, and observed that alcohol-dependent subjects receiving topiramate were significantly more likely to quit smoking at weeks 9 and 12 than placebo recipients. Thus, among alcohol-dependent persons, anti-smoking medication as a single intervention to assist in smoking cessation may be effective. However, different approaches to anti-smoking medication, such as higher than usual doses or off-label use, may be needed compared to anti-smoking medication approaches for the general population.

Perhaps the only single component, non-pharmacological, anti-smoking intervention thus far among substance abusers is a contingency management intervention for methadone-maintained tobacco smokers (Shoptaw et al., 1996). Yet results from previous research demonstrate that substance-abusing patients may be particularly sensitive to the systematic application of behavioral contingencies (Higgins et al., 1993 and 1994; Silverman et al., 1996), and the effectiveness of anti-smoking behavioral strategies has been well-established in studies of persons other than substance abusers (Hall et al., 1985; Sirota et al., 1985; Stitzer and Bigelow, 1985; Stitzer et al., 1986; Bowers et al., 1987; Risser and Belcher, 1990; Cinciripini et al., 1995; Crowley et al., 1991 and 1995). However, the study by Shoptaw et al., (1996) appears to be one of the first using contingency management, without anti-smoking pharmacotherapy, to reduce smoking among patients dependent on nicotine and another addictive substance. Methadone-maintenance subjects were able to earn up to $73 in vouchers for breath samples with carbon monoxide (CO) values less than or equal to 4 parts per million (ppm). Most of the subjects were able to produce breath CO levels below 4 ppm, which is comparable to the level of non-smokers, indicating that specific single component, non-pharmacological, anti-smoking interventions may be effective in subtypes of dually-dependent patients. Thus, this contingency management intervention, by itself, resulted in reduced breath CO levels in the subtype "methadone-maintained tobacco smokers."

Multi-component interventions have varied widely in the specific combinations of non-pharmacological and pharmacological techniques (Joseph, 1993; Hurt et al., 1994; Richter et al., 2005). In a sample of 319 substance-abusing inpatients, Joseph (1993) found that more of the inpatients who successfully quit smoking were admitted after initiation of a smoke-free policy and concurrent 21-day treatment for cigarette smoking and other addictions. Anti-smoking treatment included lectures regarding the pharmacology of nicotine, films, discussion groups, and clonidine patches. Hurt et al., (1994) obtained similar results in their study of 51 substance-abusing inpatients participating in concurrent 2.5-week treatment for nicotine dependence and treatment for other addictions. Treatment for nicotine dependence consisted of ten 1-hour group therapy sessions (group sessions four times per week) and nicotine gum. The intervention group had significantly higher smoking cessation rates than the control group at a 1-year follow-up. More recently, Richter et al. (2005) utilized a combination of 7 weeks of bupropion at 300 milligrams per day, 12 weeks of nicotine gum, and 6 sessions of motivational interviewing among 28 methadone-maintained tobacco smokers. At 6 month follow-up, subjects either reported significantly fewer cigarettes smoked per day or met criteria for biochemically-verified abstinence. Thus, there are data supporting the combination of a wide range of pharmacological and non-pharmacological techniques that impact cigarette smoking among dually-dependent patients; however, the differences between interventions are extreme, since they vary in setting, type of patient, duration, intensity, type of pharmacological intervention(s), and type of non-pharmacological intervention(s). Conclusions regarding the contribution of specific interventions to the overall effectiveness of these multi-component interventions remain to be determined.

Some researchers have begun to explore the separate effects of pharmacological and non-pharmacological components of anti-smoking interventions among dually-dependent patients (Shoptaw et al., 2002; Wiseman et al., 1995 and 2005). Shoptaw et al. (2002) evaluated the effects of relapse prevention and contingency management for optimizing smoking cessation outcomes using nicotine replacement therapy in methadone-maintained tobacco smokers. During 12 weeks of treatment, subjects assigned to receive contingency management plus nicotine patches showed significantly higher rates of smoking abstinence than those assigned to patches only or to patches plus relapse prevention. In an earlier study of the effect of nicotine patches on drug craving and cigarette use among drug abusers in abstinence-based treatment (not on methadone maintenance), nicotine patches worn for 2 days significantly reduced craving for cigarettes but, compared to placebo patches, did not affect cigarette use (Wiseman and McMillan, 1995). This result was replicated with a longer period of patch application during a combined behavioral and pharmacological anti-smoking intervention (Wiseman et al., 2005). The behavioral component, a contingency management intervention in which "reinforcement" subjects were rewarded for reducing their breath CO levels, was significantly more effective than nicotine patches based on lower CO levels and on reports of fewer cigarettes smoked per day. Reductions in breath CO levels were significant for "reinforcement" subjects, but discrepancies were observed between reductions in breath CO levels concurrent with unchanged or, for a few subjects, increased serum cotinine levels; therefore, "reinforcement" subjects may have manipulated their smoking patterns relative to the fixed timing of the CO assessments, especially if this increased the likelihood of being rewarded for a low breath CO level. Different approaches to contingency management, such as modifying the interventions to minimize likelihood of manipulation of smoking patterns in order to obtain rewards, may be needed compared to contingency management approaches successful in the general population. However, the data from these three studies indicate that, for specific subtypes of drug-abusing patients, contingency management interventions, with or without nicotine patches, may impact smoking behavior more than nicotine patches by themselves and more than nicotine patches combined with relapse prevention.

BIOCHEMICAL VERIFICATION OF SMOKING STATUS

Optimal methodology for biochemical verification of smoking status has not been determined, either for the general population or for substance-abusing patients. One of the previously cited studies, with subjects sampled from patients hospitalized for substance abuse treatment (Joseph, 1993), relied entirely on self-report of smoking status without biochemical verification. Joseph's interventions did not include rewards for reducing or quitting smoking, which probably would have increased the likelihood of subjects misrepresenting their smoking status. Contingency management interventions, frequently utilized for substance-abusing populations (Higgins et al., 1993 and 1994; Silverman et al., 1996; Shoptaw et al.,

1996 and 2002; Wiseman et al., 2005) require verification of smoking status and/or verification of abstinence from alcohol/drug use to offset the likelihood of subjects misrepresenting reduced use to obtain rewards. Some contingency management interventions have linked rewards directly to a biochemical indicator of reduced smoking or of non-smoking status (Shoptaw et al., 1996 and 2002; Wiseman et al., 2005). Since personal history is not always reliable, regardless of the type of anti-smoking intervention, an objective biomarker may be needed to accurately differentiate smokers from non-smokers and/or to verify reduction of smoking (Bramer and Kallungal, 2003).

A comparison of tests used to distinguish smokers from nonsmokers demonstrated that cotinine (blood, saliva, or urine) was the measure of choice, but, for most clinical applications, exhaled CO provided an acceptable degree of discrimination and was cheaper and simpler to apply (Jarvis et al., 1987). Studies that excluded substance-abusing smokers as well as those that targeted substance-abusing smokers have utilized breath CO alone as a measure of smoking status (Stitzer and Bigelow, 1985; Stitzer et al., 1986; Bowers et al., 1987; Rand et al., 1989; Crowley et al., 1991; Shoptaw et al., 1996). Of the studies listed, all but two (Stitzer et al., 1986; Rand et al., 1989) had fixed, rather than randomly scheduled, appointments for CO sampling. With fixed appointments for CO sampling, isolated smoking could occur immediately or shortly after that day's CO measurements and not be detected by measuring CO levels on the next day. Previous research has demonstrated that CO was sensitive to short-term manipulation of smoking patterns (Wilcox et al., 1979, and Jeffery et al., 1988). Such behavior might occur if subjects wanted to earn rewards linked to specific CO levels but did not want to totally quit smoking. Wiseman et al. (2005) observed this pattern of behavior during a contingency management intervention that rewarded reduced CO levels, in which dually-dependent subjects reported continuing to smoke cigarettes despite being rewarded for reaching CO "non-smoking" targets.

Therefore, substance-abusing persons probably require modifications of the "usual" protocol for CO monitoring of smoking status which is appropriate for other clinical populations. Random CO measurements, including evening and weekend collection times, may be needed to accurately determine average results for baseline and post-intervention CO levels (Jeffery et al., 1988), since the half-life of CO is 4 to 6 hours (Ohlin et al., 1976). If a categorical outcome such as "smoker" versus "non-smoker" is desired, the CO breakpoint may differ for substance-abusing patients compared to the general population (Shoptaw et al., 1996; Wiseman et al., 2005). Fix et al. (1979) observed that, among non-substance-abusing smokers of approximately a pack-per-day, breath CO fell from 24 ppm to 7.71 ppm after at least 24 hours of reported abstinence, supporting a CO breakpoint for "non-smoker" of 8 ppm or less in the general population. However, Wiseman et al. (2005) observed that substance-abusing smokers could achieve CO levels of 8 ppm or less, despite reporting continued daily smoking. Shoptaw et al. (1996) chose a lower breakpoint, rewarding substance-abusing smokers who achieved CO values of less than or equal to 4 ppm. If future studies utilize CO monitoring as the sole measure of smoking status in substance-abusing subjects, protocols may need to incorporate multiple CO measurements obtained at random times, including times frequently associated with a high likelihood of smoking, combined with a comparatively low CO breakpoint, to differentiate "non-smokers" from "smokers."

Because of the potential impact of short-term changes in smoking pattern on breath CO, other studies have used different biochemical markers than CO or incorporated additional biochemical markers with longer half-lives than CO, such as cotinine, to verify smoking status at the end of treatment or at follow-up after treatment (Hall et al., 1985; Jeffery et al., 1988; Glasgow et al., 1993; Hurt et al., 1994; Crowley et al., 1995; Cinciripini et al., 1995; Johnson et al., 2005). Future studies that depend on fixed appointment times for CO measurement or on relatively high CO breakpoints for "non-smoking" in substance-abusing patients may need to incorporate a biochemical marker with a longer half-life than that of CO throughout the duration of the anti-smoking treatment, rather than just at the end of treatment or at follow-up after treatment. Otherwise, researchers may miss important data on changes in smoking patterns, in addition to changes in amount smoked, during the course of the anti-smoking treatments.

Sampling of saliva markers of smoking status that have longer half-lives than CO, such as thiocyanate or cotinine, is quicker, easier, and has fewer associated risks than drawing blood for assessment of serum cotinine. Thiocyanates are infrequently used as a marker of smoking status, since they are found in many foods including almonds, broccoli, cabbage, turnips, garlic, and horseradish; patients who ingest large quantities of such foods could produce thiocyanate levels as high as those found in smokers and yield false-positive information (Prignot, 1987). Thiocyanate also provided the poorest discrimination in a comparison of tests used to distinguish smokers from nonsmokers, in which the concentration of cotinine was the best indicator of smoking (Pojer et al., 1984; Jarvis et al., 1987). However, sugar-stimulated saliva cotinine levels were significantly lower than unstimulated saliva cotinine levels in one study (Schneider et al., 1997), suggesting that changes in salivary flow can affect saliva cotinine levels. Just as patients could manipulate their smoking patterns to lower breath CO levels, it is possible that they could increase salivary flow to lower saliva cotinine levels.

Urine measures are similarly at risk for manipulation, including purposeful ingestion of large quantities of fluid to dilute the urine and to lower the level of the marker in the urine. As serum is less vulnerable to manipulation than urine, measurement of serum cotinine may be preferable for definitive validation of smoking status (Waage et al., 1992), especially for substance-abusing patients prone to manipulative behavior and/or for those with histories of attempting to manipulate results of urine drug screens. Thus, despite the discomfort associated with drawing blood and the cost of the assay, measurement of serum cotinine may be needed for certain types of patients.

A combination of breath CO and serum cotinine may be particularly suited to future anti-smoking interventions among substance-abusing patients, such as contingency management interventions that directly link rewards to both "short-term" (breath CO) and "long-term" (serum cotinine) indicators of smoking cessation/reduction. In contrast to blood drawn for measurement of serum cotinine levels, breath samples provide immediate feedback of CO levels and can result in immediate reinforcement for patients meeting CO-specific goals. Crowley and colleagues (1991) noted that subjects may earn initial reinforcement for reduced CO from several hours of tobacco abstinence that may not influence the more persistent cotinine, and, according to learning theory, reinforcement for initial small or brief steps may best shape new behavior. However, the slow disappearance of cotinine can facilitate identifying smokers who attempt to conceal their habit by not smoking for at least several hours before CO sampling but who resume smoking between CO samples (Wilcox et al., 1979). Additional rewards linked to reduced cotinine levels might discourage manipulation of smoking to meet "short-term" CO targets, although, the time needed for laboratory analysis would mandate a delay in feedback and reinforcement of cotinine results. Thus, the feedback and reinforcement for cotinine levels would be delayed compared to that for CO, but cotinine is more resistant to manipulation of smoking patterns than CO and could provide important information about patterns of smoking reduction/cessation during and after an intervention. Relatively higher amounts of reinforcement for reduced cotinine levels, compared to amounts of reinforcement for reduced CO levels, might increase the motivation for dually-dependent subjects to achieve longer-term smoking reduction/cessation. In addition, Lerman and colleagues suggested that feedback of cotinine levels might be a motivational smoking cessation intervention as well as providing validation of smoking status in clinical trials (Lerman et al., 1993).

ADDITIONAL RECOMMENDATIONS FOR FUTURE RESEARCH

Homogeneous Samples

Homogeneous samples may be important in future research on smoking cessation treatment efficacy in dually-dependent patients, since it is possible that some patients with a specific diagnosis or specific constellation of diagnoses will improve while others will not (Barber and Lubosky, 1992). For example, data indicate that a homogeneous sample of alcohol dependent subjects in full, sustained remission may have better smoking cessation outcomes from a particular treatment than other alcohol dependent subjects (Hughes and Kalman, 2006). Results from studies of homogeneous drug-dependent populations suggest that there may be anti-smoking techniques appropriate for opiate-dependent subjects taking an opiate agonist (Shoptaw et al., 1996 and 2002) and interventions tailored to in-treatment, cocaine-dependent subjects meeting criteria for early remission in a controlled environment (Wiseman et al., 2005). Although structured and semi-structured interviews as well as testing batteries may aid in selecting on the basis of diagnosis, patients might still differ on dimensions that affect outcome of smoking cessation treatment. Obtaining within-study homogeneity on all characteristics that impact effectiveness of smoking cessation in this population is improbable, until the critical characteristics are completely catalogued.

Quantitative Variables

To accomplish this feat, researchers must quantify as many of the candidate characteristics or "explanatory variables" in dually-dependent subjects as possible, both for descriptive purposes and to predict to what extent changes in the "response variables" of smoking cessation and/or reduction depend on changes in the explanatory variables (Greenhouse and Junker, 1992). Exploratory regression analyses are needed to clarify the extent of the relationship between smoking cessation/reduction and explanatory variables such as age, educational level, socioeconomic status, body mass index prior to cessation, severity of dependence on a specific substance (nicotine and non-nicotine), time since last use of a specific non-nicotine substance, time spent in alcohol/drug treatment, dosage of methadone or other medications for addictive disorders, severity of psychiatric problems other than substance use disorders, severity of medical problems, severity of stressors, and level of current functioning. Instruments such as the Addiction Severity Index (McLellan et al., 1985), frequently utilized by clinical providers for treatment planning with substance-abusing patients, generate severity scores in multiple problem areas per patient. Global Assessment of Functioning scores (Tungstrom et al., 2005), numerical equivalents for patients' social and occupational functioning within a standardized range, are also readily available in clinical settings. Thus, assessments may already be in place that will assist future researchers in studying the relationship between quantifiable characteristics of substance-abusing subjects and response to anti-smoking interventions. Studies will need to incorporate measures of nicotine dependence severity, since most alcohol/drug treatment programs have not added these to routine assessments of patients. The Fagerstrom Tolerance Questionnaire has proven reliability and validity in measuring degree of nicotine dependence (Fagerstrom and Schneider, 1989). Measurement of pre-treatment serum cotinine may also function as a marker of severity of nicotine dependence and as an explanatory variable for success or failure in smoking cessation/reduction: Hall et al. (1984) observed that elevated serum cotinine level was the best predictor of treatment dropout and of smoking at the end of treatment and at follow-up assessments.

Motivation

In addition to explanatory variables that are quantifiable, investigators must explore the impact of qualitative characteristics, such as the impact of motivation to quit smoking on treatment efficacy. By incorporating "stages of change" assessments and related methodology, investigators can explore motivation to quit and perceived barriers to quitting as explanatory variables for anti-smoking treatment response among dually-dependent patients (DiClemente et al., 1991; Asher et al., 2003). Assessment of correlates of motivation, such as barriers to change, may provide targets for specific intervention efforts ranging from providing corrective information about consequences of smoking cessation to providing methods for overcoming barriers and for increasing confidence in ability to quit (Martin et al., 2006). After identifying specific barriers to quitting smoking for in-treatment substance abusers, Asher et al. (2003) recommended corrective feedback focusing on concerns about effects of smoking cessation on sobriety and on concerns about needing cigarettes to cope with feeling depressed. Motivational interviewing, rather than more intense and/or costly interventions, may be especially appropriate for dually-dependent "precontemplators" who are not interested in smoking cessation or are not ready to quit smoking (Abrams, 1995; Monti et al., 1995). However, Hurt et al. (1994) argued that results could be biased if "precontemplators" are "carved out" and only well-motivated subjects are left to participate in anti-smoking interventions other than motivational interviewing. Anti-smoking interventions that emphasize reduction of smoking biomarker levels (CO or cotinine) allow inclusion of subjects who are unmotivated to totally stop smoking (Crowley et al., 1991), and contingency reinforcement may be particularly useful in promoting and sustaining abstinence in smokers not seeking cessation treatment (Stitzer et al., 1986). Crowley and colleagues (1995) also noted that expressed motivation to change was unrelated to outcome in their smoking cessation intervention. Therefore, the effect of motivation to quit smoking on response to smoking cessation treatment remains to be clarified.

Demographic and Diagnostic Variables

Besides motivational factors, other qualitative characteristics, including demographic and diagnostic variables, could account for different responses to interventions (Glynn, 1992). Anti-smoking interventions that have been specifically successful for women versus men in the general population, such as clonidine (Perkins, 2001), have not been studied in dually-dependent women. Qualitative characteristics related to diagnosis, such as substance-related diagnostic subtype and presence or absence of a specific concurrent psychiatric disorder, also deserve study, since an intervention may be appropriate only to certain subtypes or in the presence of certain concurrent disorders. Opiate-dependent patients on opiate agonist therapy, such as methadone, may be particularly suited to an in-clinic smoking cessation intervention implemented over a long time period, an intervention that would be inappropriate for opiate-dependent patients obtaining care through sporadic emergency room and/or primary care visits. Minimal anti-smoking interventions with alcohol-dependent patients in sustained, full remission, have achieved results equal to those from non-alcoholic populations (Hughes and Kalman, 2006), suggesting that different and/or more intense anti-smoking interventions are needed for alcohol-dependent patients who do not meet diagnostic criteria for "sustained, full remission." For example, Monti et al. (1995) speculated that sequencing anti-smoking interventions after some sobriety has been established may benefit alcohol-dependent patients in "early, partial remission." More recent data do not support the recommendation to delay smoking cessation in alcohol-dependent patients: according to Durazzo et al. (2006), as continued cigarette smoking may adversely affect recovery of brain metabolite concentrations and cognition during early remission from alcohol and, per Ceballos et al. (2006), nicotine replacement for smoking cessation may improve cognitive efficiency among in-treatment alcohol and stimulant abusers. If this effect of nicotine replacement reflects facilitation of cognitive function, rather than simple alleviation of nicotine withdrawal, nicotine replacement might be especially appropriate for cognitively impaired substance abusers in early recovery.

Clarifying the importance of diagnosis-related qualitative characteristics extends beyond substance-related diagnostic subtypes, in that understanding the impact of concurrent psychiatric disorders may be critical in matching patients to the most appropriate treatments (Glynn, 1992). Different treatment strategies may be needed for substance-abusing smokers with concurrent psychiatric disorders such as depression, schizophrenia, or personality disorders. Depression has an adverse impact on smoking cessation and may be especially detrimental in persons with comorbid alcohol dependence (Glassman, 1993; Covey et al., 1993). Therefore, depressed substance-abusing patients who are attempting to stop smoking may fare better with bupropion, which may facilitate cessation in part by reducing depressive symptoms (Catley et al., 2005), or with nortriptyline, another anti-depressant recognized as a second-line treatment for smoking cessation (Schnoll and Lerman, 2006). Adherence to nortriptyline can be tracked through blood levels; however, nortriptyline is not a first-line medication for patients at high risk for self-harm, since it can be lethal in overdose (Teicher et al., 1993). Cigarette smoking by patients with schizophrenia may lead to higher dosages of anti-psychotic medication by increasing hepatic metabolism and renal excretion and possibly enhancing dopamine release (Salokangas et al., 1997). Therefore, smokers with schizophrenia who complain about having to take "too much" anti-psychotic medication may be motivated to reduce or quit smoking if providers educate them regarding the connection between smoking and higher dosages of anti-psychotic medication. Since smoking is also associated with reduced levels of Parkinsonism from anti-psychotic medications (Goff et al., 1992), clinicians may need to provide anti-Parkinsonian medication to patients on neuroleptics who quit smoking or may need to switch to neuroleptics with fewer Parkinsonian side effects, thereby avoiding potential "self-medication" of side effects through cigarette smoking. Substance-abusing patients with concurrent personality disorders may benefit more from cognitive-behavioral therapies than from medications, as has been the case for treatment of personality-disordered patients with primary psychiatric disorders other than substance abuse (Glynn, 1992).

Anti-Smoking Medication

Thus, research is needed to determine which dually-dependent patients should receive anti-smoking medication and whether they should be matched, based on qualitative and quantitative characteristics, to specific medication(s), doses of medication, and/or to specific times for medication initiation, modification, and/or duration. Boyarsky and McCance-Katz (2000) developed preliminary guidelines for a "substance abuser-treatment" matching framework, including recommendations regarding when to initiate and discontinue pharmacotherapy. They concluded that, to maximize therapeutic benefits of treatment, substance-abusing patients should be individually assessed and provided clinically-indicated medications (Boyarsky and McCance-Katz, 2000). Substance-abusing patients with more severe nicotine dependence may be more likely to require anti-smoking medication(s) and may also require non-standard use of anti-smoking medication, such as higher than usual doses matched to their severity of nicotine dependence or combinations of medications (Hughes, 1995 and 2006; Richter et al., 2005; American Psychiatric Association, 2006). Combinations of anti-smoking medications may address a combination of specific obstacles to quitting: by combining bupropion and nicotine gum, Richter et al. (2005) may have assisted subjects in avoiding depression due to nicotine withdrawal as well as providing a means for rapid alleviation of craving to smoke. Using a combination of nicotine replacement treatments, such as the longer-acting nicotine patch to protect against withdrawal combined with the shorter-acting nicotine gum to address breakthrough craving to smoke, may also improve smoking cessation outcomes (American Psychiatric Association, 2006). Substance-abusing smokers who are refractory to current treatments may benefit from newer medications, such as varenicline and rimonabant (Henningfield et al. 2005).

Clarification is needed regarding optimum times for initiation, modification, and duration of anti-smoking medication in substance abusers. Monti et al. (1995) recommended delaying anti-smoking interventions until alcohol-dependent patients had established some sobriety, but the duration of abstinence from alcohol that might be necessary prior to attempting to quit smoking is unknown. Frequent follow-up of patients attempting to quit smoking as well as on-going modification of treatment to optimize results has been recommended: Kenford et al (1994) observed that smoking during the first two weeks of nicotine patch therapy was highly correlated with longer-term inability to quit smoking and, therefore, recommended follow-up assessment within the first 2 weeks and altering treatment, if indicated. Based on these data, prescribing small amounts of anti-smoking medication may be indicated initially, until medication effectiveness is known. Receiving limited amounts of medication might encourage substance abusers, who are prone to treatment compliance problems unless they have an incentive (Higgins et al., 1993 and 1994), to adhere to follow-up smoking cessation assessments. If dually-dependent persons do not keep appointments for follow-up, limiting amount of medication initially dispensed will reduce pharmacy-related expenditures. For patients that do adhere to follow-up appointments, long-term medication therapies and harm reduction strategies may further improve outcome for approved medications (Wiseman, 1998; McLellan et al., 2000; Henningfield et al., 2005).

Tailored Treatment

Ultimately, clarification of explanatory variables, such as time abstinent from alcohol, and clarification of strategies, such as anti-smoking medication protocols for non-adherent patients, may assist clinicians in tailoring anti-smoking treatments according to each substance-abusing patient's demographic, diagnostic, motivational, and treatment profile. Specific combinations of quantitative and qualitative explanatory variables may be important in anti-smoking treatment decisions; for example, Swan et al. (1995) found that body mass index prior to cessation (quantitative variable) and "weight gain as a reason for prior relapse" (qualitative variable) were significantly related to relapse to smoking in younger (quantitative variable) women (qualitative variable) of lower socioeconomic status (quantitative variable). Abrams et al. (1995) suggested that computer technology could be used to tailor treatment for individual patients and to provide feedback regarding each patient's response to treatment over time. A recent technology transfer study supported the feasibility of a computer-assisted system to get patients needed services, excluding anti-smoking treatment, based on their Addiction Severity Index scores (Carise et al., 2005); patients randomized to computer-assisted treatment planning received significantly more and better-matched services and were more likely to complete the full course of treatment. However, explanatory variables that predict dually-dependent patients' response to anti-smoking treatment are not fully characterized, and computer-assisted systems that match profiles of these variables to the appropriate treatment remain to be developed and implemented. In the interim, a descriptive approach using flexible research methods, such as those used in naturalistic and observational studies, may provide patterns of data that will assist in generating important hypotheses about smoking cessation in dually-dependent patients (Abrams et al., 1995).

Single-Case Research and Harm Reduction

For clinician researchers interested in such flexible methods, each substance abuser who also smokes cigarettes represents the opportunity for single-case research, possibly necessitating a combination of multiple-baseline and changing-criterion designs (Hersen, 1992). Multiple-baseline designs are particularly appropriate to evaluate treatments that are not subject to clear discontinuation, such as relapse prevention for addictive substances and/or long-term addiction pharmacotherapy, and when several target behaviors are selected for modification, such as use of alcohol, illegal drugs, and cigarettes. This is consistent with a previous guideline recommending that substance abuse treatment involve multiple modalities targeted to the various problems encountered in substance-abusing patients (Crits-Christoph and Siqueland, 1996). Unanswered questions for this dually-dependent population include whether the target behaviors of alcohol/drug use and cigarette smoking are dependent on or independent of each other, whether they respond to the same types of treatment, and what degree of baseline stability is required in each of the target behaviors to reliably detect treatment effects. Changing-criterion designs parallel harm reduction techniques, by using progressively more stringent criteria (fewer days drinking or using drugs and/or smaller amounts of daily alcohol/drug/cigarette use) and seeking incremental improvements until the end point criteria (abstinence from alcohol/drugs or smoking cessation) are attained. Although the degree of reduced alcohol, drug, or cigarette use that result in clinically meaningful improvement remains to be clarified, proponents of harm reduction argue that the all-important factor is whether individual patients are making incremental progress toward their therapeutic goals.

By embracing a wide range of behavior change, harm reduction provides a realistic, pragmatic, and flexible approach that encourages repeated treatment contacts and early access to harm-reducing options (Abrams et al., 1995). Dependence on nicotine and dependence on other substances are life-long diagnoses (American Psychiatric Association, 2000), seemingly mandating a chronic illness perspective, and harm reduction facilitates the integrated management of chronic disease (Abrams et al., 1995). If harm reduction is feasible through reduced cigarette use (Wiseman, 1998), diagnostic modifiers such as "partial remission," used to describe reduction of non-nicotine substance use, may be appropriate to describe reduction of cigarette use. Descriptive terms such as "lapse" versus "relapse," used to distinguish a temporary "slip" involving relatively insignificant amounts of alcohol/drug versus an extended period of heavy use, may also be appropriate to distinguish a temporary "slip" involving a few cigarettes on a rare occasion versus smoking a significant amount on a daily basis. Instead of focusing solely on achievement of complete, sustained remission from cigarette smoking (smoking cessation), future research may need to track whether different treatments lead to different rates of partial remission from smoking and/or different rates of relapse to heavy smoking. Developing treatment strategies beyond the initial approach may benefit treatment-refractory and/or relapse-prone subjects (Hollifield et al., 2006). These might include treatments of higher intensity, including "booster" sessions at critical junctures, and/or treatments of longer duration.

Long-Term Studies

The need for long-term studies is also one of the recommendations for research with the chronically mentally ill (Glynn, 1992). Since dually-dependent persons are likely to have chronic, relapsing problems (McLellan et al., 2000), future anti-smoking research with this population may need to parallel recommendations for research with chronically mentally ill (CMI) patients. Recommendations for research with the CMI include exploration of pharmacotherapy/psychotherapy interaction issues, long-term intervention as well as long-term follow-up with multidimensional assessments, and interfacing with other service providers, (Glynn, 1992). Multiple component anti-smoking interventions, involving a combination of pharmacological and/or non-pharmacological techniques, will benefit from standardization of procedures to minimize possible confounding of interaction effects. Otherwise, the researcher must collect, record, and analyze all uncontrolled interventions to determine their effect on treatment outcome (Glynn, 1992). Researchers may need to vary combination techniques, by studying the effects of exposure to intervention components in different sequences compared to the effects of concurrent interventions (Friedman et al., 2006). Regardless of the type of intervention, research has shown that many dually-dependent smokers are unlikely to maintain long-term gains after termination of active anti-smoking treatments (Prochaska et al., 2004), often "relapsing" to pre-treatment smoking behavior. Therefore, long-term treatment success may require long-term, chronic treatment interventions (Bigelow et al., 1981; McLellan et al., 2000). Since treatment retention is a significant problem for substance-abusing patients (Crits-Christoph and Siqueland, 1996), reinforcement contingencies and payment for attendance may need to be available to increase long-term treatment retention and adherence to long-term follow-up assessments.

Special Populations

However, even if in-treatment substance abusers are followed for smoking cessation progress over long time intervals, interfacing with other service providers will be needed because out-of-treatment substance abusers may never engage in specialized treatment (Anton et al., 2006) and/or be at high risk for fragmentation of care (Schrag et al., 2006). Anton et al. (2006) recommended identification of effective interventions that could be delivered in non-specialized health care settings, thus serving substance-abusing patients who might otherwise not receive treatment. An alternative model of care targeting this population might integrate substance abuse treatment providers in primary care clinics (Oslin et al., 2006). However, lower socioeconomic, underserved, and minority populations may have significant barriers to accessing even primary care (Abrams et al., 1995). High-risk groups, such as low-income pregnant smokers, may benefit from incentive and contingency management strategies at the worksite or in community-wide "quit-and-win" programs (Donatelle et al., 2004). Homeless smokers, who have reported high levels of boredom and stress as well as smoking cigarette butts and making their own cigarettes, may require flexible and innovative interventions to address their unique needs (Okuyemi et al., 2006). Bradford et al. (2005) implemented a shelter-based intervention, including intensive outreach and availability of weekly visits with continuity of care, which increased the likelihood of homeless individuals engaging and participating in a treatment program to reduce alcohol and illegal drug use. Further research is needed to determine whether such interventions can be expanded to include anti-smoking treatment.

Adjusting for needs of special populations, such as providing shelter-based and/or other off-site care for homeless and out-of-treatment substance abusers, is consistent with Abrams' (1995) recommendation for stepped-care or "macro-level" matching of specific group quantitative/qualitative profiles to different types of interventions. He speculated that relatively healthy persons of higher socioeconomic status might benefit more from interactive computer self-help interventions, due to this population subtype's likelihood of increased computer access and technological proficiency. Since less healthy persons with lower socioeconomic status and/or more risk factors for substance abuse and tobacco use may not benefit from computer-based self-help, Abrams (1995) suggested matching this subtype to brief counseling and brief motivational interviewing by primary care providers, and he recommended more intense interventions, such as chronic disease case management, for persons exhibiting symptoms of smoking-related illness and/or experiencing major smoking-related medical events. Chronic disease case management parallels the recommendation by McLellan et al. (2005a) that treatment for addiction, like treatment for chronic illnesses such as diabetes, hypertension, and asthma, be provided for an indeterminate period with treatment effects evaluated during the course of the treatment. Unless future researchers confirm that every dually-dependent person requires life-long addiction case management, population subtypes may benefit if matched to intensity of service according to illness severity and other complicating factors. For example, patients with a pattern of receiving multiple, detoxification-only treatments are a population subtype that may have improved continuity of care with clinical case management, based on results reported by McLellan, et al. (2005b). Case managers in this study assessed patients, made appropriate referrals, and assisted with transportation; however, smoking was not a focus of the intervention. In order to identify and triage dually-dependent population subtypes into different types or levels of interventions, Abrams (1995) called for clarification regarding appropriate screening, cut-points, and benchmarks. Once stepped-care matching of population subtypes was established, he noted that individuals failing to receive benefit at one level could be "recycled" to the same level or stepped up to more intensive, specialized, or tailored treatment and that a patient-centered system could provide continuity of care by tracking the current status and past history of each individual's responses to treatments.

Cost-Effectiveness

When effectiveness is established for specific treatments matched to an individual substance abusing smoker's characteristics and/or matched to the characteristics of a subtype of the dually-dependent population, these treatments are unlikely to be implemented unless their cost-effectiveness is also established. Cost-effectiveness of smoking cessation treatment for dually-dependent persons remains to be determined. Sindelar et al. (2004) recommended that multiple outcomes of addiction treatments, such as reduced drug use, reduced crime, and increased employment, should be considered in any economic analysis, to avoid inadequate and possibly incorrect policy inferences based on a single outcome. Smoking cessation/reduction has not been specified as an outcome to monitor but could be included in future cost-effectiveness analyses. However, concerns regarding costs of smoking cessation treatments may be unwarranted (Cromwell et al., 1997; Glasgow et al., 1993; Crowley et al., 1991). In their study of the cost-effectiveness of implementing smoking cessation treatment according to a clinical practice guideline, Cromwell et al. (1997) determined that the more intensive the intervention, the lower the cost per quality-adjusted life-year saved, although few smokers appeared willing to undertake the more intensive intervention. Thus, there may be higher long-term costs for smokers who will not participate in appropriately intensive interventions, compared to the cost of intensive interventions for participating smokers. Glasgow and colleagues noted that to some extent, contingency management approaches have built-in cost-effectiveness because, in the reinforcement groups, incentives are paid only for successfully changed behavior (Glasgow et al., 1993). Similarly, Crowley and colleagues stated that payment treatments, if effective, are affordable and that it is possible that paying patients for healthy behaviors could actually save health care funds (Crowley et al., 1991).

EXPANSION OF ON-GOING INTERVENTIONS

Until future researchers establish the definitive, cost-effective treatment(s) for substance-abusing smokers, patients may benefit from naturalistic expansion of on-going interventions originally aimed at reducing alcohol and illegal drug use. Clinicians and/or clinician researchers may have expertise in techniques that are potentially effective for smoking cessation/reduction, in addition to proven effectiveness for reduced use of other substances, and they could utilize those techniques in targeting cigarette smoking as well as alcohol/drug use. Techniques that might impact cigarette smoking, based on their effectiveness in reducing use of other substances, include network therapy (Galanter and Brook , 2001), 12-step-based therapy (Hughes, 1995; Nowinski et al., 1999; Humphreys et al., 2004), addiction pharmacotherapy targeted to non-nicotine substance use (Hughes, 1995; Schnoll and Lerman, 2006; Johnson et al., 2005; Le Foll and Goldberg, 2005; Boyd and Fremming, 2005) and contingency management (Shoptaw et al., 1996 and 2002; Wiseman et al., 2005). Evidence of any effect of alternative therapies for tobacco dependence, such as hypnotherapy and acupuncture, is anecdotal (Villano and White, 2004). However, over 25 years of clinical experience has supported claims that ear acupuncture alleviates acute opiate withdrawal, reduces craving for substances, and helps retain patients in treatment (Otto, 2003). Addiction specialists using alternative and/or established therapies for alcohol and illegal drug problems could also offer these techniques for smoking cessation, as long as patients were informed about the state of the evidence.

Galanter and Brook (2001) recommended network therapy for office-based treatment of patients with non-nicotine substance problems, which uses the patient's family and peers as a therapeutic network to provide support and to promote compliance with treatment. They successfully combined network therapy techniques with medication administration, relapse prevention, and contingency contracting. Addiction specialists who already use network therapy for alcohol and illegal drug problems could include cigarette smoking and adherence to anti-smoking interventions as additional target behaviors for the patient's therapeutic network to monitor. Although there are limited, if any, data supporting efficacy of network therapy for office-based treatment of cigarette smoking in substance abusers, data support family/peer involvement for the general population of cigarette smokers (Picardi et al., 2002; Key et al., 2004). Attending group sessions with a relative or close friend was one of the main predictors of long-term abstinence from smoking, based on follow-up telephone interviews up to two years after a behavioral intervention (Picardi et al., 2002). Key et al. (2004) reported on the effectiveness of a program that combined anti-smoking medication with provider-facilitated group therapy for participants and partners. Similar to the prior study by Picardi et al. (2002), participants with partner support achieved significantly enhanced short-term abstinence from smoking compared to those without partner support (Key et al., 2004). These data indicate possible benefit from involving relatives, close friends, and partners in smoking cessation interventions for dually-dependent persons and possible benefit from expanding network therapy to include family/peer focus on cigarette smoking as well as on alcohol and illegal drug use.

Substance abuse treatment programs frequently incorporate 12-step-based therapy (e.g., Alcoholics Anonymous); therefore, Hughes (1995) hypothesized that a 12-step-based therapy program for smoking, easily integrated into existing treatment, might benefit dually-dependent patients. Substance abuse treatment providers could implement a standardized approach to nicotine dependence by using a twelve step facilitation therapy manual, similar to the one developed for alcohol dependence (Nowinski et al., 1999). Humphreys et al. (2004) noted that self-help group involvement is associated with longitudinal reductions in substance use, improved functioning, and lower health costs. They recommended making greater use of self-help group referral methods across treatment settings and developing a menu of local 12-step groups that matched patients' needs, preferences, and cultural backgrounds. Clinicians who follow these recommendations and routinely provide information regarding local meetings of Nicotine Anonymous, a 12-step program supporting those who want to quit cigarette smoking and to quit other forms of tobacco, might increase smoking cessation rates among their substance-abusing patients. Contingency management procedures that are already in place to reinforce compliance with non-drug-related activities, such as attendance at Alcoholics Anonymous meetings (Petry et al., 2001), could be expanded to include incentives for dually-dependent patients' attendance at Nicotine Anonymous meetings. However, the efficacy of 12-step therapy for smoking cessation among in-treatment and/or out-of-treatment substance abusers remains to be determined.

Addiction pharmacotherapy targeted to non-nicotine substance use, such as naltrexone for alcoholism or opiate addiction, may also reduce smoking (Hughes, 1995; Schnoll and Lerman, 2006). Clinicians will need to monitor whether patients taking naltrexone spontaneously stop smoking cigarettes. If so, naltrexone may deserve further study as a medication with effects across multiple addictions, including smoking. Other medications are being studied that may be efficacious across different classes of substances (Johnson et al., 2005; Le Foll and Goldberg, 2005; Boyd and Fremming, 2005). Topiramate, an anticonvulsant that potentiates inhibitory and antagonizes excitatory neurotransmission to the brain's "reward system," may have potential to treat alcohol, cocaine, and/or nicotine dependence (Johnson, 2005; Johnson et al., 2005). Pre-clinical studies of rimonabant, a selective cannabinoid receptor antagonist, indicate that this medication may modulate use of cannabis, opiates, alcohol, cocaine, and/or nicotine (Le Foll and Goldberg, 2005; Boyd and Fremming, 2005). Rimonabant and topiramate are both under investigation as possible pharmacotherapies for obesity (Boyd and Fremming, 2005; Palmara et al., 2006), which may make these medications particularly appropriate choices for dually-dependent patients who are concerned about weight gain from smoking cessation or who are already overweight and/or at risk for metabolic syndrome. Combining medication(s) with contingency management may improve treatment outcomes for substance-abusing patients (Shoptaw et al., 2002; Schottenfeld et al., 2005), especially for patients prone to treatment compliance problems unless they have an incentive (Higgins et al., 1993 and 1994).

McLellan (2001) recommended expansion of contingency management procedures, which have proven effectiveness to reduce non-nicotine substance use even among patients with very severe problems ((Higgins et al., 1993 and 1994; Silverman et al., 1996). Widespread introduction of contingency management interventions into the New York City Health and Hospital Addiction Treatment Service facilitated patients' therapeutic progress as well as improving the attitude and morale of many employees (Kellogg et al., 2005). Yet contingency management interventions targeting nicotine are not widespread in addiction treatment, despite their possible effectiveness in substance-abusing smokers (Shoptaw et al., 1996 and 2002; Wiseman et al., 2005). Contingency reinforcement allows inclusion of smokers unmotivated to totally quit (Crowley et al., 1991) and may assist in promoting and sustaining cessation in such smokers (Stitzer et al., 1986). Incorporating contingency management strategies outside of formal treatment settings may impact high-risk groups, such as low-income pregnant smokers (Donatelle et al., 2004). If contingency reinforcement is linked to reduction of smoking biomarkers with longer half-lives than CO, such as cotinine, dually-dependent smokers might be motivated to achieve longer-term smoking reduction/cessation. In addition to being potential single component interventions for smoking cessation/reduction (Shoptaw et al., 1996; Wiseman et al., 2005), contingency management procedures combined with network therapy and/or medication(s) may improve treatment outcomes for substance-abusing patients (Galanter and Brook, 2001; Shoptaw et al., 2002; Schottenfeld et al., 2005). Contingency management can also be combined with 12-step-based therapy by rewarding attendance at community self-help meetings (Petry et al., 2001), which could include Nicotine Anonymous meetings. Different approaches to contingency management with dually-dependent persons, such as modifying the interventions to minimize likelihood of manipulation in order to obtain rewards, may be needed compared to contingency management approaches successful in the general population. However, contingency management approaches have built-in cost-effectiveness because incentives are paid only for successfully changed behavior (Glasgow et al., 1993), and, if effective, paying patients for healthy behaviors could actually save health care funds (Crowley et al., 1991).

CONCLUSION

Most alcohol and/or illegal drug abusers also smoke cigarettes, placing them at high risk for subsequent smoking-related problems. Despite strong links between non-nicotine substance use and cigarette smoking, dually-dependent persons are often excluded from studies of anti-smoking treatments. Substance abuse treatment focused only on decreasing subsequent use of alcohol and illegal drugs may not impact cigarette smoking; however, participating in anti-smoking treatment concurrent with other substance abuse treatment may result in better outcomes for alcohol and/or illegal drug use. Although interventions have yet to be developed that achieve long-term reductions in tobacco use in the dually-dependent population, researchers have begun to evaluate the effectiveness of single and multiple component anti-smoking interventions targeting substance abusers. Different approaches, such as higher than usual doses of approved anti-smoking medication, off-label use of other medications, and modifying behavioral interventions to minimize likelihood of manipulation of smoking patterns and/or manipulation of biomarkers, may be necessary compared to anti-smoking approaches for the general population. Regardless of the type of anti-smoking intervention, an objective biomarker is needed to accurately differentiate smokers from non-smokers and/or to verify reduction of smoking. Biochemical verification of smoking status in dually-dependent smokers may require multiple breath CO measurements obtained at random times, a comparatively low CO breakpoint to differentiate "non-smokers" from "smokers," and/or a biochemical marker with a longer half-life than that of CO sampled throughout the duration of the anti-smoking treatment. Further research may assist clinicians in tailoring anti-smoking treatments according to each substance-abusing patient's demographic, diagnostic, motivational, and treatment profile; although, cost-effectiveness of smoking cessation treatment for dually-dependent persons remains to be determined. Nevertheless, there may be higher long-term costs for smokers who refuse to participate in appropriately intensive interventions, compared to the cost of intensive interventions for participating smokers. Until future researchers establish the definitive, cost-effective treatment(s) for substance-abusing smokers, patients may benefit from naturalistic expansion of already-established techniques for treatment of non-nicotine substance use. Thus, techniques with effectiveness in reducing use of alcohol and/or illegal drugs, such as network therapy, 12-step-based therapy, pharmacotherapy for non-nicotine addictions, and contingency management, might also impact cigarette smoking.

REFERENCES

Abrams, D. B. (1995). Integrating basic, clinical, and public health research for alcohol-tobacco interactions. In J. B. Fertig , and J. P. Allen (Eds.), *Alcohol and tobacco: from basic science to clinical practice. Research monograph number 30* (3-16). Bethesda, MD: National Institute on Alcohol Abuse and Alcoholism.

Abrams, D. B., Marlatt, G. A., and Sobell, M. B. (1995). Overview of section II: treatment, early intervention, and policy. In J. B. Fertig , and J. P. Allen (Eds.), *Alcohol and tobacco: from basic science to clinical practice. Research monograph number 30* (307-323). Bethesda, MD: National Institute on Alcohol Abuse and Alcoholism.

American Psychiatric Association, (2000). *(DSM-IV-TR) Diagnostic and statistical manual of mental disorders*, 4th edition, text revision. Washington, DC: American Psychiatric Press, Inc.

American Psychiatric Association, (2006). Practice guideline for the treatment of patients with substance use disorders, 2nd edition. Am. J. Psychiatry, 163(8), S48-S58.

Anton, R. F., O'Malley, S. S., Ciraulo, D. A., Cisler, R. A., Couper, D., Donovan, D. M., Gastfriend, D. R., Hosking, J. D., Johnson, B. A., LoCastro, J. S., Longabaugh, R., Mason, B. J., Mattson, M. E., Miller, W. R., Pettinati, H. M., Randall, C. L., Swift, R., Weiss, R. D., Williams, L. D., Zweben, A. and COMBINE Study Research Group. (2006). Combined pharmacotherapies and behavioral interventions for alcohol dependence: the COMBINE study: a randomized controlled trial. *JAMA, 295(17),* 2003-2017.

Asher, M. K., Martin, R. A., Rohsenow, D. J., MacKinnon, S. V., Traficante, R. and Monti, P. M. (2003). Perceived barriers to quitting smoking among alcohol dependent patients in treatment. *J. Subst. Abuse Treat., 24(2),* 169-174.

Barber, J. P., and Lubosky, L. B. (1992). Psychotherapy research issues to consider in planning a study. In L. K. G. Hsu, and M. Hersen, (Eds.), *Research in Psychiatry: Issues, Strategies, and Methods* (331-357). New York, New York: Plenum Press.

Bigelow, G. E., Stitzer, M. L., Griffiths, R. R. and Liebson, I. A. (1981). Contingency management approaches to drug self-administration and drug abuse: efficacy and limitations. *Addictive Behaviors, 6,* 241-252.

Bowers, T. G., Winett, R. A. and Frederiksen, L. W. (1987). Nicotine fading, behavioral contracting, and extended treatment: effects on smoking cessation. *Addictive Behaviors, 12,* 181-184.

Boyarsky, B. K. and McCance-Katz, E. F. (2000). Improving the quality of substance dependency treatment with pharmacotherapy. *Subst. Use Misuse, 35(12-14)*, 2095-2125.

Boyd, S. T. and Fremming, B. A. (2005). Rimonabant—a selective CB1 antagonist. *Ann. Pharmacother., 39(4)*, 684-690.

Bradford, D. W., Gaynes, B. N., Kim, M. M., Kaufman, J. S. and Weinberger, M. (2005). Can shelter-based interventions improve treatment engagement in homeless individuals with psychiatric and/or substance misuse disorders?: a randomized controlled trial. *Med. Care, 43(8)*, 763-768.

Bramer, S. L. and Kallungal, B. A. (2003). Clinical considerations in study designs that use cotinine as a biomarker. *Biomarkers, 8(3-4)*, 187-203.

Brody, A. L., Mandelkern, M. A., London, E. D., Childress, A. R., Lee, G. S., Bota, R. G., Ho, M. L., Saxena, S., Baxter, L. R. Jr., Madsen, D. and Jarvik, M. E. (2002). Brain metabolic changes during cigarette craving. *Arch. Gen. Psychiatry, 59(12)*, 1162-1172.

Brown, L. M. (2005). Epidemiology of alcohol-associated cancers. *Alcohol, 35(3)*, 161-168.

Carise, D., Gurel, O., McLellan, A. T., Dugosh, K. and Kendig C. (2005). Getting patients the services they need using a computer-assisted system for patient assessment and referral—CASPAR. *Drug Alcohol Depend., 80(2)*, 177-189.

Catley, D., Harris, K. J., Okuyemi, K. S., Mayo, M. S., Pankey, E. and Ahluwahlia, J. S. (2005). The influence of depressive symptoms on smoking cessation among African-Americans in a randomized trial of bupropion. *Nicotine Tob. Res., 7(6)*, 859-870.

Ceballos, N. A., Tivis, R., Lawton-Craddock, A. and Nixond, S. J. (2006). Nicotine and cognitive efficiency in alcoholics and illicit stimulant abusers: implications of smoking cessation for substance users in treatment. *Subst. Use Misuse, 41(3)*, 265-281.

Cinciripini, P. M., Lapitsky, L., Seay, S., Wallfisch, A., Kitchens, K. and Van Vunakis, H. (1995). The effects of smoking schedules on cessation outcome: can we improve on common methods of gradual and abrupt nicotine withdrawal. *Journal of Consulting and Clinical Psychology, 63*, 388-399.

Covey, L. S., Glassman, A. H., Stetner, F. and Becker, J. (1993). Effect of history of alcoholism or major depression on smoking cessation. *Am. J. Psychiatry, 150*, 1546-1547.

Crits-Christoph, P. and Siqueland, L. (1996). Psychosocial treatment for drug abuse: selected review and recommendations for national health care. *Arch. Gen. Psychiatry, 53*, 749-756.

Cromwell, J., Bartosch, W. J., Fiore, M. C., Hasselblad, V. and Baker, T. (1997). Cost-effectiveness of the clinical practice recommendations in the AHCPR guideline for smoking cessation. *JAMA, 278*, 1759-1766.

Crowley, T. J., MacDonald, M. J., Zerbe, G. O. and Petty, T. L. (1991). Reinforcing breath carbon monoxide reductions in chronic obstructive pulmonary disease. *Drug and Alcohol Dependence, 29*, 47-62.

Crowley, T. J., Macdonald, M. J. and Walter, M. I. (1995). Behavioral anti-smoking trial in chronic obstructive pulmonary disease patients. *Psychopharmacology, 119*, 193-204.

DiClemente, C. C., Prochaska, J. O., Fairhurst, S. K., Velicer, W. F., Velasquez, M. M. and Rosse, J. S. (1991). The process of smoking cessation: an analysis of precontemplation, contemplation, and preparation stages of change. *J. Consult. Clin. Psychol., 59*, 295-304.

DiFranza, J. R. and Guerrera, M. P. (1990). Alcoholism and smoking. *J. Stud. Alcohol, 51*, 130-135.

Donatelle, R., Hudson, D., Dobie, S., Goodall, A., Hunsberger, M. and Oswald K. (2004). Incentives in smoking cessation: status of the field and implications for research and practice with pregnant smokers. *Nicotine Tob. Res., 6(suppl. 2),* S163-S179.

Durazzo, T. C., Gazdzinski, S., Rothlind, J. C., Banys, P. and Meyerhoff, D. J. (2006). Brain metabolite concentrations and neurocognition during short-term recovery from alcohol dependence: preliminary evidence of the effects of concurrent chronic cigarette smoking. *Alcohol Clin. Exp. Res., 30(3),* 539-551.

Fagerstrom, K. and Schneider, N. G. (1989). Measuring nicotine dependence: a review of the Fagerstrom Tolerance Questionnaire. *J. Behav. Med., 12,* 159-182.

Fix, A. J., Daughton, D. M., Kass, I., Bell, C. W. and Wass, A. (1979). Immediate carbon monoxide estimates and self-reported smoking. *Perceptual and Motor Skills, 49,* 675-678.

Friedman, E. S., Wright, J. H., Jarrett, R. B. and Thase, M. E. (2006). Combined cognitive therapy and medication for mood disorders. *Psychiatric Annals, 36(5),* 320-328.

Friend, K. B. and Pagano, M. E. (2005). Changes in cigarette consumption and drinking outcomes: findings from Project MATCH. *J. Subst. Abuse Treat., 29(3),* 221-229.

Frosch, D. L., Shoptaw, S., Nahom, D. and Jarvik, M. E. (2000). Associations between tobacco smoking and illicit drug use among methadone-maintained opiate-dependent individuals. *Exp. Clin. Psychopharmacol., 8(1),* 97-103.

Galanter, M. and Brook, D. (2001). Network therapy for addiction: bringing family and peer support into office practice. *Int. J. Group. Psychother., 51(1),* 101-122.

Glasgow, R. E., Hollis, J. F., Ary, D. V. and Boles, S. M. (1993). Results of a year-long incentives-based worksite smoking-cessation program. *Addictive Behaviors, 18,* 455-464.

Glassman, A. H. (1993). Cigarette smoking: implications for psychiatric illness. *Am. J. Psychiatry, 150,* 546-553.

Goff, D. C., Henderson, D. C. and Amico, E. (1992). Cigarette smoking in schizophrenia: relationship to psychopathology and medication side effects. *Am. J. Psychiatry, 149(9),* 1189-1194.

Gorelick, D. A., Simmons, M. S., Carriero, N. and Tashkin, D. P. (1997). Characteristics of smoked drug use among cocaine smokers. *Am. J. Addict., 6,* 237-245.

Greenhouse, J. B., and Junker, B.W. (1992). Basic statistical principles. In L. K. G. Hsu, and M. Hersen, (Eds.), *Research in Psychiatry: Issues, Strategies, and Methods* (158). New York, New York: Plenum Press.

Glynn, S. M. (1992). The chronically mentally ill. In L. K. G. Hsu, and M. Hersen, (Eds.), *Research in Psychiatry: Issues, Strategies, and Methods* (445-460). New York, New York: Plenum Press.

Hall, S. M., Herning, R. I., Jones, R. T., Benowitz, N. L. and Jacob, P. (1984). Blood cotinine levels as indicators of smoking treatment outcome. *Clin. Pharmacol. Ther. 35,* 810-814.

Henningfield, J. E., Fant, R. V., Buchhalter, A. R. and Stitzer, M. L. (2005). Pharmacotherapy for nicotine dependence. *CA Cancer J. Clin., 55(5),* 281-299.

Hersen, M. (1992). Single-case designs. In L. K. G. Hsu, and M. Hersen, (Eds.), *Research in Psychiatry: Issues, Strategies, and Methods* (73-105). New York, New York: Plenum Press.

Hershberger, S. L., Fisher, D. G., Reynolds, G. L., Klahn, J. A. and Wood, M. M. (2004). Nicotine dependence and HIV risk behaviors among illicit drug users. *Addict. Behav., 29(3),* 623-625.

Hertling, I., Ramskogler, K., Dvorak, A., Klingler, A., Saletu-Zyhlarz, G., Schoberberger, R., Walter, H., Kunze, M. and Lesch, O. M. (2005). Craving and other characteristics of the comorbidity of alcohol and nicotine dependence. *Eur. Psychiatry, 20(5-6),* 442-450.

Higgins, S. T., Budney, A. J., Bickel, W. K., Hughes, J. R., Foerg, F. and Badger, G. (1993). Achieving cocaine abstinence with a behavioral approach. *Am. J. Psychiatry, 150,* 763-769.

Higgins, S. T., Budney, A. J., Bickel, W. K., Foerg, F. E., Donham, R. and Badger, G. J. (1994). Incentives improve outcome in outpatient behavioral treatment of cocaine dependence. *Arch. Gen. Psychiatry, 51,* 568-576.

Hughes, J. R. (1995). Clinical implications of the association between smoking and alcoholism. In J. B. Fertig , and J. P. Allen (Eds.), *Alcohol and tobacco: from basic science to clinical practice. Research monograph number 30* (171-185). Bethesda, MD: National Institute on Alcohol Abuse and Alcoholism.

Hughes, J. R. and Kalman D. (2006). Do smokers with alcohol problems have more difficulty quitting? *Drug Alcohol Depend., 82(2),* 91-102.

Hollifield, M., Mackey, A. and Davidson, J. (2006). Integrating therapies for anxiety disorders. *Psychiatric Annals, 36(5),* 329-338.

Humphreys, K., Wing, S., McCarty, D., Chappel, J., Gallant, L., Haberle, B., Horvath, A. T., Kaskutas, L. A., Kirk, T., Kivlahan, D., Laudet, A., McCrady, B. S., McLellan, A. T., Morgenstern, J., Townsend, M. and Weiss R. (2004). Self-help organizations for alcohol and drug problems: toward evidence-based practice and policy. *J. Subst. Abuse Treat., 26(3),* 151-158.

Hurt, R. D., Eberman, K. M., Croghan, I. T., Offord, K. P., Davis, L. J., Morse, R. M., Palmen, M. A. and Bruce, B. K. (1994). Nicotine dependence treatment during inpatient treatment for other addictions: a prospective intervention trial. *Alcoholism: Clinical and Experimental Research, 18,* 867-872.

Hurt, R. D., Patten, C. A., Offord, K. P., Croghan, I. T., Decker, P. A., Morris, R. A. and Hays, J. T. (2005). Treating nondepressed smokers with alcohol dependence in sustained full remission: nicotine patch therapy tailored to baseline serum cotinine. *J. Stud. Alcohol, 66(4),* 506-516.

Jarvis, M. J., Tunstall-Pedoe, H., Feyerabend, C., Vesey, C. and Saloojee, Y. (1987). Comparison of tests used to distinguish smokers from nonsmokers. *Am. J. Public Health, 77,* 1435-1438.

Jeffery, R. W., Pheley, A. M., Forster, J. L., Kramer, F. M. and Snell, M. K. (1988). Payroll contracting for smoking cessation: a worksite pilot study. *Am. J. Prev. Med., 4,* 83-86.

Johnson, B. A. (2005). Recent advances in the development of treatments for alcohol and cocaine dependence: focus on topiramate and other modulators of GABA or glutamate function. *CNS Drugs, 19(10),* 873-896.

Johnson, B. A., Ait-Daoud, N., Akhtar, F. Z. and Javors, M. A. (2005). Use of oral topiramate to promote smoking abstinence among alcohol-dependent smokers: a randomized controlled trial. *Arch. Intern. Med., 165(14),* 1600-1605.

Joseph, A. M. (1993). Nicotine treatment at the drug dependency program of the Minneapolis VA Medical Center: a researcher's perspective. *J. Substance Abuse Treatment, 10,* 147-152.

Kellogg, S. H., Burns, M., Coleman, P., Stitzer, M., Wale, J. B. and Kreek, M. J. (2005). Something of value: the introduction of contingency management interventions into the

New York City Health and Hospital Addiction Treatment Service. *J. Subst. Abuse Treat.,* *28(1)*,57-65.

Kenford, S. L., Fiore, M. C., Jorenby, D. E., Smith, S. S., Wetter, D. and Baker, T. B. (1994). Predicting smoking cessation: who will quit with and without the nicotine patch. *JAMA,* *271*, 589-594.

Key, J. D., Marsh, L. D., Carter, C. L., Malcolm, R. J. and Sinha, D. (2004). Family-focused smoking cessation: enhanced efficacy by the addition of partner support and group therapy. *Subst. Abus., 25(1)*, 37-41.

Le Foll, B. and Goldberg, S.R. (2005). Cannabinoid CB1 receptor antagonists as promising new medications for drug dependence. *J. Pharmacol. Exp. Ther., 312(3)*, 875-883.

Lerman, C., Orleans, C. T. and Engstrom, P. F. (1993). Biological markers in smoking cessation treatment. *Seminars in Oncology, 20*, 359-367.

Martin, R. A., Rohsenow, D. J., MacKinnon, S. V., Abrams, D.B. and Monti, P. M. (2006). Correlates of motivation to quit smoking among alcohol dependent patients in residential treatment. *Drug Alcohol Depend., 83(1)*, 73-78.

McLellan, A. T., Luborsky, L., Cacciola, J., Griffith, J., Evans, F. and Barr, H. L. (1985). New data from the Addiction Severity Index. Reliability and validity in three centers. *J. Nerv. Ment. Dis., 173(7)*, 412-423.

McLellan, A. T., Lewis, D. C., O'Brien, C. P. and Kleber, H. D. (2000). Drug dependence, a chronic medical illness: implications for treatment, insurance, and outcomes evaluation. *JAMA, 284(13)*, 1689-1695.

McLellan, A. T. (2001). Moving toward a "third generation" of contingency management studies in the abuse treatment field: comment on Silverman et al. (2001). *Exp. Clin. Psychopharmacol., 9(1)*, 29-32.

McLellan, A. T., McKay, J. R., Forman, R., Cacciola, J. and Kemp, J. (2005a). Reconsidering the evaluation of addiction treatment: from retrospective follow-up to concurrent recovery monitoring. *Addiction, 100(4)*, 447-458.

McLellan, A. T., Weinstein, R. L., Shen, Q., Kendig, C. and Levine, M. (2005b). Improving continuity of care in a public addiction treatment system with clinical case management. *Am. J. Addict., 14(5)*, 426-440.

Miller, N. S. and Gold, M. S. (1998). Comorbid cigarette and alcohol addiction: epidemiology and treatment. *J Addict. Dis., 17(1)*, 55-66.

Monti, P. M., Rohsenow, D. J., Colby, S. M., and Abrams, D. B. (1995). Smoking among alcoholics during and after treatment: implications for models, treatment strategies, and policy. In J. B. Fertig , and J. P. Allen (Eds.), *Alcohol and tobacco: from basic science to clinical practice. Research monograph number 30* (187-206). Bethesda, MD: National Institute on Alcohol Abuse and Alcoholism.

Nowinski, J., Baker, S. and Carroll, K. (1999). Twelve step facilitation therapy manual: a clinical research guide for therapists treating individuals with alcohol abuse and dependence. In M. E. Mattson, (Ed.), *Project MATCH Monograph Series. Volume 1.* Bethesda, MD: National Institute on Alcohol Abuse and Alcoholism.

Ohlin, P., Lundh, B. and Westling, H. (1976). Carbon monoxide blood levels and reported cessation of smoking. *Psychopharmacology, 49*, 263-265.

Okuyemi, K. S., Caldwell, A. R., Thomas, J. L., Born, W., Richter, K. P., Nollen, N., Braunstein, K. and Ahluwalia, J. S. (2006). Homelessness and smoking cessation: insights from focus groups. *Nicotine Tob. Res., 8(2)*, 287-296.

Oslin, D. W., Grantham, S., Coakley, E., Maxwell, J., Miles, K., Ware, J., Blow, F. C., Krahn, D. D., Bartels, S. J. and Zubritsky, C. (2006). prism-e: comparison of integrated care and enhanced specialty referral in managing at-risk alcohol use. *Psychiatr Serv., 57(7),* 954-8.

Otto, K. C. (2003). Acupuncture and substance abuse: a synopsis, with indications for future research. *Am. J. Addict., 12(1),* 43-51.

Palamara, K. L., Mogul, H. R., Peterson, S. J. and Frishman, W. H. (2006). Obesity: new perspectives and pharmacotherapies. *Cardiol. Rev., 14(5),* 238-258.

Perkins, K. A. (2001). Smoking cessation in women. Special considerations. *CNS Drugs, 15(5),* 391-411.

Petry, N. M., Tedford, J. and Martin, B. (2001). Reinforcing compliance with non-drug-related activities. *J. Subst. Abuse Treat., 20(1),* 33-44.

Picardi, A., Bertoldi, S. and Morosini, P. (2002). Association between the engagement of relatives in a behavioural group intervention for smoking cessation and higher quit rates at 6-, 12- and 24-month follow-ups. *Eur. Addict. Res., 8(3),* 109-117.

Pojer, R., Whitfield, J. B., Poulos, V., Eckhard, I. F., Richmond, R. and Hensley, W. J. (1984). Carboxyhemoglobin, cotinine, and thiocyanate assay compared for distinguishing smokers from non-smokers. *Clin. Chem., 30,* 1377-1380.

Prignot, J. (1987). Quantification and chemical markers of tobacco-exposure. Eur. J. *Respir. Dis., 70,* 1-7.

Prochaska, J. J., Delucchi, K. and Hall, S. M. (2004). A meta-analysis of smoking cessation interventions with individuals in substance abuse treatment or recovery. *J. Consult. Clinic. Psychol., 72(6),* 1144-1156.

Rand, C. S., Stitzer, M. L., Bigelow, G. E. and Mead, A. M. (1989). The effects of contingent payment and frequent workplace monitoring on smoking abstinence. *Addictive Behaviors, 14,* 121-128.

Richter, K. P., McCool, R. M., Catley, D., Hall, M. and Ahluwalia, J. S. (2005). Dual pharmacotherapy and motivational interviewing for tobacco dependence among drug treatment patients. *Addict. Dis., 24(4),* 79-90.

Risser, N. L. and Belcher, D. W. (1990). Adding spirometry, carbon monoxide, and pulmonary symptom results to smoking cessation counseling: a randomized trial. *J. Gen. Intern. Med., 5,* 16-22.

Salokangas, R. K., Saarijarvi, S., Taiminen, T., Lehto, H., Niemi, H., Ahola, V. and Syvalahti, E. (1997). Effect of smoking on neuroleptics in schizophrenia. *Schizophr. Res., 23(1),* 55-60.

Schneider, N. G., Jacob, P., Nilsson, F., Leischow, S. J., Benowitz, N. L. and Olmstead, R. E. (1997). Saliva cotinine levels as a function of collection method. *Addiction, 92,* 347-351.

Schnoll, R. A. and Lerman, C. (2006). Current and emerging pharmacotherapies for treating tobacco dependence. *Expert Opin. Emerg. Drugs, 11(3),* 429-444.

Schottenfeld, R. S., Chawarski, M. C., Pakes, J. R., Pantalon, M. V., Carroll, K. M. and Kosten, T. R. (2005). Methadone versus buprenorphine with contingency management or performance feedback for cocaine and opioid dependence. *Am. J. Psychiatry, 162(2),* 340-349.

Schrag, D., Xu, F., Hanger, M., Elkin, E., Bickell, N. A. and Bach, P. B. (2006). Fragmentation of care for frequently hospitalized urban residents. *Med. Care, 44(6),* 560-567.

Sees, K. L. and Clark, H. W. When to begin smoking cessation in substance abusers. (1993*).
    J. Substance Abuse Treatment, 10*, 189-195.

Shoptaw, S., Jarvik, M. E., Ling, W. and Rawson, R. A. (1996). Contingency management for
    tobacco smoking in methadone-maintained opiate addicts. *Addictive Behaviors*, *21*, 409-
    412.

Shoptaw, S., Rotheram-Fuller, E., Yang, X., Frosch, D., Nahom, D., Jarvik, M. E., Rawson,
    R. A. and Ling, W. (2002). Smoking cessation in methadone maintenance. *Addiction*,
    97(10), 1317-1328.

Silverman, K, Higgins, S. T., Brooner, R. K., Montoya, M. D., Cone, E. J., Schuster, C. R.
    and Preston, K. L. (1996). Sustained cocaine abstinence in methadone maintenance
    patients through voucher-based reinforcement therapy. *Arch. Gen. Psychiatry*, *53*, 409-
    415.

Sindelar, J. L., Jofre-Bonet, M., French, M. T. and McLellan, A. T. (2004). Cost-effectiveness
    analysis of addiction treatment: paradoxes of multiple outcomes. *Drug Alcohol Depend.*,
    73(1), 41-50.

Sirota, A. D., Curran, J. P. and Habif, V. (1985). Smoking cessation in chronically ill medical
    patients. *J. Clin. Psychol.*, *41*, 575-579.

Stitzer, M. L. and Bigelow, G. E. (1985). Contingent reinforcement for reduced breath carbon
    monoxide levels: target-specific effects on cigarette smoking. *Addictive Behaviors*, *10*,
    345-349.

Stitzer, M. L., Rand, C. S., Bigelow, G. E. and Mead, A. M. (1986). Contingent payment
    procedures for smoking reduction and cessation. *J. Applied Behavior Analysis*, *19*, 197-
    202.

Swan, G. E., Ward, M. M., Carmelli, D., and Jack, L. M. (1995). Identification of subgroups
    with differential rates of relapse after smoking cessation: applications to alcohol research.
    In J. B. Fertig , and J. P. Allen (Eds.), *Alcohol and tobacco: from basic science to clinical
    practice. Research monograph number 30* (239-263). Bethesda, MD: National Institute
    on Alcohol Abuse and Alcoholism.

Tashkin, D. P., Gorelick, D., Khalsa, M., Simmons, M. and Chang, P. (1992). Respiratory
    effects of cocaine freebasing among habitual cocaine users. *J. Addictive Diseases*, *11*, 59-
    70.

Teicher, M. H., Glod, C. A. and Cole, J. O. (1993). Antidepressant drugs and the emergence
    of suicidal tendencies. *Drug Saf.*, *8(3)*, 186-212.

Tungstrom, S., Soderberg, P. and Armelius, B. A. (2005). Relationship between the Global
    Assessment of Functioning and other DSM axes in routine clinical work. *Psychiatr.
    Serv.*, *56(4)*, 439-443.

Villano, L. M. and White, A. R. (2004). Alternative therapies for tobacco dependence. *Med.
    Clin.. North Am.*, *88(6)*, 1607-1621.

Visscher, W. A., Feder, M., Burns, A. M., Brady, T. M. and Bray, R. M. (2003). The impact
    of smoking and other substance use by urban women on the birthweight of their infacts.
    Subst. Use Misuse, *38(8)*, 1063-1093.

Waage, H., Silsand, T., Urdal, P. and Langard, S. (1992). Discrimination of smoking status by
    thiocyanate and cotinine in serum and carbon monoxide in expired air. *International
    Journal of Epidemiology*, *21*, 488-493.

Wiesbeck, G. A., Wodarz, N., Weijers, H. G., Dursteler-MacFarland, K. M., Wurst, F. M.,
    Walter, M. and Boening, J.(2006). A functional polymorphism in the promoter region of

the monoamine oxidase A gene is associated with the cigarette smoking quantity in alcohol-dependent heavy smokers. *Neuropsychobiology, 53(4),* 181-185.

Wilcox, R. G., Hughes, J. and Roland, J. (1979). Verification of smoking history in patients after infarction using urinary nicotine and cotinine measurements. *British Medical Journal, 2,* 1026-1028.

Wiseman, E. J. and McMillan, D. E. (1995). Transdermal nicotine and drug craving. *Am..J. Addictions, 4,* 261-266.

Wiseman, E. J. and McMillan, D. E. (1996). Combined use of cocaine with alcohol or cigarettes. *Am. J. Drug Alcohol Abuse, 22,* 577-587.

Wiseman, E. J. (1998). Nicotine replacement therapy and smoking reduction as an interim goal. *JAMA, 279(3),* 194-195.

Wiseman, E. J. and McMillan, D. E. (1998a). Rationale for cigarette smoking and or mentholation preference in cocaine- and nicotine-dependent outpatients. *Comprehensive Psychiatry, 39,* 358-363.

Wiseman, E. J. and McMillan, D. E. (1998b). Relationship of cessation of cocaine use to cigarette smoking in cocaine-dependent outpatients. *Am. J. Drug Alcohol Abuse, 24,* 617-625.

Wiseman, E. J., Williams, D. K. and McMillan, D. E. (2005). Effectiveness of payment for reduced carbon monoxide levels and noncontingent payments on smoking behaviors in cocaine-abusing outpatients wearing nicotine or placebo patches. *Exp. Clin. Psychopharmacol.,* 13(2), 102-110.

In: Smoking Cessation: Theory, Interventions and Prevention   ISBN: 978-1-60021-591-9
Editor: Jerome E. Landow   © 2008 Nova Science Publishers, Inc.

Chapter 7

CIGARETTE CRAVING: EXPLORING THE ENIGMA

Gareth Roderique-Davies
Department of Psychology, Careers and Education
University of Glamorgan, Pontypridd, CF37 1DL, Wales, UK

ABSTRACT

It is believed by some scientists and lay-people that drug craving causes drug addiction, and indeed the assumption that craving is responsible for compulsive drug use is the cornerstone of many scientific and popular conceptualizations of addictive behaviour (Tiffany and Carter, 1998; Tiffany, 1990, 1992, 1997). The concept of "drug craving" has been prominent in the drug addiction literature since the 1950s. The World Health Organization held an Expert Committee meeting in 1954, in an attempt to define and clarify the concept of craving. This committee suggested that the term craving be excluded from scientific use because it has several everyday connotations which could lead to confusion (Jellinek et al., 1955). Despite this recommendation, and the continued expression of concern about the utility of the term craving in scientific explanations of addiction (e.g., Hughes, 1987; Wise, 1988) the use of the term in the scientific literature continued, and so did the debates concerning its definition. In 1992 a WHO/UNDCP committee defined drug craving as "the desire to experience the effect(s) of a previously experienced psychoactive substance" (UNDCP and WHO, 1992). Despite the intuitive appeal of this definition, it does not easily lend itself to the empirical investigation of the phenomenon of craving without further clarification of the scientific term "craving" as opposed to the popular generic understanding of the word. Further, many investigators employ the term "craving" without defining it precisely. Thus, there can be no guarantee of heterogeneity of the construct of craving across investigators, a fact that limits its utility (Kozlowski and Wilkinson, 1987; Merikle, 1999). This chapter reviews scientific conceptualizations of craving, specifically withdrawal and appetitive based concepts that have dominated the literature and the more recent conception of "incentive salience". It then considers the usefulness of these definitions in relation to cigarette addiction, and evaluate the assumption that craving *is* a key causal feature of addiction and investigate the claim that "a truly comprehensive theory of addictive disorders can ill afford to overlook this salient feature of addictive behaviour" (Tiffany 1990). Although the use of the term craving can be thought of as ambiguous for empirical research, the concept remains clinically useful. DSM-IV lists urges and cravings as part of the symptoms characteristic of some drug dependencies (American Psychiatric Association, 1994). The diagnostic usefulness of urges and cravings indicate that the behavioural manifestations of these constructs are important features of addictive disorders (Baker, Sherman and Morse 1987). Thus, the chapter concludes with a consideration of the relationship between conceptualizations of craving and relapse and an assessment the applicability of research into craving to smoking cessation strategies.

INTRODUCTION

It is believed by some scientists and lay-people that drug craving causes drug addiction, and indeed the assumption that craving is responsible for compulsive drug use is the cornerstone of many scientific and popular conceptualisations of addictive behaviour (Tiffany and Carter, 1998; Tiffany, 1990, 1992, 1997). The concept of "drug craving" has been prominent in the drug addiction literature since the 1950s. The World Health Organization held an Expert Committee meeting in 1954, in an attempt to define and clarify the concept of craving. This committee suggested that the term craving be excluded from scientific use because it has several everyday connotations which could lead to confusion (Jellinek et al., 1955). Despite this recommendation, and the continued expression of concern about the utility of the term craving in scientific explanations of addiction (e.g., Hughes, 1987; Wise, 1988) the use of the term in the scientific literature continued, and so did the debates concerning its definition. Nearly forty years on, in 1992, an Expert Committee of the World Health Organization (WHO) and the United Nations International Drug Control Programme (UNDCP) met again to discuss the concept of "craving", and to review the current scientific knowledge on this hypothetical construct (Markou et al., 1993). Despite the inherent problems of accurately defining a subjective concept, the WHO/UNDCP committee defined drug craving as "the desire to experience the effect(s) of a previously experienced psychoactive substance" (UNDCP and WHO, 1992). Despite the intuitive appeal of this definition, it does not easily lend itself to the empirical investigation of the phenomenon of craving without further clarification of the scientific term "craving" as opposed to the popular generic understanding of the word. Further, many investigators employ the term "craving" without defining it precisely. Thus, there can be no guarantee of heterogeneity of the construct of craving across investigators, a fact that limits its utility (Kozlowski and Wilkinson, 1987; Merikle, 1999). Although the use of the term craving can be thought of as ambiguous for empirical research, the concept remains clinically useful. DSM-IV lists urges and cravings as part of the symptoms characteristic of some drug dependencies (American Psychiatric Association, 1994). The diagnostic usefulness of urges and cravings indicate that the behavioural manifestations of these constructs are important features of addictive disorders (Baker, Sherman and Morse 1987). As Tiffany (1990) states, "given the ubiquity of urge responding among addicts (particularly during periods of abstinence), a truly comprehensive theory of addictive disorders can ill afford to overlook this salient feature of addictive behaviour". Concepts of craving will now be considered.

THE CONCEPTUALISATION OF "CRAVING"

Withdrawal Based Models

Withdrawal based models assume that the main motivating influence in compulsive drug use (including Cigarette smoking) is the avoidance of withdrawal symptoms, indeed most drugs that support compulsive use will produce a physiological dependence syndrome when the drug is withdrawn (Tiffany, 1990). Although these dependence syndromes are different across differing classes of drugs (Tiffany, 1990), it is a logical step to assume that urges and cravings are intimately related to drug withdrawal.

The earliest approaches to craving assumed that urges and cravings are caused by the physiological symptoms of withdrawal. Jellinek (1955), for example, suggested that craving for alcohol represented the anticipation of relief from the negative affect of withdrawal, and that it is this sort of craving which leads to compulsive alcohol consumption. Another approach suggests that urges and cravings are nothing more than a component of drug withdrawal. Such approaches are however purely descriptive in that they recognise that people withdrawing from drugs often report urges and cravings. This idea can be observed in the work of Shiffman and Jarvik (1976). These authors looked at trends in smoking withdrawal symptoms, and developed a 27-item questionnaire that was administered four times daily for 2 weeks to 35 participants in a smoking cessation clinic. A variety of symptoms were dealt with in the questionnaire. On the basis of a factor analysis, these authors identified a craving sub-scale as accounting for the largest share of the variance. Their findings suggest that urges are the primary manifestation of nicotine withdrawal in abstinent smokers.

However, people often report urges and cravings long after withdrawal symptoms have abated, and they have ceased using a particular drug. Fletcher and Doll (1969) for example, reported that over 20% of ex-smokers still report experiencing desire to smoke over 10 years after giving up. This is clearly inconsistent with the premise that cravings are a consequence of withdrawal, however one explanation for this could be that cravings and urges could be conditioned effects, and that some sort of learning has taken place. Wikler (1948) developed a classical conditioning model of drug withdrawal, and proposed that environmental stimuli paired with drug withdrawal became conditioned stimuli capable of eliciting conditioned withdrawal reactions. In other words, if abstinent addicts are exposed to situations in which they had previously suffered drug withdrawal, they should experience conditioned withdrawal symptoms that will lead to urges and cravings to take the drug. Wikler described craving as nothing more than one aspect of the unconditioned withdrawal syndrome that, like other aspects of the withdrawal syndrome, could become conditioned to environmental stimuli (Wikler 1948; Wikler and Pescor, 1967). This view was later slightly amended when Ludwig and Wikler (1974) described craving as a "psychological or cognitive correlate of a sub-clinical, conditioned withdrawal syndrome", and that craving was a desire for relief from withdrawal that was a necessary condition for relapse, but by itself was insufficient for relapse in abstinent addicts. However, a number of flaws exist with this model. Marlatt (1985), for example, pointed out that if Wikler's model is correct, then alcoholics would experience the most craving in treatment centers where they had undergone withdrawal, yet clinical experience has shown that cravings tend to be reported as low or non-existent by patients in re-habilitation centers. McAuliffe (1982) examined Wikler's theory of relapse in human opiate addicts. Forty addicts took part in structured interviews; the addicts had all had at least one period of abstinence outside of an institution. Only 11 of the addicts reported having experienced conditioned withdrawal by taking drugs, and only 1 relapsed as a result. The most common reason given for relapse (even for those who had reported experiencing conditioned withdrawal symptoms) was the desire for euphoria. In the same year, Chaney and colleagues reported that only 16% of relapse episodes reported by their sample of opiate addicts could be attributed to conditioned withdrawal (Chaney et al., 1982).

A similar conditioning model to that of Wikler's is Siegal's (1975) theory of drug tolerance. The theory states that stimuli reliably paired with taking a drug elicit conditioned responses opposite in direction to the direct effects of the drug. These compensatory responses are believed to be responsible for conditioned tolerance effects when the addict is taking the drug and the withdrawal symptoms when the addict is abstinent. An abstinent addict exposed to cues previously associated with drug administration (e.g. cigarette Lighters, cigarette packets, ashtrays) will have conditioned compensatory responses that are experienced as withdrawal and craving, which would increase the likelihood of relapse. Siegal (1983) argues that compensatory responses constitute the basis of urges or craving, which are major components of the drug withdrawal syndrome. The compensatory withdrawal model (Siegal, 1983) differs from Wikler's conditioned withdrawal model in that it states that withdrawal symptoms are elicited by the presence of cues associated with the administration of the drug, and not with drug withdrawal. This distinction is not, however, a practical way of distinguishing these models, since in reality cues paired with drug withdrawal and cues paired with drug administration overlap in the environment of an addict (Tiffany, 1990). For example, in Smoking behaviour a smoker attempting to quit may well still visit a bar that they used to smoke in. In this example, an ashtray could be a cue associated with administration when they were smoking and with withdrawal when they are not.

Subsequent models of withdrawal-based urges integrated conditioning theories of drug withdrawal tolerance with social-cognitive concepts. These theories suggest that physiological responses, produced by conditioned compensatory responses or conditioned withdrawal, are interpreted by the addict as desires to use the drug. Hence, these theories suggest that urges reflect the operation of attributional process, thus the combination of conditioned physiological arousal with a particular attribution for the source of that arousal is necessary for the production of urges and cravings to use a drug (Melchoir and Tabakoff, 1984; West and Schneider, 1987). By implication, physiological responses other than withdrawal may be incorrectly attributed to a desire to use a drug, or conversely under some circumstances some withdrawal responses, may not be attributed by the addict as urges and cravings (West and Schneider, 1987). For example, abstinent smokers often report increased levels of hunger (Buchhalter et al., 2005). It could be that increased hunger is either mis-attributed by the abstinent smoker as desire for a cigarette or conversely that desire for a cigarette may be mis-attributed as hunger. This could explain the observation of weight gain amongst smokers who have quit (e.g. Perkins, 1992), although it should be conceded that their may be a neuropharmacological explanation for this (Chen et al., 2005).

Problems exist with theories of conditioned withdrawal. Childress and colleagues (1988) found that in opiate addicts, at least a third deny that they experience conditioned withdrawal symptoms when they are exposed to drug-related cues, and that there is a poor correlation between craving and withdrawal signs. Ehrman and colleagues (1992) found that withdrawal-like physiological symptoms (e.g., skin resistance, temperature, heart rate) induced by drug-related cues are not highly correlated with reports of subjective state. More telling, many researchers have reported that self reported craving for some drugs (e.g., cocaine) is highest immediately after drug use, when a subjective "high" is being experienced, and withdrawal symptoms are eliminated or at their weakest (Childress et al., 1988; Ehrman et al., 1992; Fischman et al., 1990; Jaffe et al., 1989; Meyer, 1988). Therefore, if cravings for drugs were due to a desire to alleviate negative withdrawal symptoms, cravings should decrease or cease with the administration of the drug. In smokers it has been demonstrated that cigarette cravings can be increased even in non-abstinent smokers (Morgan et al., 1999). It is largely for these reasons that the negative reinforcing effects of drugs, by themselves are considered not sufficient for the development and maintenance of addiction (Robinson and Berridge, 1993, 2000).

Appetitively Based Models

Partly due to the limitations of models of urges that concentrated on negative reinforcement, some theorists associated urges and cravings with the positive reinforcing, appetitive or excitatory effects of drugs of abuse. McAuliffe and Gordon (1974) for example suggested that craving in opiate addicts reflects the desire for, and the anticipation of the euphoric effects of the drug. Many studies have shown that animals will self-administer drugs of abuse (e.g. opiates, alcohol, amphetamines or cocaine) at high rates, sometimes to the point of intoxication or dependence (Stewart, de Wit and Eikelboom, 1984). It should be noted however, that nicotine self-administration in animals is not so robust an observation (Stolerman, 1987). Despite this, attempts to develop theories of addiction based on positive reinforcement have often been generally applied to cigarette addiction as well. Wise and Bozarth (1987) developed a psychomotor stimulant theory of addiction. They stated that for all addictive drugs, "a common mechanism, or at least elements of a common mechanism, mediates both psychomotor stimulant actions and reinforcing actions". They also suggested that the strength of the reinforcing action of a drug could be predicted by the strength of the psychomotor stimulant properties of that particular drug. Many of the stimulating effects of abused drugs were equated with their appetitive or positively reinforcing properties and these, they argued, are all mediated by a common neural pathway located in the middle forebrain bundle. That drugs classified as stimulants (e.g. cocaine, nicotine and amphetamines) should have stimulating or excitatory effects is obvious, but excitatory effects have often been observed in drugs classified as depressants such as alcohol (Pohorecky, 1977; Tabakoff and Kiianmaa, 1982) and opiates (Zelman et al., 1985).

Marlatt (1985) proposed a social learning model of addictive behaviour that elaborated on the role of drugs as positive reinforcers. According to Marlatt three interlocking cognitive factors play significant roles in the relapse process. The first is self-efficacy; this refers to how the individual perceives their ability to cope with prospective high-risk situations. This is a cognitive process as it deals with perceived judgements or evaluations. The second mediator is outcome expectancies; positive outcome expectancies increase the temptation to take the addictive substance. The third factor is also a cognitive process and is attribution of causality; if the individual does succumb to their urges then the attribution of causality is important in determining whether the first relapse will lead to a full relapse. Outcome expectancies, as stated above, play an important role in the relapse process; these are based on the anticipated effects of engaging in a particular behaviour. It must be pointed out that the expected effects of taking a drug may not be the same as the actual effect of taking the drug. As Marlatt (1985) writes, "the expectations one holds about the effects (perceived outcome) often exert greater influence than the actual or 'real' effects of taking the drug". Marlatt (1985) defines craving as a subjective state motivated by the incentive properties of positive outcome expectancies. Although positive outcome expectancies may reflect the anticipation of relief from the negative effects of withdrawal, Marlatt's model points out that the main determinant of craving in addicts is the anticipation of euphoria or stimulation. In other words, "craving is a motivational state associated with a strong desire for an expected positive outcome" (Marlatt, 1985). It should be noted, that Marlatt (1985) makes a distinction between "urges" and "cravings", suggesting that urges reflect an intention to use a drug that is motivated by a craving for the drug.

There are a number of problems associated with the view that urges and cravings are associated with the positive reinforcing, appetitive or excitatory effects of drugs of abuse. Firstly, Robinson and Berridge (1993) point out that if the positive reinforcing effects of drugs are primarily due their ability to produce pleasurable affective states in addicts, these subjective pleasurable effects must be enormous. Nicotine for example is considered to be highly addictive yet does not produce strong euphoric states. As Robinson and Pritchard (1992) state, "there is no evidence that nicotine absorbed from cigarette smoke produces euphoria". Secondly, the positive reinforcement view of addiction fails to explain how cravings or relapse are elicited by drug-related cues. Wise and Bozarth (1987) and Stewart and colleagues (1984) suggest that drug-related cues can stimulate drug-like effects that motivate the addict to engage in further drug-seeking and drug-taking behaviour. But, as Robinson and Berridge (1992) ask, "what exactly is this drug-like process?" One possibility is that it reflects the positive state induced by the drug, and as such reflects a conditioned high. Stewart and colleagues (1984), in their conditioned incentive model of addiction, state that "Conditioned drug effects that mimic the unconditioned drug effects, as are conditioned positive affective states, are elicited by the environment where these drugs are experienced." In other words, drug-related cues trigger conditioned pleasure, which reminds the drug addict of the pleasurable aspects of using the particular drug, and motivates them to use the drug again. Stewart and colleagues presented considerable evidence for the positive incentive effects of addictive drugs motivate drug use, the strongest of this being that animals will self-administer drugs of abuse (nicotine self-administration being not so straight forward). However, human studies have found that subjective reports of conditioned highs occur far less frequently than subjective reports of conditioned cravings, or conditioned withdrawal signs (Childress et al., 1988; O'Brien et al., 1992). By implication, conditioned highs must be dissociated from conditioned craving, so how can the former be explained in the context of the latter (Robinson and Berridge, 1993)? Thirdly, studies have demonstrated the maintenance of drug taking in the absence of any pleasurable effects. Lamb and colleagues (1991) found that opiate users would work for a low dose of morphine, but not a placebo, despite the fact that four out of five of them could not distinguish between the subjective effects of the morphine and a placebo. Such evidence suggests that "drug 'wanting' is not equivalent to drug 'liking'." (Robinson and Berridge, 1993). With respect to smoking, evidence suggests that smoking is for many a pleasurable experience (Pomerleau and

Pomerleau, 1992; de Wit and Zacny, 1995), although whether this does or does not diminish the suggestion that wanting to smoke is not *necessarily* equivalent to liking smoking is debatable as there is a lack of published evidence considering this specifically for smoking. Drug liking and wanting will be considered later.

Dual Affect Model

Considering the evidence for and against withdrawal based models and appetitively based models, the logical compromise would be to present a model which saw cravings as arising from both positive and negative reinforcement mechanisms. Baker, Morse and Sherman (1987) suggested that affective processing systems control the reactivity to drug-related stimuli. These affective processing systems can be indexed by physiological, behavioural and subjective measures, and can be either appetitively or withdrawal based. Positive affect urges are hypothesized to be closely associated to an appetitive motivational system directly stimulated by drug use. Activation of this system could be through, for example, positive mood, drug-use-related cues, availability of the drug and small doses of the drug, and should produce urge reports, positive affect, physiological responses akin to the stimulating effects of the drug, and drug-seeking behaviour. Negative affective urges are hypothesized to be tied closely with withdrawal, and activated by negative mood, withdrawal-related cues, unavailability of the drug, and withdrawal itself. In this instance, the urge system should produce urge reports, negative affect, symptoms of withdrawal and drug-seeking behaviour. In addition, this model hypothesizes that the two types of urges are mutually inhibitory, and that activation of one system will increase the threshold for activation of the other.

Baker et al's (1987) model was based on a bioinformation-processing approach, where urges are assumed to be organized at a cognitive level within a propositional network that encodes information on eliciting stimuli, drug-related responses, and the interpretation or meaning of stimuli and responses. They proposed that these networks, are mobilised to the extent that the prevailing cue configurations are adequately matched for the encoded prototypical stimulus complex, and as the stimulus conditions become closer to the prototype, the magnitude of the responses within a given urge network will become greater. One feature of this model is that partial activation of the urge systems should lower the threshold for additional activation of the urge network. For example, drinking alcohol will produce a partial pharmacological priming of the appetitive motivational systems and so should lead to enhanced urge reactivity to smoking-related stimuli in dependent smokers (Tiffany, 1995). Baker and colleagues summarised the evidence for this dual affect model (see Baker et al., 1987 for full review) such as the facilitative effect of priming doses of drugs on subsequent self-administration (Stewart et al., 1984), the influence of signals of drug availability on eliciting urges (Meyer and Mirin, 1979), and the potential inhibitory relationship positive affect urges and negative affect urges (Baker and Morse, 1985; Zinser et al., 1992). More recent research has, however, challenged the dual affect model. Firstly, as pointed out by Tiffany (1995), a review of the literature shows that induction of positive mood generally has little or no impact on urge elicitation in the absence of explicit drug-related cues. Multi-item craving questionnaires which reflect both the anticipation of positive mood and relief of negative withdrawal (e.g., Tiffany and Drobes, 1991) generally show a high correlation between the two factors suggesting that they are not mutually inhibitory (Tiffany, 1995).

Thirdly, partial activation of urge systems through pharmacological manipulations or withdrawal does not necessarily prime reactivity to urge-relevant stimuli (Drobes and Tiffany, 1997; Maude-Griffin and Tiffany, 1996). Finally, an examination of the two major classes of cue reactions, subjective reports of urges and physiological activation, reveals little evidence of a relationship between the two, suggesting that there is little evidence that the coherence of various responses to urge-eliciting stimuli becomes greater as more urge-related stimuli are presented (Tiffany, 1988, 1990, 1995). In addition, Elash and colleagues (1995) found that craving imagery augmented the negative affect and Weinstein and colleagues (1997) found that drug-related imagery resulted in non-significant trends towards increased anxiety and decreased positive affect. The latter authors argued that dual affect model would predict that the induction of craving should result in an increase in positive affect rather than negative affect and not the other way around as observed (Weinstein et al., 1997). The relationship between craving and mood will be considered later.

Is Craving Independent of Reinforcement?

Some authors have argued that craving is independent of reinforcement mechanisms. Robinson and Berridge (1993) proposed an incentive-sensitisation theory of addiction. They argued that an adequate theory of addiction must be able to explain: "1) What accounts for drug craving elicited by drug-associated stimuli, if craving is not causally related to conditioned withdrawal signs, conditioned 'highs' or the explicit memory of past pleasure? 2) Why is craving sometimes highest immediately after drug administration, when subjective pleasurable effects are still predominant? 3) Why does obsessive craving for drugs persist in the face of enormous negative consequences associated with continued drug use, and relatively modest subjective pleasurable effects? 4) How can low doses of drugs, which do not produce discernible subjective pleasure or physical dependence, maintain drug-seeking and drug-taking behaviour? 5) Why is relapse such a prevalent and persistent feature of addiction, even in 'recovered' addicts? 6) Why can relapse be precipitated by so many different stimuli (drugs, environmental stimuli associated with drugs, mood changes)?" (Robinson and Berridge, 1993). These authors argued that traditional negative and positive reinforcement theories of addiction fail to provide adequate answers to these points, and proposed a neural basis for drug craving. They suggested that all addictive drugs have the ability to enhance mesotelencephalic dopamine transmission. One psychological function of this neural system, they suggested, was to attribute "incentive salience" to the perception, and mental representations of events associated with the activation of the system (e.g. drug taking, drug-related cues). Robinson and Berridge (1993) proposed that incentive salience transforms the perception of stimuli making that stimuli attractive "wanted" incentive stimuli. Repeated use of an addictive drug produces ever-increasing neuroadaptations in this system which eventually render it (perhaps permanently) sensitised to the drug and all stimuli associated with it. Excessive incentive salience is attached to the act of drug taking and drug-associated stimuli, and ordinary drug "wanting" becomes excessive drug craving. Further, these authors suggested that these changes in the neural systems for drug wanting occur independently of the neural systems for drug liking and for withdrawal. Thus, this theory proposes that drug craving can occur, even when the drug is no longer pleasurable, and the withdrawal effects have diminished.

Robinson and Berridge (1993) argued experimental evidence existed that repeated exposure to addictive drugs can produce neuroadaptations in order to meet the necessary requirements for the theory to be true. Firstly they pointed out that there is a whole body of evidence that addictive drugs all share the ability to enhance the mesotelencephalic dopamine system, and that "Although it cannot be said that there is a single neural system that is affected by all addictive drugs, dopamine systems and their associated structures are affected by most". Secondly, they presented what they claimed to be considerable evidence that the repeated administration of many types of addictive drugs produce behavioural sensitisation, which is associated with hypertensive mesotelncephalic dopamine systems. Thirdly, they presented evidence that the neuroadaptations underlying behavioural sensitisation are persistent and long lasting. Next they presented evidence that the expression of sensitisation is subject to conditioned stimulus control. Further, they presented evidence that the mesotelencephalic dopamine system plays a role in incentive motivation. Finally, they presented evidence that the effects of dopamine are on incentive salience and not on pleasure. For a full review see Robinson and Berridge (1993).

However, the incentive-sensitisation model has not proved to be useful in the measurement of urges and cravings, and this is perhaps reflected in the lack of published evidence considering cigarette smoking in this context. It is difficult to assess whether this model truly does provide an account of craving that is independent of reinforcement mechanisms due to it's reliance on the positive incentive-motivational aspects of drug use. Further, recent evidence suggests that one of the central tenets of incentive-sensitisation theory does not hold true for alcohol or amphetamines. Willner and colleagues (2005) observed increases in levels of both wanting and liking for these substances, so while not necessarily refuting the theory this observation is certainly contrary to one of its predictions. There is evidence to suggest that a more cognitive approach to craving, as opposed to a psychobiological approach may be more appropriate (Tiffany, 1990, 1992; Tiffany and Conklin, 2000).

Does Craving Drive Addiction?

In 1990, Stephen Tiffany stated that one notable feature of the studies that he had reviewed (Tiffany, 1988) in which dependent smokers or alcoholics were exposed to drug-related or neutral stimuli while their physiological responses and self-reported urges were monitored, was that many of the correlations between physiological responses and urges were not reported. In his review two years earlier, Tiffany had reported that out of the 13 studies he reviewed only 17 of the approximately 48 possible correlation coefficients were reported, suggesting that those not reported were not significant (Tiffany, 1988). Those reported were mostly positive (e.g., 13 out of 17 of all reported coefficients and 8 out of 10 of the significant ones), suggesting that subjective urges tended to be associated with physiological activation or arousal (Tiffany, 1990). However, the magnitudes of the significant correlations were small, accounting for, on average, only 15% of the variance. Tiffany (1990) suggested that these low or non-significant correlations would seem to be scant evidence to support theories (e.g., Ludwig and Wikler, 1974; Poulos et al., 1981; Siegal, 1983; Wikler, 1972) which claim that conditioned physiological responses are the basis for drug urges and cravings. Indeed, such data suggests that the psychological processes involved in drug use behaviour may be only loosely associated with the processes involved in verbal reports of urges and cravings. In addition to this, Tiffany (1990) stated that the available evidence did not support the notion that cravings and urges are necessary for the initiation or maintenance of drug-use behaviour. For example, Marlatt and Gordon (1980), found that only 7% of a cross section of relapsed heroin, nicotine and alcohol addicts, described urges as major factors in their relapse. As Tiffany (1990) states, "data are revealing in that they indicate that addicts typically do not spontaneously identify urges and cravings as an important component of their relapse". Tiffany (1990) suggested that the data allowed the hypothesis that the psychological processes involved in drug-use behaviour operate independently of those processes that control subjective urge responding.

Tiffany's (1990) cognitive model of drug urges and drug use rejects the assumption that craving reflects the central motivational process responsible for drug use behaviour. According to this model, craving is assumed to play a prominent role in relapse mechanisms, rather than in the day to day maintenance of the drug use behaviours. Tiffany suggests that as a result of long-term drug use, drug use behaviour becomes automatic in the addict. In other words, like other learned skills, drug use behaviour becomes efficient, stimulus orientated, difficult to control, and most importantly cognitively effortless and capable of being initiated and completed without intention. Tiffany suggests that these automated skills are stored as action schema in the long-term memory. These action schemas are unitised, self-sufficient memory systems containing the necessary information for the initiation and coordination of complicated drug-use behaviour sequences. Urges and cravings are conceptualised as constellations of verbal, somatovisceral, and behavioural responses supported by non-automatic cognitive processes, which are utilised in situations in which automatic processes cannot be invoked to produce the appropriate responses (e.g. when the individual is attempting to over-ride the execution of an automated sequence). The non-automatic cognitive processes are cognitively effortful, slow and dependent upon intention, and according to the model, would be activated in parallel with drug use action schemata either in support of it (e.g. when a smoker runs out of cigarettes), or against it (e.g. when a smoker is deliberately attempting to quit). According to this model, the mechanisms involved in linking substance-related stimuli to substance use operate relatively independently of the processes involved in controlling craving.

Research by Sayette and colleagues supports Tiffany's cognitive processing theory. The reaction times of dependent alcoholics and smokers to auditory probes were greater in the presence of drug-related cues than in the presence of drug-neutral cues (Sayette et al 1994; Sayette and Hufford 1994). Since the drug-related cues presented in these studies activated craving processes, Sayette and colleagues findings support the idea that craving is associated with the activation of non-automatic cognitive processes. Cepeda-Benito and Tiffany (1996) provided further evidence for this theory. Smokers were asked to imagine sentences that incorporated urge or no-urge descriptors. Imagery of urge sentences produced slower probe reaction times, increased heart rate and skin conductance, and higher urge ratings. These authors suggested that the drug craving disrupts cognitive performance, and as such, "provides support for the conceptualization of craving as an effortful, nonautomatic cognitive process" (Cepeda-Benito and Tiffany, 1996).

IS IT POSSIBLE TO MEASURE CRAVING?

Objective Assessment of Craving

Operant techniques have been employed for many years to measure the motivation to respond in animals. Behavioural economic analyses of motivated behaviour assume that a lawful trade-off exists between the value of a commodity, and the effort that will be expended to obtain it (Willner et al., 1995). For example, progressive-ratio (PR) schedules have been demonstrated to be useful measures of motivational strength to use drugs of abuse in animals (Markou et al., 1993; Risner and Goldberg, 1983). It is only in recent years, however, that investigators have attempted to employ a progressive ratio procedure in human behavioural pharmacological research. A human PR procedure was developed at the University of Wales Swansea to provide a behavioural measure of the urge to smoke (Willner et al., 1995; Willner and Jones, 1996). The task requires participants to respond, by pressing a key on a computer, to earn puffs on a cigarette, on a progressive ratio basis. Reports from this laboratory (Willner et al., 1995; Willner and Jones, 1996), and others (Rusted et al., 1998), suggest that this PR task can differentiate between the urge to smoke in non-abstinent smokers and those who are abstinent for 6-8 hours on average., although other studies have failed to replicate this (Morgan et al., 1999; Davies et al., 2004).

Previous studies have reported significant correlations between PR performance maintained by a variety of reinforcers (cigarettes, chocolate, beer), and questionnaire measures of craving for these reinforcers (Willner et al., 1995, 1998a, 1998b; Morgan et al., 1999). Additionally, induction of a depressed mood state has been shown to increase both questionnaire measures of craving for each of their reinforcers and performance under a PR schedule (Willner and Jones 1996; Willner et al., 1998a, 1998b). This suggests that PR performance may provide an alternative means of measuring craving in human participants, which has the advantage of being directly comparable to the same procedure in non-human subjects (Willner, 1996), although the reliability of this procedure remains uncertain.

Subjective Assessment of Craving

As stated above, earlier models of addiction commonly suggest that cravings or urges are subjective states that reflect the primary motivation responsible for drug use in addicts (Tiffany, 1995). However, there has been considerable debate about how to measure cravings. In the past, craving has been evaluated using a simple one or two item Likert scale or visual analogue scale on the assumption that cigarette cravings are unidimensional in nature. Some investigators believed that such cravings reflected positive reinforcing (incentive) properties (Marlatt, 1985; Niaura et al. 1988; Wise, 1988), others that they reflected negative reinforcing properties (Ludwig and Wikler, 1974; Poulos et al. 1981; West and Schneider, 1987), but not both. For example, Behm and Rose (1994) assessed craving using a modification of the Shiffman-Jarvik questionnaire (Shiffman and Jarvik, 1976) which is based in the DSM-IIIR criteria for nicotine withdrawal. Participants were required to respond "not at all" (1) to "extremely" (7) to items inquiring how much they had "craved a cigarette", "missed a cigarette", "thought of a cigarette", "had urges to smoke", and (negatively scored) "would have refused a cigarette". The mean of these four items constituted the participants "craving" score. A questionnaire routinely used in the Maudsley smokers clinic in London (West et al., 1989) similarly asks participants how much they had been craving, and also contains questions relating to time spent with urges to smoke, strength of urges, and difficulty not smoking. More recently, however, Tiffany and Drobes (1991) have argued that such ways of assessing craving are unreliable since they have small validation samples, an absence of information on their psychometric properties (e.g. reliability), and are inherently limited by their assumption that urges and cravings are a manifestation of a unidimensional motivational state. Tiffany and Drobes (1991) have argued that urges and cravings should not be assumed to be reflective of the motivational processes central to drug use. These authors suggested that one consequence of this assertion is that cravings and urges should have a multi-dimensional nature.

The multi-dimensional Questionnaire of Smoking Urges (QSU) was intended to provide a measure of self-reported urge to smoke that was both reliable, and sufficient in content to address the many conceptualisations of cravings to smoke cigarettes (Tiffany and Drobes, 1991). A 32-item questionnaire was presented to 230 dependent smokers assigned to one of 3 levels of cigarette deprivation (0, 1 or 6 hours). Factor analysis of the data led Tiffany and Drobes (1991) to conclude that a two-factor structure best described the subjective experience of cravings for cigarettes. Items relating to factor 1 were mainly concerned with intention and desire to smoke and anticipation of positive outcomes, whereas items relating to factor 2 were mainly concerned with an overwhelming desire to smoke, and anticipation of relief from negative affect and withdrawal. Hence factor 1 items may be considered primarily to reflect the operation of positive reinforcement, and factor 2 items may be considered to reflect the operation of negative reinforcement. This factor structure was replicated almost exactly by Davies and colleagues (2000).

This approach to the development of psychometric instruments have been applied by several research groups in the development of instruments to measure alcohol cravings (Clark, 1994; Singleton et al., 1994a; Bohn et al., 1995, Love et al., 1998) cocaine cravings (Tiffany et al., 1993), Amphetamine Craving (James et al., 2004) and Heroin cravings (Tiffany et al., unpublished). The Alcohol Craving Questionnaire (ACQ: Singleton et al., 1994a) and the Desires for Alcohol Questionnaire (DAQ: Clark, 1994) both used the QSU as their starting point, and as such have similarities both to each other and the QSU. A comparison of the two questionnaires by Love and colleagues (1998) revealed that both questionnaires yielded a three factor structure with two of the factors ("Positive and Negative Reinforcement" and "Strong desires and intentions") similar on both questionnaires. The third factor on Love and colleagues factor analysis of the DAQ revealed a "Mild desires and intentions" factor. On the ACQ, these authors found a third "No desire to drink" factor, although they suggested that this factor was unstable and was wholly comprised of "reverse-keyed" items which are logically more difficult to answer, and thus could just be a statistical artifact (Love et al., 1998). These authors argued that the factor structure of the DAQ in particular has important implications. Firstly, the "Positive and Negative Reinforcement" factor argues against accounts of craving based upon one or other of these processes, and supports the concept of the involvement of them both (Baker et al., 1987). Secondly, the presence of a "Strong Desires and Intentions" factor which includes no items related to reinforcement, provides support for theories which suggest that urges to take drugs are dissociated from reinforcement processes (Tiffany, 1990; Robinson and Berridge, 1993).

Finally, Love and colleagues (1998) argued that the presence of a single higher order factor suggested that the three lower order factors were all representations of a single higher order construct, namely "craving". James and colleagues (2004) reported an almost identical factor structure for a Desires for Speed Questionnaire (DSQ) to that of the DAQ. Tiffany and colleagues (1993) constructed two cocaine-craving questionnaire on the basis of the QSU, with one version asking questions on current craving for cocaine (Now version), and one version asking questions on average craving over the week (General). These authors also found that a multi-dimensional factor solution best described the factor structure of both questionnaires, and the presence of a single higher-order "craving" factor.

However, not all authors have endorsed the multi-factorial approach to the subjective assessment of cravings and urges. Kozlowski and colleagues (1996) factor-analyzed the 26 items that contribute to the scoring of the QSU, and failed to replicate the original factor structure. They were, able to extract a two-factor structure, but only when they restricted the analysis to the 12 items that had the highest factor loadings in the original study by Tiffany and Drobes (1991). Four of the six items, which contributed to their factor 1 scale, were negatively worded. This led Kozlowski and colleagues (1996) to conclude that the two-factor structure of the QSU may be an artifact that reflects the use of negatively worded items. They suggested that multi-dimensional scales and factor-analytical approaches may be unnecessarily complicated, and that a simple 2 or 3 item "desire" scale is adequate to measure urges to smoke (Kozlowski et al. 1996).

Is "Craving" a Multi-Dimensional Construct?

As discussed, there is much debate as to exactly what drug urges and cravings are, and as yet a universally acceptable definition of craving has not been found. Traditional assessment of craving has been based on unidimensional, single item questionnaires of unknown reliability and validity (Tiffany, 1992). The findings of a number of research groups discussed above, suggest that craving is not a unitary concept. One implication of this is that although different craving questionnaires may each satisfactorily measure a component of craving, they may not measure other equally important components. This may explain the lack of agreement amongst scientists and lay-people upon the definition of craving (Kozlowski and Wilkinson, 1987; Merikle, 1999).

In the factor analysis presented by Davies et al., (2000), the QSU items that referred specifically to urges or craving ("I crave a cigarette right now" and "I have an urge for a cigarette") loaded only on factor one. This would appear to contradict the notion of the multi-dimensional nature of "craving". It is inevitable that questions which use terms such as "craving" and urges" should load on the same factor since the two words are often used interchangeably (See below section). However, it should be noted that the term "craving" is being used as a term of convenience. Craving could be conceived of as a generic word encompassing a number of subjective experiences. Further support for the idea of craving as a multi-dimensional phenomenon may be found in "craving" questionnaires for other drugs of abuse as discussed above. Such evidence suggests that craving for a variety of different abused substances is multi-dimensional in nature and comprises at least two dimensions or factors. The next logical question is, "what exactly are these factors?" Tiffany and Drobes (1991) would not commit to precise definitions of their 2-factors, preferring to refer to them simply as factor 1 and factor 2 since "labels may convey an overly simplistic understanding of the meaning of these manifestations of smoking urges".

It is difficult to directly compare multi-dimensional craving questionnaires for different drugs, since they are necessarily different in construction. In the questionnaires mentioned above, the DSQ, DAQ and ACQ had a single factor reflecting positive and negative reinforcement, whereas the QSU and CCQ had separate factors for positive and negative reinforcement. However, it should be remembered that nicotine and cocaine are stimulants whereas alcohol is classed as a sedative/hypnotic. In addition, alcohol exhibits a biphasic effect, such that it acts as a stimulant in low doses, and as a depressant in higher doses. It is therefore unsurprising that the factor structure of craving differs across different classes of abused substances although this may not account for the similarity between the factor structure of the stimulant-based DSQ and the sedative-hypnotic based DAQ.

The finding that the Questionnaire of Smoking Urges exhibits two factors, one reflecting positive reinforcement and one reflecting negative reinforcement has been replicated and so may be considered fairly robust (Davies et al., 2000). It may be suggested that these two factors are important components in the subjective experience of craving, but may not necessarily be the only ones. Subtle intra-drug differences may exist. Thus, the subjective experience of craving for each class of drug may differ slightly. Nicotine shares many of the neuropharmacological properties of other abused psychostimulants (such as cocaine and amphetamine), which account for some of its addictive characteristics (Balfour et al, 2000). However, Balfour and colleagues (2000) have argued that aspects of the neuropharmacology of nicotine are also inconsistent with hypotheses that have been proposed to explain psychostimulant dependence. By implication, it would be expected that differing classes of drugs should have different types of subjective craving associated with them, reflected by the differing factor structures of psychometric urge questionnaires. For example, while amphetamine, cocaine and nicotine all act on the mesocorticolimbic dopamine system to enhance dopaminergic activity in the nucleus accumbens, nicotine acts at the level of the ventral tegmental area (VTA), while amphetamine and cocaine have an indirect agonist effects at the level of the nucleus accumbens. However, it has been demonstrated that repeated nicotine exposure (as would be expected to occur in a regular smoker) causes inactivation or desensitisation of the dopamine secreting cells of the VTA in rats (Pidoplichko et al., 1997). An explanation for why smokers continue with their habit despite the nicotine ceasing to stimulate the nucleus accumbens, which is thought to mediate reward, could be that the negative withdrawal aspects of the craving are more important than the positive reinforcement aspects in nicotine addiction, compared to other stimulant drugs. This remains a question to be answered by future research, but it is clear that multi-dimensional measures of craving have a role to play in any such investigations in humans. This issue is also further complicated by the effects of cigarette smoke on Monoamine Oxidase, and will be considered shortly. It is clear, however, that while drugs of abuse may have similar effects on the mesocorticolimbic dopamine system, in other respects they have different pharmacological properties, and as such may not result in identical forms of addiction.

What Is the Difference between "Urges" and "Craving"?

Kozlowski and colleagues (1989) reported that there was a clear lack of agreement among problem drug users as to the meaning of a "craving". These authors reported that 49.5% of participants indicated that a craving is a strong urge or desire to take a drug, and that 35.5% stated that a craving is any urge or desire to take a drug, even a weak urge. Kozlowski and Wilkinson (1987), however, suggest that urges and cravings represent qualitatively and quantitatively different constructs. They suggested that the term "urge" refers to the whole continuum of desires to use drugs, whereas "craving" refers to states of intense and urgent desire. It seems apparent from Kozlowski and Wilkinson's (1987) suggestion that the definition of a craving is dependent upon where the boundaries are set. Examination of Davies et al., (2000) reveals that items on the QSU that referred to "Urge" and "crave" loaded on the same factor (factor 1), suggesting that they are perceived as at least similar constructs. Tiffany and Drobes (1991) chose to refer to urges in the title of their questionnaire, but state that they were reporting "the development and initial validation of a questionnaire of smoking urges and cravings". From this quote it is clear that they viewed both terms as interchangeable, and did not distinguish between them. Tiffany later suggested that research, as yet, had not produced any empirical or psychometric justification for a substantive distinction between the term urge and the term craving (Tiffany et al, 1993). Similar to the findings reported by Davies et al., (2000), Tiffany and colleagues (1993) reported that items related specifically to "urge" and "craving" loaded on the same factor of their CCQ-Now cocaine-craving questionnaire. Furthermore, these authors reported that participants who identified craving as only a strong desire (as opposed to any urge or desire, even a weak one), did not rate the specific "urge" and "craving" items on the Cocaine Craving Questionnaire any differently from those who did not make this distinction (Tiffany et al., 1993). James et al., (2004) also reported items relating to urge and craving (for speed) loaded on the same factor. In other words, respondents to these authors questionnaire did not consider there to be a distinction between the term "craving" and the term "urge".

Could "Craving" Be Modulated by More than One Neurochemical System?

One implication of the hypothesis that craving has more than one component is the possibility that craving is modulated by more than one neurochemical system. Reports often suggest that the success rates of nicotine substitution therapies are low, with typically less than 20% of participating smokers still abstinent after 1 year (Balfour and Fagerstöm, 1996). Balfour and colleagues (2000) have suggested that one reason for this poor success rate may be that the neurobiology underpinning tobacco dependence is more complex than currently appreciated, and that "a more complete understanding of the neural mechanisms involved will facilitate the introduction of improved therapeutic approaches".

There is a plethora of evidence that implicates dopamine systems in the positive reinforcing and rewarding effects of drugs (Wise 1988, Robinson and Berridge, 1993). Di Chiara and Imperato (1988) demonstrated that drugs abused by humans increase dopamine neurotransmission in rats. It has been demonstrated that animals will work for injections of drugs directly into appropriate parts of the mesotelencephalic dopamine system (Wise and Hoffman, 1992). Since Wise concluded that dopamine mediates positive reinforcement (Wise

1988) it is likely that dopamine is the main mediator of the urge to smoke reflected by Tiffany and Drobes (1991) QSU factor 1. However, when considering nicotine addiction, what we are really considering is addiction to smoking. As a result, substances other than nicotine may be implicated in the habit of cigarette smoking. For example, smoking is known to inhibit monoamine oxidase (MAO) A and B. MAO is an enzyme that breaks down catecholamine neurotransmitters. As a result MAO inhibition increases dopamine levels in the brain. Indeed, it is this elevation in dopamine levels resulting from MAO inhibition that is utilised by antidepressants such as phenelzine. It has been suggested (Robinson and Berridge, 1993) that repeated nicotine administration might lead to sensitisation of the dopamine secreting cells of the VTA. However, this does not take account of the influence of MAO inhibition, and the resultant increase in dopaminergic activity. One reason why smoking is such an addictive habit could be due to heightened sensitivity to its positive reinforcing effects as a result of MAO inhibition in addition to the neuropharmacological effects of nicotine. West and colleagues (2000) report that the abuse liability of nicotine replacement treatments (NRTs) is low. In addition, participants in their study did not rate these products as satisfying. These findings could well reflect the fact that NRTs do not inhibit MAO.

Rasmussen, Kallman and Helton (1997) have presented evidence from animal studies implicating 5-HT-1A receptors in the neurophysiology of nicotine withdrawal. Indeed, Baumann and Rothman (1988) have proposed that withdrawal from cocaine, may serve as a useful animal model of depression. Balfour and Ridley (2000) have suggested that chronic nicotine exposure elicits changes in hippocampal 5-HT formation and release, which are depressogenic. It is therefore possible that 5-HT is the main modulator of the urges that are reflected by Tiffany and Drobes (1991) factor 2.

This speculation over the relative roles of dopamine and 5-HT in smoking addiction should be further investigated in the future regardless of the debates over whether a dopamine-based or 5-HT based model of depression is most appropriate. In humans, it has been demonstrated that smoking is more prevalent in people who suffer from depression (Breslau et al, 1993; Covey et al, 1998). Future research should consider investigating responding to multi-dimensional craving measures after administration of dopamine and 5-HT antagonists. Do 5-HT antagonists (such as Selective Serotonin Re-uptake Inhibitors) influence factor 2, but not factor 1 scores? Does the inverse apply to dopaminergic antagonists? Such investigations using multi-dimensional craving measures may help to substantially advance our understanding of the neuropharmacology of addiction.

What Factors Influence Craving?

Abstinence

There are only a few reports of the utility of multi-dimensional measures of craving. It is vital to the validity of any craving questionnaire that it demonstrates sensitivity to periods of drug abstinence since such acute periods of abstinence will inevitably lead to an increase in craving for the drug (although it should be noted that abstinence from drug use is not always necessary to induce drug craving – Tiffany and Drobes, 1991; Tiffany et al., 1993). All of the limited number of studies that have examined the influence of abstinence on the QSU suggest that it is sensitive to short periods of cigarette abstinence, and is thus a valid tool for measuring cigarette craving. For example, Tiffany and Drobes (1991) found the QSU to be differentially sensitive to 1, 2 and 6 hours of abstinence. In addition, Willner and colleagues have demonstrated that the QSU is sensitive to periods of abstinence of at 2-4 hours (Willner et al., 1995; Willner and Jones, 1996; Morgan et al., 1999; Davies et al., 2000; Davies et al., 2004). The research thus suggests that only very limited periods of abstinence are required for strong urges and craving for a cigarette to become apparent. Of more importance to smoking cessation is whether in the long term cravings are experienced and thus play a role in relapse. Hughes et al., (1994) reported that cravings for cigarettes can still be apparent 6 months or more after quitting. The role of craving in relapse will be considered later.

Cues

There are numerous other variables, apart from abstinence, which may stimulate subjective cravings, and enhance the reinforcing value of the drug. As considered above, a major determinant of drug-use behaviour in the natural environment is likely to be the presence of exteroceptive, drug-related, stimuli or "cues", such as a lit cigarette, or another person smoking. Tiffany (1990) suggests that such stimuli may elicit automatic action schemata and drug-use behaviour. Situational cues have been shown to be an important factor in the determination of cravings for a variety of drugs, such as alcohol (Rankin et al., 1983), and opiates (Robins et al., 1974). In addition, it has been suggested that such cues may play an important role in stimulating the urge to smoke cigarettes in abstinent individuals (Niaura et al., 1988), and in non-abstinent individuals (Rickard-Figueroa and Zeicher, 1992). Drobes and Tiffany (1997) reported that cue exposure resulted in large changes in subjective reports of craving compared with slight changes in the physiological responses of participants. Maude-Griffin and Tiffany (1996) found clear evidence of an effect of content-specific imagery on the subjective urge to smoke. In addition, Burton and Tiffany (1997) reported that both imaginal and, *in vivo,* smoking cues enhanced craving for a cigarette. Morgan et al., (1999) have reported that smoking-related paraphernalia (eg cigarette packets, lighters, ashtrays) increased subjective reports of craving in smokers, but that this effect was maximal in non-abstinent smokers. The magnitude of the effect of exteroceptive, smoking-related, cues has been found to vary for smokers. Hutchison and colleagues (1999) report that the urge response to cue exposure can be reduced by the administration of naltrexone to abstinent smokers maintained with transdermal nicotine replacement. Carter and Tiffany (1999) concluded from a meta-analysis of cue-reactivity, that drug-related cues increase subjective reports of craving, compared to neutral cues, for all classes of drugs of abuse.

Davies and colleagues (2000) have reported that cigarette-related cues can have an influence on craving in non-dependent smokers. Some smokers are able to sustain regular long-term tobacco smoking without becoming dependent (Shiffman, 1989). Shiffman (1989) compared dependent 20 – 40 cigarettes per day smokers to "tobacco chippers" who regularly smoked 5 or fewer cigarettes per day. Unlike the dependent smokers, chippers seemed unaffected by overnight cigarette abstinence, and showed no signs of withdrawal. In addition, chippers obtained low Fagerström dependency scores (Fagerström, 1978) and reported being able to abstain from smoking for days at a time. However, it was not the case that these chippers could be classified simply as "social smokers", since when Shiffman (1989) controlled for the amount smoke, the chippers were just as likely as dependent smokers to smoke when alone. Shiffman and colleagues have reported a number of comparisons between tobacco chippers and dependent smokers. They have reported that chippers are regularly exposed to nicotine, and absorb the same amount of nicotine from each cigarette as dependent smokers and that chippers' per-cigarette nicotine exposure resembles that of free-smoking dependent smokers (Shiffman et al., 1990). In addition, they have reported that chippers eliminate nicotine at comparable rates, and show similar cardiovascular responses to smoking as dependent smokers (Shiffman et al., 1992), and show no differences in their smoking topography (Brauer et al, 1996). Such evidence suggests that the smoking behaviour of chippers could be maintained by nicotine's pharmacological effects, and Shiffman and colleagues (1990), suggest that nicotine may have direct motivating reinforcing effects, besides its ability to relieve withdrawal. Shiffman and colleagues (1994) examined the smoking typology profiles of chippers and regular smokers and found that chippers' profiles de-emphasised dependence-related motives, and emphasised appetitive and sensory motives such as handling and pleasure from smoking. Davies et al., (2000) reported that when cigarette chippers were given the QSU to complete cue exposure elevated craving related to desire to smoke and anticipation of positive outcome, but had no effect on craving scores related to withdrawal and negative affect (as would be expected in non-dependent smokers). Such evidence is consistent with multi-dimensional theories of craving (Baker et al., 1987; Tiffany, 1990), provides evidence that the QSU has sound discriminative properties and reinforces the suggestion that cues can have a powerful influence on the desire to smoke.

Mood

Marlatt and Gordon (1980) reported that retrospective studies and anecdotal evidence suggest that negative moods are one of the most important precipitants of relapse in recovered alcoholics. It has often been assumed that negative moods increase the risk of relapse by eliciting cravings, and there is some evidence for a relationship between negative affect and craving. Greeley and colleagues (1992) reported that desire for alcohol in the presence of alcohol-related cues were predicted by scores on the depression adjective checklist. This evidence has been further supported by studies which experimentally manipulated mood. Cooney and colleagues have reported that hypnotic induction of a negative mood (Litt et al., 1990), and induction of negative mood by guided verbal imagery (Cooney et al., 1997) and musical mood induction (Willner et al., 1998b) elicited or increased desires for alcohol. Negative mood induced by means of a stressful task (Payne et al., 1992) guided imagery (Tiffany and Drobes, 1990) and musical mood induction (Willner and Jones, 1996) has also been shown to increase desire to smoke. Childress and colleagues (1994) reported increased craving for heroin following hypnotic induction of negative mood in opiate users.

O'Connell and Martin (1987) suggested that it is easier for smokers to successfully resist an urge to relapse if smoking-related cues are present than if negative affect is present. This implies that a negative affective state is a more powerful stimulus than physical cues alone. Marlatt and Gordon (1985) suggested that a combination of negative affect and the presence of drug-related cues would result in greater craving for the drug than when either factor is present alone. However, Payne et al., (1987) manipulated negative affect as well as smoking-related cues and found that, although both factors increased puff duration on a cigarette, there was no interaction between cues and affect, and no effect of either on self-reported urge to smoke.

A number of studies have reported that negative moods enhance cue-induced craving state in smokers (Elash et al., 1995; Maude-Griffin and Tiffany, 1996), alcoholics (Cooney et al., 1997) and recreational drinkers (Greeley et al., 1992; Willner et al., 1998b). However, other investigators have failed to find that negative moods enhance cue-induced craving states in alcoholics (Litt et al., 1990), smokers (Tiffany and Drobes, 1990; Shadel et al., 1998) and opiate users (Childress et al., 1994).

From the literature, it is apparent that the precise nature of the relationship between mood and craving remains unclear. There is evidence that cravings can be elicited or enhanced by cue exposure and depressed mood, but the evidence is inconsistent with respect to the extent to which these two factors interact (e.g. Willner et al., 1998b). Further, there is paradoxical evidence of the nature of the increases in cravings elicited by depressive mood induction. Willner and colleagues have reported that depressive mood induction also causes a decrease in subjective reports of hedonic capacity (Willner and Healy, 1994; Willner et al., 1998a; Willner et al., 1998b). This is consistent with the view that anhedonia is a central feature of depression (American Psychiatric Association, 1994). Although it would be reasonable to assume that more valued rewards would be more highly craved, and that unwanted rewards would be little valued, evidence such as that from Willner and his colleagues suggests that drug wanting and liking are not necessarily the same thing. The clarification of this issue is important to theories of addiction which state that that the psychological processes involved in drug-use behaviour operate independently of those processes that control subjective urge responding (Tiffany, 1990).

Combating Cigarette Cravings - Nicotine Replacement Therapies (NRTs)

Nicotine replacement therapies are widely available over the counter, as a method of aiding smokers attempting to quit. They function by replacing plasma nicotine that would normally have been derived from smoking a cigarette, on the assumption that this should reduce the severity of withdrawal, and so allow the smoker to abstain from smoking more easily. The two most commonly used nicotine replacement therapies are transdermal nicotine patches, which deliver nicotine through the skin, and nicotine chewing polacrilex gum, which delivers nicotine through the mouth and stomach. Such therapies are designed to deliver nicotine at a constant rate in order to achieve stable plasma nicotine concentrations.

Research generally suggests that nicotine replacement therapies improve cessation rates among smokers. For example, Lam and colleagues (1987) meta-analysis of 14 randomised, placebo controlled trials of the efficacy of nicotine gum in smoking cessation, reported cessation rates of 27% after 6 months with nicotine gum, compared to 18% with placebo gum. Similarly, Palmer and colleagues (1992) in their review of the pharmacodynamic and pharmacokinetic properties of transdermal nicotine have reported improved cessation rates with nicotine patches when compared to placebo patches. For example, Abelin and colleagues (1989) reported 22% cessation rates with nicotine patches after 6 months compared to 12.2% cessation with placebo patches.

However, it is clear from the meta-analyses of Abelin and colleagues (1989) and Lam and colleagues (1987), that nicotine replacement therapies are by no means completely successful. This suggests that craving is a far more complex phenomenon than simply being the result of withdrawal from a given substance, and that the nature of craving and its relationship to relapse is not a simple one.

So, What Is the Relationship between Craving and Relapse?

The clinical importance of precisely defining craving lies in the potential role of craving in relapse amongst abstinent drug users. Many investigators argue that craving is a powerful predictor of relapse amongst dependent drug users (e.g. Swan et al, 1996). If craving is not a significant predictor of relapse, there seems to be little clinical purpose in precisely defining and measuring it. However, Tiffany's (1990) cognitive processing model of drug urges and drug use appears, on the surface, to cast doubt on the importance of conscious craving for relapse. Tiffany argues that the mechanisms linking drug-related stimuli to drug-use behaviour operate independently of the processes that control craving. Hence, according to this model, drug use-behaviour is an automatic, non-conscious behaviour much akin to other automated skills such as driving a car. However, further explanation of this model has revealed that, under certain conditions, craving, and physiological and behavioural responses to cues, could be predictive of relapse (Tiffany, 1995). Most cue-reactivity research is based upon the assumption that physiological reactions to drug stimuli are mediated primarily through the process of classical conditioning. Tiffany's model, however, rejects this assumption and suggests instead that many of the physiological responses associated with urge reports represent reactions to the cognitive demands of craving, and are not classically conditioned withdrawal or appetitive effects (Tiffany, 1995). In addition, Tiffany's model suggests that somatovisceral responses invoked by cue manipulations, may have multiple determinants, possibly reflecting elements of physiological reactions encoded within the action schema that has been impeded (Tiffany, 1995). An implication of this theory is that the relationship between craving and relapse may not be a straightforward one.

Empirical evidence for a relationship between craving and relapse is not as clear cut as would be intuitively expected, and may be even more complex than Tiffany's (1990) model implies. Studies have demonstrated dissociations between drug craving and drug use. Gawin and colleagues (1989), for example, reported that desipramine (an antidepressant drug that blocks noradrenaline reuptake) decreased cocaine usage after two weeks of medication, but that it was several weeks until craving was reduced. Nemeth-Coslett and Henningfield (1986) reported that nicotine gum decreased actual smoking, but not self-reports of desire to smoke. Foltin and Fishman (1994) reported a similar result with cocaine users given Buprenorphine (mixed opioid agonist-antagonist). Other studies have reported the opposite effect of reductions of craving without any effect on drug self-administration, for example, in a sample of cocaine users given desipramine (Fishman et al., 1990) and the SSRI fluoxetine (Grabowski et al., 1995). A similar finding has been reported in smokers given the opioid receptor antagonist naltrexone (Sutherland et al., 1995; Houtsmuller et al., 1996). Houtsmuller and Sitzer (1999) have reported that the rapid smoking technique (Tiffany et al., 1986), a procedure designed to promote cigarette-related nausea, suppressed craving scores, but that craving scores were not predictive of actual smoking behaviour.

Whether or not craving is a part of withdrawal is also up for debate. DSM-IV for example has excluded craving for the description of withdrawal because there is doubt over the compatibility of the two at different stages of abstinence and may well be controlled by different processes (Teneggi et al., 2002).

Research only allows us to speculate on the nature of the relationship between craving and relapse. The findings of Morgan et al., (1999) demonstrated that although cigarette-related cues elevated factor 1 and factor 2 scores on the QSU, this effect was maximal in non-abstinent smokers. The findings of Davies et al., (2000) demonstrated that in non-dependent smokers, cue's significantly raised appetitive but not withdrawal based craving. These findings are consistent with the view that craving and associated responses to cues may be predictive of relapse under certain conditions. In addition, these findings suggest that reactivity to smoking-related cues (possibly as a result of physiological responses encoded within blocked action schema) may be a better predictor of relapse than the ability to remain abstinent. However, it should be kept in mind that these two studies were designed to assess the reliability and validity of the Questionnaire of Smoking Urges, and not to specifically examine the relationship between craving and relapse.

CONCLUSION

What is apparent is that craving is an extremely difficult concept to pin down. In the various guises that we understand it appears to be influenced by numerous other factors and its relationship to withdrawal and relapse is not understood despite assumptions that there must be one. Interventions designed to minimize cigarette craving and thus minimize withdrawal are based upon this assumption, but are seemingly not terribly successful. As such, after decades of research into a concept that we can't define, it can only be concluded that craving research can at best only have a speculative role in informing smoking cessation strategies and that current strategies that focus exclusively on craving may be well-intentioned but ultimately misguided until we finally establish what craving is and what role it plays in the acquisition, maintenance and relapse of a smoking habit.

REFERENCES

Abelin Th, Ehrsam R, Buhler-Reichart A Imhof PR and Muller Ph (1989). Effectiveness of a transdermal nicotine system in smoking cessation studies. *Methods and Findings in Experimental Clinical Pharmacology*, 11: 205-214.

American Psychiatric Association (1994). Diagnostic and statistics manual of mental disorders (4th ed.). Washington, D.C.

Baker TB and Morse E (1985). The urge as affect. Paper presented at the convention of the Association for the Advancement of Behaviour Therapy, Houston. Cited in Tiffany (1995).

Baker TB, Sherman JE and Morse E (1987). The motivation to use drugs: a psychobiological analysis of urges. In Rivers C (Ed.), *The Nebraska symposium on motivation: alcohol use and abuse*, 257-323 (Lincoln, NE, University of Nebraska Press).

Balfour DJK and Fagerstöm KO (1996). Pharmacology of nicotine and its therapeutic use inn smoking cessation and neurodegenerative disorders. *Pharmacological Therapy*, 72: 1-81.

Balfour DJK and Ridley DL (2000). The effects of nicotine on neural pathways implicated in depression: A factor in nicotine addiction? *Pharmacology Biochemistry and Behavior*, 66: 79 – 85.

Balfour DJK, Wright AE, Benwell EM and Birrell CE (2000). The putative role of extra-synaptic mesolimbic dopamine in the neurobiology of nicotine dependence. *Behavioural Brain Research*, 113: 73-83.

Baumann MH and Rothman RB (1988) Alterations in serotonergic responsiveness during cocaine withdrawal in rats: similarities to major depression in humans. *Biological Psychiatry*, 44: 578-591.

Behm FM. and Rose, JE (1994). Reducing craving for cigarettes while decreasing smoke intake using capsaicin-enhanced low tar cigarettes. *Experimental and Clinical Psychopharmacology*, 2: 143-153

Bohn MJ, Krahn DD and Staehler BA (1995) Development and initial validation of a measure of drinking urges in abstinent alcoholics. *Alcoholism: Clinical and Erxperimental Research*, 19: 600-606.

Brauer LH, Hatsukami D, Hanson K, Shiffman S (1996) Smoking topography in tobacco chippers and dependent smokers. *Addictive Behavior*, 21: 233-8.

Breslau N, Kilber MM and Andreski P (1993). Nicotine dependence and major depression. *Archives of General Psychiatry*, 50: 31-35.

Buchhalter AR, Acosta MC, Evans SE, Breland AB and Eissenberg T (2005). Tobacco abstinence symptom suppression: the role played by the smoking-related stimuli that rae delivered by denicotinized cigarettes. *Addiction*, 100: 550-559.

Burton SM and Tiffany ST (1997). The effect of alcohol consumption on craving to smoke. *Addiction*, 92: 15-26.

Carter BL and Tiffany ST (1999). Meta-analysis of cue-reactivity in addiction research. *Addiction*, 94: 327-340.

Cepeda_Benito A and Tiffany ST (1996). The use of a dual-task procedure for the assessment of cognitive effort associated with smoking urges. *Psychopharmacolgy* 117: 110-115.

Chaney EF, Roszell DK and Cummings C (1982). Relapse in opiate addicts: a behavioral analysis. *Addictive Behaviors*, 7: 291-297.

Chen H., Vlahos R., Bozinovski S., Jones J., Anderson G.P. and Morris M.J. (2005). Effect of short-term cigarette exposure on body-weight, appetite and brain neuropeptide Y in mice.

Neuropsychopharmacology, 30: 713-719.

Childress AR, McLellan A, O'Brien T, Charles P and Ehrman R (1988) Classically conditioned responses in opioid and cocaine dependence: A role in relapse? *National Institute on Drug Abuse: Research Monograph Series*, 84: 25-43.

Childress AR, Ehrman R, McLennan AT, MacRae J, Natale M and O'Brien CP (1994). Can induced moods trigger drug-related responses in opiate abuse patients? *Journal of Substance Abuse Treatment*, 11: 17-23.

Clark D (1994). Craving for alcohol. *Journal of Psychopharmacology* 9: 73.

Cooney NL, Litt MD, Morse PA, Bauer LO and Gaupp L (1997). Alcohol cue reactivity, negative mood reactivity, and relapse in treated alcoholic men. *Journal of Abnormal Psychology*, 106: 243-250.

Covey LS, Glassman AH and Stetner F (1998). Cigarette smoking and major depression. *Journal of Addiction Research*, 17: 35-46.

Davies G, Morgan M and Willner P (2000) Smoking-related cues elicit craving in tobacco "chippers": a replication and validation of the two-factor structure of the Questionnaire of Smoking Urges. *Psychopharmacology*, 152: 334-342.

Davies GM, Willner P, James DL and Morgan MJ (2004) Influence of nicotine gum on acute cravings for cigarettes. *Journal of Psychopharmacology*, 18 (1): 83-87.

de Wit H. and Zacny J. (1995). Abuse potential of nicotine replacement therapies. *CNS Drugs*, 4: 456-468.

Di Chiara G and Imperato A (1988). Drugs abused by humans preferentially increase synaptic dopamine concentrations in the mesolimbic system of freely moving rats. *Proceedings of the National Academy of Science, USA*, 85: 5274-5278.

Drobes T and Tiffany ST (1997). A comparison of imaginal and cue-exposure manipulations of smoking urge: the effect of nicotine deprivation. *Journal of Abnormal Psychology*, 106: 15-25.

Ehrman R, Ternes J, O'Brien CP and McLellan AT (1992). Conditioned tolerance in human opiate addicts. *Psychopharmacology*, 108: 218-224.

Elash CA, Tiffany ST and Vrana SR (1995). Manipulation of smoking urges and affect through a brief-imagery procedure: Self-report, psychophysiological, and startle probe responses. *Experimental and Clinical Psychopharmacology* 3: 156-162.

Fagerstöm KO (1978). Measuring degree of physical dependence to tobacco with reference to individualization of treatment. *Addictive Behavior*, 3: 235-241.

Fischman MW, Foltin RW, Nestadt G and Pearlson GD (1990). Effects of desipramine maintenance on cocaine self-administration in humans. *Journal of Pharmacology and Experimental Therapeutics*, 253: 760-770.

Fletcher C and Doll R (1969). A survey of doctors' attitudes to smoking. *British Journal of Preventative and Social Medicine*, 23: 145-153.

Foltin RW and Fischman MW (1994). Effects of buprenorphine on the self administration of cocaine by humans. *Behavioural Pharmacology*, 5: 79-89.

Gawin FH, Kleber HD, Byck R, Rounsaville BJ, Kosten TR, Jatlow PI and Morgan C (1989). Desipramine facilitation of initial cocaine abstinence. *Archives of General Psychiatry*, 46: 107-113.

Grabrowski J, Rhoades H, Elk R, Schmitz J, Davis C, Creson D and Kirby K (1995). Fluoxetine is ineffective for treatment of cocaine dependence or concurrent opiate and cocaine dependence: two placebo-controlled, double-blind trials. *Journal of Clinical Psychopharmacology*, 15: 163-174.

Greeley J, Swift W and Heather N (1992). Depressed affect as a predictor of increased desire for alcohol in current drinkers of alcohol. *British Journal of Addiction*, 87: 1005-1012.

Houtsmuller EJ, Clemmey PA, Sigler LA and Stitzer ML (1996). Effects of naltrexone on smoking and abstinence. *National Institute on Drug Abuse: Research Monograph Series*, 174: 68.

Houtsmuller EJ and Stitzer ML (1999). Manipulation of cigarette craving through rapid smoking: efficacy and effects on smoking behavior. *Psychopharmacology*, 142: 149-157.

Hughes J (1987). Craving as a psychological construct. *British Journal of Addiction* 82: 38-39.

Hughes JR, Higgins ST and Bickel WK (1994). Nicotine withdrawal versus other drug withdrawals syndromes: similarities and dissimilarities. *Addiction*, 89: 1461-1470.

Hutchinson KE, Monti PM, Rohsenow DJ, Swift RM, Colby SM, Gnys M, Niaura RS and Sirota AD (1999). Effects of naltrexone with nicotine replacement on smoking cue reactivity: preliminary results. *Psychopharmacology*, 142, 139-143.

James D, Davies G and Willner P (2004) The development and initial validation of a questionnaire to measure craving for amphetamine. *Addiction*, 99: 1181-1188.

Jellinek EM (1955). The "craving" for alcohol. *Quarterly Journal of Studies on Alcohol*, 16: 41-49.

Kozlowsi LT and Wilkinson DA (1987). Use and misuse of the concept of craving by alcohol, tobacco, and drug researchers. *British Journal of Addiction,* 82: 31-36.

Kozlowski LT Mann RE Wilkinson DA and Poulos CX (1989). "Cravings" are ambiguous: ask about urges or desires. *Addictive Behaviors*, 14: 443-445.

Kozlowski LT, Pillitteri JL, Sweeney CT, Whitfield KE and Graham JW (1996). Asking Questions About Urges or Cravings for Cigarettes. *Psychology of Addicitive Behaviors,* 10: 248-260

Lam W, Sze PC, Sacks HS and Chalmers TC (1987). Meta-analysis of randomized controlled trials of nicotine chewing-gum. *Lancet*, 2: 27-29.

Lamb RJ, Preston KL, Schindler C, Meisch RA, Davis F, Katz JL, Henningfield JE and Goldberg SR (1991). The reinforcing and subjective effects of morphine in post-addicts: a dose response study. *Journal of Pharmacology and Experimental Therapeutics*, 259: 1165-1173.

Litt MD, Cooney NL, Kadden RM and Gaupp L (1990). Reactivity to alcohol cues and induced moods in alcoholics. *Addictive Behavior*, 15: 137-146.

Love A, James D and Willner P (1998) A comparison of two alcohol craving questionnaires. *Addiction*, 93: 1091-1102.

Ludwig AM and Wikler A (1974). "Craving" and relapse to drink. *Quart. J. Stud. Alcohol*, 35, 108-130.

Markou A, Weiss F, Gold, LH, Caine SB, Schulteis G and Koob GF (1993). Animal models of drug craving. *Psychopharmacology*, 112, 163-182.

Marlatt, G.A. (1985). Cognitive factors in the relapse process. In: *Relapse Prevention*, Marlatt GA and Gordon JR (Eds.). Guildford Press, NY: 128-200.

Marlatt GA and Gordon JR (1980). Determinants of relapse: Implications for the maintenance of behavior change. In Davidson PO (Ed.), *Behavioural medicine: Changing health lifestyles* 410-452. New York: Brunner/Mazel.

Marlatt GA and Gordon JR (Eds) (1985).Relapse Prevention: Maintenance Strategies in the Treatment of Addictive Behaviors. New York: Guilford Press.

Maude-Griffin PM and Tiffany ST (1996). Production of Smoking Urges Through Imagery: The Impact of Affect and Smoking Abstinence. *Experimental and Clinical Psychopharmacology*, 4, 198-208.

McAuliffe WE (1982). A test of Wikler's theory of relapse: The frequency of relapse due to conditioned withdrawal sickness. *Int J Addict,* 17, 19-33.

McAuliffe WE and Gordon RA (1974). A test of Lindensmith's theory of addiction: The frequency of euphoria among long-term addicts. *American Journal of Sociology*, 79: 795-840.

Melchoir CL and Tabakoff B (1984). A conditioning model of alcohol tolerance. In Galanter M (Ed.) *Recent Developments in Alcoholism*, Vol. 2: 5-16. New York: Plenum Press.

Merikle EP (1999). The subjective experience of craving: An exploratory analysis. *Substance Use and Misuse* 34: 1101-1115.

Meyer R.E., Mirin S.M. (1979). *The Heroin Stimulus: Implications for a Theory of Addiction.* New York, Plenum Medical Book Company

Morgan MJ, Davies GM_and Willner P (1999) The Questionnaire of Smoking Urges is sensitive to abstinence and exposure to smoking-related cues. *Behavioural Pharmacology*, 10: 619-626.

Nemeth-Coslett R and Henningfield JE (1986). Effects of nicotine chewing gum on cigarette smoking and subjective physiological effects. *Clinical Pharmacology and Therapy*, 39: 625-630.

Niaura RS, Rohsenow DJ, Binkoff JA, Monti PM, Pedraza M and Abrams DB (1988). Relevance of cue reactivity to understanding alcohol and smoking relapse. *Journal of Abnormal Psychology*, 97, 133-152.

O'Brien CP, Childress AR, McLellan AT and Ehrman R (1992). A learning model of addiction. In O'Brien CP and Jaffe JH (Eds) *Addictive States* 157-177. New York: Raven Press.

O'Connell KA and Martin EJ (1987). Highly tempting situations associated with abstinence, temporary lapse, and relapse among participants in smoking cessation programs. *Journal of Consulting and Clinical Psychology*, 55: 367-371.

Palmer KJ, Buckley MM and Foulds D (1992). Transdermal Nicotine. A review of its pharmacodynamic and pharmacokinetic properties, and therapeutic efficacy as an aid to smoking cessation. *Drugs,* 44: 498-529.

Payne TJ, Schare ML, Levis DJ and Colletti G (1987) Cue responsivity in smokers: The effects of environmental stimuli and negative affective state on topographical changes in smoking behavior. Paper presented at the Eighth Annual Convention of the Society of

Behavioral Medicine. Cited in Tiffany (1990).

Payne TJ, Rychtarik, RG, Smith, PO, Rappaport, NB, Etscheidt M, Brown TA and Johnson CA (1992) Reactivity to alcohol-relevant beverage and imaginal cues in alcoholics. *Addictive Behaviors*, 17: 209-217.

Perkins K.A. (1992). Effects of tobacco smoking on caloric intake. Br J *Addiction*, 87, 193-205.

Pidoplichko V, De Bias M, Williams JT and Dani J (1997). Nicotine activates and desensitizes midbrain dopamine neurons. *Nature* (390): 401-404.

Pohorecky LA (1977) Brain catecholamines and ethanol: involvement in physical dependence and withdrawal. *Advances in Experimental and Medical Biology*, 85A: 495-513.

Pomerleau CS and Pomerleau OF (1992). Euphoriant effects of nicotine in smokers. *Psychopharmacology*, 108, 460-465.

Poulos CX, Hinson R and Siegal S (1981). The role of Pavlovian processes in drug tolerance and dependence: Implications for treatment. *Addictive Behaviors*, 6, 205-211.

Rasmussen K, Kallman MJ and Helton DR (1997) Serotonin-1A antagonists attenuate the effects of nicotine withdrawal on the auditory startle response. *Synapse*, 27, 145-152.

Rankin H, Hodgson R and Stockwell T (1983). Cue exposure and response prevention in alcoholics: a controlled trial. *Behavior Research and Therapy*, 21, 435-446

Rickard-Figueroa K and Zeichner A (1992). Assessment of smoking urge and its concomitants under an environmental smoking cue manipulation. *Addictive Behaviors*, 10, 240-256.

Risner ME and Goldberg SR (1983). A comparison of nicotine and cocaine self-administration in the dog: fixed ratio and progressive ratio schedules of intravenous drug infusion. *J Pharmacol Exp Ther*, 224, 319-326

Robins LN, Davis DH and Goodwin DW (1974). Drug use by US army enlisted men in Vietnam: a follow-up on their return home. *American Journal of Epidemiology*, 99, 235-249.

Robinson JH and Pritchard WS (1992). The role of nicotine in tobacco use. *Psychopharmacology*, 108: 397-407

Robinson TE and Berridge KC (1993). The neural basis of drug craving: an incentive-sensitization theory of addiction. *Brain Research Reviews*, 18: 247-291.

Robinson TE, Berridge KC. (2000). The psychology and neurobiology of addiction: an incentive-sensitization view. *Addiction, 95*(Suppl. 2), S91–117.

Rusted JM, Mackee A, Williams R and Willner P (1998). Deprivation state but not nicotine content of the cigarette affects responding by smokers on a progressive ratio task. *Psychopharmacology*, 140, 411-417.

Sayette MA and Hufford MR (1994). Effects of cue exposure and deprivation on cognitive resources in smokers. *Journal of Abnormal Psychology*, 103: 812-818.

Sayette MA, Monti PM, Rosenhow DJ, Gulliver SB, Colby SM, Sirota AD, Niaura R and Abrams DB (1994). The effects of exposure on reaction time in male alcoholics. *Journal of Studies on Alcohol*, 55: 629-633.

Shadel WG, Niaura R, Abrams DB, Goldstein MG, Rohsenow DJ, Sirota AD, Monti PM (1998) Scripted imagery manipulations and smoking cue reactivity in a clinical sample of self-quitters. *Experimental and Clinical Psychopharmacology*, 6: 179-86.

Shiffman S (1989) Tobacco "chippers" – individual differences in tobacco dependence. *Psychopharmacology,* 97: 539-547

Shiffman SM and Jarvik ME (1976) Smoking withdrawal symptoms in two weeks of abstinence. *Psychopharmacology*, 50: 35-39

Shiffman S, Fischer LA, Zettler-Segal M and Benowitz (1990). Nicotine exposure in non-dependent smokers. *Archives of General Psychiatry*, 47, 333-336.

Shiffman S, Zettler-Segal M, Kassel J, Paty J, Benowitz NL and O'Brien G (1992) Nicotine elimination and tolerance in non-dependent cigarette smokers. *Psychopharmacology* 109: 449-456

Shiffman S., Kassel J.D., Paty J., Gnys M. and Zettler-Segal M. (1994). Smoking typology profiles of chippers and regular smokers. *Journal of Substance Abuse*, 6, 21-35.

Siegal S (1975). Evidence from rats that morphine tolerance is a learned response. *Journal of Comparative and Physiological Psychology*, 89: 498-506.

Siegal S (1983). Classical conditioning, drug tolerance and drug dependence. In Israel Y, Glaser FB, Kalant H, Popham RE, Schmidt W and Smart RG (Eds), *Research Advances in Alcohol and Drug Problems*, Vol. 7: 207-246. New York: Plenum Press.

Singleton EG and Tiffany ST (1994a). Alcohol Craving Questionnaire: ACQ-now: background and administration manual. Baltimore, (NIDA Addiction Research Centre).

Stewart J, deWit H and Eikelboom R (1984). Role of unconditioned and conditioned drug effects in self-administration of opiates and stimulants. *Psychological Review*, 91: 251-268.

Stolerman IP (1987). Psychopharamcology of Nicotine. Stimulus effects and receptor mechanisms. In L.L. Iverson, S.D. Iverson and S.H. Snyder (Eds). *Handbook of Psychopharmacology: New directions in psychopharmacology* (Vol. 19, pp 241-265). NY: Plenum Press.

Sutherland G, Stapleton JA, Russell MA and Feyerabend C (1995). Naltrexone, smoking behaviour and cigarette withdrawal. *Psychopharmacology*, 120: 418-425.

Swan GE, Ward MM and Jack LM (1996) Abstinence effects as predictors of 28-day relapse in smokers. *Addictive Behaviors*, 21: 481-490

Tabakoff B and Kiianmaa K (1982). Does tolerance develop to the activating, as well as the depressant, effects of ethanol? Pharmacology, Biochemistry and Behavior, 17: 1073-1076.

Teneggi V, Tiffany ST, Squassante L, Milleri S, Ziviani L and Bye A (2002). Smokers deprived of cigarettes for 72 h: effect of nicotine patches on craving and withdrawal. *Psychopharmacology*, 164, 177-187.

Tiffany ST and Carter BL (1998). Is craving the source of compulsive drug use? *Psychopharmacology*. 12: 23-30.

Tiffany ST (1997). New perspectives on the measurement, manipulation and meaning of drug craving. *Human Psychopharmacology*, 12 (Supp): S103-S113.

Tiffany ST (1990). A cognitive model of drug urges and drug use behaviour: Role of automatic and non-automatic processes. *Psychological Review*, 97, 147-168.

Tiffany ST and Conklin CA (2000). Human models in craving research. A cognitive processing modle of alcohol craving and compulsive alcohol use. *Addiction*, 95, S145-S153.

Tiffany ST and Drobes DJ (1990). Imagery and smoking urges: The manipulation of affective content. *Addictive Behaviors*, 15: 531-539.

Tiffany S (1995) The role of cognitive factors in reactivity to drug cues. In Drummond DC, Tiffany ST, Glautier S and Remington B (Eds.), *Addictive behaviour: Cue exposure theory and practice*. New York: Wiley.

Tiffany ST (1992). A critique of contemporary urge and craving research: Methodological, psychometric, and theoretical issues. *Advances in Behavior Research and Therapy*, 14, 123-129.

Tiffany ST (1988). Contemporary theories of drug urges, conflicting data, and an alternative cognitive framework. Paper presented at the Conference on Theory and Research in Psychopathology, Performance, and Cognition, Gainsville, FL. Cited in Tiffany (1995).

Tiffany ST and Drobes DJ (1991). The development and initial validation of a questionnaire of smoking urges. *British Journal of Addiction*, 86, 1467-1476.

Tiffany ST, Singleton E, Haertzen CA and Henningfield JE (1993). The development of a cocaine craving questionnaire. *Drug and Alcohol Dependence*, 34: 19-28.

Tiffany ST, Martin EM and Baker TB (1986). Treatment for cigarette smoking: an evaluation of the contributions of aversion and counseling procedures. *Behaviour Research and Therapy*, 24: 437-452.

Tiffany ST, Fields L, Singleton E, Haertzen C and Henningfield JE (unpublished). The development of a Heroin craving questionnaire.

UNDCP and WHO informal expert committee on the craving mechanism: Report (1992). United Nations International Drug Control Programme and World Health Organisation technical report series (No. V. 92-54439T).

Weinstein A, Wilson S, Bailey J, Myles J and Nutt D (1997). Imagery of craving in opiate addicts undergoing detoxification. *Drug and Alcohol Dependence*, 48: 25-31.

West RJ and Schneider N (1987). Craving for Cigarettes. *British Journal of Addiction*, 82, 407-415.

West RJ, Hajek P and Belcher M (1989). Time course of cigarette withdrawal symptoms while using nicotine gum. *Psychopharmacology*, 99: 143-145.

West R, Hajek P, Foulds J, Nilsson F, May S and Meadows A (2000). A comparison of the abuse liability and dependence potential of nicotine patch, gum, spray and inhaler. *Psychopharmacology*, 149: 198-202.

Wikler A (1948). Recent progress in research on the neurophysiological basis of morphine addiction. *American Journal of Psychiatry*, 105: 329-338.

Wikler A and Pescor FT (1967). Classical conditioning of a morphine abstinence phenomenon, reinforcement of opioid drinking behaviour and relapse in morphine addicted rats. *Psychopharmacologia*, 10: 255-284.

Wikler A (1972). Sources of reinforcement for drug using behavior – a theoretical formulation. Pharmacology and the Future of Man. *Proceedings of 5th International Congress of Pharmacology*, 1: 18-30.

Willner P and Healy S (1994) Decreased hedonic responsiveness during a brief depressive mood swing. *Journal of Affective Disorders*, 32: 13-20.

Willner P (1996) Homology in behavioural pharmacology: an example from operant behaviour. *Behavioural Pharmacology*, 7 (supplement 1), 121.

Willner P, Benton D, Brown E, Cheeta S, Davies G, Morgan J and Morgan MJ (1998a) "Depression" increases "craving" for sweet rewards in animal and human models of depression and craving. *Psychopharmacology*, 136, 272-283.

Willner P, Field M, Pitts K, Reeve G (1998b) Mood, cue and gender influences on motivation, craving and liking for alcohol in recreational drinkers. *Behavioural Pharmacology*, 9, 631-42.

Willner P and Jones C (1996). Effects of mood manipulation on subjective and behavioural measures of cigarette craving. *Behavioural Pharmacology*, 6, 1-9.

Willner P, Hardman S and Eaton G (1995). Subjective and behavioural evaluation of cigarette cravings. *Psychopharmacology*, 118, 171-177.

Willner P, James D. and Morgan M. (2005). Excessive alcohol consumption and dependence on amphetamine are associated with parallel increases in subjective ratings of both 'wanting' and 'liking'. *Addiction*, 100, 1487-1495.

Wise RA and Bozarth MA (1987). A psychomotor stimulant theory of addiction. *Psychological Review*, 94: 469-492

Wise RA and Hoffman DC (1992). Localization of drug reward mechanisms by intracranial injections. *Synapse*, 10: 247-263.

Wise RA (1988). The neurobiology of craving: Implications for understanding and treatment of addiction. *Journal of Abnormal Psychology*, 97, 147-168.

Zelman DC, Tiffany ST, Baker TB (1985). Influence of stress on morphine-induced hyperthermia: relevance to drug conditioning and tolerance development. *Behavioral Neuroscience*, 99:122-44.

Zinser MC, Baker, Sherman JE and Cannon DS (1992). Relation between self-reported affect and drug urges and cravings in continuing and withdrawing smokers. *Journal of Abnormal Psychology*, 101: 617-629.

In: Smoking Cessation: Theory, Interventions and Prevention   ISBN: 978-1-60021-591-9
Editor: Jerome E. Landow   © 2008 Nova Science Publishers, Inc.

Chapter 8

SMOKING CESSATION IN PATIENTS WITH CARDIOVASCULAR DISEASES AND COPD

Petter Quist-Paulsen[*]

Medical Department, Soerlandet Sykehus Kristiansand, Norway

ABSTRACT

Background: Approximately 1/3 of the adult population in industrial countries and 70% in several Asian countries are daily smokers. Tobacco is the greatest preventable cause of death worldwide. Smoking is an important risk factor for developing cardiovascular disorders, and smoking causes about 90% of COPD

Methods: The literature on smoking and smoking cessation in patients with cardiovascular diseases and COPD was reviewed, and original investigations were presented.

Results: Smoking cessation is associated with an approximately 50% risk reduction for death five years after myocardial infarction or unstable angina. With longer follow up periods the benefit of smoking cessation increases even further. In COPD, smoking cessation is the only action that improves the long-term prognosis. In patients with cardiovascular diseases and COPD, smoking cessation programs with behavioral support over several months combined with nicotine replacements significantly increases quit rates. Such programs can probably be delivered by personnel without special education in smoking cessation using simple intervention principles. A long follow up period is probably the most important element in the programs. In patients with coronary heart disease smoking cessation interventions are extremely cost effective compared to all other treatment modalities. In COPD, cost effectiveness analyses have not been performed, but a smoking cessation program has shown improved survival compared to usual care.

Conclusion: In patients with cardiovascular diseases and COPD smoking cessation interventions with several months of follow up combined with nicotine replacements are

---

[*] Petter Quist-Paulsen: E-mail: petterqp@online.no; Address: Department of Hematology, St Olavs Hospital, 7006 Trondheim, NORWAY; Telephone: +4799383765 (private), +4708600 (work). Fax nr: +4773869399

effective and easily applicable in clinical practice. Wider implementation of such programs would be a cost effective way of saving lives.

THE PREVALENCE OF SMOKING

Although smoking have been slowly declining in the western Europe and north America during the last thirty years, it increases rapidly throughout the developing world, and up to 70% of the population in several Asian countries are now daily smokers [1]. In the United States, approximately 20% are smoking, and in western Europe around 1/3 of the adult population are smokers [1] . Especially in western Europe and north America smoking is now most prevalent among people with a low level of education [2].

THE HEALTH PROBLEMS OF SMOKING

Approximately 5 million people die each year because of smoking world wide [1, 3]. Tobacco is regarded as the greatest single preventable cause of death [3], and is one of the biggest threats to the world health [3]. It causes much more deaths than obesity and HIV [1]. Lifelong smoking shortens the life expectancy with about 10 years [4], and it has been estimated that smoking one cigarette on average reduces life expectancy with 11 minutes [5]. A survey of British male physicians showed that the chance of reaching 73 years of age in life long smokers were 42% compared to 78% in life long non-smokers [6]. Pulmonary and cardiovascular diseases are the most frequent causes of death, causing approximately 50% and 35% of smoking related deaths, respectively [1, 3]. Further, in smokers about a third of deaths are attributed to cancer, of which 4/5 are lung cancers [1]. It has been estimated that smoking accounts for at least 30% of cancer deaths and most lung cancer deaths (approximately 90%) [7].

Several observational studies have shown that smoking is an important risk factor for the development of coronary heart disease [8-11]. Current smokers have a two- to four-fold higher risk of coronary heart disease and sudden death than non-smokers [9-11]. The mean number of cigarettes smoked per day is positively associated with this risk, but even as few as one to four cigarettes per day increase the likelihood of developing a myocardial infarction [12]. Smokers are on average ten years younger than non-smokers when they develop myocardial infarction [13].

Regarding chronic obstructive pulmonary diseases (COPD), smoking is the principle cause in approximately 90% of cases, and 10-20% of life long smokers will develop this disease [14].

Smoking increases both the mortality and frequency of cerebral strokes [15]. A meta-analysis of 32 studies found an overall relative risk to be 1.5 in smokers versus non-smokers [16].

Studies in patients with peripheral vascular disease have shown a doubling of the risk of intermittent claudication in smokers compared to non-smokers [17]. In this patient group there are a strong dose-response relationship. In heavy smokers the relative risk is up to nine times that of non-smokers [17].

THE PATHOGENESIS OF SMOKING RELATED CARDIOVASCULAR DISEASE AND COPD

The tobacco smoke is composed of over 4000 components. The pathogenic mechanisms explaining why these components increase the risk of cardiovascular diseases are not fully understood. Nicotine itself does not seem to increase the risk significantly [18]. Experiments have shown the following effects of cigarette smoking, all of which could contribute to coronary heart disease:

- Impaired endothelial function [19], which may be the cause of the increased atherosclerosis found in smokers [8].
- Vastly increased platelet activity, which arises acutely after smoking one cigarette [20].
- Acutely increased vascular resistance with decreased coronary flow velocity [21]. In some cases this may cause vasospasm, including vasospastic angina [22].

The increased risk of cardiovascular events associated with smoking declines rapidly after cessation, and after two years of abstinence the relative risk nearly equals the risk of non-smokers [23], suggesting that factors other than atherosclerosis per se are involved in the pathogenesis.

In COPD, smoking injures the epithelium and stimulates the macrophages. The ciliar function of the epithelium is impaired, and the mucus production increased. Further, an inflammatory response is set up with infiltration of lymphocytes and neutrophils. The neutrophils release proteolytic enzymes (elastases and proteases) which cause protease and antiprotease imbalance. This results in destruction of collagen and elastin in the airways, and chronic bronchitis or emphysema develops [24].

WHY IS IT IMPORTANT THAT PATIENTS WITH CARDIOVASCULAR DISEASES AND COPD QUIT SMOKING?

Patients with Coronary Heart Disease

Smoking cessation after an acute coronary event is associated with an approximately 50% relative mortality reduction after five years compared to sustained smoking [25, 26]. With a longer follow up period, the positive effect of smoking cessation increases further, as shown in figure 1 adopted from Daly et. al. [27]. Thirteen years after myocardial infarction or unstable angina only 18% were still alive among those who continued to smoke, compared to 63% among the quitters [27].

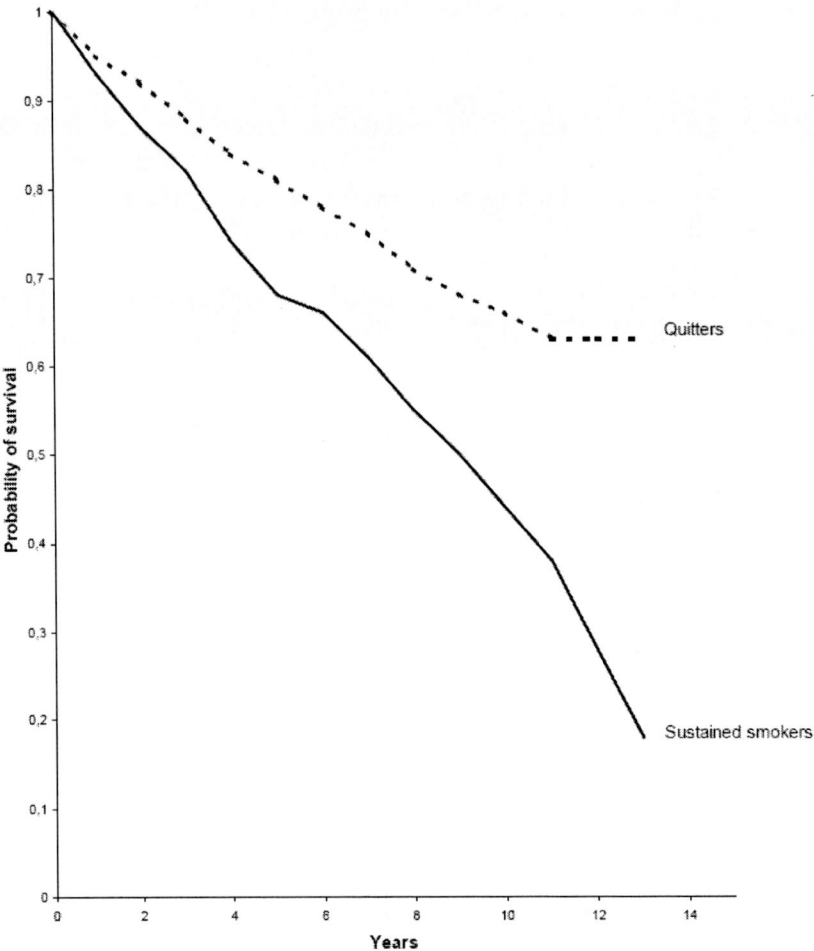

Figure 1. The probability of staying alive after admission for acute myocardial infarction or unstable angina in sustained smokers and quitters. Adopted from Daly et. al. [27].

It is both unethical and impossible to randomise patients to sustained smoking or smoking abstinence after a coronary event. Therefore, we are left with observational data which are often misleading. Smokers with an acute myocardial infarction tend to be younger and with fewer concomitant cardiac risk factors than non-smokers [13]. Therefore, their initial prognosis have been shown to be more favourable than non-smokers ("smokers paradox") [13]. Thus, differences in mortality between quitters and persistent smokers may take several years to develop. Further, most investigations have not verified quitters biochemically despite the fact that as many as 10-20% do not tell the truth about their smoking behaviour [28], and that many return to smoking within a year [29]. All these biases tend to underestimate the effect of smoking cessation. Hence, the benefit of quitting smoking after a coronary event might be even greater than reported.

Patients with COPD, Stroke and Peripheral Vascular Disease

From the large North American Lung Health Study, Anthonisen et. al. showed that smoking cessation in patients with mild obstructive pulmonary disease was very effective regarding the rate of decline in forced expiratory volume (FEV) [30]. At 11 years, approximately 40% of continuing smokers had an FEV_1 less than 60% of the predicted normal value compared with only 10% among the sustained quitters [30]. In the same investigation, nearly a doubling of the death rate was observed in continued smokers versus quitters [31]. At 14.5 years follow up there were 6.0 deaths per 1000 person-years in the group that stopped smoking versus 11.1 per 1000 person-years among the sustained smokers (figure 2) [31].

In the general population, the excess risk of stroke decreases after smoking cessation, becoming indistinguishable compared to non-smokers after some years of cessation [32]. The effect of smoking cessation in patients already suffering from stroke has to the author's knowledge not been properly investigated.

In patients with peripheral vascular disease, smoking cessation improves the symptoms from claudication, reduces the rate of amputation and increases the overall survival [32].

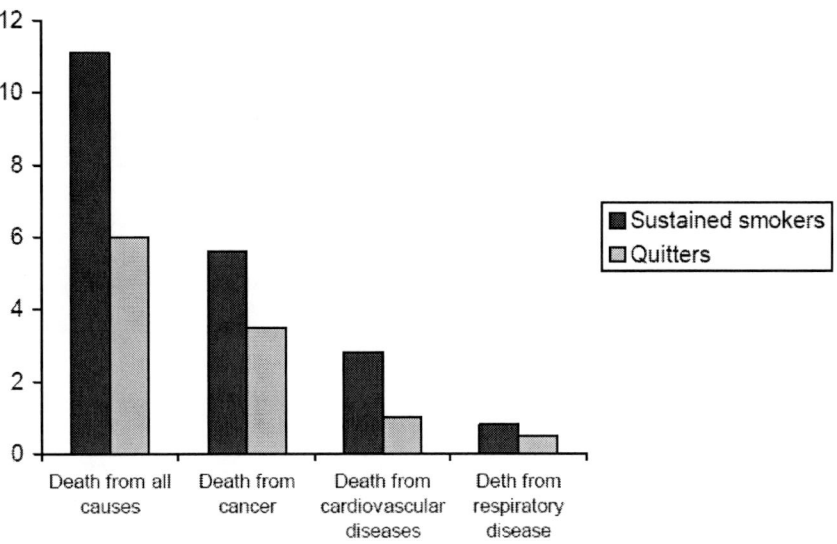

Figure 2. Rate of death per 1000 person-years in sustained smokers and quitters at 14.5 years follow up of 5887 patients with mild COPD. Adopted from Anthonisen et al. [31].

DOES SMOKING CESSATION HAVE ANY IMPACT ON QUALITY OF LIFE?

As mentioned, quitting smoking is the most effective single action to reduce mortality in patients with coronary heart disease and COPD. However, improvement in Quality of Life (QoL) may be equally important [33]. Due to the impossibility of randomising patients to either smoking cessation or continued smoking, assessments of QoL improvements in quitters versus sustained smokers are difficult to perform. The results may be biased by unmeasured confounders (i.e. patients not able to quit smoking may be a negatively selected group with low potential for QoL improvements). Multiple regression analyses have commonly been performed in order to adjust for differences in baseline characteristics in non-randomised groups. However, adjustment for all confounders is not possible [34], as exemplified by observational data showing that estrogns and vitamins reduce cardiovascular mortality, both which have later been refuted by randomised trials [35, 36]. Despite some authors claim that smoking cessation improves QoL [1], there are little evidence that this is true. Only a few studies have assessed this question. In the general population, studies have obtained mixed results [37, 38].

In patients with coronary heart disease, two investigations have been performed on this topic [39, 40]. Taira et al found that patients who managed to give up smoking after percutaneous coronary intervention improved their health-related QoL to a greater extent than sustained smokers [39]. However, this study included patients without motivation to stop smoking and adequate adjustments for confounders may have been difficult to perform. We did not find that the health-related QoL improved with smoking cessation in a one year perspective, even when applying a questionnaire especially designed to be sensitive for changes in patients with coronary heart disease [40]. Further, the QoL was not a significant predictor of smoking cessation [40]. In contrast to Taira et al, we only included patients motivated to quit smoking. Therefore, we may have been more successful in adjusting for differences in baseline characteristics, and this could explain why our results contradict the findings by Taira et. al. Thus, whether smoking cessation in patients with coronary heart disease has impact on QoL is still a matter of debate. Studies with a longer follow up period than one year are warranted.

In COPD, Toennesen et al showed significantly improvement in health related QoL as measured by the St George Respiratory Questionnaire in quitters compared to sustained smokers in a 12 months follow up study [41], indicating that smoking cessation increase health related QoL i patients with COPD. But again, more studies are needed confirm this finding.

WHY IS IT SO DIFFICULT TO QUIT SMOKING?

Each year approximately one third of the smokers try to quit, but only about 3% of the quit attempts result in sustained (12 months) cessation [42]. Ten seconds after inhalation, a very high level of nicotine reaches the brain, and stimulates the nicotine acetylcholine receptors [42]. In response, dopamine is released which speeds reaction times, and improves attention, concentration and problem-solving capabilities [18, 42]. However, this system adapts after a few hours, and becomes downregulated [18, 42]. But after a night sleep the system partly upregulates, and the first cigarette in the morning often produces arousal and relaxation. Regular smokers experience withdrawal symptoms some hours after the last cigarette, which consist of irritability, restlessness, feeling miserable, and impaired concentration [42]. These symptoms affect behaviour and are a strong impetus to start smoking again, as all symptoms disappear immediately after inhalation of a cigarette [18, 42]. Thus, the withdrawal symptoms are an important cause of the addiction [18, 42].

POPULATION STRATEGIES TO PREVENT SMOKING

Public intervention is the most effective way to reduce the prevalence of smoking [43]. Evidence exists for a significant positive effect of the following initiatives: Abandoning smoking in public places and work places, prohibiting tobacco advertisement, educating people about the health hazards of smoking, providing cessation clinics/telephone counselling, and increasing the prices of the tobacco products [43].

WHAT KIND OF SMOKING CESSATION MODALITIES ARE EFFECTIVE AMONG THE GENERAL POPULATION?

In people without a special incitement for stopping smoking, the sustained quit rates are rather low (i.e. 5%-10%), regardless of the type of intervention. Still, several treatment modalities have proven their efficacy: Individual behavioural counselling [44], group behavioural therapy [45], telephone counselling [46], and self-help materials (i.e. booklet, video) [47]. Regarding pharmaceutical products, nicotine replacement therapy has been shown to almost double the cessation rates [48]. The antidepressant bupropion and the new nicotine acetylcholine receptor agonist varenicline might be of similar efficacy [49, 50].

A stage based transtheoretical model has been recommended in smoking cessation, especially in guidelines from the USA [51]. This model separates individuals into five different stages (precontemplation, contemplation, preparation, action, and maintenance), and different interventions are used in each stadium. Accurate investigation and treatment have to be applied as the individuals progressively go through the different stages [51]. This process is rather complicated, and often needs psychologically trained personnel. Why this complicated method has gained so much popularity is somewhat difficult to understand as a systematic review did not find evidence that this method was superior to simpler cessation programs [52]. Whether thorough planning of the quit attempt is necessary is also not documented. On the contrary, an investigation found that most successful quit attempts may be unplanned [53]!

WHAT KIND OF SMOKING CESSATION MODALITIES ARE EFFECTIVE AMONG HOSPITALISED PATIENTS?

Intensive intervention started at hospital plus follow-up for at least one month was found to significantly increase quit rates in a meta analysis of 17 randomised trials [54]. Nicotine replacements alone did not seem to have any significantly effect, but adding nicotine replacements to intensive behavioural support seemed to increase the quit rates further [54]. Applying both intensive intervention and nicotine replacements might double the cessation rates compared to usual care [54], but the evidence supporting this is somewhat scarce. Brief interventions during hospitalisation have not shown significant effect [54, 55]. The kind of provider does not seem to matter, as smoking cessation programs delivered by psychologists, physicians, and nurses are all of similar efficacy [56].

INVESTIGATIONS ON SMOKING CESSATION INTERVENTION IN PATIENTS WITH CORONARY HEART DISEASE

Despite the vast mortality benefit of smoking cessation in patients suffering an acute coronary event only about a third stop smoking spontaneously [57]. Randomised trials on smoking cessation methods in patients with coronary heart disease have obtained mixed results. Several studies of interventions to change lifestyle, where smoking cessation was only part of the program, have been performed [58-64]. Unfortunate, most of them did not show any significant effect on quit rates [58-61].

Regarding investigations only addressing smoking cessation, brief interventions during hospitalisation have been ineffective [55, 65, 66]. Such brief interventions usually include a firm advice from a physician to stop smoking, information about the health hazards of continued smoking, and self help materials. It is this kind of smoking cessation intervention that is recommended from the Joint European Societies, which includes the European Society of Cardiology [67]. It is also the most widely used method to increase cessation rates among coronary heart patients [67]. Therefore, it is very disappointing that this method does not seem to be of any significant effect [55, 65, 66]. In a recent paper [67], and in a companion news report in the BMJ [68], more efficient ways to improve quit-rates were asked for.

Five randomised studies have investigated whether a smoking cessation program with several months of intervention is able to increase the quit rates [57, 69-72]. The first was a Lancet paper showing 62% abstainers in the intervention group compared to 28% in the usual care group [69]. The intervention principles were rather simple: Patients in the intervention group were told that continued smoking could lead to further heart attacks because it would narrow the arteries in a manner similar to furring in a pipe, sometimes with complete blockage. Some information on how to quit were sometimes given. The article does not describe the length of the intervention, and unfortunately no biochemically verification of the quitters were performed. Another investigation in patients after coronary arteriography randomised patients to a behavioural smoking cessation program with a mean of four telephone calls during four months, or usual care [70]. After 12 months there was a trend toward increased quit-rates in the intervention group, but not reaching standard level of statistical significance (57% versus 48% cessation rates in the intervention and the usual care group, respectively, p0.06). However, the intervention seemed effective in the subgroup with more severe disease. A third study showed a 71% cessation rate in the intervention group compared to 45% in the usual care group one year after admission for myocardial infarction [71]. The intervention was delivered by especially trained nurses using social learning theory combined with addiction models. The patients were followed regularly for 4 months. The main drawback of this study was the application of a rather complicated psychological approach, which may be difficult to implement in clinical practice. Dornelas et. al. randomised 100 patients after myocardial infarction [72]. The intervention was delivered by a psychologist implementing the transtheoretical model, and consisted of bedside counselling followed by regular telephone calls during 6 months. After 12 months 34% and 55% were abstinent in the usual care group and intervention group, respectively (p<0.05). There were no biochemical verification of the quitters in this study, and using the transtheoretical model is unnecessary as most patients stop smoking while hospitalised [57]. In other words, they already are in the maintenance stadium of the transtheoretical model, and focusing only on relapse prevention seems more logical.

The fifth paper is our own paper, and it is the largest so far [57]. Two hundred and fifty patients admitted for acute myocardial infarction, unstable angina or coronary bypass surgery were randomised to either a smoking cessation intervention program or usual care.

Physicians were not involved in the program. All cardiac patients, independent of study participation, were offered group sessions conducted by cardiac nurses twice per week, in which the importance of smoking cessation was mentioned. A video shown during these sessions and a booklet handed out to all patients contained general information on coronary heart disease, which included advice to give up smoking. Besides this, the control group received no specific instructions on how to stop smoking. One of three cardiac nurses consulted the patients in the intervention group one or two times during the hospital stay. The intervention was based on a 17 page booklet especially made for the purpose of the trial (figure 3). This manual emphasised the health benefits of quitting smoking after a coronary event. Two figures showed the mortality differences between those who continued smoking and those who stopped smoking after myocardial infarction or unstable angina. One of the figures was a bar chart showing 60% risk reduction for death after 5 years if quitting [73], and the other was a linear chart showing that after 13 years 18% of continued smokers were alive compared to 63% of the quitters [27]. On the basis of these figures the participants were told that they most probably would suffer a new heart attack if they continued smoking, and that their risk of death would be markedly increased if they continued smoking (fear arousal message). The booklet also contained chapters on how to prevent relapse, how to stop smoking for those who either continued smoking or relapsed, and how to use nicotine replacements. How to identify and cope with high risk situations for relapse was explained, and action plans for coping with these situations were suggested. The patients were strongly advised not to smoke during hospitalisation. Those with strong withdrawal urges were advised nicotine replacements (gum or patch). If spouses smoked, they also were asked to quit. The study nurses initiated telephone contacts two days, one week, three weeks, three months, and five months after hospital discharge. Those with special needs were telephoned monthly thereafter. At six weeks, at the same day they were scheduled for the follow up appointment with a physician, all participants in the intervention group had a consultation with the study nurses at the outpatient clinic. The outpatient contacts included positive feedback (e.g. "Congratulations, you are still free of smoking. That means that you already have a much lesser chance of suffering a new heart attack.") and relapse prevention. The health benefits of quitting were repeated, and if necessary a fear arousal message was given. Those who either continued smoking or relapsed were offered additional support and advice. Apart from a one-day course in smoking cessation counselling, the study nursed had no special training in smoking cessation intervention. Patients who claimed to be quitters and had a urinary nicotine metabolite concentration below a cut of value consistent with non-smoking were counted as quitters. Most patients (85%) received more telephone calls than the intended minimum of five. The mean total time devoted to each patient was approximately 2.5 hours, including time to fill in questionnaires for the purpose of the trial. A third of the participants used nicotine replacements. At 12 months follow up, the intervention group had a statistically significant 20% increased cessation rate compared to the control group (NNT 5). Due to a higher drop out rate in the intervention group, in an intention to treat analysis the difference in quit rates between the groups was 13% (NNT 8, still statistically significant).

The groups showed similar smoking cessation rates while in hospital and at six weeks' follow up, suggesting that a long follow up period was the most important element in the program. The patients were in general very satisfied with the cessation program, indicating that giving a fear arousal message is a feasible method [74].

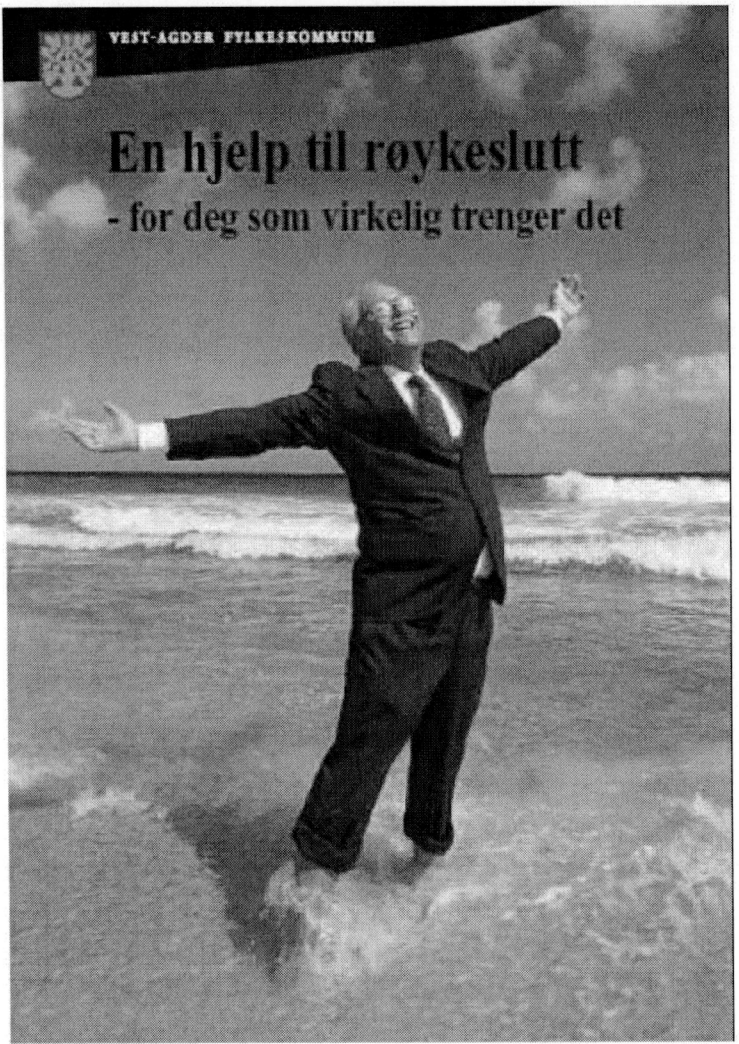

Figure 3. The front cover of a booklet used in helping patients with coronary heart disease to stop smoking. The English version of the booklet can be provided by contacting the author (petterqp@online.no).

Regarding pharmaceuticals, there are no studies with a long follow up period only investigating the effects of nicotine replacements in patients with coronary heart disease [54]. On the other hand, they have been incorporated in many of the studies mentioned above [55, 60, 62, 66, 71], and have been found to be safe [75]. In a Cochrane review, the authors concluded that nicotine replacements probably increase quit rates if combined with high intensity behavioural intervention [54]. In the last few years bupropion has gained popularity. This psychopharmaceutical product has been shown to be safe and effective in patients with coronary heart disease, with a continuos cessation rate of 22% in the bupropion group compared to 9% in the placebo group at 12 months follow up (p<0.01) [76]. However, its effect in combination with behavioural therapy in patients with heart disease is still unknown.

In conclusion, smoking cessation interventions given briefly during hospitalisation or given as part of a life style intervention program are ineffective regarding quit rates in cardiac patients. There are strong evidence that individual smoking cessation intervention with several months of follow up significantly increase quit-rates, and that such therapy should be combined with nicotine replacements. Further, our investigation showed that such a program could be delivered by personnel without special education in smoking cessation, and that simple intervention principles applicable in an ordinary clinical setting could be used.

WHO MANAGE TO QUIT SMOKING AFTER A CORONARY EVENT?

Several investigations have assessed the predictors of smoking cessation in patients with coronary heart disease [55, 71, 72, 77-80]. The results have been mixed, but the following predictors have rather consistently been found to be positively associated with smoking cessation:

- Low level of nicotine addiction [55] (most often as assessed by the Fagerstrom index [81]).
- High level of self confidence in smoking cessation [71, 72, 77] (as assessed by the total self efficacy score [82]).
- The severity of the coronary event, i.e. having myocardial infarction as reason for admission [55, 78, 79].
- Having no previous heart disease [80].
- Low level of hostility and depression [78].

We found that a high level of nicotine addiction, a low level of self confidence in quitting, and having previous coronary heart disease all were significant negative predictors of smoking cessation in a multivariate analysis [83]. A high level of nicotine addiction was the strongest negative predictor in our study [83]. We have further shown that the level of nicotine addiction can be assessed with one simple question; are you smoking the first cigarette in the morning within 30 min of waking [83]? This is easier than applying the Fagerstrom Questionnaire which covers eight items of various aspects of smoking behaviour. If the answer to the question is yes, the patient has a high level of nicotine addiction and may benefit from highly intensive behavioural support and high strength of nicotine replacement therapy.

INVESTIGATIONS ON SMOKING CESSATION INTERVENTION IN PATIENTS WITH COPD

A very large randomised smoking cessation intervention study in patients with mild COPD included nearly 6000 patients [84]. Patients were allocated to usual care or intensive smoking cessation counselling combined with nicotine chewing gum. The counselling consisted of advice to quit from a physician (one cession), group counselling (12 sessions in 10 weeks) and regular follow up by telephone contacts (duration and frequency not stated). At 12 months follow up 34% were abstainers in the intervention group compared to 9% in the usual care group (p<0.01), and at five years follow up the cessation rates were 21% and 5%, respectively (p<0.01) [84]. A cochrane review from 2001 found evidence that a combination of psychosocial intervention and pharmacological intervention is superior to no treatment or to psychosocial intervention alone [85]. Three other studies are worth mentioning [86-88]. The first is an investigation of from 43 general practices in the Netherlands [86]. Three hundred and ninety-two patients with COPD were randomised to usual care or an intensified minimal intervention strategy consisting of information from a physician, a booklet about smoking and COPD, a video, two consultations by physicians, and maximum three telephone contacts by nurses. They also received information about nicotine replacements. At 6 months follow up, significantly more smokers had quitted smoking in the intervention group than in the usual care group (16% versus 9%). Two other investigations have failed to show any long term benefit of bupropion alone regarding quit rates in patients with COPD [87, 88]. It is presently unknown whether the combination of intensive counselling and bupropion is effective.

ARE SMOKING CESSATION PROGRAMS IN PATIENTS WITH CARDIOVASCULAR DISEASES AND COPD COST EFFECTIVE?

Despite smoking cessation programs with several months of intervention significantly increases smoking cessation rates in patients with smoking related disease, many hospitals do not provide such programs as part of routine care [67]. One possible explanation for this may be that the cessation programs are thought not to be worth their costs. As the therapeutic arena becomes more crowded, and in times of health economic constraints, analyses of treatment costs relative to healthcare benefits are important. Cost effectiveness analyses in terms of cost per year of life saved or gained provide this opportunity, enabling us to compare the various treatment modalities [89]. Several cost effectiveness analyses have been published on secondary prevention strategies for cardiovascular disease [90]. Regarding smoking cessation intervention, only two studies have been performed [91, 92]. One 13 year old analysis was based on a study of patients suffering myocardial infarction in the sixties [91], and showed that a smoking cessation program was very cost effective compared to other treatment modalities. We recently published a paper about the cost effectiveness of a cessation program in a low risk setting (i.e. patients with stable coronary disease) [92]. Due to the vast uncertainties associated with cost effectiveness analyses we aimed to do conservative assumptions, thereby calculating a maximum cost per life year gained by the program. The only important cost of the program was the 2.5 hours of a nurse's working time. This one time investment gave a very much lower cost effectiveness ratio than all other treatment modalities in patients with coronary heart disease (i.e. 1/25 the cost per life year gained of statins in patients with stable coronary heart disease) (figure 4).

To the author's knowledge there are no cost effectiveness analysis regarding smoking cessation intervention in patients with COPD or non-coronary cardiovascular diseases.

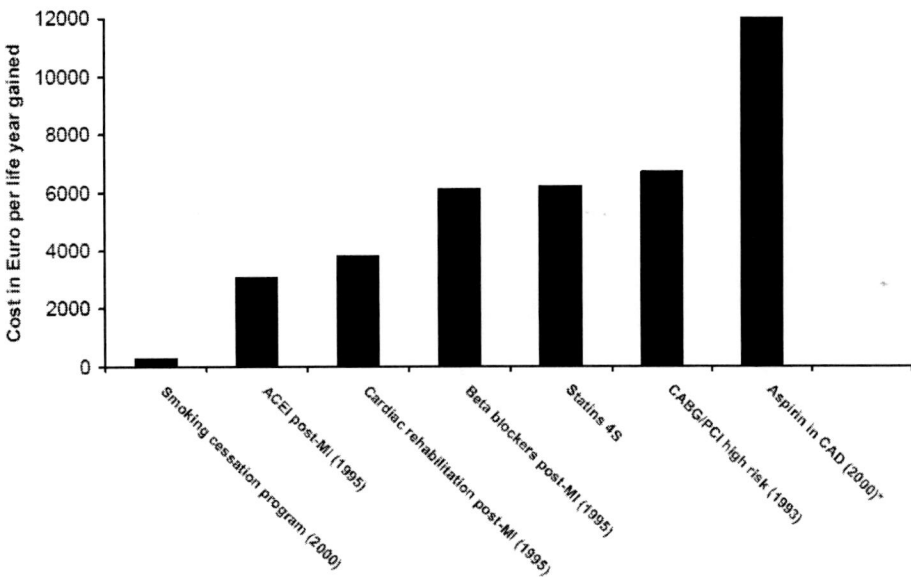

Figure 4. Comparison of the cost effectiveness of a smoking cessation program in patients with stable coronary heart disease with other treatment modalities [92]. Estimates are in the lifetime perspective.

METHODS TO CONFIRM SMOKING CESSATION

In clinical trials biochemical validation of the smoking status is important because some patients do not tell the truth about their smoking behaviour [28]. There are several methods to validate smoking status [93, 94]. CO measurements in breath or blood are inadequate in detecting occasional and light smokers because of the low sensitivity and relatively short half life [95]. Cotinine measurements in serum, saliva or urine is a widely used method. Cotinine is a metabolite from nicotine, and all nicotine products (i.e. patches, gum, snuff) will increase the cotinine concentration above the cut-off value for non-smokers. The half life of cotinine is approximately 20 hours, and a person who uses nicotine replacements may have an increased cotinine concentration for several days after cessation [93, 94]. Thus, patients using snuff or nicotine replacements must stop this ideally 10 days before the test. This may be difficult to accomplish and false positive results are likely to occur. Thiocyanate measurements can abolished this bias, because thiocyanate is not increased in patients using snuff or nicotine replacements as it derives from the cyanide in the tobacco smoke. However, thiocyanate measurements has been reported to have a relatively low specificity due to its presence in various nourishment [96]. After smoking cessation its concentration remains elevated for up to a month [97], but in cessation trials with 12 months follow up period this would not pose problems since most of the quitters stop smoking in the first few weeks [57].

It could be debated whether continuos abstinence rather than point prevalence cessation rates, and whether a longer follow up period than 12 months should be performed when assessing cessation rates in patients. In hospitalised patients, the vast majority stop smoking early (i.e. while hospitalised) [57], and return to smoking after one year of abstinence is very rare [29]. Therefore, point prevalence cessation rates at 12 months follow up seems adequate in assessing quit rates in patients with smoking related diseases.

CONCLUSION

"Everything should be made as simple as possible, but not simpler." Albert Einstein.

In this article several lines of evidence have been presented that support the following important elements in a smoking cessation program in patients with cardiovascular diseases and COPD:

1. You have to inform on the health hazards of continued smoking, thereby increasing the patients' motivation to stay free of smoking ("fear arousal message"). It may be important to repeat this information as patients may forget and deny.
2. You have to follow-up the patients for several months. This is probably the most important factor in the program. Someone has to care about the patients and their smoking behaviour. The patients need to know that someone is going to call them, and ask whether they are still free of smoke.
3. Most patients, especially those smoking within 30 min of waking, should be offered nicotine replacements and/or bupropion.

In hospitalised patients with smoking related disease, and especially in coronary heart patients, most do not smoke during hospitalisation. Thus, smoking cessation programs in these patients only have to focus on relapse prevention. Complicated approaches, such as the stage based transtheoretical model, are probably not necessary.

In patients with coronary heart disease, even highly intensive smoking cessation programs have been shown to be extremely cost effective compared to all other treatment modalities. In patients with COPD, such analysis have not been performed, but no other intervention than smoking cessation have been shown to improve the long term prognosis.

Why is the easiest, cheapest and most effective method to reduce mortality in patients with smoking related diseases not part of routine care in many hospitals? Is working with this topic too "low technology", and associated with too low prestige? Is it due to too few resources in marketing compared to the pharmaceutical industry? Anyway, we hope the results presented in this article will be helpful in increasing the implementation of effective smoking cessation programs, and thereby saving lives world-wide.

REFERENCES

[1] Schroeder SA. What to Do With a Patient Who Smokes. *JAMA* 2005;294:482-87.
[2] Statistisk Sentral Byrå: www.ssb.no/emner/03/01/royk. Accessed March 13, 2006.
[3] Edwards R. The problem of tobacco smoking. *BMJ.* 2004;328:217-19.
[4] Doll R, Peto R, Boreham J, Sutherland I. Mortality in relation to smoking: 50 years' observations on male British doctors. *BMJ.* 2004;329:1519

[5]   Shaw M, Mitchell R, Dorling D. Time for a smoke? One cigarette reduces your life by 11 minutes. *BMJ.* 2000; 320: 53.

[6]   Philips AN, Wannamethee SG, Walker M, Thomson A, Smith GD. Life expectancy in men who have never smoked and those who have smoked continuously: 15 year follow up of large cohort of middle aged British men. *BMJ.* 1996;313:907-908.

[7]   Lerman C, Patterson F, Berrettini W. Treating tobaco dependence: State of the science and new directions. *J. Clin. Oncol.* 2005;23:311-23.

[8]   Rigotti NA, Pasternak RC. Cigarette smoking and coronary heart disease. *Cardiology clinics.* 1996;14:51-68.

[9]   Jonas MA, Oates JA, Ockene JK, *et.al.* Statement on smoking and cardiovascular disease for health care professionals: AHA Medical/Scientific Statement. *Circulation.* 1992;86:1664-1669.

[10] Doll R, Peto R, Wheatley K, Gray R, Sutherland I. Mortality in relation to smoking: 40 years' observations on male British doctors. *BMJ.* 1994;309:901-11.

[11] Phillips AN, Wannamethee SG, Walker M, Thomson A, Davey Smith G. Life expectancy in men who have never smoked and those who have smoked continuously: 15 year follow up of large cohort of middle aged British men. *BMJ.* 1996;313:907–908.

[12] Willet WC, Green A, Stampfer MJ, *et. al.* Relative and absolute excess risk of coronary heart disease among women who smokes cigarettes. *N. Engl. J. Med.* 1987;317:1303-9.

[13] Jorgensen Stig, Kober L, Ottensen M, Torp-Pedersen C, Videbaek J, Kjoller E. The Prognostic Importance Of Smoking Status At The Time Of Acute Myocardial Infarction In 6676. *J. Cardiovasc. Risk.* 1999; 6:23–27. .

[14] Devereux G. ABC of chronic obstructive pulmonary disease. Definition, epidemiology, end risk factors. *BMJ.* 2006;332:1142-44.

[15] US Department of Health and Human Services. The health consequences of smoking: a report of the surgeon general. Atlanta, GA; 2004.

[16] Shinton R, Beevers G. Meta-analysis of relation between cigarette smoking and stroke. *BMJ.* 1989;298:789-94.

[17] Tonstad S, Johnston JA. Cardiovascular risks associated with smoking: a review for clinicians. *Eur. J. Cardiovasc. Prev. Rehab.* 2006;13:507-14.

[18] Benowitz NL. Cigarette smoking and nicotine addiction. *Med. Clin. North. Am.* 1992;76:415-37.

[19] Celermajer DS, Sorensen KE, Georgakopoulos D. Cigarette smoking is associated with dose-related and potentially reversible impairment of endothelium-dependent dilatation in healthy young adults. *Circulation.* 1993;88:2149-55.

[20] Pittilo RM, Clarke JM, Harris D, *et al*. Cigarette smoking and platelet adhesion. *Br. J. Haematol.* 1984;58:627-32.

[21] Quillen JE, Rossen JD, Oskarsson HJ, *et al*. Acute effect of cigarette smoking on the coronary circulation: Constriction of epicardial and resistance vessels. *J. Am. Coll. Cardiol.* 1993;22:642-47.

[22] Sugiishi M. Cigarette smoking is a major risk factor for coronary spasm. *Circulation.* 1993;87:76-9.

[23] Rosenberg L, Kaufman DW, Helmrich SP, *et al*. The risk of myocardial infarction after quitting smoking in menn under 55 years of age. *N. Engl. J. Med.* 1990;322:213-17.

[24] MacNee W. ABC of chronic obstructive pulmonary disease. Pathology, pathogenesis, and pathophysiology. *BMJ.* 2006;332:1201-4.

[25] Wilson K, Gibson N, Willan A, Cook D. Effect of smoking cessation on mortality after myocardial infarction: meta-analysis of cohort studies. *Arch. Intern. Med.* 2000;160:939-44.

[26] Critchley JA, Capewell MD. Mortality risk reduction associated with smoking cessation in patients with coronary heart disease. *JAMA.* 2003; 290(1): 86-97.

[27] Daly LE, Mulcahy R, Graham IM, Hickey N. Long term effect on mortality of stopping smoking after unstable angina and myocardial infarction. *BMJ.* 1983;287:324-6.

[28] Woodward M, Tunstall-Pedoe H. Biochemical evidence of persistent heavy smoking after a coronary diagnosis despite self-reported reduction: analysis from the Scottish Heart Health Study. *Eur. Heart J.* 1992; 13:160-165

[29] Hunt W, Barnet L, Branch L. Relapse rates in addiction programs. *Journal of Clinical Psychiatry.* 1977;(27):455.

[30] Anthonisen NR, Connett JE, Murray RP. Smoking and lung function of lung health study. *Am. J. Respir. Crit. Care Med.* 2002;166:675-9

[31] Anthonisen NR, Skeans M, Wise RA, et. al. The effects of a smoking cessation intervention on 14.5-year mortality. *Ann. Intern. Med.* 2005;142:233-39.

[32] US Department of Health and Human Services. The health consequences of smoking: a report of the surgeon general. Atlanta, GA; 1990.

[33] Probstfield JL. How cost-effective are new preventive strategies for cardiovascular disease? *Am. J. Cardiol.* 2003;91:22G-27G.

[34] Brotman DJ, Walker E, Lauer MS, O'Brien RG. In search of fewer independent risk factors. *Arch. Intern. med.* 2005;165:138-45

[35] Hulley S, Grady D, Bush T, Furberg C, Herrington D, Riggs B, Vittinghoff E. Randomized trial of estrogen plus progestin for secondary prevention of coronary heart disease in postmenopausal women. Heart and Estrogen/progestin Replacement Study (HERS) Research Group. *JAMA.* 1998;280:605-13.

[36] Bønaa K. H., Njølstad I., Ueland P. M., Schirmer H., Tverdal A., Steigen T., Wang H., Nordrehaug J. E., Arnesen E., Rasmussen K., the NORVIT Trial Investigators. Homocysteine Lowering and Cardiovascular Events after Acute Myocardial Infarction. *N. Engl. J. Med.* published at www.nejm.org on Mar 12, 2006.

[37] Mitra M, Chung MC, Wilber N, Klein Walker D. Smoking status and quality of life: a longitudinal study among adults with disabilities. *Am. J. Prev. Med.* 2004;27:258-60.

[38] Tillmann M, Silcock J. A comparison of smokers' and ex-smokers' health-related quality of life. *J. Public Health Med.* 1997;19:268-73.

[39] Taira DA, Seto TB, Ho KK, Krumholz HM, Cutlip DE, Berezin R, Kuntz RE, Cohen DJ. Impact of smoking on health-related quality of life after percutaneous coronary revascularization. *Circulation.* 2000;102:1369-74.

[40] Quist-Paulsen P, Bakke PS, Gallefoss F. Does smoking cessation improve Quality of Life in patients with coronary heart disease? *Scandinavian Cardiovascular Journal.* 2006; 40: 11-16.

[41] Tønnesen p, Mikkelsen K, Bremann L. Nurse-conducted smoking cessation in patients with COPD using nicotine sublingual tablets and behavioral support. *Chest.* 2006;130:334-42.

[42] Jarvis MJ. Why people smoke. *BMJ.* 2004;328:277-9.

[43] Jamrozik K. Population strategies to prevent smoking. *BMJ.* 2004;328:759-762.

[44] Lancaster T, Stead LF. Individual behavioural counselling for smoking cessation. *The Cochrane Databse of Systematic Reviews.* 2005;(2): CD001292.

[45] Stead LF, Lancaster T. Group behavioural therapy programmes for smoking cessation. *The Cochrane Databse of Systematic Reviews.* 2002;(3): CD001007.

[46] Stead LF, Lancaster T, Perera R. Telephone counselling for smoking cessation. *The Cochrane Databse of Systematic Reviews.* 2001;(2): CD002850.

[47] Lancaster T, Stead LF. Self-help interventions for smoking cessation. *The Cochrane Databse of Systematic Reviews.* 2005;(3): CD001118.

[48] Silagy C, Lancaster T, Stead L, Mant D, Fowler G. Nicotine replacement therapy for smoking cessation. *The Cochrane Databse of Systematic Reviews* 2004;(3): CD000146.

[49] Jorenby D. Clinical efficacy of bupropion in the management of smoking cessation. *Drugs.* 2002;62 Suppl 2:25-35.

[50] Jorenby DE, Taylor Hays J, Rigotti NA, et al. Efficacy of varicline, an alfa4beta2 nicotinic acetylcholine receptor partila agonist, vs placebo or sustained release bupropion for smoking cessation. A randomised controlled trial. *JAMA.* 2006;296:56-63.

[51] Prochaska JO, DiClemente CC, Norcross JC. In search of how people change. Applications to addictive behaviors. *Am. Psychol.* 1992;47:1102-14

[52] Riemsma RP, Pattenden J, Bridle C, Sowden AJ, Mather L, Watt IS, Walker A. Systematic review of the effectiveness of stage based interventions to promote smoking cessation. *BMJ.* 2003;326:1175-77.

[53] West R, Sohal T, "Catastrophic" pathways to smoking cessation: findings from national survey. *BMJ.* 2006;332:458-69.

[54] Rigotti NA, Munafo MR, Murphy MF, Stead LF. Interventions for smoking cessation in hospitalised patients. *The Cochrane Databse of Systematic Reviews.* 2001;(2): CD001837.

[55] Hajek P, Taylor TZ, Mills P. Brief intervention during hospital admission to help patients to give up smoking after myocardial infarction and bypass surgery: randomised controlled trial. *BMJ.* 2002;324:87-9.

[56] Mojica WA, Suttorp MJ, Sherman SE, Morton SC, Roth EA, Maglione MA, *et.al.* Smoking-cessation interventions by type of provider: a meta-analysis. *Am. J. Prev. Med.* 2004;26:391-401.

[57] Quist-Paulsen P, Gallefoss F. Randomised controlled trial of smoking cessation intervention after admission for coronary heart disease. *BMJ.* 2003; 327: 1254-1257.

[58] Van Elderen-van Kemenade T, Maes S, van den Broek Y. Effects of a health education programme with telephone follow-up during cardiac rehabilitation. *Br. J. Clin. Psychol.* 1994;33:367-78.

[59] Jolly K, Bradley F, Sharp S, Smith H, Thompson S, Kinmonth AL, et al. Randomised controlled trial of follow up care in general practice of patients with myocardial infarction and angina: final results of the Southampton heart integrated care project (SHIP). The SHIP Collaborative Group. *BMJ.* 1999;318:706-11.

[60] Campbell NC, Ritchie LD, Thain J, Deans HG, Rawles JM, Squair JL. Secondary prevention in coronary heart disease: a randomised trial of nurse led clinics in primary care. *BMJ.* 2002;324:87-9.

[61] Murchie P, Campbell NC, Ritchie LD, Simpson JA, Thain J. Secondary prevention clinics for coronary heart disease: four year follow up of a randomised controlled trial in primary care. *BMJ.* 2003;326:84-90.

[62] DeBusk RF, Miller NH, Superko HR, Dennis CA, Thomas RJ, Lew HT, et al. A case-management system for coronary risk factor modification after acute myocardial infarction. *Ann. Intern. Med.* 1994;120:721-9.

[63] Carlsson R, Lindberg G, Westin L, Israelsson B. Influence of coronary nursing management follow up on lifestyle after acute myocardial infarction. *Heart* 1997;77:256-9.

[64] The Vestfold Heartcare Study Group. Influence on lifestyle measures and five-year coronary risk by a comprehensive lifestyle intervention programme in patients with coronary heart disease. *Eur. J. Cardiovasc. Prev. Rehabil.* 2003;10:429-37

[65] Moreno Ortigosa A, Ochoa Gomez FJ, Ramalle-Gomara E, Saralegui Reta I, Fernandez Esteban MV, Quintana Diaz M. Efficacy of an intervention in smoking cessation in patients with myocardial infarction.. *Med. Clin. (Barc)* 2000;114:209-10. (In Spanish.)

[66] Rigotti NA, McKool KM, Shiffman S. Predictors of smoking cessation after coronary artery bypass graft surgery. Results of a randomized trial with 5-year follow-up. *Ann. Intern. Med.* 1994;120:287-93.

[67] Reimer W S, de Swart E, de Bacquer D, Pyørælæ K, Keil U, Heidirch J, *et. al.* Smoking behaviour in European patients with established coronary heart disease. *Eur. Heart J.* 2006;27:35-41.

[68] Kmietowicz Z. More than half of smokers go on smoking after coronary events. *BMJ.* 2005;331:862.

[69] Burt A, Thornley P, Illingworth D, White P, Shaw TR, Turner R. Stopping smoking after myocardial infarction. *Lancet.* 1974;1:304-6.

[70] Ockene J, Kristeller JL, Goldberg R, Ockene I, Merriam P, Barrett S, et al. Smoking cessation and severity of disease: the coronary artery smoking intervention study. *Health Psychol.* 1992;11:119-26.

[71] Taylor CB, Houston-Miller N, Killen JD, DeBusk RF. Smoking cessation after acute myocardial infarction: effects of a nurse-managed intervention. *Ann. Intern. Med.* 1990;113:118-23.

[72] Dornelas EA, Sampson RA, Gray JF, Waters D, Thompson PD. A randomized controlled trial of smoking cessation counselling after myocardial infarction. *Prev. Med.* 2000;30:261-8.

[73] Sparrow D, Dawber TR. The influence of cigarette smoking on prognosis after a first myocardial infarction. A report from the Framingham study. *Journal of Chronic Diseases.* 1978;31:425-32.

[74] Quist-Paulsen P, Gallefoss F. Is fear arousal message feasible in helping cardiac patients to stop smoking? Response to reference 57 at *bmj.com.* 2006

[75] Working Group for the Study of Transdermal Nicotine in Patients With Coronary Artery Disease. Nicotine replacement therapy for patients with coronary artery disease. *Arch. Intern. Med.* 1994;154:989-95.

[76] Tonstad S, Farsang C, Klaene G, Lewis K, Manolis A, Perruchoud AP, et al. Bupropion SR for smoking cessation in smokers with cardiovascular disease: a multicentre, randomised study. *Eur. Heart J.* 2003;24(10):946-55.

[77] Hasdai D, Garratt KN, Grill DE, Mathew V, Lerman A, Gau GT, *et al*..Predictors of smoking cessation after percutaneous coronary revascularization. *Mayo Clin. Proc.* 1998;73(3):205-9.

[78] Brummett BH, Babyak MA, Mark DC, Williams RB, Siegler IC, Clapp-Channing N, *et. al*.. Predictors of smoking cessation in patients with a diagnosis of coronary artery disease. *J. Cardiopul. Rehab.* 2002;22:143-7.

[79] Ockene J, Kristeller JL, Goldberg R, Ockene I, Merriam P, Barrett S. Smoking cessation and Severety of Disease: The Coronary Artery Smoking Intervention Study. *Health Psychol.* 1992, 11(2), 119-126.

[80] Attebring MF, Hartford M, Hjalmarson A, Caidahl K, Karlsson T, Herlitz. Smoking habits and predictors of continued smoking in patients with acute coronary syndromes. *J. Adv. Nurs.* 2004; 46(6):614-23.

[81] Heatherton TF, Kozlowski LT, Frecker RC, Fagerstrom KO. The Fagerstrom Test for Nicotine Dependence: a revision of the Fagerstrom Tolerance Questionnaire. *British Journal of Addiction.* 1991;86(9):1119-27.

[82] Yates AJ, Thain J. Self-efficacy as a predictor of relapse following voluntary cessation of smoking. *Addictive Behaviors.* 1985;10(3):291-8.

[83] Quist-Paulsen P, Bakke PS, Gallefoss F. Predictors of smoking cessation in patients admitted for acute coronary heart disease. *European Journal of Cardiovascular Prevention and Rehabilitation.* 2005; 5: 472-478.

[84] Anthonisen NR, Connett JE, Kiley JP, et al. Effects of smoking cessation intervention and the use of an inhaled anticholinergic brochodilator on the rate of decline of FEV1. The Lung health Study. *JAMA.* 1994;272:1497-505.

[85] van der Meer RM, Ostelo, Jacobs, et al. Smoking cessation for chronic obstructive pulmonary disease. *The Cochrane Database of Systematic Reviews.* 200, Issue 1. Art. No.: CD002999. DOI: 10.1002/14651858.CD002999.

[86] Hilberink SR, Jacobs JE, Bottema BJAM, et al. Smoking cessation in patients with COPD in daily general practice (SMOCC): Six months' results. *Prev. Med.* 2005;41:822-7.

[87] Wagena EJ, Knipschild PG, Huibers MJ, et al. Efficacy of bupropion and nortriptyline for smoking cessation among people at risk for or with chronic obstructive pulmonary disease. *Arch. Intern. Med.* 2005;165:2286-92.

[88] Tashkin DP, Kanner R, Bailey, et al. Smoking cessation in patients with chronic obstructive pulmonary disease: a double blind, placebo-controlled, randomised trial. *Lancet.* 2001;357:1571-5.

[89] Kupersmith J, Holmes-Rovner M, Hogan A, Rovner D, Gardiner J. Cost-effectiveness analysis in heart disease, part I: general principles. *Prog. Cardiovasc. Dis.* 1994; 37: 161-84.

[90] Probstfield J L. How cost-effective are new preventive strategies for cardiovascular disease? *Am. J. Cardiol.* 2003;91(suppl):22G-27G.

[91] Krumholz HM, Cohen BJ, Tsevat J, Pasternak RC, Weinstein MC. Cost-Effectiveness of a Smoking Cessation Program After Myocardial Infarction. *JACC.* 1993; 22(6): 1697-702.

[92] Quist-Paulsen P, Lydersen S, Bakke PS, Gallefoss F. Cost effectiveness of a smoking cessation program in patients admitted for coronary heart disease. *European Journal of Cardiovascular Prevention and Rehabilitation.* 2006; 13: 274-280.

[93] Gilbert DD. Chemical analyses as validators in smoking cessation programs. *Journal of Behavioral Medicine.* 1993;16:295-308.

[94] Idle JR. Titrating exposure to tobacco smoke using cotinine--a minefield of misunderstandings. *Journal of Clinical Epidemiology.* 1990;43:313-7.

[95] Lando HA, McGovern PG, Kelder SH, Jeffery RW, Forster JL. Use of carbon monoxide breath validation in assessing exposure to cigarette smoke in a worksite population. *Health Psychology.* 1991;10:296-301

[96] Foss OP, Lund-Larsen PG. Serum thiocyanate and smoking: interpretation of serum thiocyanate levels observed in a large health study. *Scand. J. Clin. Lab. Invest.* 1986;46:245-51.

[97] Støa KF. Studies on thiocyanate in serum. Doctoral thesis. University of Bergen, 1957.

In: Smoking Cessation: Theory, Interventions and Prevention   ISBN: 978-1-60021-591-9
Editor: Jerome E. Landow   © 2008 Nova Science Publishers, Inc.

Chapter 9

PREOPERATIVE SMOKING INTERVENTION

Ann M. Møller
Department of Anesthesiology,
Herlev University Hospital, Herlev, Denmark

ABSTRACT

In the last decade we have become increasing aware of the detrimental effects of smoking on surgical outcome. During more than half a century scientists have identified the relationship between smoking and different types of complications relating to surgery and anesthesia, but only recently effective preoperative smoking intervention have been researched.

This chapter sets out to identify the effects of smoking on surgical outcomes, intra- as well as postoperatively. The effects of smoking relates to duration and amount of tobacco smoking as well of the type and setting of surgery. The patophysiological background for the changes in organ function induced by tobacco smoking will be explained.

In the recent years several authors have explored the effect of preoperative smoking intervention on the risk of postoperative complications as well as on patient smoking habits in the short and long term. The chapter will include a review of these trials. In addiction the effectiveness and appropriateness of different types of preoperative smoking intervention methods will be discussed.

Finally the chapter will discuss national and international approaches to facilitate the implementation of effective preoperative smoking intervention programs.

INTRODUCTION

Until recently, lifestyle related factors such as smoking and drinking habits of patients in hospitals normally were registered in patients' charts – but otherwise considered a personal issue, that was not acted on. Slowly, but surely this is changing. Lifestyle interventions have become socially acceptable – although some health professionals still feel awkward when having to deal with issues they feel belong to the patient's private sphere. However, as we shall discuss in this chapter, intervening with lifestyle related factors is very important for reducing the risk of complications during and after surgery.

In the western world about 20-35 % of adults presenting for surgery are smokers. The rate fluctuates with the type of surgery, since some types of surgery are more common on smokers than in non-smokers. However, the link between smoking and postoperative complications is well documented across surgical specialties.

PHYSIOLOGY

Cigarette smoke contains over 4000 substances, some of which are pharmacologically active, some antigenic, some cytotoxic, some mutagenic and some others carcinogenic[1]. It consists of a gaseous phase and a particulate phase. About 85 % of cigarette smoke is gaseous, consisting mainly of nitrogen, oxygen and carbon dioxide. However, it also contains carcinogens such as hydrocyanic acid and hydrazine, and irritants such as hydrocyanotic acid, acetaldehyde, ammonia, formaldehyde, acrolein, and not least: carbon monoxide. In the particulate phase the main toxic agent is nicotine.

Cardiovascular System

The acute effect of smoking is first of all due to nicotine and carbon monoxide. Nicotine has sympathomimetic properties, and thus increases the pulse rate, blood pressure, vascular resistance and peripheral blood flow. These effects increase myocardial contractility, leading to an increase in oxygen consumption by the myocardium. The demand for oxygen is thus increased. The increase in vascular resistance, however, diminishes oxygen transport in the muscular tissue, including the myocardium, the internal organs, and the skin[2;3]. Following the smoking of one cigarette, the pressor response lasts for about 30 min.

Carbon monoxide can occupy 3-17% of the oxygen binding sites at the hemoglobin molecule in smokers to form carboxyhemoglobin (COHb). In non-smokers COHb rarely exceeds 2%[4]. The amount of COHb is dependent on the individual's tobacco consumption and the length of time that has elapsed, since the individual last smoked[5]. Carbon monoxide not only occupies the oxygen binding sites, but also shifts the oxygen dissociation curve to the left, and thereby increases the affinity of hemoglobin for oxygen with the resultant reduction in tissue oxygenation.

The short term effects of smoking are thus increased oxygen consumption due to the sympathomimetic effects of nicotine and a reduction in oxygen delivery caused by both nicotine and carbon monoxide. The effects of nicotine and carbon monoxide decline within 12-24 hours of smoking cessation due to the metabolisation of nicotine to the inactive cotinin and the washout of carbon monoxide[6].

Hemostatic System

Smoking increases the production of hemoglobin, red blood cells, and platelets and increases platelet reactivity[7]. Fibrinogen is also increased. This leads to an increase in hematocrit and increased blood viscosity, increasing the risk of thromboembolic episodes. Pulmonary embolism and deep venous thrombosis (DVT) accounts for many deaths in patients with smoking related pulmonary disease. This is due to reduced mobility in these patients and to the presence of coagulation abnormalities seen in smokers. Cigarette smoking is the strongest known environmental influence on plasma fibrinogen and has consistently been linked to elevated plasma fibrinogen levels[8]. This is likely to be the explanation for the increased rate of deep venous thrombosis and pulmonary embolisms seen in smokers. Cessation from smoking results in a rapid reduction in the plasma fibrinogen[9]. The potential influence of inflammation on coagulation and impaired fibrinolysis are other reasons for the increased incidence of DVT seen in smokers.

Arterial thromboembolic phenomena correlate very strongly to smoking and decreased platelet survival time and increased platelet aggregability has been found in smokers[10]

Respiratory System

Smoking is related to the development of acute and chronic pulmonary changes. The pathophysiology is related to

a. mucus hypersecretion
b. impairment of mucociliary clearing
c. small airway narrowing

Smoking leads to a decrease in mucociliary transport. Chronic cough, sputum production and breathlessness are much more common in smokers[11]. Smoke contains ciliostatic and ciliotoxic substances such as hydrocyanic acid, acetaldehyde, acrolein and formaldehyde. The cilia become inactive and destroyed. At the same time the mucus normally secreted in the tracheobronchial system is changed by smoke components and becomes hyperviscous and its rheologic properties changes. All together the mucociliary clearance is impaired. Laryngeal and bronchial reactivity as increased in smokers,

Even in otherwise asymptomatic smokers the closing volume test shows signs of small airway narrowing. Changes in closing capacity suggests trapping of air, and loss of elastic recoil in the peripheral airways[12;13]. Pulmonary surfactant is also decreased.[14]. These changes eventually worsen and lead to the development of chronic obstructive pulmonary disease and emphysema.

After smoking cessation the pulmonary changes will gradually improve, depending on the duration of smoking and the amount of cigarettes or other types of tobacco smoked. Ciliary activity starts to recover within 4-6 days after smoking cessation, sputum volume decreases within 2-6 weeks, and the tracheobronchial clearance usually improves within 3 month.[15;16].

Immune System

Tobacco smoking increases the inflammatory process and also has immunosuppressive effect. Smokers have an increased white cell count compared to non-smokers. Biochemically confirmed tobacco abstinence leads to a rapid and sustained decrease in white cell count and absolute neutrophil counts, possibly reflecting a decrease in an underlying state of tobacco induced inflammation[17]. Smokers have been shown to have lower Immunoglobulin levels than non-smokers[18;19]. Upon smoking cessation S-IgA may decline further for about one week, then returns to pre-cessation values. Smoking is also related to low natural killer cell activity and alterations in immunoregulatory T-cell activity. Only scarce research has been performed on the effects of smoking cessation and the return of normal immune function, but some findings suggest that about 6 weeks will normalize most of the functions.

Drug Metabolism

In general, drug metabolism is increased in smokers, due to an induction of liver enzymes[20]. The constituents of tobacco smoke, primarily nicotine, have their own pharmacological effects which may potentiate or antagonize the desired pharmacological effect. End-organ responsiveness may also be altered by tobacco. Smokers have a decreased tolerance to pain, and therefore needs larger doses, independent of the action of the analgesic drug. Some opiods are metabolized faster in smokers, whereas codeine and paracetamol are not affected. Smokers need larger doses of benzodiazepines to achieve a desired effect. The effect of neuromuscular blockers used in anesthesia is affected by nicotine, competing for the acetylcholine receptors at the neuromuscular end plates[21]. The size of this effect is rather unpredictable, but in general, the dose needed to achieve a sufficient block is larger. It is estimated that a period of 6-8 weeks is required to alter the smoking induced changes in drug metabolism, but this issue needs further research[22]

Smoking and Perioperative Complications

Smoking is related to a long list of complications relating to anesthesia and surgery. It is relevant to consider the potential hazard of the smoking patient at an early occasion.

ASPIRATION

Not many years ago, patients waiting for surgery were not allowed to smoke for a varying amount of time prior to the operation. This was due to the belief that smoking was increasing the ventricular emptying time and that abstinence from smoking would reduce the risk of aspiration. However, smoking does not increase the gastric volume or alter the pH of the gastric secretions[23] Smoking does make the gastroesophageal sphincter incompetent, and this may increase the risk of reflux from the ventricle, resulting in pulmonary aspiration[24].

Intra-Operative Cardiopulmonary Problems

Anesthesia induction is often dramatic in smokers, due to active hemodynamic reflexes and the hypersensitive airway. The incidence of laryngospasm, bronchospasm, aspiration, hypoventilation, hypoxemia and reintubation was found to be about doubled in smokers compared to non-smokers in a large survey[25]. The imbalance between myocardial oxygen supply and demand and the increased risk of atherosclerosis makes the smoker undergoing anesthesia likely to suffer from a range of cardiovascular incidents and complications[22;26;27].

Postoperative Complications

The development of postoperative complications can ruin an otherwise successful operation, causing the patient discomfort, extending their stay in hospital and potentially undermining the the surgical procedure.

Postoperative complications may cause permanent injuries to the patient, intensive care admittance or even death. Complications can also influence the patient's social life, causing dismissal from work, impair leisure time activities and thereby lessen social contact[28]. Furthermore, postoperative complications are expensive, extending stay in hospital, perhaps causing secondary surgery, intensive care therapy or other interventions[29-31]. All of these are reasons to try to avoid postoperative complications – from a patient orientated view as well as seen from the health economists view.

Postoperative complications are more common after emergency surgery than after elective surgery – probably due to a multitude of factors – such as the nature of the surgical disease, the existence of co-morbidity, medical conditions associated with the surgical disease, such as hypovolemia, and metabolic changes. In elective surgery, complications occur less frequently, but still do occur in a varying range depending on type of surgery, comorbidity - and life style induced changes in patient physiology. Complications arising in elective procedures such as hip or knee alloplasty, an operation performed in order to raise quality of life – may seem even more unreasonable to patients than those following emergency procedures.

Complications in smokers are not different from complications in non-smokers – they just occur more frequently and are often more serious. The commonest complications are pulmonary complication, cardiovascular complications, infections and complicated wound healing. These can occur separately or together in any combination.

Pulmonary Complications

Postoperative pulmonary complications are a major cause of morbidity, mortality, prolonged hospital stay and increased cost of care[32]. Pneumonia, bronchitis, lobar atelectasis, respiratory failure and prolonged mechanical ventilation are among the major pulmonary complications[33]. Along with other risk factors, smoking has been recognized as a risk factor for the development of postoperative pulmonary complications since Morton published his paper in 1944[34]. The risk conferred by cigarette smoking persists in the absence of chronic obstructive lung disease.

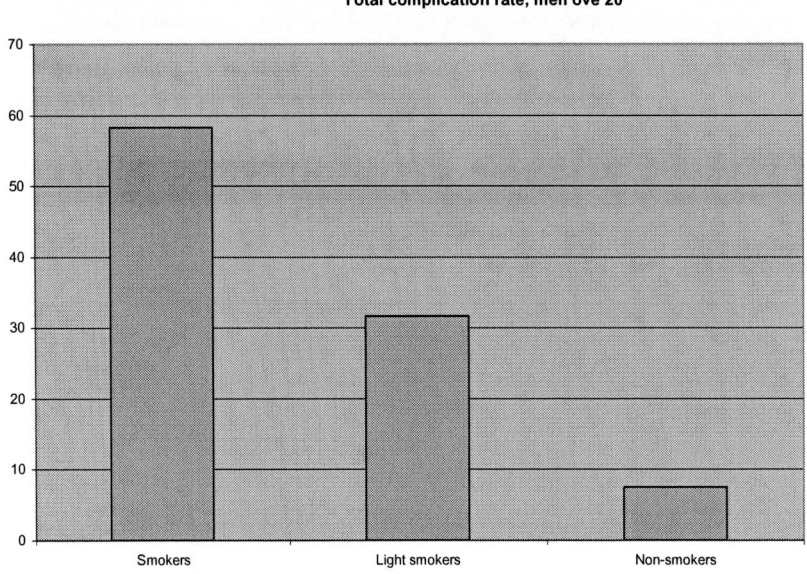

From: Morton: Tobacco Smoking and Pulmonary Complications, Lancet 1944.

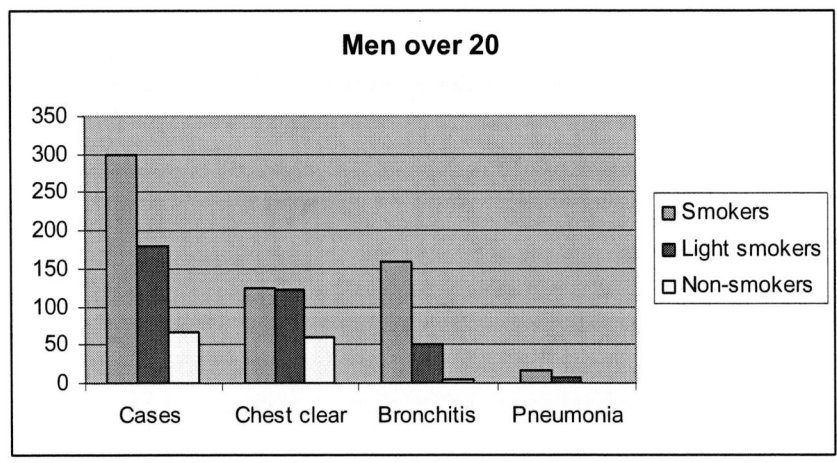

From: Morton: Tobacco Smoking and Pulmonary Complications, Lancet 1944.

The relationship between smoking and postoperative pulmonary complications has been demonstrated many times Morton first published his paper in the Lancet. In 1981, Garibaldi et al. identified smoking as one of several independent risk factors for development of pneumonia in surgical patients, with smokers having twice the risk for postoperative pneumonia as non-smokers[35]. Along with smoking other risk factors, such as low serum albumin concentration on admission, high ASA classification, longer operative procedures and thoracic or upper abdominal site of surgery were identified. Many studies of the risk factors for postoperative pulmonary complications have pointed as smoking among the most important. Figure 1. gives an overview of the studies and odd ratios.

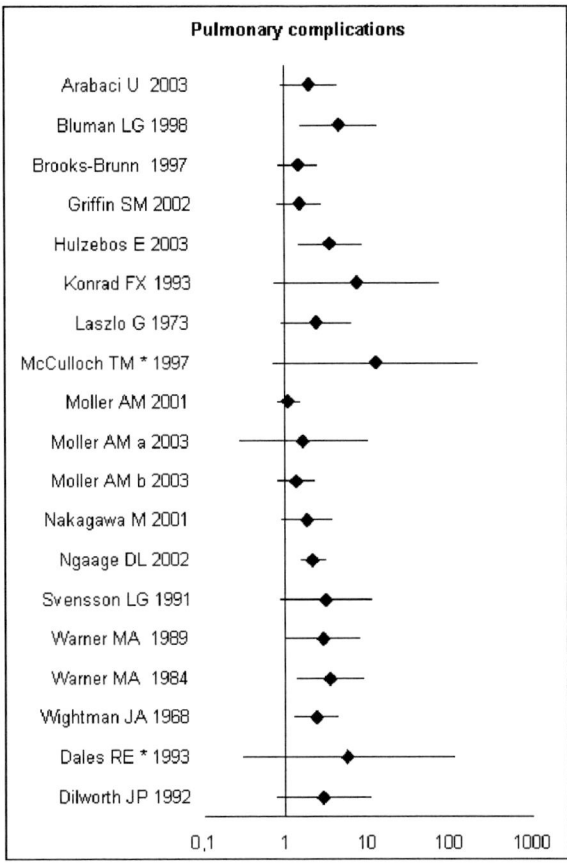

Figure 1. Association between smoking and postoperative pulmonary complications OR (95% CI).

WOUND HEALING

The most frequent complications over-represented in smokers are those related to wound healing processes. The increased incidence is most likely caused by a combination of the effects of smoking on the vascular system[36], the effect on the healing process[37], and the immune system changes seen in smokers[38;39].

Nicotine inhibits the proliferation of red blood cells, fibroblasts and macrophages[40], all of which must be present to heal injured tissue. As mentioned above, nicotine also increases platelet adhesiveness, causing micro-clots and decreased microperfusion[41;42]. This may lead to clot formation and reduced blood flow[43]. Finally, nicotine produces cutaneus vasoconstriction because of catecholamine release[44]. The presence of carbon monoxide will also inhibit the wound healing process by reduced oxygen availability in the tissue, as previously described. Smokers have impaired collagen production, resulting in less elasticity of the skin and a reduced capability of wound healing. Mature collagen is also the main determinator of strength of an operative wound.

The clinical consequences of smoking induced impaired wound healing are multiple. Studies describe unsatisfactory scarring, wound infections, wound dehiscence, impaired bone healing and a high incidence of non union[45-48]. Postmenopausal women, who smoke lose significantly more cortical bone and have a higher incidence of spinal osteoporosis and hip fractures than non-smoking women[49-51].

Plastic surgeons have been telling their patients to stop smoking before surgery for decades, due to the clinical experience of delayed wound healing and unsatisfactory scarring seen in smoking patients[52-54].

Overall, smokers suffer from impaired wound healing[55], impaired bone healing[56;57] and anastomotic dehiscence in bowel and vascular surgery[58]. Some prospective results indicate that smoking cessation for 4 weeks increased the wound healing process and reduces the risk of wound infections to the level of never smokers[59]. Figure 2 gives an overview of trials describing the relationship between smoking and wound complications.

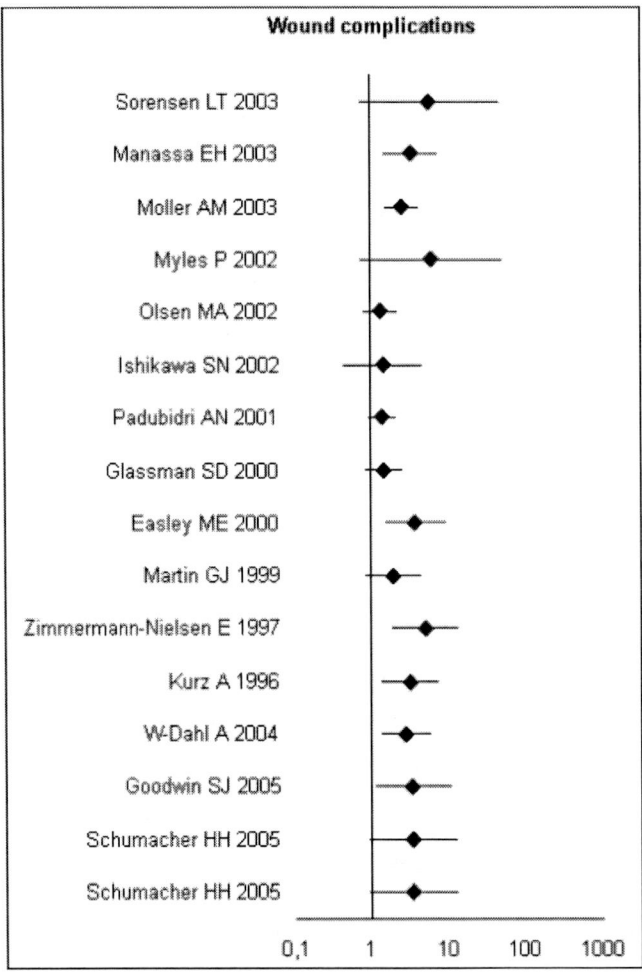

Figure 2. Association between smoking and postoperative wound complications. Odds ratio (95% CI).

TIME IN POST ANESTHESIA CARE UNIT (PACU)

Time spent in PACU is of considerable clinical and economic interest: it can become a limiting factor on the number of surgical procedures an institution can perform, and PACU services are expensive.

Handlin et al. demonstrated that 19% of smokers had prolonged stay in PACU compared to 7% of non-smokers – even after correction for type and duration of surgery[60]. Handlin also described a dose-relationship response between pack years and risk of prolonged PACU stay. The studies conclude that the perioperative care of smokers will cost an extra 20% (this is based solely on the extra time spent in the PACU. Any other costs smokers might incur would, of course, increase the figure). The reasons for smokers' prolonged PACU stay are not fully described and possible interventions also remain to be explored.

Risk of Postoperative Intensive Care Admittance

The rate of postoperative intensive care admittance is related to the type, size and site of the surgical procedure, as well as to the co-existence of medical disease. However, smoking seems to be an additional risk factor for unplanned postoperative intensive care admittance[61;62].

Very little research has been performed about smoking and the risk of postoperative intensive care admittance. However, because smoking leads to cardiovascular and pulmonary disease, impairs immune system and increases the risk of serious postoperative complications, it is not unlikely that smokers will fill the intensive care units. Smoking itself is associated with an increased risk of postoperative intensive care admittance, and also increased the risk of prolonged mechanical ventilation[63]. If smoking has resulted in chronic obstructive lung disease this risk is further increased.

Smokers also tend to stay longer in the intensive care unit. In one study the average time spent in intensive care unit was increased from 2,4 days in non-smokers to 3,2 days in smokers[64]. Another study[31] found that smokers had 10,1% risk of prolonged intensive stay after CABG compares to 6,1% of the non-smokers.

In conclusion, although only scarcely researched, is seems that smokers are in risk zone for unplanned intensive care admittance after surgery, for prolonged intensive stay after major surgery and for prolonged mechanical ventilation.

Passive Smoking

The patophysiological changes associated with passive smoking are not yet fully described. However, some evidence does imply that passive smoking – defined as the inhalation of other peoples smoke in a non-smoker (or smoker) are harmful in relation to anesthesia and surgery. Passive smoking seems to influence the course of anesthesia for adults as well as for children. Dennis[65], studied 120 adults undergoing elective surgery in general anesthesia and found an increased risk of respiratory complications in both active and passive smokers.

The effect of passive smoking, however, has been best described in children whose parents smoke. In 2003, Drongowski found that in children undergoing general anesthesia, environmental tobacco smoke exposure increased the incidence of respiratory problems during induction and emergence from anesthesia significantly[66]. Skolnick et al. demonstrated a dose relationship between the risk of airway complications in children receiving general anesthesia And the urinary cotinine concentration in 602 children[67]. Several studies have shown passive smoking to be a risk factor for respiratory event during the postoperative period. Lyons et al. demonstrated that the risk of events was related to the number of cigarettes smoked by individuals, to whom the child was exposed[68]. Children exposed to passive smoking consume less rocuronium – a non depolarizing neuromuscular blocking agent, during anesthesia. This may lead to a prolonged anesthetic course, unless taking into consideration by the anesthesiologist when administering the drug[69]. In conclusion, some evidence suggests a dose relationship between the magnitude of passive smoking and the overall risk of respiratory complications in children and adults. Furthermore, passive smoking also seems to influence drug metabolism. More research is needed within this field.

CIGARS, PIPES AND SMOKELESS TOBACCO

The research evaluating the relationship between smoking and surgical complications almost exclusively focus on cigarette smoking, probably because of the larger fraction of smokers who smoke only cigarettes. However, the question often arises: Is there any difference between cigarette smoking and other ways of tobacco use, such as cigar smoking, pipe-smoking, water-pipe or smokeless tobacco.

Cigars or cheroot smokers suffer from greater risk of impaired pulmonary function than other smokers, as do pipe smokers[70]. Cigar smoking has become increasing popular among young males in the developed countries. How this will affect the risk of surgical complications is unknown.

Water-pipe smoking is a new trend, originating from the middle east, practiced notably among youth.[71]. The aerosol of water-pipe smoke has high concentrations of carbon monoxide, nicotine, tar and heavy metals. No studies have described the relation between surgery and water-pipe smoking, but there is no reason to believe that the pattern of complications would differ much.

Smokeless tobacco has the advantage of not producing passive smoking. It also is not inhaled into the lungs of the user. Because of this, the risk of lung cancer and other smoking related lung problems is lower in the smokeless tobacco user that in the cigarette smoker[72]. Some evidence suggests that the mortality risk is lower with smokeless tobacco than with cigarette smoking. No studies explore the relation between smokeless tobacco and surgery.

In conclusion, it is unknown exactly how different smoking habits alter the increased risk of complications after surgery. More research is needed in this field.

THE EFFECT OF SMOKING INTERVENTION
ON POSTOPERATIVE COMPLICATIONS

Although evidence of the harmful effects of smoking on surgical outcome has been known for decades, only few have studied the effects of preoperative smoking intervention.

In 1984, Warner et al performed a retrospective study including 500 patients that related preoperative smoking behaviour to the risk of postoperative pulmonary complications[73]. In this study, they showed that the patients who stopped smoking more than eight weeks before cardiac bypass surgery had significantly fewer postoperative pulmonary complications than those who either smoked or had stopped less than eight weeks before surgery. These results were confirmed in 1989, where 200 patients were evaluated[74]. In this study, patients who stopped smoking more than 6 weeks before surgery had a pulmonary complication rate of 14,5% compared to 57,1% in those who did not. Patients who had stopped smoking more than 6 month before surgery had rates similar to those who had never smoked (11,1% versus 11,9%).

The results of these descriptive studies led the way for randomised controlled trials, investigating the effect of preoperative smoking intervention on the postoperative complication rate and on patients smoking habits in the perioperative period[75;76]. In one trial, patients scheduled for hip or knee alloplasty were randomised 6-8 weeks before surgery to either smoking intervention or control. The overall postoperative complication rate was significantly reduced in the intervention group compared with the controls. The largest effect of intervention was seen for wound related complications. The relative risk reduction for wound complications was 83% and the number needed to treat (NNT) was four.

In another trial, however, patients scheduled for colorectal resection were randomised to either abstinence from smoking/reducing by 50% or maintenance of smoking habits. This trial could not demonstrate any difference between the groups. The results of these two trials raise several additional questions which will be dealt with below.

Intervention

Smoking intervention can be anything from verbal information or a leaflet suggesting smoking cessation to very intensive and comprehensive programs including verbal counselling, nicotine replacement therapy weekly meetings and phone hotline. Nicotine replacement can be free of costs for the patients or not. A systematic review[77] has evaluated the efficacy of different intervention in non-hospitalized smokers and concludes that the more intensive the intervention the better the effect on smoking habits. Another systematic review(78) outlines the abundant evidence showing that nicotine replacement therapy doubles the chances of smoking cessation. So the most effective intervention would be an intensive, individual counselling with nicotine replacement therapy.

Timing of Preoperative Smoking Cessation

The optimal timing of preoperative smoking cessation intervention remains unknown. The evidence that interventions occurring 6-8 weeks before surgery is effects is fairly clear. However – physicians have had concerns that brief preoperative abstinence might actually be harmful due to excess amounts of sputum production over the first few weeks after quitting[79] On the other hand, the washout of nicotine and carbon monoxide will occur with in 24-48 hours and this may indeed be beneficial. No clinical trials have been performed on short term preoperative smoking cessation so far. In any case, abstinence within a few weeks of surgery does not significantly increase the rate of complications[74;80;81].

Effect on Patients Smoking Habits

The effect of preoperative smoking intervention on patient smoking habits has been fairly well researched. In all studies the intervention achieves a significant increase in the odds of smoking cessation in the perioperative period. The studies are, however, rather heterogeneous, which means that the populations and the interventions are quite different from study to study.

In the previously described study on patients undergoing hip or knee alloplasty, 64% stopped smoking completely in the intervention group compared to 7.7% in the control group. In this study the perioperative period was defined as six to eight weeks before surgery until 10 days after[75]. In the study on patients undergoing colorectal resections, a cessation or reduction rate of 89% in the intervention group compared to 13% in the control group in the preoperative (two to three weeks before surgery) period ($P < 0.05$) was found[76]. Wolfenden provided an intervention one to two weeks before surgery based on a computerised smoking intervention programme. The cessation rates were high in both the intervention (78%) and usual care (65%) group[82]. This intervention was quite intensive and individually designed. Ratner found 73% of the intervention group abstinent for at least 24 hours before surgery compared to 53% of controls [83].

Figure 3 summarizes the result of the existing randomised controlled trials on the effect of preoperative smoking intervention on patients smoking habits on the day of surgery.

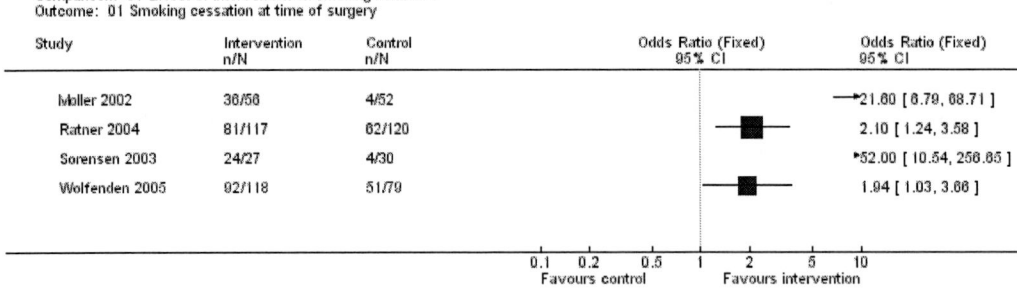

Figure 3.

Attitudes toward Smoking Intervention

Many nurses and physicians have been reluctant to even ask patients about their smoking habits – thereby confronting them with their unhealthy lifestyle. This attitude does not make smoking intervention counselling easier. And it seems that patients actually very often indeed, have a wish to stop smoking, and need professional help to do so. In a qualitative study performed in Denmark, the patients generally agreed that they welcomed the opportunity to change their smoking habits before surgery[84]. None of the patients mentioned that they felt intruded into their private life. The impeding operation was perceived as a motivating factor for changing their smoking habits. Even patients who continued to smoke explained that they were glad they had been offered the opportunity of getting help and advice. Graham-Garcia concluded that patients undergoing surgery aremore susceptible to advice about smoking cessation due to increased motivation[85]. So the time of surgery may be a window of opportunity for successful smoking intervention.

Warner examined the practices and attitudes among anesthesiologists and surgeons in a postal survey[86]. More than 90% of both groups almost always asked their patients about smoking habits and believed that surgical patients should maintain abstinence after surgery. However, only 30% of the anesthesiologists and 58% of the surgeons routinely advised their patients to quit smoking.

Barriers include lack of training regarding intervention techniques, a perceived lack of effective interventions, and insufficient time to intervene. These results may raise the question whether health care professionals should be better educated in life style intervention initiatives.

HEALTH CARE ORGANISATION

Evidence suggests that we record the smoking habits of all surgical patients and initiate smoking cessation interventions 6-8 weeks before surgery if possible or perhaps at a shorter interval.

However, even with high-quality evidence, implementing these changes can be difficult. This is because there are many barriers today in health-care systems, which makes the introduction of new interventions difficult. Even with high-quality trials published in international journals, one would be wrong to rely on the passive diffusion of knowledge into the health-care system. There can be unwillingness among the decision-makers in the health-care system, or within the medical staff. (For example, it has been shown that staff members who smoke are much less likely to discuss smoking habits with their patients[87]). Even though economic analysis has shown that the reduction of complications would save more money than an effective preoperative smoking intervention would cost hospital administrators are still reluctant to spend money on preventive initiatives.

To overcome these barriers, it is important to act on several levels. It is, of course, important that scientific results are published in different types of journals, in order to reach as many practioners as possible. This, however, may not be enough. To enable patients to benefit from these interventions we should publish national and international clinical guidelines; present results at conferences; and introduce preventive interventions into the qualifying examinations for doctors and other staff [88]. Last, but not least it is important to collaborate across disciplines: anesthesiologists and surgeons, general practioners and hospitals departments. Every country should consider developing national policies to ensure that smoking prevention initiatives are implemented throughout their health-care system, in order to improve the quality of treatments and outcomes for all patients.

Table 1. Preoperative smoking cessation for patients admitted to surgery

When	What
At admission to surgery from GP, specialist or others	Include history of present smoking (yes/no daily smoking), If yes recommend smoking cessation and give information about smoking intervention programs in the hospital / community
At first contact to the surgeon, anaesthesiologist	Obtain smoking history (yes/no) if not done yet. If yes, inform about (oral and written) the increased risk at surgery and the effect of smoking intervention before surgery. Recommend smoking cessation and offer smoking intervention program, if not done already. Motivate the un-motivated patient.
At decision of operation	Include smoking as a risk factor in the dialogue among the surgeon, anaesthesiologist and patient, in the same way as severe heart disease, unstable diabetes etc.
At discharge	Register the intervention and present smoking habits in the discharge letter
At follow up for quality improvement	Include a few indicators in the quality management program, (choose among screening for smoking, information, and recommendation, smoking intervention, smoking rate preoperatively.)

CONCLUSION

Tobacco smoking carries a major risk of the development of complications during and after surgery. The most common tobacco related complications are impaired wound healing, infections, pulmonary and cardiovascular complications. Smoking intervention is effect in reducing the complication rate and well accepted by the patients.

REFERENCES

[1]   Holbrook JH. In: Braunwald, Isselbacher KJ, Petersdorf RG, editors. *Principles of Internal Medicine.*New York: McGraw-Hill; 1987. p. 855-9.

[2]   Jensen JA, Goodson WH, Hopf HW, Hunt TK. Cigarette smoking decreases tissue oxygen. *Arch. Surg.* 1991 Oct;126(9):1131-4.

[3]   Riley RH, Davis NJ, Finucane KE, Christmas P. Arterial oxygen saturation in anaesthetised patients during transfer from induction room to operating room. *Anaesth Intensive Care.* 1988 May;16(2):182-6.

[4]   Hess W. [Affinity of oxygen for hemoglobin--its significance under physiological and pathological conditions]. *Anaesthesist.* 1987 Sep;36(9):455-67.

[5]   McDonough P, Moffatt RJ. Smoking-induced elevations in blood carboxyhaemoglobin levels. Effect on maximal oxygen uptake. *Sports Med.* 1999 May;27(5):275-83.

[6]   Davies JM, Latto IP, Jones JG, Veale A, Wardrop CA. Effects of stopping smoking for 48 hours on oxygen availability from the blood: a study on pregnant women. *Br. Med. J.* 1979 Aug 11;2(6186):355-6.

[7]   Erskine RJ, Hanning CD. Do I advice my patients to stop smoking pre-operatively? *Curr. Anaesth. Crit. Care.* 1992;3:175-80.

[8]   Tapson VF. The role of smoking in coagulation and thromboembolism in chronic obstructive pulmonary disease. *Proc. Am. Thorac. Soc.* 2005;2(1):71-7.

[9]   Feher MD, Rampling MW, Brown J, Robinson R, Richmond W, Cholerton S, et al. Acute changes in atherogenic and thrombogenic factors with cessation of smoking. *J. R. Soc. Med.* 1990 Mar;83(3):146-8.

[10] Bierenbaum ML, Fleischman AI, Stier A, Somol H, Watson PB. Effect of cigarette smoking upon in vivo platelet function in man. *Thromb. Res.* 1978 Jun;12(6):1051-7.

[11] Beckers S, Camu F. The anesthetic risk of tobacco smoking. *Acta Anaesthesiol. Belg.* 1991;42(1):45-56.

[12] Hoeppner VH, Cooper DM, Zamel N, Bryan AC, Levison H. Relationship between elastic recoil and closing volume in smokers and nonsmokers. *Am. Rev. Respir. Dis.* 1974 Jan;109(1):81-6.

[13] Just M, Monso E, Ribera M, Lorenzo JC, Morera J, Ferrandiz C. Relationships between lung function, smoking and morphology of dermal elastic fibres. *Exp. Dermatol.* 2005 Oct;14(10):744-51.

[14] Hartl D, Griese M. Surfactant protein D in human lung diseases. *Eur. J. Clin. Invest.* 2006 Jun;36(6):423-35.

[15] Kensler CJ, Battista SP. Chemical and physical factors affecting mammalian ciliary activity. *Am. Rev. Respir. Dis.* 1966 Mar;93(3):Suppl-102.

[16] Camner P, Philipson K, Arvidsson T. Withdrawal of cigarette smoking: a study on tracheobronchial clearance. *Arch. Environ. Health.* 1973 Feb;26(2):90-2.

[17] Abel GA, Hays JT, Decker PA, Croghan GA, Kuter DJ, Rigotti NA. Effects of biochemically confirmed smoking cessation on white blood cell count. *Mayo Clinic Proceedings.* 2005 Aug;80(8):1022-8.

[18] Evans P, Der G, Ford G, Hucklebridge F, Hunt K, Lambert S. Social class, sex, and age differences in mucosal immunity in a large community sample. *Brain Behav. Immun.* 2000 Mar;14(1):41-8.

[19] Barton JR, Riad MA, Gaze MN, Maran AG, Ferguson A. Mucosal immunodeficiency in smokers, and in patients with epithelial head and neck tumours. *Gut.* 1990 Apr;31(4):378-82.

[20] Miller LG. Recent developments in the study of the effects of cigarette smoking on clinical pharmacokinetics and clinical pharmacodynamics. *Clin. Pharmacokinet.* 1989 Aug;17(2):90-108.

[21] Teiria H, Rautoma P, Yli-Hankala A. Effect of smoking on dose requirements for vecuronium. *Br. J. Anaesth.* 1996 Jan;76(1):154-5.

[22] Pearce AC, Jones RM. Smoking and anesthesia: preoperative abstinence and perioperative morbidity. *Anesthesiology.* 1984 Nov;61(5):576-84.

[23] Adelhoj B, Petring OU, Frosig F, Bigler DR, Jensen BN. Influence of cigarette smoking on the risk of acid pulmonary aspiration. *Acta Anaesthesiol. Scand.* 1987 Jan;31(1):7-9.

[24] Chattopadhyay DK, Greaney MG, Irvin TT. Effect of cigarette smoking on the lower oesophageal sphincter. *Gut.* 1977 Oct;18(10):833-5.

[25] Schwilk B, Bothner U, Schraag S, Georgieff M. Perioperative respiratory events in smokers and nonsmokers undergoing general anaesthesia. *Acta Anaesthesiol. Scand.* 1997 Mar;41(3):348-55.

[26] Higham H, Sear JW, Neill F, Sear YM, Foex P. Peri-operative silent myocardial ischaemia and long-term adverse outcomes in non-cardiac surgical patients. *Anaesthesia.* 2001 Jul;56(7):630-7.

[27] Nierman E, Zakrzewski K. Recognition and management of preoperative risk. *Rheum. Dis. Clin. North Am.* 1999 Aug;25(3):585-622.

[28] Lindsay GM, Hanlon P, Smith LN, Wheatley DJ. Assessment of changes in general health status using the short-form 36 questionnaire 1 year following coronary artery bypass grafting. *Eur. J. Cardiothorac. Surg.* 2000 Nov;18(5):557-64.

[29] Berdan L, Rahr R, Spann L. Medical and lifestyle approaches to cardiovascular rehabilitation. *Physician Assist.* 1993 Dec;17(12):29-6, 38.

[30] Chang SS, Baumgartner RG, Wells N, Cookson MS, Smith JA, Jr. Causes of increased hospital stay after radical cystectomy in a clinical pathway setting. *J. Urol.* 2002 Jan;167(1):208-11.

[31] Christakis GT, Fremes SE, Naylor CD, Chen E, Rao V, Goldman BS. Impact of preoperative risk and perioperative morbidity on ICU stay following coronary bypass surgery. *Cardiovasc. Surg.* 1996 Feb;4(1):29-35.

[32] Lawrence VA, Dhanda R, Hilsenbeck SG, Page CP. Risk of pulmonary complications after elective abdominal surgery. *Chest.* 1996 Sep;110(3):744-50.

[33] Trayner E Jr, Celli BR. Postoperative pulmonary complications. *Med. Clin. North Am.* 2001 Sep;85(5):1129-39.

[34] Morton HJV. Tobacco smoking and pulmonary complications after operation. *Lancet.* 1944.

[35] Garibaldi RA, Britt MR, Coleman ML, Reading JC, Pace NL. Risk factors for postoperative pneumonia. *Am. J. Med.* 1981 Mar;70(3):677-80.

[36] Whiteford L. Nicotine, CO and HCN: the detrimental effects of smoking on wound healing. *Br. J. Community Nurs.* 2003;8(12):S22-S26.

[37] Jorgensen LN, Kallehave F, Christensen E, Siana JE, Gottrup F. Less collagen production in smokers. *Surgery.* 1998 Apr;123(4):450-5.

[38] Hersey P, Prendergast D, Edwards A. Effects of cigarette smoking on the immune system. Follow-up studies in normal subjects after cessation of smoking. *Med. J. Aust.* 1983 Oct 29;2(9):425-9.

[39] Zeidel A, Beilin B, Yardeni I, Mayburd E, Smirnov G, Bessler H. Immune response in asymptomatic smokers. *Acta Anaesthesiol. Scand.* 2002;46:959-64.

[40] Sherwin MA, Gastwirth CM. Detrimental effects of cigarette smoking on lower extremity wound healing. *J. Foot Surg.* 1990 Jan;29(1):84-7.

[41] Drexler H. Endothelial dysfunction: clinical implications. *Prog. Cardiovasc. Dis.* 1997 Jan;39(4):287-324.

[42] Mazzoni MC, Schmid-Schonbein GW. Mechanisms and consequences of cell activation in the microcirculation. *Cardiovasc. Res.* 1996 Oct;32(4):709-19.

[43] Tur E, Yosipovitch G, Oren-Vulfs S. Chronic and acute effects of cigarette smoking on skin blood flow. *Angiology.* 1992 Apr;43(4):328-35.

[44] Nolan J, Jenkins RA, Kurihara K, Schultz RC. The acute effects of cigarette smoke exposure on experimental skin flaps. *Plast. Reconstr. Surg.* 1985 Apr;75(4):544-51.

[45] Siana JE, Rex S, Gottrup F. The effect of cigarette smoking on wound healing. *Scand. J. Plast. Reconstr. Surg. Hand Surg.* 1989;23(3):207-9.

[46] Manassa EH, Hertl CH, Olbrisch RR. Wound healing problems in smokers and nonsmokers after 132 abdominoplasties. *Plast. Reconstr. Surg.* 2003 May;111(6):2082-7.

[47] Padubidri AN, Yetman R, Browne E, Lucas A, Papay F, Larive B, et al. Complications of postmastectomy breast reconstructions in smokers, ex-smokers, and nonsmokers. *Plast. Reconstr. Surg.* 2001 Feb;107(2):342-9.

[48] Kwiatkowski TC, Hanley EN, Jr., Ramp WK. Cigarette smoking and its orthopedic consequences. *Am. J. Orthop.* 1996 Sep;25(9):590-7.

[49] Cumming RG, Klineberg RJ. Case-control study of risk factors for hip fractures in the elderly. *Am. J. Epidemiol.* 1994 Mar 1;139(5):493-503.

[50] Nelson HD, Nevitt MC, Scott JC, Stone KL, Cummings SR. Smoking, alcohol, and neuromuscular and physical function of older women. Study of Osteoporotic Fractures Research Group. *JAMA.* 1994 Dec 21;272(23):1825-31.

[51] Hoidrup S, Prescott E, Sorensen TI, Gottschau A, Lauritzen JB, Schroll M, et al. Tobacco smoking and risk of hip fracture in men and women. *Int. J. Epidemiol.* 2000 Apr;29(2):253-9.

[52] Netscher DT, Clamon J. Smoking: adverse effects on outcomes for plastic surgical patients. *Plast. Surg. Nurs.* 1994;14(4):205-10.

[53] Rohrich RJ, Coberly DM, Krueger JK, Brown SA. Planning elective operations on patients who smoke: survey of North American plastic surgeons. *Plast Reconstr. Surg.* 2002 Jan;109(1):350-5.

[54] Krueger JK, Rohrich RJ. Clearing the smoke: the scientific rationale for tobacco abstention with plastic surgery. *Plast. Reconstr. Surg.* 2001 Sep 15;108(4):1063-73.

[55] Towler J. Cigarette smoking and its effects on wound healing. *J. Wound Care.* 2000 Mar;9(3):100-4.

[56] Adams CI, Keating JF, Court-Brown CM. Cigarette smoking and open tibial fractures. *Injury.* 2001 Feb;32(1):61-5.

[57] Glassman SD, Anagnost SC, Parker A, Burke D, Johnson JR, Dimar JR. The effect of cigarette smoking and smoking cessation on spinal fusion. *Spine.* 2000 Oct 15;25(20):2608-15.

[58] Fawcett A, Shembekar M, Church JS, Vashisht R, Springall RG, Nott DM. Smoking, hypertension, and colonic anastomotic healing; a combined clinical and histopathological study. *Gut.* 1996 May;38(5):714-8.

[59] Sorensen LT, Karlsmark T, Gottrup F. Abstinence from smoking reduces incisional wound infection: a randomized controlled trial. *Ann. Surg.* 2003 Jul;238(1):1-5.

[60] Handlin DS, Baker T. The effects of smoking on postoperative recovery. *Am. J. Med.* 1992 Jul 15;93(1A):32S-7S.

[61] Moller AM, Pedersen T, Villebro N, Schnaberich A, Haas M, Tonnesen R. A study of the impact of long-term tobacco smoking on postoperative intensive care admission. *Anaesthesia.* 2003 Jan;58(1):55-9.

[62] Moller AM, Maaloe R, Pedersen T. Postoperative intensive care admittance: the role of tobacco smoking. *Acta Anaesthesiol. Scand.* 2001 Mar;45(3):345-8.

[63]   Jayr C, Matthay MA, Goldstone J, Gold WM, Wiener-Kronish JP. Preoperative and intraoperative factors associated with prolonged mechanical ventilation. A study in patients following major abdominal vascular surgery. *Chest.* 1993 Apr;103(4):1231-6.

[64]   Arabaci U, Akdur H, Yigit Z. Effects of smoking on pulmonary functions and arterial blood gases following coronary artery surgery in Turkish patients. *Jpn. Heart J.* 2003 Jan;44(1):61-72.

[65]   Dennis A, Curran J, Sherriff J, Kinnear W. Effects of passive and active smoking on induction of anaesthesia. *Br. J. Anaesth.* 1994 Oct;73(4):450-2.

[66]   Drongowski RA, Lee D, Reynolds PI, Malviya S, Harmon CM, Geiger J, et al. Increased respiratory symptoms following surgery in children exposed to environmental tobacco smoke. *Paediatric Anaesthesia.* 2003 May;13(4):304-10.

[67]   Skolnick ET, Vomvolakis MA, Buck KA, Mannino SF, Sun LS. Exposure to environmental tobacco smoke and the risk of adverse respiratory events in children receiving general anesthesia. *Anesthesiology.* 1998 May;88(5):1144-53.

[68]   Lyons B, Frizelle H, Kirby F, Casey W. The effect of passive smoking on the incidence of airway complications in children undergoing general anaesthesia. *Anaesthesia.* 1996 Apr;51(4):324-6.

[69]   Reisli R, Apilliogullari S, Reisli I, Tuncer S, Erol A, Okesli S. The effect of environmental tobacco smoke on the dose requirements of rocuronium in children. *Pediatric Anesthesia.* 2004 Mar;14(3):247-50.

[70]   Lange P, Groth S, Nyboe J, Mortensen J, Appleyard M, Jensen G, et al. Decline of the lung function related to the type of tobacco smoked and inhalation. *Thorax.* 1990 Jan;45(1):22-6.

[71]   Knishkowy B, Amitai Y. Water-pipe (narghile) smoking: an emerging health risk behavior. *Pediatrics.* 2005 Jul;116(1):e113-e119.

[72]   Daniel RH, Roth AB, Liu X. Health risks of smoking compared to Swedish snus. *Inhal. Toxicol.* 2005 Dec 1;17(13):741-8.

[73]   Warner MA, Divertie MB, Tinker JH. Preoperative cessation of smoking and pulmonary complications in coronary artery bypass patients. *Anesthesiology.* 1984 Apr;60(4):380-3.

[74]   Warner MA, Offord KP, Warner ME, Lennon RL, Conover MA, Jansson-Schumacher U. Role of preoperative cessation of smoking and other factors in postoperative pulmonary complications: a blinded prospective study of coronary artery bypass patients. *Mayo Clin. Proc.* 1989 Jun;64(6):609-16.

[75]   Moller AM, Villebro N, Pedersen T, Tonnesen H. Effect of preoperative smoking intervention on postoperative complications: a randomised clinical trial. *Lancet.* 2002 Jan 12;359(9301):114-7.

[76]   Sorensen LT, Jorgensen T. Short-term pre-operative smoking cessation intervention does not affect postoperative complications in colorectal surgery: a randomized clinical trial. *Colorectal. Dis.* 2003 Aug;5(4):347-52.

[77]   Lancaster T, Stead L. Physician advice for smoking cessation. *Cochrane Database Syst. Rev.* 2004;(4):CD000165.

[78]   Silagy C, Lancaster T, Stead L, Mant D, Fowler G. Nicotine replacement therapy for smoking cessation. *Cochrane Database Syst. Rev.* 2004;(3):CD000146.

[79]   Bluman LG, Mosca L, Newman N, Simon DG. Preoperative smoking habits and postoperative pulmonary complications. *Chest.* 1998 Apr;113(4):883-9.

[80] Moores LK. Smoking and postoperative pulmonary complications. An evidence-based review of the recent literature. *Clin. Chest. Med.* 2000 Mar;21(1):139-x.

[81] Kuri M, Nakagawa M, Tanaka H, Hasuo S, Kishi Y. Determination of the duration of preoperative smoking cessation to improve wound healing after head and neck surgery. *Anesthesiology.* 2005 May;102(5):892-6.

[82] Wolfenden L, Wiggers J, Knight J, Campbell E, Rissel C, Kerridge R, et al. A programme for reducing smoking in pre-operative surgical patients: randomised controlled trial*. *Anaesthesia.* 2005 Feb;60(2):172-9.

[83] Ratner PA, Johnson JL, Richardson CG, Bottorff JL, Moffat B, Mackay M, et al. Efficacy of a smoking-cessation intervention for elective-surgical patients. *Res. Nurs. Health.* 2004 Jul;27(3):148-61.

[84] Moller AM, Villebro NM. [Preoperative smoking intervention: What do patients think? A qualitative study]. *Ugeskr Laeger.* 2004 Nov 11;166(42):3714-8.

[85] Graham-Garcia J, George-Gay B, Heater D, Butts A, Heath J. Application of the Synergy Model with the surgical care of smokers. *Crit. Care Nurs Clin. North Am.* 2006 Mar;18(1):29-xii.

[86] Warner DO, Sarr MG, Offord KP, Dale LC. Anesthesiologists, general surgeons, and tobacco interventions in the perioperative period. *Anesthesia and Analgesia.* 2004 Dec;99(6):1766-73.

[87] Willaing I, Jorgensen T, Iversen L. How does individual smoking behaviour among hospital staff influence their knowledge of the health consequences of smoking? *Scandinavian Journal of Public Health.* 2003;31(2):149-55.

[88] Haynes B, Haines A. Getting research findings into practice - Barriers and bridges to evidence based clinical practice. *British Medical Journal.* 1998 Jul 25;317(7153):273-6.

[89] Ngaage DL, Martins E, Orkell E, Griffin S, Cale AR, Cowen ME, et al. The impact of the duration of mechanical ventilation on the respiratory outcome in smokers undergoing cardiac surgery. *Cardiovasc. Surg.* 2002 Aug;10(4):345-50.

[90] Nigrovic V, Wierda JM. Post-succinylcholine muscle pain and smoking. *Can. J. Anaesth.* 1994 May;41(5 Pt 1):453-4.

[91] Teiria H, Yli-Hankala A, Neuvonen PJ, Olkkola KT. Cigarette smoking does not affect thiopentone pharmacodynamic or pharmacokinetic behaviour. *Can. J. Anaesth.* 1997 Dec;44(12):1269-74.

In: Smoking Cessation: Theory, Interventions and Prevention   ISBN: 978-1-60021-591-9
Editor: Jerome E. Landow   © 2008 Nova Science Publishers, Inc.

Chapter 10

NICOTINE USE AND WEIGHT - RELATED ISSUES IN WOMEN

*Amy L. Copeland[1], Gerald S. Hecht[2]
and Meredith A. Terlecki[1]*
[1] Louisiana State University, Shreveport, Louisiana, USA
[2] Southern University and A and M College, Shreveport, Louisiana, USA

ABSTRACT

Cigarette smoking has been linked to eating and weight-related issues in numerous basic and clinical studies. Typically, smoking and weight issues, such as weight concern, dietary restraint, and clinically significant eating disorders like Bulimia Nervosa have been positively correlated with smoking among women. Existing literature suggests that women smokers are less likely to quit smoking, are less successful in initial cessation attempts, and relapse at higher rates than male smokers (Grunberg, Winders, and Wewers, 1991). Female smokers are also more likely to report smoking cigarettes to manage negative mood and to control weight—factors that have been identified as influencing women's smoking patterns and success in quitting (Solomon and Flynn, 1993). Women are more concerned about postcessation weight gain, tend to get more weight-control benefits from smoking, and suffer more postcessation weight gain than men (Perkins, Mitchell, and Epstein, 1995; Pirke and Laessle, 1993). Women are also more likely to experience increased appetite as a nicotine withdrawal symptom than are men (e.g., Perkins et al., 1995). This chapter contains information about the relationship between smoking and weight/eating-related issues, ranging from basic laboratory studies with animals and humans, to clinical applications and smoking cessation treatment.

1. OVERVIEW OF SMOKING AND SMOKING-RELATED PROBLEMS

Cigarette smoking is the leading cause of preventable death in the United States (US). Approximately 430,000 deaths each year (CDCP, 1997) are attributed to smoking. Smoking is known to cause cancer, heart disease, stroke, chronic obstructive pulmonary disease, and other serious smoking-related illnesses. Successful smoking cessation efforts have reduced the prevalence of cigarette smoking in the US by about half since 1960 (Breslau and Peterson, 1996; Fiore et al., 1989; Pierce et al., 1989). About 47 million Americans (25% of the adult US population) smoke cigarettes (CDCP,1997; Giovino, 2002).

Despite the fact that about 33% of tobacco smokers will die prematurely from smoking-related diseases, smoking cessation has not received adequate attention in the US health care system. The majority of cigarette smokers seek smoking cessation and related advice from a primary care provider (Ockene, 1987; Pederson, Baskerville, and Wanklin, 1982); however, the assessment and treatment of tobacco dependence has not been implemented consistently or effectively in this setting. Thorndike, Rigotti, Stafford, and Singer (1998) reported that only 21% of smokers presenting at a primary clinic were provided smoking cessation information and related advice. Furthermore, efficacious smoking cessation treatments are not routinely available in the primary care setting. General care providers report that they are ineffective in the treatment of tobacco dependence, unless the patient is already suffering from a tobacco-related disease.

In many respects, tobacco dependence is considered a chronic disease that requires repeated intervention. Although some smokers maintain abstinence after the first quit attempt, the majority of smokers cycle through continuous patterns of relapse and remission. This cyclical pattern has been conceptualized in contemporary models of addictive behaviors, such as the Stages of Change (Prochaska, DiClemente, and Norcrosse, 1992), in which smokers are seen as progressing through stages of preparedness or "readiness" to stop smoking, take action to actually change smoking behavior, maintain those changes, relapse, and consider quitting again once they decide there are more cons than pros to smoking. Within this model, it is critical that intervention efforts are consistent with the smoker's stage of change.

Research indicates that approximately 60% of current smokers wish to quit smoking (Fava, Velicer, and Prochaska, 1995), but that very few request or receive professional assistance. Epidemiological studies report that approximately 70% of smokers have made at least one quit attempt (CDCP, 1997). Unfortunately, most individual cessation efforts are unsuccessful and result in a relapse. In fact, two-thirds of self-quitters relapse within 2 days (Hughes, Gulliver, Fenwick, et al., 1992). Of the reported 46% of smokers who have tried to quit smoking in the last year, only 7% were abstinent one year later (CDCP, 1993; Fiore and Baker, 1995; Hatziandreu et al., 1990). A failure to recognize the chronic nature of tobacco dependence and the critical physiological and cognitive factors maintaining smoking, may affect how smoking cessation programs are developed and implemented.

2. APPROACHES TO SMOKING CESSATION

2.1. Motivating Smokers to Quit

The US Public Health Service's (USPHS) Clinical Practice Guidelines on treating tobacco dependence highlights the essential role of clinicians and other health care providers in the process of identification, prevention, and cessation of tobacco use in the US (Fiore et al., 2000). The USPHS guideline recommend that clinicians provide cigarette smokers with basic information on smoking cessation and offer a brief screening intervention regardless of their expressed interest to quit smoking. Brief interventions, often shorter than 5 minutes, can elicit motivation to quit smoking, even in patients who do not express an interest in quitting (Fiore et al., 1995; Glynn, Manley, and Pechacek, 1995; Russell, Wilson, Taylor, and Baker, 1979). Brief interventions including a motivational interviewing component have been effective in smoking cessation efforts.

Miller and Rollnick's (1991) motivational interviewing uses a client-centered, directive method to elicit motivation to change by developing discrepancy between the current and desired behavior. Motivational enhancement might be more effective than emphasizing the adverse health effects of smoking because it offers social support, enhances motivation to quit smoking, increases self-efficacy, and provides advice on reducing withdrawal symptoms (Lennox and Taylor, 1994). It is also likely that the patient is aware of general adverse health effects related to smoking. If the patient is unwilling to quit smoking, the USPHS guideline recommends using motivational techniques to enhance the smoker's motivation to quit smoking.

2.2. Behavioral Approaches to Smoking Cessation

For patients who are willing or have expressed an interest to quit smoking, clinicians should be prepared to intervene. According to the USPHS guideline, smoking cessation interventions in a primary clinic should follow 5 major steps (5 A's) to systematically assess for tobacco dependence and encourage smoking cessation: 1) ask about tobacco use; 2) advise the patient to quit; 3) assess the patient's willingness to quit smoking; 4) assist the quit attempt; and 5) arrange for follow-ups. The steps can be delivered in a matter of minutes. Although the clinician should not expect the smoker to make immediate changes, simply providing this type of brief advice and motivation can help move smokers closer to quitting (Fiore et al., 2000). Follow-up contact does not necessarily need to occur in person. Contacts that occur by phone or by mail have been shown to be effective in relapse prevention (Brandon, Collins, Juliano, and Lazev, 2000).

Three types of counseling and behavioral therapies have also been effective in the treatment of nicotine dependence including psychosocial treatment, practical counseling (skills training and problem solving), and supportive therapy. Practical counseling includes providing basic information about smoking and successful quitting, teaching coping skills, and recognizing situations that may trigger relapse. Supportive treatment includes encouraging the patient to quit smoking, talk about the quitting process, and communicating with empathy and concern. Supportive treatment also involves social skills training, cigarette refusal, establishing a support network from friends/family, as well as initiating supporting behaviors outside the therapy setting.

2.3. Pharmacological Approaches to Smoking Cessation

In addition to brief interventions for smoking cessation, effective pharmacotherapies for smoking cessation can be provided in the primary care setting or purchased directly by the patient (the nicotine transdermal patch and nicotine gum). The following five cessation aids are typically offered as a first-line pharmacotherapy for smoking cessation: Bupropion, nicotine gum, oral nicotine inhaler, nicotine nasal spray, and nicotine transdermal patch (Fiore et al., 2000). These pharmacotherapies have been shown to significantly increase the duration of smoking abstinence. Pharmacotherapies include nicotine replacement therapy (NRT) and non-nicotine medications such as bupropion. Nicotine replacement therapy typically comes in the form of chewing gum, transdermal patch, nasal spray, lozenge, or oral inhaler. To date, nicotine chewing gum and nicotine transdermal patches are the only types of NRT available over-the-counter. Bupropion is a non-nicotine medication initially approved by the Federal Drug Administration (FDA) as an antidepressant (marketed as Wellbutrin) and, subsequently, as an aid to smoking cessation (Zyban). Bupropion has been shown to reduce the efffects of nicotine withdrawal and related symptoms as well as decrease craving for cigarettes. It is also associated with decreased postcessation weight gain, but weight gain tends to occur once the medication regimen is discontinued. Other non-nicotine drugs used for smoking cessation are clonidine, mecamylamine (a nicotine antagonist), Nortriptyline, and most recently verinicline (Chantix). However, the FDA issued an Early Communication in 2007 that Chantix had been associated with adverse events related to changes in behavior, agitation, depressed mood, suicidal ideation, and actual suicidal behavior, and is therefore used great caution and close monitoring. It should be noted that the best outcomes for smoking cessation are the result of combined behavioral counseling and pharmacotherapy (Fiore et al., 2000).

3. SMOKING CESSATION AND WOMEN

An important question regarding smoking cessation is whether there should be different interventions for men and women. Women may be at an increased risk of smoking-related diseases and tend to have more difficulty than men with smoking cessation. The Surgeon General's most recent publication on women and smoking reported that smoking-related diseases have reached epidemic levels in women (USDHHS, 2001). In the last 50 years, the percentage of female cancer deaths attributed to lung cancer has increased 600%. In 2000, it was estimated that more women died of lung cancer than breast, uterus, and ovary cancers combined. More recently, studies have found that serious smoking-related illnesses such as myocardial infarction (MI) might be greater for women than men (Prescott et al., 1998). The increased risks of MI and stroke are further intensified in women who use oral contraceptives (USDHHS, 1989). Finding efficacious smoking cessation programs is a current world-wide public health agenda, especially among women (World Health Organization, 1999).

Smoking cessation rates have been remarkable in men and relatively unchanged in women (Fiore et al., 1989; Giovino et al., 1995; Kandel et al., 1997). In the 1960s, approximately 52% of men and 34% of women smoked cigarettes regularly (USDHHS, 2001), which decreased to 43% of men and 31% of women in the 1970s (Pierce et al., 1989). Smoking prevalence curves of comparable birth cohorts indicate that women consistently report lower rates of smoking cessation (Escobido and Peddicord, 1996). Since 1990, the prevalence of cigarette smoking decreased less substantially in women than in men. Some studies even found an increase in smoking initiation among certain female minority and age groups. In fact, the Center for Disease Control and Prevention reported a dramatic increase in cigarette smoking among teenage girls. If the smoking prevalence rate continues to follow this trajectory, some researchers predict that the US will become the first nation where women will be the majority of smokers (Pierce et al., 1989).

A potential explanation of the differential smoking prevalence rate in men and women could be related to the fact that women appear to have more difficulty than men quitting smoking. The National Household Survey on Drug Abuse ($n = 87, 915$) found that women were more likely to meet nicotine dependence as defined by the Diagnostic and Statistical Manual for Mental Disorders, Fourth Edition (DSM-IV: American Psychiatric Association, 1994; Kandell, Chen, Warner, Kessler, and Grant, 1997). Clinical studies have examined sex differences in smoking cessation outcomes and have found considerably poorer outcomes in women (i.e., greater relapse) (Ockene, 1993; Swan, Ward, Carmelli, et al., 1993). Smoking cessation aids such as nicotine replacement therapy also appear to be less efficacious in women than in men (Perkins, 1996).

Although women may benefit from the same smoking cessation interventions as men, women appear to face different obstacles in smoking cessation including depression, weight concern, and hormonal cycles (Benowitz and Hatsukami, 1998). There may also be sex differences in nicotine self administration, nicotine discrimination, nicotine's effects on mood, smoking-related cognitions, the reinforcing effects of nicotine, and smoking expectancies including beliefs about weight suppression. It seems obvious that gaining a better understanding of the sex differences that do exist could help researchers develop smoking cessation programs that are better suited to help women quit smoking.

4. SMOKING BEHAVIOR IN WOMEN

Determining why the smoking prevalence rate has remained relatively unchanged in women while increasing markedly in teenage girls is also an important area of research. More females smoke cigarettes to control weight, improve affect, and reduce stress. For example, Vidrine, Anderson, Pollak, and Wetter (2006) examined self-generated smoking outcome expectancies in adolescents and found that boys endorsed several positive smoking expectancies including finding smoking pleasurable and enjoying the taste or smell of cigarettes, whereas, girls consistently generated a single positive outcome expectancy: weight control. Even very young girls/children have beliefs about smoking's appetite and weight control properties (Kendzor, Copeland, Stewart, Businelle, and Williamson, 2007). However, it remains unclear at what age this belief starts being viewed as a positive outcome of smoking, versus a negative outcome associated with adverse health consequences (Copeland, Diefendorff, Kendzor et al., 2007).

Tobacco use and body weight are inversely related and more women than men report smoking cigarettes to control body weight (Gritz, Klesges, and Meyers, 1989). Women's beliefs about smoking and appetite control also appear to be more salient relative to men's beliefs (Brandon and Baker, 1991; Copeland, Brandon, and Quinn, 1995; Wetter, Smith, Kenford, et al., 1994). In fact, even women who have successfully quit smoking, or exsmokers, maintain strong expectancies that cigarettes control appetite and weight (Brandon and Baker, 1991; Copeland et al., 1995). Younger women are more likely to report weight gain as a factor contributing to smoking relapse (Swan et al., 1993), although prospective studies have not yielded consistent results. Furthermore, female smokers who have more weight concerns are less likely to enter smoking cessation treatment (Ogden and Fox, 1994) and are more likely to drop out of treatment prematurely (Copeland, Martin, Geiselman, Rash, and Kendzor, 2006; Namenek Brouwer and Pomerleau, 2000).

There have been a number of studies that have contributed to our understanding of the relationship between weight control/dieting and nicotine use. These include studies that have linked smoking with clinically significant disordered eating among women, as well as subclinical, yet significantly elevated weight concerns. The latter behaviors and attitudes have often been conceptualized as dietary restraint (i.e., intention to control body weight by restrictive eating; Herman and Mack, 1975; Herman and Polivy, 1975) or weight concern. As a construct, dietary restraint has distinguished women especially vulnerable to smoking to control appetite and weight (Ogden, 1994). Disinhibition (i.e., loss of control eating resulting from a temporary disruption of dietary restraint due to emotional reactions or environmental events; Heatherton and Polivy, 1992), in addition to dietary restraint, has been indicative of postcessation weight gain among smokers (Hall, Ginsberg, and Jones, 1986). Interestingly, the relationship between restrained eating and smoking was found to be mediated by smoking outcome expectancies for appetite and weight control among college women smokers (Copeland and Carney, 2003).

A related construct, weight concern, has also been associated with smoking among women. Jeffery et al. (2000) points out an important distinction between two types of weight concern in the study of weight-concerned smokers, especially as pertains to smoking cessation outcomes. One type is weight concern specifically related to smoking and anticipated postcessation weight gain. A second type of weight concern is not related to smoking, but rather a more general concern. Although the two types of weight concern have been positively correlated with each other, smoking-related weight concern was associated with poor smoking cessation outcomes, whereas weight concern unrelated to smoking (e.g., dieting) was associated with more smoking cessation attempts (Jeffery et al., 2000).

Cigarette smoking has also been found to be prevalent among women with clinically significant eating disorders, especially those with Bulimia Nervosa. Females with Bulimia Nervosa have been found to endorse the belief that smoking decreases appetite, and that they smoked to avoid eating or to control weight (Bulik et al., 1992; Welch and Fairburn, 1998). With comorbidity rates reported to be as high as 50% between smoking and eating disorders in some studies, this relationship further underscores the significance of weight control and cigarette smoking among women.

Although there do not appear to be sex differences in the subjective effects of pure nicotine (Perkins, 2002), there may be contextual differences in smoking behavior between men and women. When confronted with a stressful situation or while experiencing a negative affect, smokers typically report a greater desire to smoke cigarettes (Perkins and Grobe, 1992). Women are more likely than men to smoke in response to a stressful situation, to relief negative affect, and for nicotine's sedative effects (Livson and Leino, 1988; Sorenson and Pechacek, 1987). Smoking to relax or cope with depressive symptoms and negative affect is more common among women than men (Oakley, Brannen, and Dodd, 1992).

Furthermore, mood fluctuations with the menstrual cycle might affect cigarette smoking in women. Symptoms such as depression and irritability are common during the premenstrual phase of the menstrual cycle and women may smoke more during this phase to relieve premenstrual symptoms. Smoking behavior has been found to vary significantly over the course of the menstrual cycle in women who endorse severe premenstrual symptoms; where they are more likely to increase smoking behavior during this phase of the menstrual cycle (Perkins, Donny, and Caggiula, 1999; Pomerleau, 1996). However, generally speaking smoking behavior has not been found to vary significantly across the menstrual cycle phases.

Nicotine may have differential reinforcing properties in men and women (Benowitz and Hatsukami, 1998; Perkins, 1999), whiah may affect smoking cessation outcomes. Perkins (1999) found that women may rely on psychosocial cues related to cigarette smoking more so than pure nicotine. For example, when women smoke cigarettes they achieve similar blood levels of nicotine as men; however, women do not report pure nicotine to be as reinforcing as men do (Perkins et al., 1996). Instead, women also appear to rely on the nonpharmacological factors of nicotine use including contextual and social cues (Perkins et al., 2006). Other cues that are associated with smoking such as particular moods or social settings might elicit the urge to smoke and cue smoking behavior during abstinence (Shiffman et al., 1996). Niaura and colleagues (1998) found that women's self-rated confidence in their ability to quit smoking significantly decreased when presented with imaginal exposure situations that were associated with smoking (e.g., occupational stress). Smoking cessation treatment in women might need to address environmental coping skills to improve smoking abstinence rates in this population.

In 2001, the Surgeon General highlighted the importance of determining whether gender-tailored smoking cessation interventions may increase smoking abstinence in specific groups of girls and women (USDHHS, 2001). In the last decade, numerous controlled laboratory studies on sex differences in the subjective and physiological effects of smoking have helped to dissimulate sex specific differences in smoking behavior. A greater understanding of the sex differences in smoking behavior and smoking-related concerns in women may enhance smoking cessation interventions for women. Smoking cessation interventions may need to incorporate gender specific topics such as weight concern, particular moods (e.g., negative affect, stress), and contextual factors to improve smoking abstinence rates in women. Future research is needed to evaluate the efficacy of tailored smoking cessation programs for women.

5. THE EFFECTS OF NICOTINE

In many ways nicotine, and its primary delivery vehicle-- preparations of the tobacco plant, presents itself as a paradox among drugs of abuse. Even an initial, cursory database search will yield, depending upon whether one has chosen tobacco as opposed to nicotine as a search term will yield information concerning a deadly mix of carcinogenic and hypoxia inducing poisons in the case of the former or a potentially highly effective therapeutic medication for a variety neurodegenerative conditions.

In everyday life, we know that despite the well known ability of nicotine to dramatically alter both neurochemical and neurophysiological proccesses in the central nervous system (CNS) as well as hormonal and neuromodulatory activity in the endocrine system – there are no reflections of this in criminal justice and public policy edicts regulating acceptable patterns of nicotine self-administration per se. In the United States there are currently no federal or state statutes prohibiting, for example, operation of a motor vehicle while under under the influence of psychoactive doses of nicotine. To the best of the author's knowledge the same cannot be said for any other behaviorally reinforcing psychoactive substance whose most common administration route is direct inhalation of the vaporous form of the drug –widely regarded as the most rapid administration route for penetration into the CNS.

Nicotine in tobacco brings illness and death to millions of people. Yet nicotine when extracted from the tobacco plant and purified has the potential to be a valuable pharmaceutical agent. Nicotine fairly specifically binds to the cholinergic nicotinic gating site on cationic ion channels in receptors throughout the body. This action initiates the release of a variety of neurotransmitters including biogenic amines such as the catecholamines norepinephrine and dopamine as well as indolamines such as serotonin. Pure nicotine has no known carcinogenic properties (refs) and can be administered in numerous ways including transdermal patches and tablets. Evidence exists that chronic administration of nicotine may result in: (1) positive reinforcement, (2) negative reinforcement, (3) reduction of body weight, (4) enhancement of information processing performance (eg. vigilence, information retrieval, reduced influence of distractive environmental stimuli on measures of sustained attention, etc.). Additionally, evidence exists that nicotine may offer protection against: (5) Parkinson's disease (6) Tourette's disease and (7) Alzheimers disease. Although the reliability of these effects are highly variable, the relevant data continue to generate both laboratory and clinical research studies geared to find more therapeutic applications for this interesting compound.

In an an acute, placebo-controlled double-blind of the actions of nicotine on various measures of mood and attention (Levin Connors, Sparrow, Hinton, Erhardt, Meck, Rose, and March, 1995), six smokers and 11 nonsmokers were assessed with the Clinical Global Impressions (CGI) scale, Hopkins' symptom check list (SCL-90-R), the Profile of Mood States (POMS), Conners' computerized Continuous Performance Test (CPT), the Stroop test, and an interval-timing task. The smokers underwent overnight deprivation from smoking and were given a 21 mg/day nicotine skin patch for 4.5 h during a morning session. The nonsmokers were given a 7 mg/day nicotine skin patch for 4.5 h during a morning session. Active and placebo patches were given in a counterbalanced order approximately 1 week apart. Nicotine caused a significant overall nicotine-induced improvement on the CGI. This effect was significant when only the nonsmokers were considered, which indicated that it was not due merely to withdrawal relief. Nicotine caused significantly increased vigor as measured by the POMS test. Nicotine caused an overall significant reduction in reaction time (RT) on the CPT. Nicotine improved accuracy of time estimation and lowered variability of time-estimation response curves. Because improvements occurred among nonsmokers, the authors concluded that the nicotine effects were not merely reflecting a relief of withdrawal symptoms.

5.1. Sex Differences in the Effects of Nicotine

Interestingly, it is becoming clear that marked sex differences mediate many of the psychoactive effects of nicotine. A laboratory animal study (Donny et al., 2000) in which male and female Sprague-Dawley rats were allowed to self-administer nicotine at one of four doses (0.02-0.09 mg/kg, free base) on both fixed and progressive ratio schedules of reinforcement found that acquisition of self-administration at the lowest dose was faster in females than males. However, few sex differences were found in the number of active responses, number of infusions, or total intake of nicotine during stable fixed ratio self-administration. In contrast, females reached higher break points on a progressive ratio. For both schedules, females had shorter latencies to earn their first infusion of each session and demonstrated higher rates of both inactive and timeout responding.

A recent human study of male and female nonsmokers (File, Fluck, and Leahy, 2001)--a double-blind, placebo-controlled study—examined the effects of nicotine (2 mg administered by inhalator) on the cognitive performance of male and female non-smoking students and on mood changes following a moderately stressful task. The groups were matched for age and IQ, and did not differ in pre-test measures of anxiety, depression, extroversion and neuroticism or in their weekly alcohol or daily caffeine intake. Results showed that exposure to moderate stress significantly increased ratings of anxiety, discontent and aggression and nicotine blocked these mood changes in females, but enhanced them in males. This suggests that young women may start regular smoking as a form of stress self-medication, which implies that preventative and smoking cessation programs would be more successful in women if they addressed issues of stress and anxiety, which may be core factors underlying initiation and maintenance of regular smoking.

5.2. Nicotine and Appetite/Weight-Related Effects in Females

Women often report that they smoke cigarettes to avoid weight gains and that they relapse after abstaining from tobacco because of weight gains. Men also report these concerns but to a lesser extent. This gender difference may reflect sociological and cultural pressures about physical appearance, or it may reflect sex differences in the effects of nicotine. However, women actually get more weight-control benefits from smoking, and are more likely to experience postcessation weight gain than men (Perkins, Mitchell, and Epstein, 1995; Pirke and Laessle, 1993), and they are also more likely to experience increased appetite during nicotine withdrawal than are men (e.g., Perkins et al., 1995).

Behavioral studies of laboratory animals have indicated that food deprivation and caloric restriction may result in increased self-administration of nicotine (De La Garza and Johanson, 1987; Lang, Latiff, McQueen, and Singer, 1977). A laboratory study using female rats (Grunberg, Bowen, and Winders, 1986) showed that nicotine administration decreased normal body weight gains and cessation of nicotine was accompanied by significant increases in body weight compared to controls. In contrast to previous studies of male rats, the nicotine-related changes in body weight were accompanied by changes in bland food and water consumption. These findings indicate that females are more sensitive than males to the effects of nicotine on body weight and feeding during and after drug administration.

6. SUGGESTIONS FOR ASSISTING WOMEN WITH WEIGHT CONCERN QUIT SMOKING

Studies attempting to prevent postcessation weight gain and smoking cessation have yielded mixed results, and some have even indicated that weight gain was associated with successful smoking cessation (Hall, Turnstall, Vila, and Duffy, 1992). More recently, cognitive-behavioral therapy to reduce weight concerns improved smoking cessation outcomes in weight-concerned women, whereas behavioral weight control counseling did not (Perkins et al., 2001), indicating that addressing cognitions about perceived significance of weight gain may be more beneficial than acquiring and using specific weight control skills.

Typical weight gain following smoking cessation is 6-9 pounds (e.g., Perkins, 1993). Individuals who smoke heavily are at greatest risk to gain weight during a cessation attempt. There is also some evidence that women using cigarettes for weight control to prevent disinhibited eating, may be at risk for excessive weight gain once they stop smoking. The current guidelines suggest making patients aware of the possibility of weight gain and letting them know that modest weight gain poses a much less risk to health than does continued smoking. According to research findings, women should be highly encouraged to avoid extreme weight control measures and dietary restriction while attempting to quit smoking. This will likely put them at risk of being unsuccessful at both smoking cessation and weight control. Use of bupropion (Zyban) should be encouraged, since it is associated with less postcessation weight gain than the other pharmacotherapies. However, this advantage appears to last only as long as individuals are taking bupropion, therefore women should be prepared and counseled in advance for how to best cope with what may be a high risk for relapse when weight gain occurs. Research also seems to suggest that women who quit smoking in the follicular phase of their menstrual cycle may have better outcomes, since increased desire to smoke and to alleviate negative affect have been associated with the late luteal phase (Allen, Hatsukami, Christianson, and Nelson, 1999).

Future Directions

We have reviewed literature regarding females' use of nicotine in relation to weight-related issues and concerns. There appear to be social/environmental, physiological, including hormonal influence, and cognitive variables that influence smoking in women in ways that are different from men. The following issues in particular should be addressed in the near future in order to increase our understanding of the clinical course of smoking in women and to improve the outcomes for women in smoking cessation interventions.

1. Gender-specific clinical interventions should be developed, implemented, and assessed at various follow-up intervals to examine outcomes (i.e., abstinence rates);
2. These interventions should specifically target factors that have been shown to be problematic for women during cessation attempts. These factors include, mood, outcome expectancies regarding appetite and weight control and mood management, and the effects of hormonal fluctuations on nicotine withdrawal symptoms, such as appetite and desire to smoke;

3. Follow-up assessments should continue for significant length of time postcessation. This would help to inform relapse prevention efforts specific to women smokers;

4. Controlled, laboratory studies that examine the influence of the menstrual/estrous cycle on nicotine self-administration and withdrawal in female humans and animals should continue to be conducted. The results of these studies seem particularly promising in understanding the unique process of nicotine use, dependence, withdrawal and cessation in women;

5. Cessation intervention protocols that are specific to women with eating disorders, namely Bulimia Nervosa, need to be developed and tested. The comorbid diagnosis of nicotine dependence and Bulimia Nervosa likely complicates the treatment of either disorder on its own. Such interventions would be aided by investigations of possible common etiologies underlying the two disorders.

REFERENCES

Allen, S. S., Hatsukami, D. K., Christianson, D., and Nelson, D. (1999). Withdrawal and premenstrual symptomatology during the menstrual cycle in short-term smoking abstinence: Effects of menstrual cycle on smoking abstinence. *Nicotine and Tobacco Research, 1*, 129-142.

Benowitz, N. L. and Hatsukami, D. (1998). Gender differences in the pharmacology of nicotine addiction. *Addiction Biology, 3*, 383-404.

Brandon, T.H. and Baker, T.B. (1991). The Smoking Consequences Questionnaire: The subjective expected utility of smoking in college students. *Psychological Assessment, 3*, 484-491.

Brandon, T. H., Collins, B. N., Juliano, L. M. and Lazev, A. B. (2000). Preventing relapse among former smokers: a comparison of minimal interventions through telephone and mail. *Journal of Consulting and Clinical Psychology, 68*, 103-113.

Breslau N. and Peterson, E. L. (1996). Smoking cessation in young adults: Age at initiation of cigarette smoking and other suspected includes. *American Journal of Public Health, 86*, 253-256.

Brownell, K. D. and Cohen, L. R. (1995). Adherence to dietary regimens 2: Components of effective interventions. *Behavioral Medicine, 20*, 155-164.

Bulik, C. M., Sullivan, P. F., Epstein, L. H., McKee, M., Kaye, W. H., Dahl, R. E. et al.

(1992). Drug use in women with anorexia and bulimia nervosa. *International Journal of Eating Disorders, 11*, 213-225.

Center for Disease Control and Prevention (1997). Perspectives in disease prevention and health promotion smoking-attributable mortality and years of potential life lost - United States, 1984. *Morbidity and Mortality Weekly Reports, 46(20)*, 444-451.

Center for Disease Control and Prevention (1993). Smoking cessation during previous year among adults – United States, 1990 and 1991. *Morbidity and Mortality Weekly Reports, 42*, 504 507.

Copeland, A.L., Brandon, T.H., Quinn, E.P. (1995). The Smoking Consequences Questionnaire-Adult: Measurement of smoking outcome expectancies of experienced smokers. *Psychological Assessment, 7*, 484-494.

Copeland, A. L. and Carney, C. E. Smoking expectancies as mediators between dietary restraint and disinhibition and smoking in college student women. *Experimental and Clinical Psychopharmacology, 11*, 247-251.

Copeland, A. L., Diefendorff, J. M., Kendzor, D. E., Rash, C. J., Businelle, M. S., Patterson, S. M. and Williamson, D. A. (2007). Measurement of smoking outcome expectancies in children: Development of the Smoking Consequences Questionnaire-Child. *Psychology of Addictive Behaviors, 21*, 469-477.

Copeland, A. L., Martin, P. D., Geiselman, P. J., Rash, C. J., and Kendzor, D. E. (2006). Predictors of pretreatment attrition from smoking cessation among pre- and postmenopausal, weight-concerned women. *Eating Behaviors, 7*, 243-251.

De La Garza, R. and Johanson, C. E. (1987). The effects of food deprivation on the self-administration of psychoactive drugs. *Drug and Alcohol Dependence, 19*, 17-27.

Donny, E. C., Caggiula, A. R., Rowell, P. P., Gharib, M. A., Maldovan, V., Booth, S., Mielke, M. M, Hoffman, A. and McCallum, S. (2000). Nicotine self-administration in rats: estrous cycle effects, sex differences, and nicotinic receptor binding. *Psychopharmacology, 151*, 392-405.

Fairburn, C. G. (1995). *Overcoming binge eating*. New York: Guilford Press.

Fava, J. L., Velicer, W. F., and Prochaska, J. O. (1995). Applying the transtheoretical model to a representative sample of smokers. *Addictive Behaviors, 20*, 189-203.

File, S. E., Fluck, E. and Leahy, A. (2001). Nicotine has calming effects on stress-induced mood changes in females but enhances aggressive mood in males. *International Journal of Neuropsychopharmacology, 4*, 371-376.

Fiore, M. C., Jorenby, D. E., Schensky, A. E., Smith, S. S., Bauer, R. R., and Baker, T. B. (1995). Smoking status as the new vital sign: effect on assessment and intervention in patients who smoke. *Mayo Clinic Proceedings, 70*, 209-213.

Fiore, M. C., and Baker, T. B. (1995). Smoking cessation treatment and the good doctor club. *American Journal of Public Health, 85*, 161-163.

Fiore, M. C., Bailey, W. C., Cohen, S. J., Dorfman, S. F., Goldstein, M. G., Gritz, E. R., et al. (2000). *Treating tobacco use and dependence. Clinical Practice Guideline*. Rockville, MD: U.S. Department of Health and Human Services. Public Health Service.

Fiore, M. C., Novotny, T. E., Pierce, J. P., Hatziandreu, E. J., Patel, K. M., Davis, R. M. (1989). Trends in cigarette smoking in the United States. The changing influence of gender and race. *Journal of the American Medical Association, 261*, 49-55.

French, S. A., Jeffery, R. W., Klesges, L. M., and Forster, J. L. (1995). Weight concerns and change in smoking behavior over two years in a working population. *American Journal of Public Health, 85*, 720-722.

French, S. A., Jeffery, R. W., Pirie, P. L., and McBride, C. M. (1992). Do weight concerns hinder smoking cessation efforts? *Addictive Behaviors, 17*, 219-226.

Giovino, G. A. (2002). Epidemiology of tobacco use in the United States. *Oncogene, 21*, 7326-7340.

Giovino, G. A. (1995). Epidemiology of tobacco use and dependence. *Epidemiological Reviews, 17*, 48-65.

Glynn, T. J., Manley, M. W., and Pechacek, T. F. (1990). Physician-initiated smoking cessation program: the National Cancer Institute trials. *Progress in Clinical Biological Research, 339*, 11-25.

Gritz, E. R., Klesges, R. C., and Meyers, A. W. (1989). The smoking and body weight relationship: implications for intervention and postcessation weight control. *Annals of Behavioral Medicine, 11,* 144-153.

Grunberg, N. E., Bowen, D. J., and Winders, S. E. (1986). Effects of nicotine on body weight and food consumption in female rats. *Psychopharmacology, 90,* 101-105.

Hall, S. M., Ginsberg, D., and Jones, R. T., (1986). Smoking cessation and weight gain. *Journal of Consulting and Clinical Psychology, 54,* 342-346.

Hall, S. M., Turnstall, C. D., Vila, K. L. and Duffy, J. (1992). Weight gain prevention and smoking cessation: Cautionary findings. *American Journal of Public Health, 82,* 799-803.

Hatziandreu, E. J., Pierce, J. P., Lefkopoulou, M., et al. (1990). Quitting smoking in the United States in 1986. *Journal of the National Cancer Institute, 82,* 1402-1406.

Heatherton, T. F. and Polivy, J. (1992). Chronic dieting and eating disorders: a spiral model. In Crowther, J. H., Tannenbaum, D. L., Hobfoll, S. E., Stephens, M. P. (Eds.), *The etiology of bulimia nervosa: the individual and family context.* Washington: Hemisphere Publishing Corp. p. 133-155.

Herman, C. P. and Mack, D. (1975). Restrained and unrestrained eating. *Journal of Personality, 43,* 647-660.

Herman, C. P. and Polivy, J. (1975). Anxiety, restraint, and eating behavior. *Journal of Abnormal Psychology, 84,* 666-672.

Hughes, J. R., Gulliver, S. B., Fenwick, J. W., et al. (1992). Smoking cessation among self-quitters. *Health Psychology, 11,* 331-334.

Jeffery, R. W., Hennrikus, D. J., Lando, H. A., Murray, D. M., and Liu, J. W. (2000). Reconciling conflicting findings regarding postcessation weight concerns and success in smoking cessation. *Health Psychology, 19,* 242-246.

Kandel, D., Chen, K., Warner, L. A., Kessler, R. C., Grant, B. (1997). Prevalence and demographic correlates of symptoms of last year dependence on alcohol, nicotine, marijuana and cocaine in the U.S. population. *Drug and Alcohol Dependence, 44,* 11-29.

Kendzor, D. E., Copeland, A. L., Stewart, T. M., Businelle, M. S., Williamson, D. A. (2007). Weight-related concerns associated with smoking in young children. *Addictive Behaviors, 32,* 598-607.

Lang, W. J., Latiff, A. A., McQueen, A., and Singer, G. (1977). Self administration of nicotine with and without a food delivery schedule. *Pharmacology, Biochemistry, and Behaviour, 7,* 65-70.

Levin Connors, Sparrow, Hinton, Erhardt, Meck, Rose, and March (1995).

Livson, N., and Leino, E. V. (1988). Cigarette smoking motives: factorial structure and gender difference in a longitudinal study. *International Journal of Addiction, 23,* 535-544.

Miller, W. R., and Rollnick, S. (1991). Motivational interviewing: Preparing people to change addictive behavior. New York: Guilford Press.

Namenek Brouwer, R. J. and Pomerleau, C. S. (2000). "Prequit attrition" among weight-concerned women smokers. *Eating Behaviors, 2,* 145-151.

Niaura, R., Shadel, W. G., Abrams, D. B., et al. (1998). Individual differences in cue reactivity among smokers trying to quit: effects of gender and cue type. *Addictive Behaviors, 23,* 209-224.

Oakley, A., Brannen, J., and Dodd, K. (1992). Young people, gender and smoking in the United Kingdom. *Health Promotion International, 7,* 75-88.

Ockene, J. K. (1987). Smoking intervention: The expanding role of the physician. *American Journal of Public Health, 77,* 782-783.

Ockene, J. K. (1993). Smoking among women across the lifespan: prevalence, interventions, and implications for cessation research. *Annals of Behavioral Medicine, 15,* 135-148.

Ogden, J. (1994). Effects of smoking cessation, restrained eating, and motivational states on food intake in the laboratory. *Health Psychology, 13,* 114-121.

Ogden, J. and Fox, P. (1994). Examination of the use of smoking for weight control in restrained and unrestrained eaters. *International Journal of Eating Disorders, 84,* 1818-1820.

Pederson, L. L., Baskerville, J. C., and Wanklin, J. M. (1982). Multivariate statistical models for predicting change in smoking behavior following physician advice to quit smoking. *Preventative Medicine, 11,* 536-549.

Perkins, K. A. (1993). Weight gain following smoking cessation. *Journal of Consulting and Clinical Psychology, 61,* 768-777.

Perkins, K. A. (1996). Sex differences in nicotine vs. non-nicotine reinforcement as determinants of tobacco smoking. *Experimental and Clinical Psychopharmacology, 4,* 166-177.

Perkins, K. A. (1999). Nicotine discrimination in men and women. *Pharmacology, Biochemistry, and Behavior, 64,* 295-299.

Perkins, K. A., Donny, E., Cagguila, A. R. (1999). Sex differences in nicotine effects and self-administration: human and animal evidence. *Nicotine and Tobacco Research, 1,* 301-305.

Perkins, K. A., and Grobe, J. E. (1992). Increased desire to smoking during acute stress. *British Journal of Addiction, 87,* 1037-1040.

Perkins, K. A., Jacobs, L., Sanders, M., Caggiula, M. (2002). Sex differences in the subjective and reinforcing effects of cigarette nicotine dose. *Psychopharmacology, 163,* 194-201.

Perkins, K. A., Doyle, T., Ciccocioppo, M., Conklin, C., Sayette, M., Caggiula, A. (2006). Sex differences in the influence of nicotine dose instructions on the reinforcing and self-reported rewarding effects of smoking. *Psychopharmacology, 184,* 600-607.

Perkins, K. A., Marcus, M. D., Levine, M. D., D'Amico, D., Miller, A., Broge, M., Ashcom, J., and Shiffman, S. (2001). Cognitive-behavioral therapy to reduce weight concerns improves smoking cessation outcome in weight-concerned women. *Journal of Consulting and Clinical Psychology, 69,* 604-613.

Perkins, K. A., Mitchell, S. L., Epstein, L. H. (1995). Physiological and subjective responses to food cues as a function of smoking abstinence and dietary restraint. *Physiology and Behavior, 58,* 373-378.

Pierce, J. P., Fiore, M. C., Novotny, T. E., Hatziandreu, E. J., and Davis, R. M. (1989). Trends in cigarette smoking in the United States. *Journal of the American Medical Association, 261,* 61-65.

Pirke, K. M. and Laessle, R. G. (1993). Restrained eating. In A. J. Stunkard and T. A. Wadden (Eds.), *Obesity: Theory and therapy, 2nd Edition,* pp. 151-162. Raven Press: New York.

Pomerleau, C. S. (1996). Smoking and nicotine replacement treatment issues specific to women. *American Journal of Health Behavior, 00,* 291-299.

Prochaska, J.O., DiClemente, C.C., and Norcross, J.C. (1992). In search of how people change: Applications to addictive behaviors. *American Psychologist, 47,* 1102-1114.

Russell, M. A., Wilson, C., Taylor, C., and Baker, C. D. (1979). Effect of general practitioners' advice against smoking. *British Medical Journal, 2,* 231-235.

Shiffman, S., Gnys, M., Richards, T. J. et al. (1996). Temptations to smoke after quitting: a comparison of lapsers and maintainers. *Health Psychology, 15,* 455-461.

Sorenson, G., and Pechacek, T. F. (1987). Attitudes toward smoking cessation among men and women. *Journal of Behavioral Medicine, 10,* 129-137.

Swan, G. E., Ward, M. N., Carmelli, D. et al. (1993). Differential rates of relapse in subgroups of male and female smokers. *Journal of Clinical Epidemiology, 46,* 1041-1053.

Thorndike, A. N., Rigotti, N. A., Stafford, R. S., and Singer, D. E. (1998). National patterns in the treatment of smokers by physicians. *Journal of the American Medical Association, 279,* 604-608.

US Department of Health and Human Services (2001). *Women and smoking: a report of the Surgeon General.* Rockville, MD. US Department of Health and Human Services, Public Health Service, Office of the Surgeon General; Washington, D. C.

Vidrine, J. I., Anderson, C. B., Pollak, K. I., and Wetter, D. W. (2006). Gender differences in adolescent smoking: mediator and moderator effects of self-generated expected smoking outcomes. *American Jmurnal od Health Promotion, 20,* 383-387.

Welch, S. L. and Fairburn, C. G. (1998). Smoking and Bulimia Nervosa. *International Journal of Eating Disorders, 23,* 433-437.

Wetter, D. W., Smith, S. S., Kenford, S. L., et al. (1994). Smoking outcome expectancies: factor structure, predictive validity, and discriminant validity. *Journal of Abnormal Psychology,103,* 801-811.

World Health Organization (1999). WHO International Conference on Tobacco and Health, Kobe, *Making a Difference in Tobacco and Health: Avoiding the Tobacco Epidemic in Women and Youth.* Kobe, Japan, 14-18 November, Kobe Declaration; http://tobacco-.who.int/en/fctc/kobe/declaration.html.

In: Smoking Cessation: Theory, Interventions and Prevention   ISBN: 978-1-60021-591-9
Editor: Jerome E. Landow   © 2008 Nova Science Publishers, Inc.

Chapter 11

WISHING AND ACCOMPLISHING: MOTIVATIONS FOR SMOKING CESSATION

Éva Susánszky, Zsuzsa Szántó and Mária Kopp
Institute of Behavioral Sciences, Semmelweis University, Budapest, Hungary

ABSTRACT

Introduction: The aim of our study was to bring to light the motivational differences between the successful quitters and the smokers who just contemplate on quitting. We analyzed self-reported motivations of ex-smokers' smoking cessation and the reasoning of current smokers who consider quitting.

Material and methods: The study is based on the Hungarostudy Health Panel (HHP) which is the second wave of the Hungarostudy 2002, a national representative health survey of the adult Hungarian population. The Hungarostudy Health Panel was completed in 2006. In the follow-up study data of 3701 persons were analyzed. Cessation motivations were examined on the basis of various self-reported health status indicators, education, self-rated economic situation, and sources of social support. To the original questionnaire some new blocks were added; comparing to base-line, smoking habits have been deeper investigated with further inquiries.

Results: About half of the respondents are never smokers, 21 percent have quitted and 28 percent reported thoughts about giving up smoking. More than half of the current smokers contemplate on smoking cessation. Among the people with a smoking history, ex-smokers and contemplating current smokers alike (38-40 %), disease prevention was mentioned as the single most important reason of cessation. Financial reasons were mostly mentioned by current smokers; ex-smokers were more likely to explain their decision with deteriorating health, especially with the occurrence of certain diseases. Cardio-vascular morbidity played the most important role in smoking cessation. Cancers, respiratory disease and diabetes also increased significantly the odds of quitting. High blood pressure stimulated quitting considerations but not cessation. Social pressure was an underlying reason of quitting among women and among older persons. Among current smokers, the cohabitants and the better-off tended to entertain thoughts of quitting.

Conclusion: Our study confirmed the great importance of the experience of cardiovascular diseases in the smoking cessation: although people emphasize preventive purposes of their cessation efforts, existing circulatory and heart problems play the major role both in actual cessation and in quitting considerations. The odds of having serious thoughts about quitting are almost three times higher among smokers who developed cardiovascular disease; ex-smokers also attribute their quitting to treated circulatory illnesses.

1. INTRODUCTION

In the Hungarian population which shows a high and relatively permanent prevalence of smoking, the use of tobacco causes a multitude of avoidable disease. Similarly to other developed countries, smoking is the leading preventable cause of disease and death in Hungary.

Smoking may induce harm to nearly every organ of the body. Active smokers are at higher risk of several diseases that are either lethal or lead to permanent disabilities such as cancers, diseases of the respiratory and circulatory systems, organs of the vision, and an impaired general health [Edwards 2004, Peto 2000]. On the other hand, quitting smoking has been proved to result in benefits reducing health risks and improving health in general. Smoking cessation is one of the most effective ways to enhance the chances of improving one's health and prolonging one's life [Edwards 2004, Godfredsen 2003, Ostbye 2002, Peto 2000, Wilson 2000]. The earlier people stop smoking, the higher the chance of the increase of life expectancy [Taylor 2002]. However, it is harder to quit smoking in younger age [Ockene 2000], probably because younger people are less likely to encounter the most important motivating factor, the deterioration of health. Another demographic factor, gender, also predicts success of the cessation attempts: some studies suggest that women have more difficulties quitting smoking than men [Mackay, Amos 2003].

Starting and maintaining smoking are complex behaviors with genetic, personality, psychological and environmental factors contributing their variance. Data suggest that individual differences in susceptibility to nicotine dependence may be mediated by genetic factors [Batra 2003, Perkins 2001, Surgeon General 2001, Lerman 2000], for example the potential role of olfactory receptor genes were implicated [Fürst 2004]. In twin studies the heritability estimates for smoking have ranged from 46 to 84 percent, indicating a substantial genetic component to smoking. Personality traits such as novelty seeking, harm avoidance, and reward dependence, psychological characteristics like attitudes, expectations, coping strategies, and self-efficacy, and some mental disorders, for example depression and anxiety are documented to have an impact on the development of the smoking habit [Kremer at al 2005, Urbán 2005]. The most important environmental factors that have also been found to contribute to the risk of initiation and persistence of smoking are certain forms of social learning, social cohesion, and sets of models concerning smoking [Urbán 2005]. In adolescence, good peer relations can have both negative and positive effects on starting and maintaining smoking, depending on the norm system and behavioral models of the peer group.

In spite of the fact that the harmful consequences of smoking are well known in the population, tobacco use, especially cigarette smoking is a widely acceptable social behavior of adults in Hungary. Early initiation and habituation is commonly disapproved but it is often rewarded by peers as a symbol of bravery, independence and maturity in fairly young ages. The social tolerance toward smoking weakens the quitting intentions and reduces the chances of successful cessation. On the other hand, various legislative and governmental measures of tobacco control – most importantly increasing the taxes and price of tobacco products and banning or restricting smoking in public and work places – encourage quitting among those who are considering it.

1.1. Prevalence of Smoking in Hungary

For the estimation of the number and proportion of smokers in the population several representative population surveys can be of use. Based on the data available from the latest survey, 38-42 percent of adult men and 23-29 percent of adult women are regular smokers in Hungary [KSH 2002, HUNGAROSTUDY 2002, OLEF 2003, WHO 2006]. Surveys repeated in different times show that the proportion of male smokers is somewhat decreasing or at least stagnating while smoking is increasing among women and young people. According to the Hungarian data of the Global Youth Tobacco Survey [Németh 2003] in the age group of 13-16, the prevalence of smoking is 33 percent (both for girls and boys). Habituation starts at younger and younger age. Both Hungarian men and women acquired the habit of smoking in their teens; women started to smoke somewhat earlier than men. Women often suspend smoking when they become pregnant but later they return to their habit. However, smoking is relatively frequent even among pregnant women: 16 percent of the general female population and 26 percent of gypsy women are regular smokers. Men usually quit smoking at an older age, especially when they have already developed circulatory disease. When this happens many of them lastingly, often permanently, cease to smoke. With increasing age, the proportion of smokers is decreasing in the Hungarian population: it is only 6.3 percent among people aged 65 and older [HUNGAROSTUDY 2002]: 7 percent among women and 17 percent of men [OLEF 2003].

1.2. Extent of Cigarette Consumption

The per capita cigarette consumption is prominently high for decades. The average consumption per adult per year (the number of cigarettes purchased, divided by the population aged 15 and above) was 2151.4 cigarettes, or slightly more than 6 cigarettes consumed daily. This is much higher than the EU average of 1654.2 cigarettes per year or 4.5 per day [WHO HFA]. According to official commercial statistics the consumption has been decreasing during the last couple of years; however, because of the growing illegal cigarette market, these statistics cannot be accepted without certain reservation. Self-administered population surveys that rely on self reports estimate the daily average consumption as significantly higher, somewhere between half and one package a day [Csoboth 2006]. The CINDI health survey conducted in 2002 in Hungary found that 42 percent of current smoker men and 44 percent of current smoker women consumed at least 20 cigarettes per day; 21 percent of men and 35 percent of women reported smoking about 10 cigarettes daily [WHO CINDI 2002]. According to the more moderate figures of the OLEF 2003 survey which was conducted by the Hungarian health administration, about one quarter of men and one tenth of women smoked al least one whole package of cigarettes every day [OLEF 2003].

1.3. Passive Smoking

Forty percent of adult Hungarians and among them 20 percent of non-smokers live in their household together with current smokers, according to questionnaire surveys. A 2002 survey found that every fifth active worker spends more than five hours per day together with smokers in the workplace. Almost three quarter (73 %) of the smokers and 38 percent of non-smokers share their workplace with smoking individuals [Antmann 2005]. These data direct the attention to the insufficiency of law-enforcement concerning the protection of the work force from passive smoking and keeping the workplaces smoke-free.

1.4. Smoking-Attributed Morbidity

The inter-county comparative statistical analysis of the WHO concluded that smoking places the greatest burden of disease on the Hungarian population. The burden was estimated using the prevalence of oral tobacco use and the current levels of smoking impact (such as lung cancer morbidity and mortality). The comparison was based on the DALY indicator which represents the years of healthy life lost because of being in states of poor health or disability and the time lost due to premature mortality (table1).

Table 1. Ten leading risk factors as causes of disease burden measured in DALYs in Hungary (2002)

	Males		Females	
Rank	Risk factors	DALY (%)	Risk factors	DALY (%)
1.	Tobacco	25.5	Tobacco	15.2
2.	Alcohol	22.8	High blood pressure	11.8
3.	High blood pressure	12.6	High BMI	9.1
4.	High cholesterol	9.5	High cholesterol	8.1
5.	High BMI	6.7	Alcohol	6.8
6.	Low fruit and vegetable intake	6.2	Low fruit and vegetable intake	5.0
7.	Physical inactivity	3.8	Physical inactivity	3.9
8.	Lead	1.1	Unsafe sex	2.1
9.	Iatrogenic causes	1.0	Indoor smoke from solid fuels	1.2
10.	Illicit drugs	1.0	Childhood sexual abuse	1.0

Source: WHO.

1.5. Smoking-Attributed Mortality

About one third of the Hungarian population aged 15 and above is regular smoker and one out of two, an estimated 1.3 million people, will die because of a tobacco-attributed cause. The indicators of smoking-related mortality place Hungary in the upper third of the

European countries. The Standard Mortality Ratio (SDR) was 491.02 per 100.000 in 2003, while in the EU member countries (members before May 2004) the SDR was 216.7, i.e. less than half of the Hungarian value. Even the ten countries that become EU members in May 2004 have a much lower average SDR, 368.65 per 100.000. Only other former Communist countries show higher smoking related mortality rates [WHO HFA 2005].

In 2003, 16 percent of total mortality was attributed to smoking: 23 percent of male mortality and 9 percent of female mortality in all ages. The average number of years lost because of smoking was 21 years for adult males and 16 years for females. On the other hand, during the last 13 years the smoking-attributed mortality has dropped (table 2) and indeed it decreased faster than that of the total mortality while the proportion of smokers has not changed. This positive tendency appears in the female population as well despite the increasing number of female smokers.

**Table 2. Changes in the proportion of smoking-attributed deaths
in total mortality, all ages, between 1999 and 2003 in Hungary (%)**

	1990	2000	2003
Males	29	31	23
Females	9	11	9
All	20	21	16

Sources: WHO HFA and KSH.

1.6. Age Structure of the *Smoking-Attributed Mortality*

Smoking-attributed mortality is not characteristic in the population below 35 years. After that, tobacco-related deaths appear and the number steadily increases with age. Around 60, the rate of mortality attributable to smoking starts to decrease. By the latest available data in 1999, 35 percent of total mortality was tobacco-related in the 35-64 age group of males and 17 percent in the same age group of females. In the age group 65 and older, 27 percent of males and 8 percent of females died in a smoking related disease.

1.7. Prevention

Although pulmonologists tried to raise the public awareness concerning the dangers of the widespread heavy smoking and the consequent passive smoking as early as in the 1960s, the Hungarian Parliament passed the legislation of restrictions on smoking in the workplace and other public places as the protection of non-smokers only in 1999 ["Act XLII, n.d.]. The Act and the programs that followed it enhanced the social acceptance of the efforts aimed to establish and maintain a smoke free-environment and thus decrease involuntary passive smoking. The restrictions were further facilitated by the preparations for joining the European Union because the harmonization of legislation required new or modified regulations of the taxation, production, promotion, and trade of tobacco products. As a consequence of the scarce resources and the insufficient governmental commitment, the anti-smoking regulations have not yet changed into an integrated high priority public health initiative.

Since the 1990s each public health program has set the objective of controlling and restricting smoking, especially at the workplaces and other public places. However, according to the data available, no significant success has been achieved so far: the proportion of smokers remained about the same [OLEF 2000, 2003] although the amount of cigarettes in legal trade has decreased considerably.

In 2003 the Parliament approved the National Public Health Program for a 10 year term. The program's main objective is to improve the health of the population to a level more adequate to the social and economic status of Hungary. The most important requirement is to bring Hungarian life expectancy at birth closer to the EU average; the minimal objective is to reach the level of 71 years for males and 79 years for females. The main emphasis is on the prevention, especially in the field of smoking-related health problems. Anti-smoking actions become high priority in the programs planned for 2005. In that year the National Action Plan against Smoking was launched. The five year Action Plan intends to decrease cigarette consumption by 8 percent, cut the prevalence of regular smoking by 10 percent, to increase the proportion of never-smokers reducing initiation and habituation among children and adolescents, and reduce the exposition of the population to environmental tobacco smoke by multiplying the number of smoke-free public places.

1.8. Aims of the Study

Our present study analyses the motivations behind smoking cessation. We examined the considerations of current smokers who contemplate about quitting, and also explanations of the ex-smokers on why they stopped smoking. Our previous studies showed that in the Hungarian population poor health, age, and family situation (cohabitation) influence primarily the intention to quit. Different symptoms and diseases produce distinctive stimuli in different ages as well as among people who live alone or together with others [Szanto 2003, 2005]. In the present study we compare the quitting motivations of current smokers and successful quitters. Our hypothesis is that "wishing" is not the same as "accomplishing", in other words, those who plan to quit smoking at great length but continue smoking and those who made the decision and succeeded in quitting differ significantly from each other in age, health status, and family position. On the other hand, we do not anticipate differences in other demographic and social characteristics.

2. DESIGN AND STUDY POPULATION

The study is based on data from the Hungarostudy Health Panel (HHP). The purpose of the HHP is to monitor the changes in the health status of the Hungarian population and to find, describe, and analyze the associations between psychosocial characteristics and the physical, mental, and emotional health status.

The baseline survey (Hungarostudy 2002) was conducted in 2002 on a randomly selected national sample that represented the Hungarian adult population (18 years and over) by age, gender, and place of settlement (i. e. the 150 sub-regions of Hungary)[Kopp 2006]. Out of the participants of the baseline study, 62 percent agreed in a written consent to be included into the follow-up. The second wave was organized and conducted with the participation of 3701 individuals from the baseline study in 2005. The original questionnaire was used again but certain fields were expanded by adding new blocks or additional questions to the previously used blocks. The group of questions that focused on the smoking habits was also developed further by certain new questions. The original questionnaire block was extended in the direction of the possible motivating forces that initiated cessation plans or facilitated the actual quitting. The questionnaire was filled by specially trained district nurses who interviewed the participants in their homes. The average duration of completing the questionnaire was about one hour.

3. METHODS

3.1. Variables

The health status measures were constructed from the participants' self-reported health problems and their self-evaluation of overall health.

General health: The respondents indicated their satisfaction or dissatisfaction with their general health status on a five-grade scale where 1 indicated very poor health status and 5 indicated excellent health.

Incidence of chronic illnesses: The respondents were asked to indicate diseases they received medical care for in the past three years on a list of chronic diseases. The list contained the following diseases and disease groups: cancer, diabetes, diseases of the liver and kidney, psychiatric diseases, respiratory, digestive, and cardiovascular morbidity, cerebral-vascular disease, muscular-skeletal diseases, and allergies.

Smoking: The questionnaire contained the following categories: never smoker, quitter, and current smoker. The motivations of smoking cessation were analyzed both in the groups of those who contemplated on quitting but continued to smoke and of those who had successfully stopped smoking.

Socio-economical status: Socio-economic status was represented by education and economic situation. Education was measured by the completed level of schooling (elementary school, vocational training, high school, or higher education). Economic status was characterized by the perception of one's economic situation as compared to a perceived country average, and was assessed using a ten-grade Lickert-scale.

Family situation was measured by the indicator of cohabitation: living alone or together with a spouse or partner.

3.2. Statistical Analysis

Continuous variables were compared using Student's t-test and categorical variables were analyzed with the chi-square test or the Fisher exact test, as appropriate. Binomial regression was used to explain the characteristics of the motivation types of smoking cessation. We used the method of logistic regression to examine the significance and direction of the linear relationships between the independent (continuous and categorical) variables or predictors on the binary dependent variable. The choice of a given type of motivation (1 = mentioned, 0 = not mentioned) was considered as the dependent variable. Gender, age, education level, cohabitation (1 = lives in cohabitation, 0 = lives alone), and the continuous variable measuring economic situation were used as primary predictors; the binary indicator of general health (1 = satisfactory, 0 = not satisfactory) and the incidence of certain diseases (1 = treated, 0 = not treated) were included as modifying factors. The analysis was performed using the statistical software package SPSS, version 11.

4. RESULTS

The follow-up study provided questionnaire data of 3701 individuals to analyze. Slightly more than half of the sample (51 %) has never smoked, one fifth of the respondents (21 %) ceased to smoke, and 28 percent was a current smoker. Table 3 shows the distribution of the sample by age, gender, education and cohabitation.

**Table 3. Distribution of smoking status in the sample by age,
gender, education and cohabitation (%)**

	Never smoker (N=1895)	Ex-smoker (N=786)	Current smoker (N=1020)
Average age (years)	54.2±17,8	52.9±15,3	44.4±13,4
Female	72.2	42.6	50.7
Elementary or less education	38.2	24.1	30.5
Vocational training school	21.3	33.0	34.8
High school	25.6	28.7	26.9
Higher education	14.9	14.3	7.8
Cohabitant	63.2	80.1	73.1
Economic situation (score mean)	4.99±1,70	4.96±1,78	4.62±1,98

There are significant differences between the groups so each of them has a unique characteristic. On the average, ex-smokers are higher educated, and more typically live together with a partner or spouse than members of the other two groups. Current smokers are significantly younger than non-smokers, and the proportion of people having university or college degree is about half of those who are not smoking. Never smokers more likely live alone, are women, and are older, than people with a history of smoking. Non-smokers (ex-smokers and never smokers similarly) evaluate their economic situation more favorable than smokers. The group of never smokers is the most heterogeneous one concerning the levels of education: the proportions of both the least and the most educated are the highest in this group.

Table 4 shows that the health status of the respondents – indicated both by the value of self-rated general health and by the self-reported prevalence of treatment received for certain disorders – differs significantly by the history of smoking. The groups of the non-smokers (i.e. never smokers and ex-smokers) have similar disease structure. Judging by the indicators of health presented here, current smokers have a more favorable health status than non-smokers; however, it should be noticed that on the average they are 8-10 years younger than the members of the other two groups.

After establishing the demographic, social and health profile of the sample, we analyzed of the motivation of the quitting intentions reported by respondents who had a smoking history. Both the ex-smokers and the current smokers who planned to quit were asked about their reasons using the same fixed-alternative questions. Respondents were requested to point out the dominant reason in case they had more than one possible motivation.

Table 4. Distribution of smoking status in the sample by general health status and the prevalence of certain diseases and disease groups (%)

	Never smoker (N=1895)	Ex-smoker (N=786)	Current smoker (N=1020)
Unsatisfactory health status (SRH)**	20.3	22.6	16.1
Diabetes**	10.5	11.5	4.4
Hepatic disorder**	1.5	3.6	2.0
Respiratory disorder *	6.2	8.1	5.0
Allergy*	9.1	8.5	6.4
Disease of the digestive system**	8.2	12.0	7.8
Kidney disease	4.8	4.6	4.0
Musculo-skeletal disease**	29.4	27.1	23.7
High blood pressure**	35.3	32.1	18.3
Cancer*	3.2	5.0	2.6
Psychiatric disease	5.7	6.5	5.3
Cardiovascular disease **	18.4	18.4	7.9
Cerebro-vascular disease	3.6	4.2	2.5

*p<0.05, **p<0.01.

From all people who had a history of smoking, 97 percent of the respondents (N = 759) identified their motivation for quitting or considering cessation. Among the current smokers, only 4 individuals hesitated when asked about future plans to quit smoking; 52 percent of smokers (N = 528) clearly expressed their wish to stop smoking somewhere in the future, and with the exception of only three persons they also specified their reasons to do it.

Table 5 displays the motivation choices of those who contemplate to stop and those who have already stopped smoking.

Table 5. Motivation choices of contemplating current smokers and ex-smokers (%)

	Ex-smokers (N=759)	Smokers (N=525)
Present illness	26.9	18.7
Prevention of future illness	38.1	39.8
Social pressure	21.3	16.2
Financial reasons	13.7	25.3

Prevention as the dominant motivation is mentioned in the same proportion by the two groups. For ex-smokers, present illnesses and pressures from family, friends and other agents of the social environment played important roles in their decision to quit. Smokers who are thinking of smoking cessation rather considered financial reasons – the high and rising price of tobacco products – as the potential cause to give up smoking.

How and in what extent did demographic and social characteristics and the general and specific features of health status influence the cessation motivations of smokers and ex-smokers? First we constructed dichotomous variables based on the individual categories of motivation. Then using the method of binomial regression we analyzed the influence of factors that may strengthen or reduce the probability of choosing a given motivation category separately in the two groups of smokers and quitters. The indicators of the general health as well as treatments for specific diseases were considered as explanatory variables. Since there was no significant difference in the prevalence of psychiatric, cerebral-vascular, and kidney disease in the two groups we did not include these health problems into the examination. On the other hand, each socio-demographic variable (shown in table 3) demonstrated certain explanatory potential and was consequently included into the analysis. Regression analysis was performed stepwise in both groups. The results are presented in table 6 and 7. The tables include each variable that was entered in the model but the values of the odds ratio –Exp (B) – and the 95 percent confidence intervals for odds ratio – CI for Exp (B) – will only be presented where the effect of the variable is significant. Both in table 6 and table 7 the results of four regression models are shown together: factors that increase or decrease the chance of mentioning a motivation category are present illness, prevention of future illness, perception of social pressure, or financial reasons.

Table 6. Odds ratios for increasing or decreasing ex-smokers' motivations for quitting

	model OR (CI) Present illness (N=204)	model OR (CI) Prevention (N=289)	model OR (CI) Social pressure (N=162)	model OR (CI) Price (N=104)
Unsatisfactory general health (SRH)	.58 (.37-.90)	1.57 (1.01-2.45)	NS	NS
Diabetes	NS	NS	NS	2.13 (1.12-4.05)
Hepatic disorder	NS	NS	NS	NS
Respiratory disorder	1.94 (1.04-3.61)	NS	NS	NS
Allergy	NS	NS	NS	NS
Disease of the digestive system	NS	NS	NS	NS
Muscular-skeletal disease	NS	NS	NS	NS
High blood pressure	NS	NS	NS	NS
Cancer	3.59 (1.62-7.95)	NS	NS	NS
Cardiovascular disease	4.28 (2.74-6.67)	.51 (.32-.81)	.53 (.29-.96)	.41 (.20-.84)
Gender	NS	NS	1.92 (1.29-2.87)	NS
Age	NS	NS	2.37 (1.38-4.06)	NS
Education	.76 (.62-.93)	NS	NS	NS
Cohabitation	NS	.64 (.43-.95)	NS	NS
Financial situation	NS	NS	NS	NS

4.1. Ex-Smokers – Analysis of Motivations of Those Who Have Successfully Quitted

4.1.1. Model 1: The Main Reason for Quitting Is Present Disease

Comparing the models it can be observed at first sight that for the ex-smokers it was cardiovascular disease that triggered cessation. The present illness that prompted quitting was most likely cardiovascular disease: those who reported treatment for cardiovascular problems were four times more likely to mention illness as the reason for quitting (OR = 4.28) than those who had not been treated for this problem. The effects of cardiovascular disease are present in the other three models as well in so far as the occurrence of such illnesses halves the odds of explaining cessation with other reason than illness.

Besides heart disease, cancer and respiratory illness also have significant motivational power. Treatment for cancer almost quadruples (OR = 3.59), respiratory disease nearly doubles (OR = 1.94) the chances of cessation. The presence of a serious illness and the negative assessment of one's health are usually closely related so it is not surprising that the self-report of satisfactory health halves the odds of explaining quitting with health-related reasons.

4.1.2. Model 2: The Main Reason for Quitting Is Prevention of Future Disease

Satisfaction with one's general health is the best indicator of the prevention-motivated smoking cessation. The chances of explaining quitting with preventive purposes are one and a half times as great among those with satisfactory health (OR = 1.57) than among those who described their health as unsatisfactory. The presence of cardiovascular illness and cohabitation also showed significant relationships with preventive considerations: both factors decrease the odds of such motivations.

4.1.3. Model 3: The Main Reason for Quitting Is Social Pressure

In the indication of social pressure as motivating factor age plays the most important role (OR = 2.37). As age increases, the chances of referring to environmental demands as an explanation of cessation are also increasing. Gender seems to be another important aspect: comparing to men, women are almost twice as likely to quit smoking because of social – especially familial – pressure (OR = 1.92).

4.1.4. Model 4: The Main Reason for Quitting Is Financial Cause

It is not easy to interpret the model of financial motivations because two illnesses seem to determine the choice of economic reasons. The presence of diabetes significantly increases (OR = 2.13), heart disease decreases the explanatory role of financial factors.

4.2. Current Smokers – Analysis of Motivations of Those Who Contemplate On Quitting

Table 7. Odds ratios increasing or decreasing current smokers' motivations for quitting

	2.1 model OR (CI) Present illness (N=98)	2.2 model OR (CI) Prevention (N=209)	2.3 model OR (CI) Social pressure (N=85)	2.4 model OR (CI) Price (N=122)
Unsatisfactory general health	.53 (.28-.99)	NS	NS	NS
Diabetes	NS	NS	NS	NS
Liver disease	NS	NS	NS	NS
Respiratory disease	NS	NS	NS	NS
Allergy	NS	NS	NS	NS
Disease of the digestive system	NS	NS	NS	NS
Muscular-skeletal disease	NS	NS	NS	NS
High blood pressure	2.00 (1.11-3.62)	NS	NS	.35 (.17-.72)
Cancer	NS	NS	NS	NS
Cardiovascular disease	2.44 (1.17-5.08)	.30 (.12-.72)	NS	NS
Gender	NS	NS	NS	NS
Age	1.03 (1.00-1.05)	NS	.97 (.95-.99)	NS
Education	NS	1.31 (1.07-1.61)	NS	.66 (.51-.86)
Cohabitation	NS	NS	2.82 (1.37-5.78)	.55 (.34-.89)
Financial situation	NS	NS	1.19 (1.04-1.36)	.80 (.71-.91)

4.2.1. Model 1: The Main Reason of Quitting Plans Is Present Disease

From disease experiences, heart disease and high blood pressure implicate a motivating force of quitting considerations. Self-reported satisfactory health halves the odds of explaining contemplating cessation for health-related reasons (OR = 0.53).

4.2.2. Model 2: The Main Reason of Quitting Plans Is Prevention of Future Disease

Prevention as reason for thoughts about giving up smoking becomes more and more characteristic along the increase of levels of education. A one-unit change in the education results in a 1.31 unit change of the odds of preventive considerations. The presence of cardiovascular illness – similarly to the ex-smokers – decreases the odds of preventive purposes (OR = 0.30).

4.2.3. Model 3: The Main Reason of Quitting Plans Is Social Pressure

Quitting plans triggered by social pressures is influenced most significantly by the cohabitation variable. Cohabitants (those living with a spouse or partner) are almost three times more likely to consider stopping smoking (OR = 2.82) than those who live alone. The same is true in relation to the financial situation: the more favorable the assessment of the respondents' financial situation the more likely they mention social-familial pressure as the dominant motivation. Age plays an adverse effect on this motivation category as younger people are more likely to identify social-environmental forces as the purpose of quitting considerations.

4.2.4. Model 4: The Main Reason of Quitting Plans Is Financial Cause

In accordance with our expectations, unfavorable assessment of one's financial situation increases the chances of giving explanatory values to financial factors. Domination of this reason is also influenced by education, cohabitation, and by the prevalence of high blood pressure. Higher education and cohabitation decreases the odds of identifying financial causes. High blood pressure also decreases the chances of placing financial situation on the top of the list of motivations (OR = 0.35).

5. CONCLUSION

The aim of our study was to bring to light the motivational differences between successful quitters and smokers who just contemplate about quitting. We assumed that (1) ex-smokers and the current smokers who considered stopping smoking had similar considerations for quitting, but (2) the motivating power of these considerations is influenced significantly by demographic and social background variables as well as by indicators of general health and specific health problems.

We expected to find the same structure of motivations in the two groups. Based on our previous results, we assumed that deteriorating health and the presence of diagnosed and treated diseases would constitute the most frequent type of motivation. We also assumed that motivations would be significantly modified by demographic and social factors.

Our results show that people with a smoking history emphasized the role of preventive reasons in their quitting considerations and not the role of deteriorating health or disease experiences. About two-fifths of both the ex-smokers and currents smokers who think about quitting gave this explanation. This apparently stable attitude toward smoking is probably the consequence of the last decades' anti-smoking campaigns. Health educators seem to be successful in conveying the importance of behavioral factors in health and illness. Disease prevention and health promotion agencies point out the health damaging effects of smoking on the one hand and the benefits of quitting such as the increase of disability-free life years and the savings resulting from the discontinuation of expenses related to tobacco products[1] on the other hand.

Although the high costs of smoking obviously presents a considerable inconvenience for current smokers, this aspect is not generally the main cause for quitting. Those who contemplate quitting tend to mention economic reasons almost twice as frequently as those who actually stopped. It seems that financial factors do not play as vital a role as one might assume. The purchase statistics which indicate no significant association between the increasing tobacco costs and the unchanging proportion of smokers further undermine such expectations.

The intention to preserve one's health appears in the testimonies of smokers and ex-smokers alike. However, while only around one fifth of the current smokers indicated actual

---

[1] An average Hungarian smoker who smokes 20 cigarettes a day manages to smoke away a car's worth in 10-years.

disease or declining health status as the reason of quitting plans, the proportion of ex-smokers who explained quitting with health problems was significantly higher.

Not all diseases influenced cessation considerations in the same way. The most important result of our study is the demonstration of the role of cardiovascular disease both in planning and actually stopping to smoke. Cardiovascular disease increases the chances of successful quitting by more than four times, and the frequency of thoughts about quitting more than doubles when the disease is present. Quitting is also significantly influenced by cancer and respiratory disease; quitting plans are stimulated by high blood pressure.

General health status is also important when the changes of health behavior are explained by preventive considerations. Contrary to our expectations, however, these changes were associated with favorable self evaluation of health.

While the preventive explanations were found among both planners and quitters in the same proportion, socio-demographic background variables affected the separate motivational models differently. Women and older people were twice as likely to mention environmental – mostly familial – pressure than men and younger people. Presumably this is connected to the considerations encouraged by pregnancy and caring for young children in the case of women; and existing health problems – perhaps the needs of other people in the household – in the case of older people. As apposed to these groups, non-cohabitant ex-smokers tended to rank their own health as the motivation for quitting higher.

Gender was shown not to be a decisive factor in the planning of cessation which was apparently much more affected by the economic situation and cohabitation. In the group contemplating cessation the motivating power of environmental pressure tended to be ranked higher by better-off cohabitants. Respondents with higher education were more likely to mention prevention, while lower educational levels increased the chance of economic considerations.

To summarize we can confirm that the Hungarostudy Health Panel enabled us to perform a more detailed analysis and was therefore a useful device for acquiring a deeper understanding of the population's attitudes toward smoking. Contrary to our expectations, the motivations of ex-smokers and current smokers contemplating cessation do not coincide. Current smokers characteristically find their health to be satisfactory and are motivated mainly by future-oriented primary prevention as well as economic and social environmental factors. Actual cessation on the other hand, is usually not influenced by such rational considerations but by necessity: occurrence of certain – primarily cardiovascular – disease and unsatisfactory health conditions.

ACKNOWLEDGMENTS

This study was supported by the Hungarian State Founds NKFP 1b/020/2004 and OTKA TS 049785 (2004).

REFERENCES

Act XLII 1999 on the Protection of Non-Smokers (n.d.) Retrieved Nov 15, 2006, from http://www.complex.hu/kzlcim/tv999.htm (In Hungarian)

Antmann K., Oroszi B., Oszlár J., Forrai J., Sima Á. and Morava E. (2005). A Representative Health Study 2001-2002. *Report on Smoking. Medicus Universalis,* 38 (1), 29-36. (In Hungarian)

Batra V., Patkar A. A., Berrettini W. H., Weinstein S. P. and Leone F. T. (2003). The Genetic Determinants of Smoking. *Chest,* 123, 1730-1739.

Csoboth Cs. (2006). Relationship between Smoking and the Quality of Life in the Hungarian Population. In M. Kopp and M. E. Kovács (Ed.). The Quality of Life of the Hungarian Population in the Turn of the Millennium (203-209.) *Budapest: Semmelweis Kiadó.* (In Hungarian)

Edwards R. (2004). The Problem of Tobacco Smoking. British Medical Journal, 328, 217-219.

Füst G., Gudmundur J. A., Kramer J., Szalai Cs., Duba J., Yang Y., Chung E. K., Zhou B., Blanchong C. A., Lokki M. L., Bödvarsson S., Prohászka Z., Karádi I., Vatay Á., Kovács M., and Romics L. (2004). Genetic Basis of Tobacco Smoking: Strong Association of a Specific Major Histocompatibility Complex Haplotype on Chromosome 6 with Smoking Behavior. *International Immunology,* 16 (10),1507-1514.

Godfredsen N. S., Osler M., Vestbo J., Andersen I. and Prescott E. (2003). Smoking Reduction, Smoking Cessation, and Incidence of Fatal and Non-Fatal Myocardial Infarction in Denmark 1976-1998: A Pooled Cohort Study. *Journal of Epidemiology and Community Health,* 57, 412-416.

HUNGAROSTUDY 2002. Statistical Summary. Retrieved Nov 20, 2006, from http://www.behsci.sote.hu/szechenyiterv/statbook_2002.htm (n.d.) (In Hungarian)

Kopp M. S., Skrabski Á., Szántó Zs. and Siegrist J. (2006). Psychosocial determinants of premature cardiovascular mortality differences within Hungary. *Journal of Epidemiology and Community Health,* 60, 782-788.

Kremer I., Bachner-Melman R., Reshef A., Broude L., Nemanov L., Gritsenko I., Heresco-Levy U., Elizur Y., and Ebstein R. P. (2005). Association of the Serotonin Transporter Gene With Smoking Behavior. *American Journal of Psychiatry,* 162, 924-930.

Lerman C., Caporaso N. E., Audrain J., Main D., Boyd N. R., and Shields P. G. (2000). Interacting Effects of the Serotonin Transporter Gene and Neuroticism in Smoking Practices and Nicotine Dependence. *Molecular Psychiatry,* 5, 189–192.

Mackay J. and Amos A. (2003).Women and tobacco. *Respirology,* 8, 123-130.

Németh Á (2003). Global Youth Tobacco Survey. Hungary National Report. Retrieved Nov 17, 2006, from http://www.cdc.gov/Tobacco/global/gyts/reports/pdf/hungary.pdf

Ockene J. K., Emmons K. M., Mermelstein R. J., Perkins K. A., Bonollo D. S., Voohees C. C. and Hollis J. F. (2000). Relapse and Maintenance Issues for Smoking Cessation. *Health Psychology,* 19 (1), 17-31.

OLEF National Health Interview Survey 2003. Executive Update. (2004). Melles M. (Ed.). Johan Béla National Center for Epidemiology, Budapest, 2004. Retrieved Nov 19, 2006, from http://www.oek.hu/oek.web?to=,8,722,711 and nid=203 and pid=1 and lang=hun

Ostbye T., Taylor D. H. and Jung S. H. (2002). A Longitudinal Study Of The Effects Of Tobacco Smoking and other Modifiable Risk Factors on Ill Health in Middle-Aged and Old Americans: Results from the Health and Retirement Study and Asset and Health Dynamics among the Oldest Old Survey. *Preventive Medicine,* 34, 334-345.

Perkins K. A. (2001). Smoking Cessation in Women: Special Considerations. *CNS Drugs* 15 (5), 391-411.

Peto R., Darby S., Deo H., Silcocks P., Whitley E. and Doll R. (2000). Smoking, Smoking Cessation, and Lung Cancer in the UK since 1950: Combination of National Statistics with Two Case-Control Studies. *British Medical Journal,* 321, 323-329.

Statistical Yearbook 2002. Budapest: Hungarian Central Statistical Office.

Surgeon General Office on Smoking and Health (2001). Women and Smoking. Retrieved Nov 17, 2006, from www.cdc.gov/tobacco. (n.d.)

Szántó Zs. and Susánszky É. (2003). Relationships between Health Status and Cessation Initiative among Smokers of Different Age Groups. *Lege Artis Medicinae,* 13 (8), 682-685. (In Hungarian)

Szántó Zs., Susánszky É. and Kopp M. (2005): Relationships Between Unfavorable Health Status and Smoking Cessation Attempts in Hungary. *Social and Preventive Medicine,* 50 (5), 324-33.

Szilágyi T. (2004). Tobacco Control in Hungary: Past, Present, Future. Health 21 Hungarian Foundation. Retrieved Nov 17, 2006, from http://www.policy.hu/ tszilagyi/content.html

Taylor D. H., Hasselblad V., Henley S. J., Thun M. and Sloan F. A. (2002). Benefits of smoking cessation for longevity. *American Journal of Public Health,* 92, 990-996.

Surgeon General's Report: The Health Consequences of Smoking. 2004. U.S. Department of Health and Human Services, Centers for Disease Control and Prevention, National Center for Chronic Disease Prevention and Health Promotion, Office on Smoking and Health. Retrieved Nov 20, 2006 from http://www.cdc.gov/tobacco/sgr/sgr_2004/ sgranimation/ flash/index.html

The World Health Report 2003 – Shaping the future. Retrieved Nov 20, 2006 from http://www.who.int/whr/2003/en. (n.d.)

Urbán R., Kugler Gy., Oláh A. and Szilágyi Zs. (2005). Relationships between smoking, psychological well-being, and level of education among young adult males. A cross-sectional survey. *Pszichológia,* 25(1), 71-90. (In Hungarian).

Urbán, R., Kugler, Gy., Oláh, A, and Szilágyi, Zs. (2006). Smoking And Education: Do Psychosocial Variables Explain The Relationship Between Education And Smoking Behavior? *Nicotine and Tobacco Research,* Vol. 8 (4) 1-9.

WHO CINDI (Countrywide Integrated Noncommunicable Disease Intervention) Programme 2006. Retrieved Nov 22, 2006 from http://www.who.dk/CINDI (n.d.)

WHO HFA (Health for All Database) 2006. Retrieved Nov 20, 2006 from http://www.euro.who.int/hfadb

WHO Regional Office for Europe Hungary 2006. Retrieved Nov 20, 2006 from http://www.who.dk/Document/E80607.pdf

Wilson K., Gibson N., Willan A. and Cook D. (2000). Effect of Smoking Cessation on Mortality after Myocardial Infarction. Meta-analysis of Cohort Studies. *Archives of Internal Medicine,* 60, 939-944.

In: Smoking Cessation: Theory, Interventions and Prevention   ISBN: 978-1-60021-591-9
Editor: Jerome E. Landow   © 2008 Nova Science Publishers, Inc.

Chapter 12

IMPACT OF SMOKING AND SMOKING CESSATION ON SUCCESSFUL AGING

*Hui-Chuan Hsu**

Department of Healthcare Administration, Asia University, Tokyo, Japan

ABSTRACT

Purpose: Past research has emphasized the impact of smoking on physical health; however, the impact on mental and social health has been less explored. The purpose of this prospective study is to estimate the risks of smoking and cessation to successful aging for the elderly in Taiwan.

Methods: The data came from face-to-face interviews in Taiwan that used an elderly population-based probability sample provided by the Population and Health Research Center, Bureau of Health Promotion. Data were followed from baseline 1993 to 1999, and only the survivor samples (n=2,525) were selected for analysis. Smoking status was separated into 'never smoked,' 'quit,' 'light smoker' and 'heavy smoker' categories. Successful aging indicators included activities of daily living, cognitive function, depressive symptoms, and social support. Hierarchical logistic regression models were used for analysis of the 6-year prediction of failing in successful aging, by controlling for demographics, co-morbidities, and successful aging state at baseline.

Results: The sample was made up of 53.6% elderly nonsmokers, 21.4% ex-smokers, 10.0% light smokers and 15.0% heavy smokers at the baseline year. Heavy smokers had a higher risk of depressive symptoms. Influences of smoking status on other successful aging losses were not significant though. Ex-smokers had higher physical disability and cognitive impairment, and heavy smokers had lower social support.

Conclusion: Elderly are more likely to be aware of the smoking risks to physical health which can help them quit smoking. They are, however, less likely to appreciate the risks of smoking to mental health. Smoking cessation projects should consider the holistic health

---

* Correspondence: Hui-Chuan Hsu, Ph.D. Department of Healthcare Administration, Asia University. No. 500, Lioufeng Road, Wufeng Township, Taichung 413, Taiwan. Email: gingerhsu@seed.net.tw.

problems of the elderly and develop strategies to eliminate the smoking risk to successful aging.

Key words: smoking, smoking cessation, successful aging, health promotion.

INTRODUCTION

Numerous prospective studies have identified cigarette smoking as a major risk factor for cardiovascular diseases, chronic bronchitis, several types of cancers, and others (Carstensen et al, 1987; Christen et al., 2000; Freund et al., 1993; He et al., 2001; Hsu and Pwu, 2004; Hu and Lanese, 1998; Mclaughlin et al., 1995; Ruigrok et al., 2001; Sauer et al., 2002; Suminori and Hirayama, 1990; Wald and Watt, 1997; Yuan et al., 1996). Smoking cessation has an effect on reducing heart disease, possibility of death, relative risk of death after acute myocardial infarction, or increase in lung function (Cheng et al., 1999; Liaw and Cheng 1998; Lee et al., 1997; Pelkonen et al., 2001; Rea et al., 2002; Wilson et al., 1998). However, fewer past studies have explored the impact of smoking or smoking cessation on health with a comprehensive view.

Since the concept of "successful aging" (Rowe and Kahn, 1987, 1998) has become the new paradigm in gerontology, the recent trend of health promotion for the elderly focuses more on positive and comprehensive measures and is not only limited to morbidity or mortality. According to Rowe and Kahn's definition (1997), successful aging is defined as a three-component model, which includes the absence and low risk of disease, high psychological and physical function, and engagement with life. In the consideration of holistic health and also cultural variation, in our previous study we have modified the concept of successful aging to physical, mental and social dimensions (Hsu and Chang, 2004), including basic and advanced physical function, mental function (cognitive function and absence of depressive symptoms), and social health (good social support and engagement in productive activities).

Many risk factors have been found to be related to one indicator or multiple indicators of successful aging, including age, gender, educational level, marital status, mastery of aging, self efficacy, self-rated health, diabetes, COPD, hearing problems, arthritis, depression, social contacts, regular exercise, social network and support, financial status, life satisfaction, etc. (Abraham and Hanasson, 1995; Albert et al., 1995; Chou and Chi, 2002; Garfein and Herzog, 1995; Glass et al., 1995; Strawbrdige et al., 1996; Schaie, 1990; Seeman et al., 1994; Seeman et al., 1995; von Faber et al., 2001). In our previous studies in Taiwan, age, gender, education, marital status, personal income, ethnic group, and previous successful aging status were related to current successful aging (Hsu and Chang, 2004; Hsu, 2005; Hsu, 2006), but a geographic level difference was not found (Hsu and Chang, 2004).

Among those risk or protective factors to successful aging, the effect of smoking was not confirmed, and whether smoking cessation has an effect on successful aging is still unknown. The reasons may be that it needs longitudinal data to confirm the causal effect of smoking to successful aging, and that using the successful aging indicators as the health outcome is not widespread. If we could find the relationship between smoking behavior and different dimensions of successful aging, it would be helpful in promoting successful aging for the elderly and making suggestions for quit smoking projects in health policy.

The purpose of this chapter is to determine differences between different smoking status regarding social status indicators and changes in successful aging using a longitudinal study designed to follow groups of the elderly in Taiwan. The impact of smoking and smoking cessation to successful aging is discussed. The research questions are:

1. Is smoking related to longitudinal successful aging?
2. Can smoking cessation help in successful aging?

METHODS

Data

Data were obtained from the 1993, 1996, and 1999 waves of the "Survey of Health and Living Status of the Elderly in Taiwan". The sample was nationally representative of persons' aged 60 years and above in the year 1989, and was drawn from the household register which included institutionalized populations. The sampling was a three-stage equal probability sampling method: the first stage consisted of stratified samples of the administrative units (townships); the second stage consisted of blocks (Lin) in the selected townships as clusters; and the third stage consisted of two respondents selected systematically from the register in each selected Lin. A total of 4,049 people completed the interview in 1989. The samples included in this chapter were the initial cohort during 1989 and its follow-ups in 1993, 1996, and 1999 with sample sizes of 3,155 (77.9%), 2,669 (65.9%), and 2,310 (57.0%) people respectively (figure 1). The participants' deaths were also recorded and verified with official death registration records. By examining the goodness-of-fit test of gender and age, the death or lost follow-up cases were older and more of males.

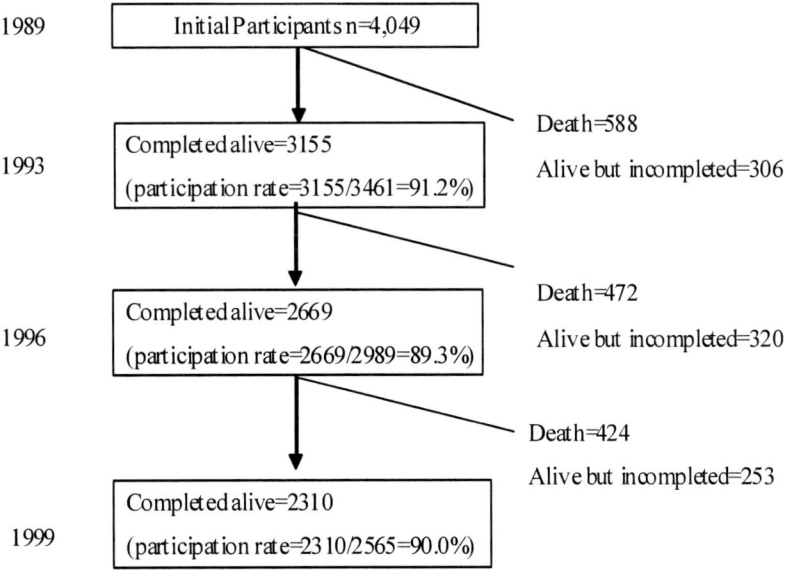

Figure 1. The cohort samples and follow-ups.

MEASURES

Smoking

Two kinds of smoking behavior were defined. In the cross-sectional status, smoking behaviors were categorized as non-smokers (never smoked, ex-smokers (quit), light smokers (smoking one pack of cigarettes or less per day), and heavy smokers (smoking more than one pack of cigarettes per day). In the longitudinal analysis, smoking behaviors were observed during 1993 to 1999, and categorized as never smoked, quit successfully (since 1993 or earlier, and quit after 1993 to 1999), new smokers (did not report smoking at 1993 but began to smoke at 1996 or 1999), swing quitters (reported quitting in 1993 but resumed smoking at 1996 or 1999), and current smokers (reported continuously smoking during 1993 to 1999).

Successful Aging

Successful aging indicators provided the framework used to measure the health of the elderly. These indicators were adapted from Rowe and Kahn's successful aging framework (Rowe and Kahn, 1997; 1998) and the WHO's active aging (WHO, 2002) concept. Accordingly, activities of daily living (ADL), cognitive function, depressive symptoms, and social support were consolidated into physical, mental and social dimensions to measure successful aging. The cut-off criteria of the successful aging indicators have been discussed in other research (Hsu and Chang, 2004).

1. Physical function was assessed primarily by measurements of ADL. Six items of ADL were assessed: eating, dressing, transferring from a bed or chair, walking in the house, going to the toilet, and taking a bath. The concept of normal physical function was determined when there was no difficulty present, or impairment was temporary for less than 3 months. Normal function was defined as having no difficulty or having only temporary difficulty for less than 3 months.

Mental health (maintenance of high mental function):

2. Cognitive function was measured with the Short Portable Mental Status Questionnaire (SPMSQ) using 10 items in 1993 and 6 items in 1996 and 1999. The items of SPMSQ are slightly different among the surveys. The measures included: where are you located now; your home address; what are the day, month, year; how old are you; who is the current president and the last president; count backward from 20 by 3's, reiterate some words or reiterate numbers in reverse, what is your mother's maiden name. Normal cognitive functioning or impairment was adjusted for educational level, according to the rule of interpolation (Wu and Chang, 1997).

3. Symptoms of depression were assessed with the Center for Epidemiologic Studies Depression Scale (CES-D), scoring each item from 0 to 3. The CES-D scale measured 11 items in 1993 and by 10 items in 1996 and 1999. The cutoff point for depressive symptoms was determined by converting it to a score of 16 on a 20-item scale (Radloff, 1977), and using

T-transformation (Kohout et al., 1993) to determine the cutoff points in 1993 and 1996. The cutoff point for depressive symptoms was a score of 9 or greater in 1993 (11 items), and a score of 8 or greater in 1996 and 1999 (10 items).

4. Social support was assessed as the giving and taking of emotional support and instrumental support, which included satisfaction derived from the emotional care of family/friends, satisfaction with care received when ill and financial support received when ill, consultation for family/friends concerning problems or worries, helping family/friends with child care, helping with activities of daily living, and establishment of financial or material support. Each variable was scored 0 or 1, yielding a possible total score of the four variables ranging from 0 to 4. Next, a score of 4 was defined as "high" social support; a score of 3 was "medium"; and a score of 2 or below was "low" social support. High or medium social support was defined as "successful".

CONTROL VARIABLES

Demographics and self-reported chronic disease were used for controlling variables. Demographic variables used in this chapter included age, gender, educational level, ethnic group, and marital status. Ethnic groups included Fuchien, Hakka, Mainlanders, and others, each of which has a distinct dialect and a slightly different culture. Marital status was recorded as either living with a spouse (married or living together) or living without a spouse (never married, divorced, separated, or widowed). Education is categorized as illiterate, literate but no formal education or elementary school, primary high school, and senior high school or beyond. The prevalence of self-reported chronic diseases were included in analysis, such as hypertension, diabetes, heart disease, stroke, respiratory disease, digestive disease, kidney disease, and cancer. The number of prevalent chronic diseases above was used in the model. The successful aging status at baseline (1993) was also used for controlling variables to predict the 1999 status.

Analysis

Descriptive analysis and the Chi-square test were used. Logistic regression analysis was conducted for the risk (odds ratio, OR) of smoking status at baseline to predict the failure in successful aging indicators 6 years later.

RESULTS

Table 1 shows the demographic characteristics of the study samples at baseline year 1993. About 26.0% aged 75 or more; 43.% were female and 56.4% were male; 40.4% were illiterate, 41.0% were of elementary school level, and 18.6% were junior high school or higher. Fuchien group comprised 61.1%, Hakka 15.6%, Mainlanders were 21.7%, and 1.6% were aboriginals or others. About 68.5% have a spouse (married or living together), and 31.5% have no spouse.

Table 2 shows the cross-sectional smoking status and longitudinal smoking behaviour. At the baseline, there were 53.6% non-smokers, 16.4% ex-smokers, 7.7% light smokers and 11.4% heavy smokers. When separated by gender, most of the female elderly were non-smokers (92.5%). In the male elderly, only 22.8% were non-smokers, 35.9% were ex-smokers, 15.8% and 25.5% were light and heavy smokers respectively.

In the longitudinal view, there were 33.6% never smoked, 11.6% who successfully quit and 3.6% were new quitters, 0.5% were new smokers after 1993, 1.1% swing quitters announced quitting in 1993 but started to smoke again after, and 11.7% kept smoking for 6 years, 4.5% were missing their data, and 33.4% were dead during the follow-up. It shows that most of the participants maintained their smoking habit during the follow-up, and only a few of the elderly would change their smoking behaviour. Further, to analyze by gender, only 14.7% of the male men elderly never smoked, and 20.2% quit smoking before 1993; 20.1% of the men kept smoking from 1993-1999.

Table 1. Demographic characteristics of samples at baseline 1993

Baseline characteristics	%
Age	
60-64	6.1
65-69	40.7
70-74	27.1
75-79	15.0
80+	11.0
Gender	
Men	56.4
Women	43.6
Education	
Illiteracy	40.4
Elementary school /non-formal education	41.0
Junior high school	8.2
Senior high school or over	10.4
Ethnic groups	
Fuchien	61.1
Hakka	15.6
Mainlanders	21.7
Others	1.6
Marital Status	
With spouse	68.5
No spouse	31.5

n=3,155.

Table 2. Cross-sectional and longitudinal smoking status by gender (%)

	Total	Male	Female
Cross-sectional 1993			
Non-smokers	53.6	22.8	92.5
Ex-smokers	16.4	35.9	3.0
Light smokers	7.7	15.8	2.8
Heavy smokers	11.4	25.5	1.7
Longitudinal 1993-1999			
Never smoked	33.6	14.7	61.7
Quit successfully			
Since 1993 or earlier	11.6	20.2	1.7
Since during 1993-1999	3.6	5.9	0.9
New smokers	0.5	0.3	0.9
Swing quitters	1.1	2.0	0.1
Current smokers	11.7	20.1	2.1
Death/loss in follow-up	33.4	36.8	32.6

N=3155

Note 1. Non-smokers are those who never smoked. Ex-smokers are those who smoked before but now have quit. Light-smokers are the current smokers who consumed no more than 1 pack of cigarettes per day; heavy-smokers are those who consumed more than 1 pack of cigarettes per day.

Note 2. Since the quitting question in 1999 was unavailable, several assumptions are made: (1) the non-smokers in 1996 were still non-smokers in 1999; (2) if the case was ex-smokers in 1996 and non-smokers in 1999, the case was defined as ex-smoker in 1999. (3) If the case was a smoker in 1996 and did not report smoking consumption in 1999, the case was defined as ex-smokers in 1999.

Note 3. The longitudinal smoking status was defined: "Never smoked" means those who never smoked during 1993-1999 and in the past. "Quit successfully" means those who had smoked before but quit, and did not report smoking during 1993-1999; it is also categorized as quit before 1993 and quit after 1993. "New smokers" means those who did not report being a smoker at baseline 1993, but started to smoke in 1996 or 1999. "Swing" means those who quit smoking but began to smoke again during 1993-1999. "Current smokers" indicates those continuous and also current smokers.

Table 3 shows a continuously successful aging rate during 1993-1999 by baseline smoking status. When observing the 6 year continuity, non-smokers had a lower rate of normal physical function (72.5%), lower normal cognitive function (63.3%), and lower absence of depressive symptoms (45.9%). Ex-smokers showed a higher rate of absence in depression (59.6%) than other smoking status people. Social support was not significantly related to smoking status. Further, when the male and female elderly separated into the analysis, the smoking relationship only showed significantly in the physical function of the male elderly, which indicates the male ex-smokers had poorer physical function. The influence of smoking on women elderly's successful aging was not found.

Table 4 showed the successful aging in 6 years by longitudinal smoking behaviour. Smoking behaviour was significantly related to longitudinal physical function, cognitive function, and depressive symptoms, but the relationships were inconsistent. Current smoker elderly had higher physical function (87.6%) and cognitive function (81.2%). New smokers and swing quitters show a low rate of absence in depressive symptoms, i.e., they had higher probability to be depressive. New smokers also had the lowest rate of normal cognitive function (50.0%). Swing quitters had the lowest rate of good social support (21.6%) as well, but it was not significantly different. Among the successful quitters, the earlier quitters showed similar physical function to new quitters (quit after 1993), but earlier quitters showed more mental successful aging in normal cognitive function and absence of depressive symptoms.

Table 3. Successful aging rate by smoking status at three waves

1993 smoking status	1993-1999 continuous successful aging	1993-1999 Male	1993-1999 Female
Normal physical function %	***	*	
Non-smokers	72.5	86.5	68.1
Ex-smokers	78.3	79.9	52.0
Light smokers	85.6	86.9	76.0
Heavy smokers	85.5	86.8	64.7
Normal cognitive function %	***		
Non-smokers	63.3	77.4	58.5
Ex-smokers	74.3	75.1	61.9
Light smokers	77.5	80.6	54.5
Heavy smokers	79.1	79.1	77.8
Absence of depressive symptoms %	***		
Non-smokers	45.8	65.8	39.8
Ex-smokers	59.6	61.5	28.6
Light smokers	51.3	55.7	20.8
Heavy smokers	57.4	58.8	25.0
Good social support %			
Non-smokers	35.8	46.0	32.6
Ex-smokers	38.6	38.7	34.8
Light smokers	38.4	37.0	48.0
Heavy smokers	42.4	40.3	26.7

Note 1: Only survivors are included in the analysis. Deaths during 1993-1999 were 1103 persons.

Note 2: Smoking status was according to the baseline year (1993).

Note 3: The successful aging criteria are as follows: Normal physical function is defined as normal in all ADL/IADL items (without disability or disabled less than 3 months). Normal cognitive function was indicated by a SPMSQ score cut-off by education (for example at 1993, score more than 6 for illiterate elderly, score more than 7 for elementary school educated elderly, score more than 8 for junior high school or higher educated elderly). "No depressive symptoms" was indicated by the CES-D score less than 9 at 1993 and less than 8 at 1996 and 1999. Good social support was indicated by a score equal or more than 3 in four items of social support.

Note 4. Analysis examined by Chi-square test, *p<0.05, **p<0.01, ***p<0.001.

Table 4. Successful aging during 1993-1999 by longitudinal smoking behavior types

Longitudinal smoking behavior	Normal physical function %	Normal cognitive function %	Absence of depressive symptoms %	Good social support %
Never smoked	72.5	63.5	46.0	35.7
Quit successfully				
Since 1993 or earlier	78.5	74.7	61.8	40.2
Since during 1993-1999	78.8	69.5	53.8	38.2

New smokers	72.2	50.0	35.3	41.2
Swing quitters	75.7	70.6	38.9	21.6
Current Smokers	87.6	81.2	55.2	39.4
Chi-square test	***	***	***	

Note: The longitudinal smoking status was defined: "Never smoked" means those who never smoked during 199-1999 and in the past. "Quit successfully" means those who had smoked before but quit, and did not report smoking during 1993-1999; it is also categorized as quit before 1993 and quit after 1993. "New smokers" means those who did not report a smoker being at baseline 1993, but started to smoke in 1996 or 1999. "Swing quitters" means those who quit smoking but began to smoke again during 1993-1999. "Current smokers" indicates those continuous smokers. *p<0.05, **p<0.01, ***p<0.001.

The result of logistic regression of smoking status to predict the 6-year failure in successful aging indicators is shown in table 5. Since most of the elderly did not change their smoking behaviour during follow-up, the smoking behaviour in the logistic regression was according to the 1993 status. The result showed that smoking status at baseline did not show a significant relationship to the successful aging 6 years later by controlling demographics and health variables. However, compared to non-smokers, ex-smokers had slightly higher possibility of impaired physical function (OR=1.420), impaired cognitive function (OR=1.194), having depressive symptoms (OR=1.200). Light and heavy smokers had lower odds ratio in impaired physical function and cognitive function, but had higher risk in having depressive symptoms (OR=1.250 and 1.560) as well as poor social support (OR=1.211 and 1.251).

Table 5. Odds ratios of failure in successful aging in 6 years by smoking status at baseline

1993 characteristics	1999 successful aging status			
	Impaired physical function	Impaired cognitive function	Having depressive symptom	Poor social support
Smoking				
Ex-smokers	1.420	1.194	1.200	1.035
Light smokers	0.961	0.986	1.250	1.221
Heavy smokers	0.777	0.790	1.560	1.251
Age at 1993				
Age 75 or over	3.305***	2.889***	1.446*	1.406*
Gender				
Female	0.977	1.834**	1.748**	1.046
Education				
Elementary school	0.717	0.571**	0.626***	0.552***
Primary high school	0.558*	1.296	0.437***	0.378***
Ethnic groups				
Hakka	0.738	0.915	0.776	0.905
Mainland provinces	0.697	0.779	1.136	1.254
Others	3.336	2.449	2.181	0.653
Marital status				
With spouse	0.826	1.066	0.958	0.524***
Chronic disease no.	1.348***	1.094	1.192**	1.092
Physical function disabled	5.255***	1.715	2.928**	2.464*
Cognitive impaired	1.266	4.646***	1.236	1.529*
Depressive symptoms	1.517*	1.081	2.450***	1.552***

Table 5. (Continued)

1993 characteristics	1999 successful aging status			
	Impaired physical function	Impaired cognitive function	Having depressive symptom	Poor social support
Poor social support	1.650**	1.223	1.154	1.857***
-2 LL without covariates	1411.578	1426.455	2237.283	2400.683
-2LL with covariates	1215.532	1294.310	2023.971	2181.441
Model χ^2 (d.f.=16)	203.477	153.280	226.621	225.851

Note 1: Proxy or missing cases were excluded by case wise. Deaths cases were also excluded.

Note 2: The dependent variable was according to the 1999 successful aging status. The reference groups of independent variables are: age (<75), gender (male), education (illiterate), ethnic group (Fuchien), marital status (without spouse), chronic disease numbers (as continuous variable), physical function 1993 (normal), cognitive function 1993 (normal), depressive symptoms 1993 (no symptoms), social support 1993 (high).

Note 3: -2LL means -2 Log Likelihood. Estimation of constant is omitted in the table.

Being older and female resulted higher risk in failing of successful aging. The more highly educated persons had lower risks in physical disability, depressive symptoms and poor social support. Having a spouse showed less risk in poor social support (OR=0.524), but marital status had no relationship to the other three indicators. Having more chronic diseases resulted in higher risks in physical disability and depressive symptoms. The baseline successful aging indicators also predicted the 6-years-later successful aging status. Physical function disability strongly related to the 6-years-later after physical disability (OR=5.255) and related to depressive symptoms and social support. Cognitive impairment at baseline predicted well in poor cognitive function 6-years later (OR=4.646) and related to later poor social support (OR=1.529). Showing depressive symptoms meant a higher risk in physical disability (OR=1.517), later depressive symptoms (OR=2.450), and poor social support (OR=1.552). Poor social support at baseline also significantly related to later social support (OR=1.857).

CONCLUSION

Unlike the past research which usually focused on the impact of smoking or smoking cessation to morbidity, this longitudinal study contributed to examining the relationship of smoking behaviour and successful aging. At the baseline 1993, there were 53.6% non-smokers, 16.4% ex-smokers (quit smoking), 7.7% light smokers (consuming 10 or less cigarettes per day) and 11.4% heavy smokers (consuming more than 10 cigarettes per day). By analyzing the multiple logistic regressions to control for demographic and health related variables, the baseline smoking status did not significantly influence the 6-years-later successful aging status. However, compared to non-smokers, ex-smokers showed a higher risk of failing in successful aging indicators, and current smokers had a higher risk for depressive symptoms or poor social support.

Longitudinal smoking behaviour and its impact on health as well was less explored in the past research. Results in this chapter showed that most of their smoking habit remains the same during the follow-up, but there were still some new smoking quitters, new smokers, and swing quitters. Since many ex-smokers arouse their motivation for smoking cessation related to their physical health problems (Hsu and Pwu, 2004), the earlier they realize the smoking impact on health, the more easily for the smokers to quit their smoking behaviour. This study showed that 3.6% survivors reported to be new quitters (quit during follow-up), and the elderly who kept smoking for 6 years were only 11.7%, if including the 33.5% of deaths in the samples. In table 4, the "never smoked" group was not the healthiest group in four successful aging indicators; even the "kept smoking" samples displayed a highest percentage in normal physical function and normal cognitive function.

Several possible explanations are as follows. First, smoking cessation is more likely to be a response to impoverished health, also in some way to reflect their health belief. In other words, for the smoking population, the smoking habit may start in early adulthood. If some health problems arose in the smokers such as cancer or respiratory diseases (Hsu and Pwu, 2004), it would make them decide to quit smoking. But at that time, they had already failed in successful aging and probably would be unable to recover anymore. Also, this study used strict criteria toward continuous successful aging, which means if one person has ever failed in any of the three waves follow-up, he/she was categorized to be "unsuccessful". The criteria would be insensitive enough to detect the dynamic health improvement for the quit smokers. And only the survivors were in the longitudinal study and the smoking impact on the deaths was excluded in the analysis. Second, for the current smokers, if they were less vulnerable in genetics or healthier in other life style dimensions, they may still achieve successful aging criteria and they don't see the causal relationship of smoking and their health. And therefore they will not have any motivation to quit smoking either.

Third, most of the smokers or ex-smokers were male, and females occupied most of the "never smoke" group. It has found that there was inequality in successful aging in women and men (Hsu, 2005). This chapter also found that females had poorer cognitive function (OR=1.834) and a greater possibility of showing depressive symptoms (OR=1.748). When the men and women samples were analyzed separately (table 3), gender was not significantly related to the longitudinal successful aging except for ex-smokers who had poorer physical function. Fourth, the samples of swing quitters or new quitters were limited, so no further analysis was done to explore the relationship of these changing behaviour and health. And the most challenging part of conducting smoking or smoking cessation research is that the smoking behaviour may change over time, and among the elderly longitudinal study some of them may die or may not be available for a follow-up. Therefore, the cumulative impact of smoking is difficult to estimate by limited data waves.

The influence of smoking cessation on different dimensions (physical, mental, and social) of health is quite interesting. In table 4, we found that successful quitters have higher proportion of success in physical function, cognitive function, and absence of depressive symptoms than new smokers or swing quitters. Earlier ex-smokers were also better than current smokers in depressive symptoms (61.8% versus 55.2%), but worse in physical function and cognitive function. Social support was not significantly related to smoking behaviour. By controlling other confounders in the multiple logistic regression model (table 5), smoking behaviour was insignificantly related to the four successful aging indicators, but ex-smokers did show a higher risk than non-smokers in four indicators, and ex-smokers also had less risk than current smokers in depressive symptoms and poor social support. The smoking cessation is possibly the response to impoverished health. Through comparing the different impacts of smoking cessation to four indicators of successful aging, it indicates that the response to poor health was only limited to physical health, and unfortunately, the smoking cessation may not definitely reverse the disabled physical health back to normal again. The good news is that smokers who quit had better emotional health (absence of depressive symptoms) or possible better social support than current smokers.

The effect of smoking on mental health, both cognitive and emotional health, needs further investigation. The conclusion of tobacco effects on cognitive health in past research was inconsistent (Bäckman et al., 2001), and the researchers think that the safe suggestion is to limit smoking behaviour. It was also reported that smokers have more major depression than non-smokers or higher anxiety (Glassman et al., 1990; Patton, et al., 1996). It also found the relationship between suicide and smoking (Miller et al., 2000), which was criticized because confounders were not controlled (Sheikh, 2000). In fact, past studies found that Nicotine has an effect to relieve stress and bring relaxation (Balfour, 1991; Silverstein, 1982). It means that the smoking behaviour may be the adjustment to relieve their depression or anxiety, and thus it would be hard for smokers to quit smoking, and so the depression rate is higher in smokers than non-smokers. Similarly, we also found that Taiwanese women were more likely to adjust their depressive symptoms by talking to family or friends or attending religious activities, while the men were more likely to attend group activities to drink (Hsu et al., 2003). If most of the smokers were men and the men were more likely to adjust their depression or stress by unhealthy lifestyles such as drinking and smoking, this would not be helpful in dealing with their mental health problem. Since the failure in physical function is more likely to be observed and noticed, it makes people more willing to take action to do health promotion at the onset of disease or disability. However, the cognitive or emotional dimension of health is likely to be neglected as a health problem for the elderly, and this may be worse for the current smokers. The impact of smoking and smoking cessation to depression and other mental health problems is suggested to be one of the tobacco research topics.

There are some limitations in this chapter. First, the deaths and those unable to be followed up were excluded in the analysis. It may underestimate the smoking impact of successful aging, because the deaths or lost cases were more likely to be frail and disabled. Second, the dynamic change of health was unavailable to observe because of only three waves of data. If smoking cessation has an effect on successful aging which may need a cumulative time, it is unable to detect these small changes by only limited waves of data. The smoking or quitting behaviour is changing with time as well, and we can only estimate the effect of smoking or cessation according to the baseline. Fortunately, most of the cases of swing smokers or new smokers were few in the samples, and the bias should be limited. Third, other health behaviours were included in the analysis, such as drinking, chewing betel nuts, or diet habits, which may be confounders to successful aging. It is suggested that researchers study the impact of a combination of health behaviours on successful aging in future studies.

Although many studies have found the smoking risks to health, smoking cessation programs are still working hard to convince the population. Changing people's lifestyles or health beliefs is never an easy work. In this chapter, the smoking impact on successful aging was not significant, and smoking cessation represents more a response to failure in successful aging than a preventive behaviour, especially a response to physical disability or diseases. Elderly are more likely to be aware of the smoking risks to physical health which can help them quit smoking. However, they are less likely to appreciate the risks of smoking to mental and social health, and even adjust their mental distress by smoking, which may delay the diagnosis and care for the mental problems among the elderly. Smoking cessation projects should consider the holistic health problems of the elderly and develop strategies to eliminate the smoking risk to successful aging.

ACKNOWLEDGMENTS

This research was supported by grants from the National Science Council, the project of "Successful aging of the elderly in Taiwan" (NSC 92-2320-B-468-001). I thank the Population and Health Research Center, Bureau of Health Promotion, Department of Health, Taiwan, for providing the data. The interpretation and conclusions contained herein do not represent those of the Bureau of Health Promotion. I also thank Mr. Gerald Irby for editing the manuscript draft.

REFERENCES

Abraham, J.D., Hansson, R.O. (1995). Successful aging at work: an applied study of selection, optimization, and compensation through impression management. *Journal of Gerontology: Psychological Sciences* 50B(2), P94-P103.

Albert, M.S., Jones, K., Savage, C.R., Berkman, L., Seeman, T., Blazer, D., Rowe, J.W. (1995). Predictors of cognitive change in older persons: MacArthur studies of successful aging. *Psychology and Aging* 10(4), 578-589.

Bäckman, L., Small, B.J., Wahlin, Åke, W. (2001). Aging and memory: cognitive and biological perspective. In: Birren, J.E., Schaie, K.W. (eds.) *Handbook of the Psychology of Aging*. San Diego, Academic Press, 349-377.

Balfour, D.J. (1991). The influence of stress on psychopharmacological responses to nicotine. *British Journal of Addiction* 86(5),489-93.

Carstensen, J.M., Pershagen, G.., Eklund,G. (1987). Mortality in relation to cigarette and pipe smoking: 16 years observation of 25,000 Swedish men. *Journal of Epidemiology Community Health* 41, 166-172.

Cheng, Y.J., Hildesheim, A., Hsu, M.M., Chen, I.H., Brinton, L.A., Levine, P.H., Chen, C.J., Yang, C.S. (1999). Cigarette smoking, alcohol consumption and risk f nasopharyngeal carcinoma in Taiwan. *Cancer Causes and Control* 10(3), 201-207.

Chou, K.L., Chi, I. (2002). Successful aging among the young-old, old-old, and oldest-old Chinese. *International Journal of Aging and Human Development* 54, 1-14.

Christen WG. Glynn RJ. Ajani UA. Schaumberg DA. (2000). Buring JE. Hennekens CH. Manson JE. Smoking cessation and risk of age-related cataract in men. *Journal of American Medical Association* 284(6), 713-6.

Freund, K.M., Belanger, A.J., D'Agostino, R.B., et al. (1993). The health risk of smoking: the Framingham study: 34 years of follow-up. *Annual Epidemiology.* 3, 417-424.

Garfein, A.J., Herzog, R. (1995). Robust aging among the young-old, old-old, and oldest-old. *Journal of Gerontology: Social Sciences.* 50B(2), S77-S87.

Glass, T.A., Seeman, T.E., Herzog, A.R., Kahn, R., Berkman, L.F. (1995). Change in productive activity in late adulthood: MacArthur studies of successful aging. *Journal of Gerontology: Social Sciences.* 50B(2), S65-S76.

Glassman, A.H., Helzer, J.E., Covey, L.S., et al. (1990). Smoking, smoking cessation, and major depression. *Journal of American Medical Association.* 264, 1546-9.

He, J., Oogden L.G., Bazzano, L.A., Vupputuri, S., Loria, C., Whelton, P.K. (2001). Risk factors for congestive heart failure in US men and women: NHANES I Epidemioilogic Follow-up Study. *Archives of Internal Medicine.* 161(7), 996-1002.

Hsu, H.C. (2006). Does social participation by the elderly reduce mortality and cognitive impairment? *Aging and Mental Health.* (revision in review).

Hsu, H.C. (2005). Gender disparity of successful aging in Taiwan. *Women and Health.* 42(1), 1-21.

Hsu, H.C., Chang, M.C. (2004). Successful aging and active aging in Taiwan: a multi-level analysis. *Taiwanese Journal of Social Welfare.* 3(2), 1-36. [in Chinese]

Hsu, H.C., Pwu, R.F. (2004). Too late to quit? Smoking and smoking cessation on morbidity and mortality among the elderly in a longitudinal study. *Kaohsiung Journal of Medical Sciences.* 20(10), 484-491.

Hsu, H.C., Ho, C.S., Kung, P.J. (2003). Research project report of "Research demonstration in health care issues in Taichung County, the Knowledge, Attitude, and Practice for National Health Promotion Survey in Taiwan". Granted by Bureau of Health Promotion, Department of Health. (BHP-CPHSR-92-1)

Hu, S.C., Lanese, R.R. (1998). The applicability of the theory of planned behavior to the intention to quit smoking across workplaces in southern Taiwan. *Addictive Behaviors.* 23(2), 225-37.

Kohout, F.J., Berkan, L., Evans, D.A., and Cornohi-Huntley, J. (1993). Two shorter forms of the CES-D depression symptoms index. *Journal of Aging and Health,* 5(2), 179-193.

Lee, L.T., Chen, C.J., Suo, J., Luh, K.T., Lin, R.S. (1997). Pulmonary tuberculosis and long cancer: a case-control study. *Formosan Journal of Medicine.* 2,176-84.

Liaw, K.M., Cheng, C.J. (1998). Mortality attributable to cigarette smoking in Taiwan: a 12-year follow-up study. *Tobacco Control.* 7(2), 141-148.

Mclaughlin, J.K., Hrubez, Z., Blot, W.J., et al. (1995). Smoking and cancer mortality among U.S. veterans: a 26-year follow-up. *International Journal of Cancer.* 60,190-193.

Miller, M., Hemenway, D., Bell, N.S., Rimm, E. (2000). Cigarettes and suicide: a prospective study of 50,000 men. *American Journal of Public Health.* 90, 768-773

Patton, G.C., Hibbert, M., Rosier, M.J., Carlin, J.B., Caust, J., Bowes, G. (1996). Is smoking associated with depression and anxiety in teenagers?. *American Journal of Public Health.* 86(2), 225-30.

Pelkonen, M., Notkola, I.L., Tukiainen, H., Tervahauta, M., Tuomilehto, J., Nissinen, A. (2001). Smoking cessation, decline in pulmonary function and total mortality: a 30 year follow up study among the Finnish cohorts of the Seven Countries Study. *Thorax.* 56(9), 703-7.

Radloff, L.S. (1977). The CES-D scale: a self-report depression scale for research in the general population. *Applied Psychological Measurement.* 1: 385-401.

Rea, T., Heckbert, S.R., Kaplan, R.C., Smith, N.L., Lemaitre, R.N., Psaty, B.M. (2002). Smoking status and risk for recurrent coronary events after myocardial infarction. *Annals of Intern Medicine.* 137(6), 494-500.

Roget, E., Murray, J.L. (1980). Smoking and cause of death among U.S. veterans: 16 years of observation. *Public Health Report.* 95, 213-222.

Rowe, J.W., Kahn, R.L. (1997). Successful aging. *The Gerontologist.* 37, 433-440.

Rowe, J.W., Kahn, R.L. (1998). The structure of successful aging. In: J.W. Rowe, and Kahn, R.L., (eds) *Successful Aging.* NY: Dell Publishing, 36-52.

Ruigrok, Y., Buskens, E., Rinkel, G.J.E. (2001). Attributable risk of common and rare determinants of subarachnoid hemorrhage. *Stroke.* 32(5), 1173-1175.

Sauer, W., Berlin, J.A., Strom, B.L., Miles, C., Carson, J.L., Kimmel, S.E. (2002). Cigarette yield and the risk of myocardial infarction in smokers. *Archives of Internal Medicine.* 162(3), 300-306.

Schaie, K.W. (1990). The optimization of cognitive functioning in old age: predictions based on cohort-sequential and longitudinal data. In: Baltes, P.B. and Baltes, M.M. (eds.) *Successful aging: perspectives from the behavioral sciences.* Cambridge: Cambridge University Press, 94-117.

Seeman, T.E., Berkman, L.F., Blazer, D., Rowe, J.W. (1994). Social ties and support and neuroendocrine function: the MacArthur studies of successful aging. *Annals of Behavioral Medicine.* 16(2), 95-106.

Seeman, T.E., Berkman, L.F., Charpentier, P.A., Blazer, D.G., Albert, M.S., Tinetti, M.E. (1995). Behavioral and psychosocial predictors of physical performance: MacArthur studies of successful aging. *Journal of Gerontology: Medical Sciences.* 50A(4), M177-M183.

Sheikh, K. (2000). Depression and the association of smoking and suicide. *American Journal of Public Health.* 90(12), 1952-1953.

Silverstein, B. (1982). Cigarette smoking, nicotine addiction, and relaxation. *Journal of Personality and Social Psychology.* 42(5), 946-50.

Strawbridge, W.J., Cohen, R.D., Shema, S.J., Kaplan, G.A. (1996). Successful aging: predictors and associated activities. *American Journal of Epidemiology.* 144(2), 135-41.

Suminori, A., Hirayama, T. (1990). Cigarette smoking and cancer mortality risk in Japanese men and women: results from reanalysis of the six-prefecture cohort study data. *Environmental Health Perspective.* 87, 19-26.

von Faber, M., van der Wiel, A.B., van Exel, E., Gussekloo, J., Lagaay, A.M., van Dongen, E., Knook, D.L., van der Geest, S., Westendorp, R.G.J. (2001). Successful aging in the Oldest old: who can be characterized as successful aged? *Archives of Internal Medicine.* 161, 2694-2700.

Wald, N.J., Watt, H.C. (1997). Prospective study of effect of switching from cigarettes to pipes or cigars on mortality from three smoking related diseases. *British Medical Journal.* 314,1860-1863.

Wilson, P., D'Agostino, R.B., Levy, D., Belanger, A.M., Silbershatz, H., Kannel, W.B. (1998). Prediction of coronary heart disease using risk factors categories. *Circulation.* 97(18), 1837-1847.

World Health Organization. (2002). *Active Ageing: a Policy Framework.* Ageing and Life Course Program, Second United Nations World Assembly on Ageing, Madrid, Spain, April 2002.

Wu, S.C., Chang, M.C. (1997). *Health care for the elderly in Taiwan. Series of Taiwan Elderly Research, book series (6).* Institute of Taiwan Family Planning. Taipei, Institute of Public Health, National Taiwan University. [in Chinese]

Yuan, J.M., Ross, R.K., Wang, X.L., et al. (1996). Morbidity and mortality in relation to cigarette smoking in Shanghai, China: a prospective male cohort study. Journal of American Medical Association 275, 1646-1650.

In: Smoking Cessation: Theory, Interventions and Prevention   ISBN: 978-1-60021-591-9
Editor: Jerome E. Landow   © 2008 Nova Science Publishers, Inc.

Chapter 13

BIOCHEMICAL FEEDBACK TO IMPROVE SMOKING CESSATION INTERVENTIONS – RESULTS FROM A POINT-OF-CARE TEST FOR NICOTINE METABOLITES IN URINE OR SALIVA

Graham F. Cope[*]
Institute of Research and Development, University of Birmingham,
Birmingham, B15 2TH, UK

ABSTRACT

Background: Feedback is an important mechanism to bring about behavioural change. Printed and computer-generated information, either generic or targeted, has been used extensively to improve smoking cessation. Biochemical feedback provides personalised information, which gives a source of comparison for the individual among their cohort and gives an assessment of risk, establishes the current status and provides a platform for a change opinion of the smoker. Carbon monoxide monitoring, although primarily used to verify smoking habit, it can provide feedback, which can encourage smokers to quit. However, lack of specificity and sensitivity of this test limits its suitability. Cotinine testing, the preferred method to verify and monitor smoking habit, is primarily laboratory based, which has problems of delay and data accessibility.

Aim: To provide a simple point-of-care test for cotinine and other nicotine metabolites, which retain the sensitivity and specificity of laboratory testing, yet provides an immediate result. To demonstrate that feedback from the test can improve smoking cessation advice.

Method: A urine test was developed and used in an antenatal care setting. Immediate feedback about smoking levels increased awareness of tobacco intake on foetal development. A saliva test was also developed and used in general dental practice to interact with patients to improve understanding why smoking causes oral disease.

---

[*] G.Cope.mermaid@ukonline.co.uk

Results: During the antenatal study in the case group there was a significant reduction in test-verified smoking (p<0.001), with 16% quitting and 33% significantly reducing their cigarette usage. There was a significant reduction in urinary nicotine metabolite concentration (NMC) by the end of pregnancy compared to the control group. In the dental study a similar pattern emerged, with 23% of the case group quitting compared to 7% in the control group.

Conclusion: Biochemical feedback from a rapid, point-of-care test for smoking can significantly improve smoking cessation interventions and bring about behavioural change.

BACKGROUND

Smoking cessation advice concentrates on initiating behavioural change to overcome the addictive nature of nicotine. Helping to focus the individual on his or her responses to their addiction, and understanding the harm produced by it are important and successful approaches to smoking cessation.

Personalised feedback of information about the effects of smoking on health has been the focus of numerous studies. It provides important information about the risks and the levels of risk involved, with the hope to increase the engagement in the message promoted. Feedback should aim to increase awareness of the message and enhanced interaction with the educational materials [1].

Feedback can be broken down into different approaches. At one end of the spectrum there is the generic information which is relevant to a population. This may be the whole population, such as information about the risks of smoking and lung cancer, or specifically to a part of the populace, such as the dangers of smoking in pregnancy. Information can be more targeted to specific individuals, such as addressed tailored printed material has been shown to enhance its ability to attract notice and readership[2].

Personalized interventions, generated by computer-based or web-based expert systems, which take into account numerous variables, such as baseline smoking status, readiness to change, perceived barriers to quitting and past quit attempts, can generate thousands of different individualised messages [3]. The tailored personalized letters, often followed by monthly email reminders, contain health risk information and coping strategies, have large scale population impact and achieve impressive reported cessation results [4, 5].

Most interventions attempt to motivate an individual to adopt a healthier lifestyle, by providing the information and the skills necessary to do this, and also to reinforce the benefits and motivation to maintain the changes. It has been established that providing feedback about a smoker's biological markers of harm is a useful way to motivate or reinforce quit attempts. Biochemical feedback provides personalised information, which gives a source of comparison for the individual among their cohort and establishes the current status and provides a platform for a change opinion of the smoker. These markers educate smokers about their potential risk of disease or the actual physical damage they may incur. These markers can also initiate or help maintain a change in behaviour [6].

BIOMARKERS

Biomarkers are biological or biochemical indicators of smoking or are related to past smoking behaviour, which gauge harm exposure or genetic susceptibility to smoking-related disease [7]. There are markers related to harm exposure, for example carbon monoxide (CO), either in expired-air or carboxyhaemoglobin, and cotinine, the major metabolite of nicotine, measured in serum, saliva or urine. These gauge levels of short term smoking, but may indicate the degree of exposure over a longer period of time. Pulmonary functioning measurements, such as pulmonary function tests, notably spirometry and x-rays, can indicate harm due to past exposure. And there is genetic testing for lung cancer susceptibility, particularly the presence of the CYP2D6 enzyme [6].

Risser and Belcher studied smokers and provided them with expired-air CO values, together with spirometry readings together with brief counselling and self-help literature. The result was an increase in their intention to quit, raising to 51% compared to 44% of controls who did not receive the intervention; thus indicating a change in attitude [8]. Wallace et al investigated the use of spirometry to improve smoking cessation in chronic obstructive pulmonary disease (COPD) in a primary care setting. He found that this simple, immediate test result was able to identify the disease in its early stages, so reducing the individual's risk of debilitating morbidity, but the feedback supplemented the smoking cessation advice, by providing objective data to improve patient motivation[9]. Along similar lines Bovet et al studied smokers with peripheral atherosclerosis and showed the experimental group ultrasound photographs of their own arterial plaques, thus indicating the harm caused by smoking. This feedback increased smoking cessation significantly when assessed at 6 months, with 22% quitting compared to 6% in the control group [10]. Lerman et al extended the intervention from marker of a tobacco intake (CO) and a marker of physiological effect (pulmonary function test), by incorporating a test for genetic susceptibility to lung cancer (CYP2D6) [11, 12]. However, the results were disappointing, with no significant effect on cessation when measured after a 12-month period. Although the pairing of CO and counselling did have a short-term effect, it was concluded that incorporating genetic susceptibility could be counter productive, in increasing anxiety about future disease development, which may have an adverse effect by reinforcing the smoking behaviour.

COTININE TESTING

One biomarker for harm exposure which has received considerable attention is cotinine testing. This is a major metabolite of nicotine and unlike CO is specific to tobacco intake and has a long half-life, such that it monitors smoking over a number of days, rather than just a few hours. Cotinine is one of approximately 8 metabolites of nicotine, and can be measured with a range of laboratory based techniques, most involving expensive equipment and requiring trained laboratory staff [13, 14]. Cotinine is the marker of choice to verify smoking habit and there have been attempts to use laboratory cotinine results to provide feedback to reduce smoking habit.

Haddow and his group in one multi-site randomised controlled trial in pregnancy measured cotinine levels in serum samples collected by a number of physicians. The cotinine was assayed in a centralised laboratory and the results were interpreted and relayed back to the woman via her physician. This was followed up 1 month later by another measurement; while a control group had no knowledge of the study. The results were that the intervention group had an increase in birth-weight and the conclusions drawn were that cotinine could be used to provide valuable feedback, but it required the co-operation of a large number of physicians and the central laboratory to rapidly relay the results for the protocol to have any effect [15]. In another study Frank et al collected urine samples from pregnant smokers at each pre-natal visit and had them analysed for cotinine. The results were graphically displayed along with a drawing and description of foetal development at that particular gestational age. Later, within 24-48 hours, the results were made available to the pregnant women and her smoking cessation counsellor. The results were that the intervention group had a much greater decrease in cotinine levels by the end of pregnancy, compared to the control group who did not receive the feedback until the end of pregnancy. There was a confirmed quit rate of 18% compared to 2% in the control group. It was concluded that that visual graphic feedback of cotinine levels was cost efficient and a possible method to decrease smoking during pregnancy [16]. The drawbacks of this approach were the impracticality of laboratory cotinine testing and relaying the result to the counsellor within a short period of time, and having them available for the next consultation.

The inference from these and other studies was that personalized biomarker feedback may increase motivation for quitting smoking. Assessment of the literature shows that three variables appear to be especially important: namely the type of biomarker feedback used, the level of accompanying treatment or counselling and the repetition of the feedback. For biomarker interventions to be credible they must be understood, accepted and acted upon. It is important to ensure that smokers understand the purpose of the biological testing, what is being measured, how this applies to their own smoking behaviour and to their health, and in the case of pregnancy the health of the foetus. Providing written hand-outs and graphic displays of changes in biomarker values with time was suggested as an important way of increasing smoking comprehension of the test results. People are more responsive to messages structured in positive terms of the potential gain rather than the negative effects or disadvantages of continuing the habit. It is also important to considered is how the message is conveyed and by whom [6].

With these recommendations in mind the author embarked on a course of investigation to develop a point-of-care cotinine test which could provide an alternative to laboratory-based analysis, yet retain the suitability of instantaneous CO monitoring. This, in the case of a urine test, could be used in a hospital-based antenatal setting to provide feedback to reduce smoking in pregnancy, and in the case of a saliva test in a general dental practice setting to reduce smoking-related oral disease.

SMOKESCREEN

A technology was developed based on a previously published colorimetric assay, based on the König reaction [17, 18]. The assay detected the pyridine ring, common to nicotine and all its metabolites, utilizing diethyl-thiobarbituric acid as the complexing agent. This was incorporated into a patented testing device called SafeTube™, which comprises of a plastic testing device made in 2-parts: a liquid measuring device in the shape of a syringe, and a clear plastic tube where the reaction or test takes place. The device can safely hold chemical reagents apart, which would prematurely react, and bring them together immediately prior to the addition of the liquid sample. The enclosed device post-sample addition also minimizes operator contamination [19].

A 2ml urine sample is measured by the syringe and injected onto the reagents, which once dissolved turn pink if cotinine or other metabolites are present; the higher the concentration the darker the colour. The SmokeScreen® test (Mermaid Diagnostics Limited, Stourbridge, UK) provides a 5-minute assay, which can be carried out in any extra-laboratory situation by healthcare professionals with a minimum of training, with the added advantage of cost savings over laboratory analysis, to which it is analytically comparable[20].

The test can be used as a stand-alone, whereby the sample if it turns pink then it is from a smoker. Alternatively, it can be used with a colour chart for a semi-quantitative assessment of smoking habit, or finally with a dedicated portable instrument or colorimeter with absorbance reading at 510nm for a quantitative result of nicotine metabolite concentration (NMC) produced by comparison to a cotinine standard curve. The results from a laboratory evaluation correlate with self-reported cigarette consumption (r=0.69, p<0.0001) and nicotine yield of cigarettes smoked (r=0.14, p<0.001), and independent cotinine measurements by gas chromatography (r=0.89, p<0.001) [19]. A recent independent evaluation compared the test with CO monitoring and laboratory-based creatinine-corrected cotinine measurements. The smokescreen test was found to have a sensitivity and specificity of 100% and 98% respectively, in its ability to detect active smoking [20].

SMOKESCREEN IN PREGNANCY

The test provides feedback, both visually, by virtue of a variable colour change indicating smoking level and also numerically, when the result can be expressed graphically, when an individual's result be compared with others from the same cohort. The impact of this feedback was first gauged in an antenatal setting in an attempt to reduce smoking in pregnancy.

New referrals to a hospital antenatal clinic, smokers and non-smokers alike, were randomized into the case group, those receiving feedback from the smoking test, or controls who were only relayed their test result at the end of pregnancy. After a brief verbal explanation of the test and the aims of the research, they were asked for a sample of urine, which had invariably been brought to clinic for routine testing. The volunteers were interviewed in a private room and the 5-minutes test was carried out in their presence, during which time a questionnaire was completed by interview, detailing current and previous smoking habit, co-habitation with a smoker and other social and demographic details.

On completion the volunteers were shown the resultant colour of the test and given the numerical result, illustrated as a point on a graph plotted against reported daily cigarette consumption. Current smokers and those with a positive result were followed through the study, while the non-smokers were further excluded. A specific 'quit date', usually within the next 14 days, was chosen by mutual agreement, and this was written on the test result sheet. They were given a printed self-help leaflet and invited to return for measurement at their next and subsequent visits. A positive attitude was taken to smoking, with emphasis on trying to empower the smoker, with information, feedback and encouragement, to change her smoking behaviour. This protocol was repeated whenever the patient returned to the clinic, up to and including the 36 week visit, with measurement, questioning about changes in smoking, specific events on the 'quit date', and reinforcement of advice.

For comparison the control group was not seen at their initial visit, but their urine measured, consequently they did not have the benefit of the feedback. They received routine counseling about smoking in pregnancy as part of usual care. Control patients were traced throughout pregnancy and interviewed at their 36-week visit. Like the case women they were interviewed, and the nature of the study explained. They were asked about changes to their smoking throughout pregnancy, and about the frequency and source of any anti-smoking advice throughout pregnancy.

The study involved 109 smokers in the case group who were followed through to delivery and 83 smokers in the control group. When the case group were questioned about changes to smoking habit 16 (16.2%) reported quitting smoking, 33 (33.3%) reported significantly reduced their cigarette consumption, leaving 50.5% who reported being unable to change, and had maintaining their usual smoking habit. In the control group, none reported quitting during their pregnancy, 30 (47.6%) reported cutting down, and 33 (52.4%) reported maintaining their usual habit.

Collectively, there was a highly significant fall in nicotine metabolite concentration (NMC) results in the case group, from 'booking' to 36 weeks gestation (p<0.0001), whereas in the control group there was no significant difference between the two points. The smoking test results in the intervention group at 36 weeks were significantly lower than the control group (p<0.003). Indicating the smoking habit in the case group had changed following the intervention.

Smoking habits at 36 weeks, as determined by the smoking test, showed that of those in the case group 22.2% had below detectable levels, 5.1% had a positive, but very low result (indicating exposure to environmental tobacco smoke or occasional cigarette use); 42.4% had a significantly lower result than at 'booking'; and 11.1% had elevated values, indicating increased nicotine intake. This included 3 women who had a result more than doubled their initial result. The changes in the control group were very different, with only 6.8% negative and 33.9% having a significantly lower result. However, the greatest difference was that 45.7% had a higher result than at their initial visit, with 17 women having a result more than double, indicating a much higher nicotine intake.

The feedback from the test contributed to the brief counseling and self-help materials, but the nature of the test was used to increase the understanding of the detrimental effects of smoking in pregnancy. It was explained that if nicotine products could be detected in the urine, then that implied that the same chemicals were present in the blood stream and during pregnancy the blood was nourishing the foetus, and thus exposing it to the harmful effects of smoking. This realization also contributed to the feedback effect of the test.

When asked to subjectively evaluate the influence of the smoking test on changes in their smoking behaviour, a majority thought the test had helped them to appreciate more about their smoking. The control group was asked to recall any questions or advice they were given by hospital staff while attending the hospital. A majority (66.7%) could not recount any questions or information being given, even though questions were routinely included as part of the 'booking' procedure. This implies that the feedback did improve engagement with the counseling and information given.

Analysis of birth parameters and comparison with test results showed that test levels at the 'booking' were not related to any post-partum parameters or other delivery assessments, while at the end of pregnancy the test results inversely correlated with birthweight ($p<0.01$), body length ($p<0.05$), and that with head circumference approached significance ($p=0.056$). There was no significant relationship between the smoking test result and gender, gestation, type of delivery or Apgar scores.

Adjustment for test results revealed a significant difference in birthweight between the case group (3.26 Kg) and the control group (3.08 Kg, $p<0.03$). This would suggest the intervention had an overall effect of improving birthweight [21].

The study was structured to provide as many of the desirable factors previously advocated, notably personalized biomarker feedback, an understanding of the purpose of the testing, what was being measured and how it applied to the woman's own smoking behaviour. We provided written hand-outs and graphic displays of the biomarker value. We were aware that people are more responsive to messages structured in positive terms, and this was the emphasis on the message.

It is accepted that pregnancy is a special case, in that women are more likely to quit for the duration of their pregnancy, but relapse shortly after giving birth. We wished to address a chronic condition to determine whether the same approach could be applied. Based on a similar protocol we attempted to address the effects of smoking on oral health, an area which has not received a great deal of attention. Our aim was to develop the SmokeScreen test to analyse saliva and to use this as a chair-side test to provide feedback to smokers with oral disease.

SMOKESCREEN IN DENTISTRY

The levels of nicotine metabolites in saliva are approximately one fifth that found in urine for a similar level of cigarette consumption. We improved the sensitivity of the assay by utilizing 2,2-dimethyl-1,3 dioxane-4,6-dione (Meldrum's acid) as the complexing agent [22]. This produced a yellow derivative if nicotine metabolites were present, again in a concentration-dependent manner. However, due to the reduced concentration the test development time was extended to 10 minutes and resultant colour read against a 6 point scale $(0 - 6)$ colour chart to give a semi-quantitative assessment of nicotine metabolite concentration [23].

In an operator-blinded randomised controlled trial 100 smoker were recruited from patients registered from a general dental practice. They were randomised to either the case group (n=50) or the control (n=50) group. All volunteers were attracted by a free and comprehensive oral examination. Each was given verbal smoking cessation counselling and literature packs. Each then provided a 2ml saliva sample by expectoration. Control subjects were informed that their result would be relayed to them at their next visit and immediately discharged. Case subjects were shown the test procedure and their test result, with a full interpretation of the result in relation to the findings in the in oral examination, with particular emphasis on disease states of the gums prior. All volunteers were recalled after 8 weeks for repeat testing. At recall, the operator repeated the saliva sampling and testing procedure and the all case group subjects who re-attended for the 8-week re-assay completed a questionnaire to assess their opinion, on a visual-analogue scale, of the smoking test to evaluate its value in aiding their smoking cessation counselling.

The primary oral examination assessed a series of periodontal parameters. The results showed a significant correlation between the SmokeScreen test results and incidence of caries ($r=0.25$, $p<0.01$), Community Periodontal Index Treatment Needs scores ($r=0.4$, $p<0.001$), probing pocket depths ($r=0.26$ $p<0.01$), tooth mobility, ($r=0.34$, $p<0.001$) and the presence of adverse oral mucosal changes ($r=0.26$, $p<0.01$). These findings confirmed that smoking has an adverse effect on oral health, but this was the first report of a biochemical marker and unfavourable periodontal outcome [24].

At the original presentation there was no significant difference between baseline NMC test results for the case group and the controls. However, at the 8-week recall there was a significant reduction in smoking habit in the case group, with a reduction in test results from the baseline value of 4.2 to 2.58 compared with no change in the controls ($p<0.0001$). For case group subjects 10 (23%) patient quit smoking, 20 (45%) had reduced their verified smoking habit and there was a significant reduction in test results from baseline to follow-up ($p<0.00001$). For the control subjects 3 (7%) had quit and 9 (21%) had reduced their nicotine intake. There was no reduction in test results in the control group during the 2 month study period ($p=0.72$).

The case group evaluated the SmokeScreen test as part of the intervention and 88% felt that the test provided clear results that were easy to interpret. Thirty three percent felt that the combination of observing the test, talking with the primary care dental practitioner and reading the anti-smoking literature pack was the most informative and supportive method. The results from the visual-analogue scale demonstrated that 9% found the test to be of 'no use', whereas 27% felt it was a 'very useful' aid to the smoking cessation counseling. Overall, the majority believed the test to be beneficial. There was a significant correlation between the degree of change in smoking habit as measured by the test and the perceived benefit of using the test, ($r=0.64$, $p<0.001$) [25].

Although this was a smaller study, the smoking test was only semi-quantitative and only for a 2-month period. The results reinforced the findings of feedback, with additional materials and counseling produced an effective smoking cessation intervention.

CONCLUSION

Behavioural change is the main objective of smoking cessation interventions. The computer and web-based expert systems, providing personalized letters or email messages, have the potential to interact with a large number of smokers. However, there is a need for procedures to interact with smokers in clinical settings, when they are receiving treatment for smoking-related illness or condition. The healthcare professional needs to expand on the National Practice Guidelines which calls for all health care providers to "ask" all patients about tobacco use, and to "advise, assess, assist and arrange" when smokers want to quit smoking (the "5 As"), by assessing more accurately the level of nicotine intake and to use that information to personalize the assistance offered.

The biomarkers for smoking related illness are many [26], and only two, relating to tobacco intake, namely CO and cotinine have been described here in detail. Each has its own advantage, in that CO monitoring can give instantaneous results and provide information to verify cessation but also provide feedback to assess the level of risk. However, anecdotally many healthcare professionals who use this technique recognise that false positives often occur due to exposure from CO non-tobacco sources. But more important is the fact that expired-air CO only detects smoking habit over a matter of 6 to 8 hours. Many smokers are aware of this and have to abstain for a relatively short period of time, for example over night, and they can be rewarded with a negative result.

Cotinine, on the other hand, is specific to tobacco intake and the half-life of 18 hours (compared to 3 hours for CO) means that it is monitoring smoking habit over a number of days. Also, cotinine levels have been shown to be a good indicator of nicotine dependence and are related to the Fagerstrom Test for Nicotine Dependence [27]. Therefore, theoretically assessment of cotinine levels, with counseling, can be used to provide the smoker with information for them to judge their level of risk for smoking-related disease and if the result is graphically displayed as an individual point and others obtained from the same population then this provides a means to establish their current status and a comparison among their cohort. This information could provide a platform for a change opinion of the smoker.

It was this hypothesis combined with the availability of the SmokeScreen test formed the basis of the interventions described above. In the pregnancy study the expectation of greater interaction with the educational materials and counseling with biomarker feedback appeared to be successful, and on occasions this approach was extended from the pregnant smoker to her partner, who accompanied her to the antenatal visit. The low cost and availability of the test allowed smoking partners to be tested at the same time. This often had encouraging results, engaging the partner into a smoking cessation process, whereby they formed a collaboration to quit smoking together. This can also be extended to repeat testing. This provides ongoing feedback, in a similar way to the psychological methods employed in the Weight Watchers programme. It has been suggested that incorporate behavioural treatment, with dietary change and increased physical activity, can improve the psychological state, including mood. These changes may help motivate overweight people to maintain the physical activity and nutritional practices necessary to lose and maintain weight [28]. Similar psychological advantage can be achieved by obtaining lower cotinine testing during a smoking cessation programme.

So, in conclusion biomarker feedback has been used in many studies to improve smoking cessation interventions, however, the lack of large scale, well designed studies prevented a definitive statement on the effectiveness of biomarker risk assessment as an aid to smoking cessation [29]. Clearly, larger studies with greater scientific rigour are required but the evidence provided above indicates that SmokeScreen could provide a suitable tool for such investigations.

REFERENCES

[1]   DiClemente CC, Marinilli AS, Singh M, Bellino LE. The role of feedback in the process of health behaviour change. *Am. J. Health Behav.* 2001; 25: 217-227.

[2]   Skinner CS, Campbell MK, Rimer BK, Curry S, Prochaska JO. How effective is tailored print communication? *Ann. Behav. Med.* 1992; 21: 290-98.

[3]   Stretcher VJ, Kreuter M, Den Boer D, Kobrin S, Hospers HJ, Skinner CS. The effects of computer-tailored smoking cessation messages in family practice settings. *J. Fam. Pract.* 1994; 39: 262-68.

[4]   Velicer WF, Prochaska JO, Redding CA. Tailored communications for smoking cessation: past successes and future directions. *Drug Alcohol Rev.* 2006; 25: 49-57.

[5]   Prochaska JO, Velicer WF, Redding C, Rossi JS, Goldstein M, DePue J et al. Stage-based expert systems to guide a population of primary care patients to quit smoking, eat healthier, prevent skin cancer and receive regular mammograms. *Prev. Med.* 2005; 41: 406-416.

[6]   McClure JB. Are biomarkers a useful aid in smoking cessation? A review and analysis of the literature. *Behav. Med.* 2001; 27: 37-47.

[7]   McClure JB. Are biomarkers useful treatment aids for promoting health behaviour change? An empirical review. *Am. J. Prev. Med.* 2002: 22: 200-207.

[8]   Risser NL, Belcher DW. Adding spirometry, carbon monoxide and pulmonary symptom results to smoking cessation counselling: a randomised trial. *J. Gen. Intern. Med.* 1990; 5: 16-22.

[9]   Wallace LD, Troy KE. Simple office spirometry for primary care practitioners. *J. Am. Acad. Nurse Practitioners.* 2006; 18: 414-421.

[10]   Bovet P, Perret F, Cornuz J, Quilindo J, Paccaud F. Improved smoking cessation in smokers given ultrasound photographs of their own arthosclerotic plaques. *Prev. Med.* 2002; 34: 215-220.

[11]   Lerman C, Orleans CT, Engstrom PF. Biological markers in smoking cessation treatments. *Seminars Oncol.* 1993; 20: 359-367.

[12]   Lerman C, Gold K, Audrain J, et al. incorporating biomarkers of exposure to genetic susceptibility into smoking cessation treatments: effects on smoking-related cognitions, emotions, and behaviour change. *Health Psychol.* 1997; 16: 87-99.

[13]   Jarvis MJ, Tunstall-Pedoe H, Feyerabend C, Vesey C, Saloojee Y. Comparison of tests used to distinguish smokers from non-smokers. *Am. J. Public Health.* 1987; 77: 1435-1438.

[14]   Benowitz NL. Biomarkers of environmental tobacco smoke exposure. *Environ Health Perspectives.* 1999; 107 (suppl 2) 349-355.

[15]   Haddow JE, Knight GJ, Kloza EM, Palomaki GE, Wald NJ. Cotinine-assisted intervention in pregnancy to reduce smoking and low birthweight delivery. *Br. J. Obst. Gynae.* 1991; 98: 859-865.

[16]   Frank JE, Hoffman DS, Flanagan V. Use of repeated cotinine determinations as a motivational and educational tool in smoking cessation counselling for pregnant women. *Paed Res.* 1999; 45: 1153.

[17] Barlow RD, Stone RB, Wald NJ, Puhakainen EVJ. The direct Barbituric acid assay for nicotine metabolites in urine: a simple colorimetric test for the routine assessment of smoking status and cigarette smoking intake. *Clin. Chim. Acta.* 1987; 165: 45-52.

[18] Peach H, Ellard GA. Jenner PJ, Morris RW. A simple, inexpensive urine test of smoking. *Thorax.* 1985; 40: 351-357.

[19] Cope G, Nayyar P, Holder R, Gibbons J, Bunce R. A simple near-patient test for nicotine and its metabolites in urine to assess smoking habit. *Clin. Chim. Acta.* 1996; 256: 135-149.

[20] Hobbs SD, Wilmink ABM, Adam DJ, Bradbury AW. Assessment of smoking status in patients with peripheral arterial disease. *J. Vasc. Surg.* 2005; 41: 451-456.

[21] Cope GF, Nayyar P, Holder R. Feedback from a point-of-care test for nicotine intake to reduce smoking during pregnancy. *Ann. Clin. Biochem.* 2003; 40: 674-679.

[22] O'Doherty S, Cook M, Roberts DJ. Enhancing the LC analysis of nicotine and its metabolites in urine using Meldrum's acid as a complexing *agent J. High Resolution Chromatr.* 1990; 13: 74-77.

[23] Cope G, Nayyar P, Holder R, Brock G, Chapple I. Near-patient test for nicotine and its metabolites in saliva to assess smoking habit. *Ann. Clin. Biochem.* 2000; 37: 666-73.

[24] Barnfather KDP, Cope G, Chapple ILC. Salivary cotinine and indices of periodontal health in general practice. *J. Dental Res.* 2002; 81: A203.

[25] Barnfather KDP, Cope G, Chapple ILC. Effect of incorporating a 10 minute point of care test for salivary nicotine metabolites into a general practice based smoking cessation programme: randomised controlled trial. *Br. Med. J.* 2005; 331: 999-1001.

[26] Hatsukami DK, Benowitz NL, Rennard SI, Oncken C, Hecht SS. Biomarkers to assess the utility of potential reduced exposure tobacco products. *Nic. Tob. Res.* 2006; 8: 600-622.

[27] Prokhorov AV, De Moor C, Pallonen UE, Hudmon KS, Koehly L, Hu SH. Validation of the modified Fagerstrom Tolerance Questionnaire with salivary cotinine among adolescents. *Add. Behav.* 2000; 25: 429-433.

[28] Miller-Kovach K, Hermann M, Winick M The psychological ramifications of weight management. *J. Women's Health Gender Med.* 1999; 8: 477-482.

[29] Bize R, Burnard B, Mueller Y, Cornuz J. Biochemical risk assessment as an aid for smoking cessation,. *Cochrane Database of Systematic Reviews.* 2005; Issue 4. art No. CD004705.

In: Smoking Cessation: Theory, Interventions and Prevention   ISBN: 978-1-60021-591-9
Editor: Jerome E. Landow   © 2008 Nova Science Publishers, Inc.

Chapter 14

THE ROLE OF ORAL HEALTH PROFESSIONALS IN TOBACCO CESSATION

Giuseppe Pizzo[*][1], *Maria R. Piscopo*[1],
Maria E. Licata[1] *and Joan M. Davis*[2]

[1] Department of Oral Sciences, University of Palermo, Italy
[2] Department of Dental Hygiene, College of Applied Sciences and Arts,
Southern Illinois University, Carbondale, Illinois, USA

ABSTRACT

Tobacco is the major independent risk factor for the development of oral cancer and potentially malignant lesions. It is also involved in the pathogenesis of periodontal disease. The members of the dental team can play an effective role in tobacco preventing and cessation as they provide preventive and therapeutic services to a basically healthy population on a regular basis.

In this paper, the authors present specific strategies to guide oral health professionals (i.e. dentist and dental hygienist) providing smoking cessation interventions.

The "Five A's" strategic approach represents a brief and effective protocol for smoking cessation that members of dental team can use with all patients in their office practice. This protocol involves *asking* each patient about tobacco use, *advising* users to quit, *assessing* their willingness to make a quit attempt, *assisting* them with the quitting process and *arranging* follow-up to prevent relapse. Intensive interventions, more effective than brief ones, can be further adopted with any smokers willing to make a quit attempt. Patients not ready to quit may be motivated to make a quit attempt by employing the "Five R's" approach. Dental professionals can encourage their patients to identify reasons why quitting is personally *relevant* and the oral health *risks* of tobacco use; dental professionals can also *rewards* that patients can experience from quitting and help the patients to identify *roadblocks* to quitting. All patients attempting to quit should also be encouraged to use the pharmacotherapy agents.

---

[*]   Dipartimento di Scienze Stomatologiche, Università di Palermo; Via del Vespro 129; 90127 Palermo, Italy; phone: +39-091-6552231 fax: +39-091-6552203; email: giuseppepizzo@unipa.it ; secondary email: giuseppepizzo@odonto.unipa.it

The "Stages of Change" model may be helpful to assist the clinician in assessing readiness to make a quit attempt. Tobacco users are categorised as belonging at any one time to one of five stages: Pre-contemplation (not thinking about stopping); Contemplation stopping; Preparing to stop; Action-making a quit attempt; Maintaining abstinence or relapsing. The intention is to help tobacco users move through the stages by using different interventions at different stages.

Growing evidence supports the efficacy of smoking cessation counselling by oral health professionals. Dentists and dental hygienists, therefore, should be trained on smoking cessation counselling and dental offices should incorporate this service into routine patient care. While the approach to smoking intervention provides a useful framework from which to begin, special considerations need to be given when treating various categories of tobacco users such as smokeless tobacco users, adolescents and women.

1. TOBACCO AND ORAL HEALTH

Tobacco Users Worldwide

Tobacco-use, specifically smoked tobacco, is the leading preventable cause of premature morbidity and mortality worldwide. Because of tobacco's diffusion into both industrialized and developing countries, tobacco-use represents a profound global public health problem [1, 2]. Recent United States (U.S.) surveys estimate around 46 millions, or almost 21.6% of adults, smoke cigarettes. Cigarette smoking is the most widely used and dangerous of the tobacco products available with an additional 10 million Americans smoking cigars and 12 million use smokeless tobacco. Adult smoking rates world-wide are estimated at 27% in the United Kingdom (UK), 38% in Australia, and 63% in China. Across the European Union (EU), the prevalence of smoking among adults varies considerably and ranges from 17% in Sweden to 45% in Greece, with an average of 29% [1, 3, 4].

As a direct result of the widespread use of tobacco globally, approximately five million people will die each year of tobacco-related diseases with more than 440,000 of these being U.S. adults. Sadly, this number will double within the year 2020 without aggressive preventive community interventions. By the year 2030, the World Health Organization (WHO) estimates that tobacco-use will be the primary important cause of preventable death worldwide with 70% of deaths occurring in developing countries among people aged 35-69 years [1-3]. The increase of educational programs and activities aimed at tobacco cessation, taxes on tobacco products, policy and legislative efforts, prevention programs in schools and interventions providing community tobacco cessations strategies, have contributed over the past several years in the decline of tobacco use among adults in U.S., Canada, Australia, and Europe. However, only 5% of the world's population is covered by comprehensive smoke-free laws and the state of global tobacco control implementation of effective measures is just at beginning [4-7].

Tobacco-use in any form, both smoked and smokeless, has the potential to cause systemic and oral diseases which are summarized in table 1 [8]. It has been estimated that tobacco-use causes 35% of all cancers, 33% of all heart strokes, and 90% of chronic obstructive pulmonary disease, including emphysema. Moreover, an estimated 38,000 U.S. adults die each year from secondhand smoke related diseases (lung cancer cardiovascular diseases). Children with one or both parents who smoke in the home or car, have a higher incidences of pulmonary diseases [8-10].

Table 1. Tobacco-related Systemic Diseases

Cancer Lung, mouth, esophagus, pharynx, larynx, pancreas, breast, stomach, uterine and bladder, cervical, kidney, leukemia
Chronic obstructive pulmonary and other respiratory diseases Chronic bronchitis and emphysema, pneumonia
Cardiovascular diseases Coronary and peripheral arterial diseases
Complications of pregnancy Intrauterine growth retardation, low birth weight and preterm birth babies, miscarriage, sudden infant death syndrome and early menopause
Other effects Impotence, peptic ulceration, facial wrinkling, cataracts, hip fractures, low bone density

Adverse Oral Health Effects of Tobacco Use

Tobacco, when is smoked, produces and releases a combination of hundreds of potentially toxic chemicals, including carbon monoxide, tar, free radicals, nicotine (a psychoactive drug that induce dependence), nitrosamines (potent carcinogens, the principal of which is benzopyrene), and oxidant gases [11-13].

The toxins contained in tobacco smoke as well as the release of tobacco specific nitrosamines, nicotine and other toxins in smokeless tobacco, produce numerous adverse effects on not only general health but the development of oral diseases due to both local and systemic exposure of chemicals.

The damaging effects of smoked tobacco (cigarettes, cigars, pipes, hookahs) on oral health are well recognized, which the major of them are summarized in table 2 [3, 11, 14].

A substantial number of studies have indicated smoking cigarettes poses a significant risk factor for the development and progression of periodontitis with an overall estimated 50% of periodontitis attributable to current and past cigarette smoking. It has been shown that the degree and severity of periodontitis is directly related to the number of cigarettes smoked daily and the number of years the patient has smoked. Moreover, cigarette smoking was strongly and consistently associated with a dose-dependent increase in the risk for incident tooth loss. Smokers are three to six times more likely than non-smokers to develop periodontitis, whereas localized gingival recession is primarily associated with smokeless tobacco use [15-17]. The mechanism by which tobacco products may influence the development and progression of periodontitis may include alteration of microbial composition of plaque, impairment of immune and inflammatory response to the plaque, and alteration of the healing processes [11, 16, 18].

Table 2. Tobacco-related Oral Diseases and Conditions

Periodontal disease, gingival recession
Reduction of response to periodontal therapy
Oral, pharyngeal and esophageal cancers
Pre-cancerous lesions (leucoplakia, erythroplakia, dysplasia)
Delayed wound healing after oral surgery
Failure of osseointegration of dental implants, peri-implantitis
Hairy brown tongue
Nicotine stomatitis
Halitosis, xerostomia
Discoloration of teeth
Altered sense of smell and taste

As oral tissues are exposed to several carcinogens found in smoked tobacco, the risk for oral cancer is very high, especially if it is combined with the consumption of alcohol. Oral cancer and precancerous lesions occur much more frequently among smokers than among non-smokers with 5-25% of precancerous lesions going on become dysplastic or invasive carcinoma and approximately 70% of oral cancers are associated with smoking. Smokeless tobacco use significantly increases the risk for oral, pharyngeal and esophageal cancers, and other oral precancerous lesions, such as Snuff dipper's pouch [3, 19].

Many other oral diseases and conditions are directly related to and aggravated by smoking, such as nicotine stomatitis (smoker's palate), necrotizing ulcerative gingivitis, halitosis, failure of osseointegration of dental implants, discoloration of teeth, altered sense of smell and taste, hairy brown tongue, delayed wound healing after oral surgery. Therefore, it is important to stress to the patient how important tobacco cessation is in the promotion of a general health and oral health [8, 14].

2. TOBACCO CESSATION INTERVENTIONS

Brief Clinical Intervention

People who use tobacco on a regular basis often develop not so much a 'bad habit' but rather 1) chemical dependence 2) daily habitual rituals 3) use in a social context which supports their tobacco use. Health professionals can and should play a key role in treating this chronic relapsing disease and thus be a part of reducing the number of tobacco-related deaths and related diseases. Tobacco cessation interventions are the most important, cost-effective, preventive maintenance that health professionals can offer to all their patients [20-23].

In developed countries, approximately 70% want to quit and 30-40% of smokers make a quit attempt in any year with an average of two to four quit attempts made before they are successful [3]. In many western countries, at least 70% of smokers consult a physician each year with more visiting a dental office than their physician. Brief advice and encouragement to quit offered at each visit from oral health care professionals can substantially increase cessation rates from 3-5% on their own to 10-15% with a brief intervention [24-31]. Therefore, all oral health care providers have the potential to have a profound impact on tobacco morbidity and mortality by offering cessation interventions on all patients who use tobacco [3, 18, 22, 23, 32-34].

A Brief Intervention

The United States Public Health Service (PHS), in collaboration with numerous experts in the tobacco cessation field, developed guidelines for clinicians to use when providing cessation interventions. The evidence-based interventions recommended the use of a system that included the 5A's (ask, advise, assess, assist arrange) to help people in their quit attempt and the 5R's (relevance, advice, rewards, risks, repetition) for patients unwilling to quit [20].

A brief clinical intervention should be incorporate into practice by every member of the dental team, offering every tobacco users a minimum of 3-4 counseling sessions of 3-5 minutes of time each [20]. Several studies reported that brief advice on smoking cessation given by a dentist or a dental hygienist at every appointment resulted in smoking cessation rate of about 5-12% [25]. Though the percent of a long term successful quit is low due to the highly addictive nature of nicotine, this kind of strategic approach is able to reach a large number of people and thus decrease the long-term prevalence of morbidity and mortality related to tobacco use [3].

Tobacco cessation interventions should be individualized and account for the reasons the person uses tobacco, the environment in which the use occurs, availability of resources to quit and individual preferences on how to quit. The oral health professional should always remember that cessation can be very difficult to achieve, and is important to be patient and persistent when developing, implementing and providing each patient with an individual cessation intervention.

The use of the PHS guidelines, involves asking each patient about tobacco use, advising users to quit, assessing their willingness to make a quit attempt, assisting them with the quitting process and arranging follow-up to prevent relapse (figure 1) [20, 35, 36].

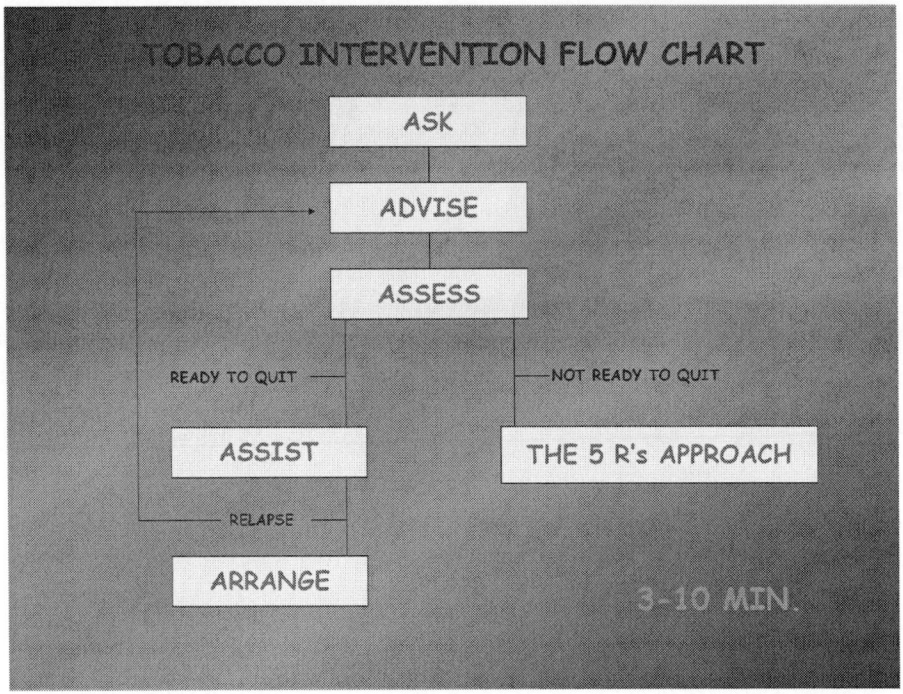

Figure 1.

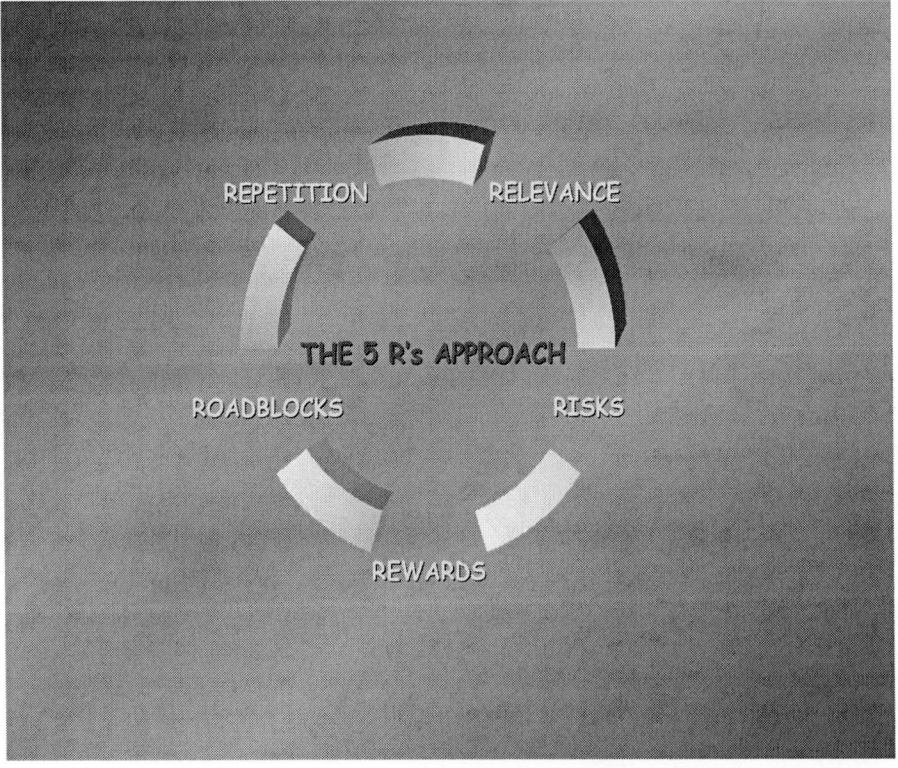

Figure 2.

The 5 A's

1. Ask

The first step in providing a tobacco intervention involves systemically identifying all tobacco users, at every visit, then documenting their patterns of consumption and history of use. It is important to ask every patient, using simple questions or by inclusion of these questions on a health history form, about their current smoking status (e.g., "Do you ever smoke or use any type of tobacco?"), considering it as one of the "vital signs". The smoking status might be asked at every following appointment and for those who have stopped in the past year. The health care provider should also determine the patient's attitude towards tobacco use to better understand his or her willingness to make a serious quit attempt. This can also be collected by specific questions on the health history form filled out at the initial visit and subsequent health history up-dates. This will institutionalize tobacco use information and prompt the clinician to inquire about the patient's use.

2. Advise

All tobacco users should be strongly advised to make a quit attempt. Advice given by healthcare providers should be clear (providing an unambiguous message to stop and remember the patient that the goal is a complete cessation of all forms of tobacco use), strong and direct (emphasize the importance and the benefits of quitting), and personalized (e.g., "I need you to know that quitting smoking is the most important thing you can do to protect your current and future health"). It is very important to relate the tobacco use to the patient's own current health or illness and his or her oral clinical situation, social and economic costs, and the impact of tobacco use on children and other members of his or her family.

Finally, the oral health care provider should take into account the patient's interest in stopping tobacco use. The patient's unwillingness in quitting, despite clinical advice, can be due to the fact that tobacco users are often uninformed about benefits of quitting or discouraged by previous episodes of relapses.

3. Assess

The third step of the protocol involves assessing the patient's motivation and interest to make a quit attempt within the next 30 days, by simple and clear questions (e.g., "Are you interest in making a quit attempt of tobacco use?"). It may be useful assessing patient's willingness to quit and their personal concerns surrounding their tobacco use before they are encouraged to make a quit attempt. It is thought there may be less resistance on the patient's part if they feel the clinician understands their situation and may encourage further thought of quitting. No one can make a tobacco user quit – they need to make the decision and do the difficult work to beat the addiction. Healthcare providers can encourage, support and provide resources in order to increase a successful quit attempt. Therefore a 'successful' intervention may mean helping someone consider quitting or getting more information or ultimately setting a quit date.

Dentists or dental hygienists have available an effective model to assess a tobacco user's readiness to change smoking behavior: the Transtheoretical Model ("Stages of Change" Model) [37]. It will be described in a subsequent section.

Moreover, it is essential to determine the patient's level of nicotine dependence which will assist the clinician in determining the level of intervention that will be needed for a specific patient. The Fagerström test for nicotine dependence (FTND) is the most widely used quantitative method to assess the degree of nicotine dependence (table 3), the severity of withdrawal symptoms, difficulty in achieving abstinence and possible relapse [38]. Although this test was designed for smokers, it can be adopted to all tobacco users [3].

If the patient is not ready to make a quit attempt, the members of dental team may provide a brief motivational intervention to increase the willingness of future attempts, and the interest in tobacco adverse effects as well as the benefits of quitting by utilizing the 5 R's – covered in the next section [20].

Table 3: FAGERSTRÖM TEST FOR NICOTINE DEPENDENCE

	Scoring			
	0	**1**	**2**	**3**
1. How soon after you wake up do you smoke your first cigarette?	More than 1 hour	31 to 60 minutes	6 to 30 minutes	5 minutes or less
2. Do you find it difficult to refrain from smoking in places where it is forbidden?	No	Yes		
3. Which cigarette would you most hate to give up?	Any other	First one in the morning		
4. How many cigarettes do you smoke per day?	Less than 10	11 to 20	21 to 30	More than 31
5. Do you smoke more frequently during the first hours after waking than during the rest of the day?	No	Yes		
6. Do you smoke when you are so ill that you are in bed most of the day?	No	Yes		

Scoring: 0-2 low; 3-4 medium; 5-6 high; 7-10 very high level of nicotine dependence.

4. Assist

The dentist or dental hygienist should support and assist all tobacco users ready to quit by formulating a quit plan. This might include assisting the patient to set a quit date preferably within the next 2 weeks. In addition to setting a quit date, encourage them to obtain external sources of social support and help from family, friends and coworkers, discuss nicotine withdrawal symptoms, and, if necessary, recommending and prescribing the use of pharmacotherapy (nicotine replacement therapy or non-nicotine replacement theory) [39]. All of these components are very important in order to increase the patient chance of successfully quitting.

The dental professional should make patients aware of how to anticipate life activities or 'cues' that may prompt them to smoke or use smokeless. Behavioral strategies, such as encouraging patients to remove tobacco products from his or her environment and plan alternative daily activities, will address habitual and social elements on a behavioral level. It is very important that the clinicians communicate, at every visit, the appreciation of patient's effort of the quit attempt, emphasizing that the most people find it difficult and need several attempts before succeeding.

If the patient is seriously motivated to quit, the health care provider may extend the Assist step by providing or referring for a more intensive clinical intervention, characterized by higher percent of success (15-25%) [40].

5. Arrange

The fifth and final step of the 5A's involves arranging a follow-up contact for all patients attempting to quit within the first week after the quit date. Moreover, a second appointment should be arranged again within the first month after the quit date as a follow-up. During the visits, members of dental team should congratulate the patient underling the positive outcomes (reduction or disappearance of cough, improvement of sense of taste and smell, reduction of halitosis and discoloration of teeth). If the patient indicates they have started using tobacco again, they should be remind that nicotine dependence is a chronic relapsing disease. It should be stressed that relapse is not a failure, but rather a learning experience and that most people require several attempts before succeeding.

During the initial period of tobacco abstinence and for up one year after the quit date, there is a high risk of relapse. So, it is important to provide a relapse preventive intervention by reinforcing patient's decision to quit, reminding him or her the benefits of cessation, and identifying possible problems arising form the process. But, if necessary, the oral health care provider should consider the possibility for the patient of an intensive clinical intervention.

The 5 R's for those Not Ready to Quit

The tobacco user not interest in quitting may lack information about the adverse health effects of tobacco use and benefits of quitting (such as improved health and financial savings), may be demoralized by previous episodes of relapses or enjoys the perceived 'benefits' of being able to concentrate, relaxation and calm as well as a weight reduction tool that nicotine induces biochemically when used [20, 35, 36, 41].

1. Relevance

The first step clinicians should take is to encourage the patient to identify reasons why quitting would be personally important to them such as personal health concerns (uncontrolled periodontitis, leukoplakia), or the health effects of secondhand smoke to children and family members.

2. Risks

Oral health care providers should encourage the patient to identify potential short or long-term negative health effects of tobacco use that are important to them. Moreover, patients should be given information on the oral health risks of tobacco use. An appropriate pamphlet could be given to the patient at the end of the appointment to reinforce the cessation intervention and continue to provide pertinent information.

3. Rewards

It is very important to allow the patient to identify the potential rewards or benefits of quitting. Members of dental team can highlight rewards that seem most relevant to the patient (e.g., improved health, sense of taste and smell, saving money, feeling better about self, setting a good example for children, feeling better physically, performing better in physical activities, reduced wrinkling aging of skin).

4. Roadblocks

In the following phase, attention might be focused on the identification of potential barriers that may compromise the success of a quit attempt. Talking about these obstacles can help dental team in increasing patient's motivation to tobacco use cessation. Typical barriers may include: withdrawal symptoms, fear of failure, weight gain, lack of support, depression, enjoyment of tobacco.

5. Repetition

It is extremely important that the clinician repeat the motivational intervention at every office visit, remembering that most people try to quit several times before reaching the goal. A note of the tobacco intervention should be made in the chart in order to remind the clinician to ask about current tobacco use as well as reinforce previous information provided.

The "Stages of Change" Model

An effective tobacco cessation intervention requires an assessing of a smoker's readiness to change behavior. The most widely model used to examine the process of behavior change and motivation is the Transtheoretical Model commonly known as "Stages of Changes" Model. This model helps health care providers understand the stages of behavioral changes among tobacco users and identify five stages of readiness to the smoking cessation process [37].

The "Stages of Change" Model involves five stages:

Precontemplation – not interested in quitting in the next six months
Contemplation – interested in quitting in the next six months but dose not set a quit date
Preparation for action – ready to quit in the next 30 days and sets a quit date
Action – has already quit in the past six months
Maintenance – successfully quit for more than a year – but may relapse at any time

The goal of utilizing this model is to help tobacco users move through the stages by using different interventions at different identified stages. As a part of the tobacco intervention, the stage of change should be noted in the patient's chart to ensure continuity of care [35-37, 40, 42, 43].

Precontemplation Stage

The patients in precontemplation are not aware that their tobacco use is a problem and have no intention of quitting tobacco use (changing behavior) in the next six months. Smokers in this stage overestimate the benefits of smoking, underestimate the risks and are not seriously interested in quit information. The aim of the health care provider is primary to increase the awareness of adverse effects of tobacco use by encouraging personal reflection using the 5Rs. It is important the patient does not feel pressured an subsequently discontinue interaction or change healthcare providers. The sense of trust and a supportive environment is paramount in offering appropriate long-term care.

Contemplation Stage

In the second stage of change, the patient recognizes that the risks of tobacco use outweigh the benefits and is seriously thinking about smoking cessation. He also expresses the intention to quit in the next six months. However the patient in contemplation is often indecisive to change their behavior and may stay in this stage for years. Therefore, the aim of the dental professional is to encourage the patient move towards considering an actual quit date by building on their perceived benefits to quitting and any negative health effects they are personally experiencing.

Preparation Stage

In this stage, the patient has made the decision to quit tobacco within the month. Often, tobacco users at this stage have previously attempted to quit, but without success. Clinicians should work with the patient to develop a patient centered quit plan that you and the patient develop together. These motivational interventions include focusing on pharmacotherapies, specific quit information, utilizing a phone quitline or online resources, developing behavior modification skills, emphasizing the benefits of being tobacco free, encouraging the patient to receive an extra-treatment social support by family and friends, and setting a quit date.

Action Stage

In this stage, the tobacco user has already quit and been abstinent for at least six months. As a chronic relapsing disease, nicotine dependence is a very difficult addiction to beat. The possibility of relapse is ever present for former tobacco users. Therefore, support should be offered to manage withdrawal symptoms, weight gain, and negative moods experienced as a result of the quitting process, and to prevent relapse. In fact, this is the most frequent stage for relapse, which can occur mainly during the first 2 to 3 weeks. Therefore, it is important to provide support and make suggestions for relapse prevention. The dental professional should maintain frequent contact with the patient, encouraging their success and offering support and strategies to remain tobacco free.

Maintenance Stage

This is the stage in which the tobacco user had maintained tobacco free for six continuous months. Although users have achieved a successful behavior change, they may be at risk of relapse and can cycle through the stages on average of 3 to 4 times before maintaining a successful quit. Therefore, continued efforts should be made to prevent future relapse even with patients who have been quit for many years.

Intensive Clinical Intervention

There is substantial evidence that demonstrates higher abstinence rates (15-25%) with an intensive clinical intervention than a brief intervention [40]. This kind of intervention consists in 4-6 sessions of personalized counseling of about 10-15 minutes of intervention at each visit. The overall duration of the intensive clinical intervention might be distributed over 4-6 weeks [20]. A personalized quit plan can be developed with the patient and used as a map for a successful quit. There are four types of counseling and behavioral therapies that may be included in smoking cessation interventions [3, 20].

1. Provide practical counseling and problem solving and skill training: In this phase it is the patient should be encouraged to adhere to total abstinence. The personalized quit plan should include the development of patient specific strategies on how to address withdrawal symptoms by identifying and anticipate high risk situations, suggesting simple resistance strategies such as keeping busy, changing routines associated with tobacco use and dedicate more time for hobbies. Discussion on healthy eating habits, exercise and adequate water intake will also help address withdrawal and cravings that occur during the quit process for many tobacco users.

2. Provide intra-treatment social support: the patient should be encouraging in hi or her quit attempt at each visit as well encouragement to use phone quitlines and online quit support programs. These have been show to increase quit attempts for those who use them.

3. Help patients to obtain extra-treatment social support for the quit attempt by involving family and friends. A smoke-free home environment should be encouraged, especially if a family member is continuing to smoke.

4. Discuss and prescribe appropriate pharmacotherapy: though pharmacotherapy available for tobacco cessation is safe and effective, many tobacco users do not know how to properly utilize the products often resulting in the discontinuance of use. Patients should be carefully monitored and doses adjusted as treatment proceeds.

3. THE ROLE OF ORAL HEALTH PROFESSIONALS

Evidences suggest that oral health professionals (e.g., dentist and dental hygienist) have the opportunity to reduce the prevalence of tobacco use among their patients and to promote awareness of tobacco-related oral conditions and diseases [25, 30, 31, 34, 44]. The dental team, has in fact, the opportunity to provide tobacco cessation counseling to a large proportion of tobacco users since many visit a dental office annually for conditions such as halitosis, discoloration of teeth, altered sense of taste, which may be directly related to tobacco use. When patient's bring-up their concern of halitosis, discolorations of teeth, periodontal disease, oral cancer, the members of dental team can use this 'teachable moment' to provide an effective brief clinical counseling highlighting the negative impact of their tobacco use in the mouth [29, 32, 33, 35, 36, 45-47].

Though dental professionals are ideally placed to promote tobacco cessation interventions, many practitioners still do not offer this potentially life-saving service [44, 48-53]. Disappointingly, only 30-50% of U.S. dentists and 25% of dental hygienists routinely ask their patients about tobacco use and advice them to quit. Only 24% assess patient's willingness to make a quit attempt, and less than 5% assist them in the quitting process [29, 41, 42, 54]. Some studies report that almost 89% of dentists think they should promote tobacco cessation, but fever than 10% reported that they had adequate knowledge of tobacco cessation techniques. In fact, many members of dental team report that they lack the knowledge and training to provide a comprehensive intervention [33, 41, 44, 50, 54]. Moreover, they fear patients will leave their dental practice or cause discord in the dentist/dental hygienist-patient relationship if tobacco cessation is provided. Others fundamental barriers limiting involvement in smoking cessation include perceived lack of relevance of smoking cessation to dentistry, and organizational factors within the practice setting [33, 36, 53, 55].

Because of these barriers, it is important to introduce systematic tobacco cessation training in dental and dental hygiene school undergraduate curricula as a standard for practice didactic and clinical tobacco use assessment. The assessment should target both knowledge base of the public health impact of tobacco use and the necessary skills for behavioral change counseling and communication [34, 41, 42, 56, 57, 58]. Collected data by the Global Health Professionals Survey (GHPS) on tobacco use and cessation counseling among health professional students estimate that 87-99% of students believed they should promote smoking cessation with only 5-37% of them received training in how to conduct such interventions [22]. In the U.S., nearly half of dental schools include didactic training in tobacco cessation counseling with less than half of dental and dental hygiene schools providing practical clinical training [59, 60]. Because of the potential role in tobacco cessation interventions by the dental team, dental and dental hygiene schools should implement didactic and clinical training on tobacco cessation interventions [28, 34, 44, 58].

4. SPECIAL NEED PATIENTS

Smokeless Tobacco Users

Smokeless tobacco (ST) is tobacco that is not burned when used and is usually placed in the buccal mucosal area in the oral cavity. There are two main types of ST: oral snuff and chewing tobacco-also known as spit tobacco. In the U.S., ST has increased since the 1970's, especially the use of moist snuff among young males [61, 62]. Several epidemiological studies have found associations between ST use and negative oral health effects, due to the direct contact with the oral mucosa for prolonged periods of carcinogens delivered from ST. These effects include an increased risk for oral cancer, gingival recession, dental erosion and a potential for dental caries. ST use is also associated with risk factors for cardiovascular disease, such as elevated blood pressure and cholesterol levels [21, 63, 64].

Health professionals need to implement a protocol for the identification and treatment of ST users in their practice. Because of the evident oral health effects, the dental team has an ideal opportunity to identify ST users and provide a tobacco cessation intervention. There is documented evidence indicating that such interventions may increase tobacco abstinence rates in ST users, especially when the oral damage of ST is evident [30, 31, 45, 65]. Since pharmacotherapies have not been shown to affect long-term abstinence, multicomponent approaches, including telephone counselling, may also be used to help ST users to quit [34, 65].

All tobacco users, including ST users, should be routinely identified at each visit (Ask), encouraged to quit (Advise, Assess), and as with cigarette smokers, follow-up of the patients is essential (Assist, Arrange). Members of dental team, moreover, should inform the patient of the oral health risks in order to motivate them to quit (5R's), and include information about smoking, as many ST users also smoke cigarettes. For those ST users ready to quit, clinicians should help the patient develop an individualized quit plan utilizing behavioral change techniques and available resources [30, 45, 66]. If a basic intervention is inadequate for the level of addiction, the clinician can refer to an outside resource that provides nicotine dependence counseling or seek more advanced training themselves in order to provide more intensive care.

Adolescents

Despite the major gain made to reduce smoking among adults, tobacco use remains highly prevalent in the youth population [67].

It is estimated that almost 3 million adolescents in the world use tobacco and nearly 17% of youth started smoking before age 18. The 2006 U.S. National Youth Tobacco Survey reports that 23% of high school students are current smokers, and it has been estimated that every day approximately 4,000 American adolescents try a tobacco product for the first time. Similarly, ST users often begin using smokeless tobacco in their youth. A recent U.S. National Survey (2006) found that ST was the third most prevalent form of tobacco ever used among adolescents and young adults (8.2%) [62, 68, 69]. Numerous factors may determine the use of tobacco by adolescence such as family behavior (e.g., parents who smoke or do not smoke), cultural, religious (U.S. American Indians and ceremonial use *vs* habitual use), school norms, the availability of tobacco products, and community tobacco control strategies creating a tobacco-free environment [5, 67, 70, 71].

It is very important to stress how critical is to encourage the prevention of tobacco use as well as offering cessation services among young people to reduce tobacco-related diseases. In fact, frequently adolescents often underestimate their risk of tobacco-related diseases and overestimate the easy of make a quit attempt in the future their ability to quit. Moreover, research shows that brief interventions by clinicians can effectively impact on the use of tobacco by youth [67, 72-75].

Women

It is estimated that rates of smoking in women have actually increased in several countries with almost 22% in developed countries, and almost 9% in developing countries. Moreover, exposure to tobacco smoke seems to pose an increase risk of disease in women as compared to men. In fact, women who use tobacco in any form have twice the risk of cardiovascular diseases and lung cancer than men as well as an increased risk of breast cancer, an increased risk of colorectal cancer mortality, greater variability of menstrual cycle length, and in reaching early menopause [76-79].

Unfortunately, many women are not aware of the health risks of smoking cigarettes during prenatal and postnatal periods to the fetus of pregnant women and themselves and continue to smoke during their pregnancy [76-78]. Several studies have suggested that smoking during pregnancy increases the risk of low birth weight, miscarriage, and sudden infant death syndrome [8, 20].

The rates of smoking cessation before and during pregnancy are low. Between 9% and 45% of women report stopping smoking on their own in preparation for pregnancy or quit after they know they are pregnant. These women are more likely to have support and encouragement at home for quitting or to have stronger belief about the dangerous effects of smoking on their unborn child's health. Moreover an additional 6% of women who are still smoking during pregnancy and are in precontemplation or contemplation stage may be receptive to an effective intervention delivered as part of prenatal care. However, similar survey data also suggest that most women who stop during pregnancy return to smoking after they have given birth. Between 50% and 80% return to smoking in the first year after delivery. This is much higher than would be predicted by the relapse rates of people who have been quit continuously for more than 6 months. A possible explanation for the high quit rate and high relapse rate might be because pregnant women often stop for the sake of their fetus and subsequently relapse due to post partum depression, stress of a new child and cravings related to previous tobacco use [80]. Therefore, health providers, including members of the dental team, should offer an effective tobacco cessation intervention before or during pregnancy to increase motivation to quit and reduce risks of smoking to the fetus. Health providers should also encouraging pregnant patients to continue in abstain after the delivery and information on how to reduce the potential for relapse.

Oral health care provider advice and encouragement to quit is very effective with this population and has been found that a brief clinical intervention improves smoking cessation rates and smoking abstinence up to 1 year postpartum. Moreover, since women present for more dental office visits than males, female patients are more accessible to the oral health provider tobacco intervention message, and gender specific strategies may be most successful [78, 81].

REFERENCES

[1]   Centers for Disease Control and Prevention (CDC). Cigarette smoking among adults-United States, 2003. *MMRW Morb Mortal Wkly Rep.* 2007;56:1157-1161.

[2]   World Health Organization (WHO). Why is tobacco a public health priority? Geneva: WHO, 2005. Available at: http://www.who.int/tobacco/health_priority/en/index.html. Accessed May 26, 2008.

[3]   Warnakulasuriya S, Sutherland G, Scully C. Tobacco, oral cancer, and treatment of dependence. *Oral. Oncol.* 2005;41:244-260.

[4]   Joossens L. Effective tobacco control policies in 28 European countries. European Network for Smoking Prevention, 2004. Available at: http://www.ensp.org/ publications/ enspreports. Accessed May 26, 2008.

[5]   Aquilino ML, Lowe JB. Approaches to tobacco control: the evidence base. *Eur. J. Dent. Educ.* 2004;8:11-17.

[6]   Watt RG, Benzian H, Binnie V, Gafner C, Hovius TJ, Mecklenburg RE. Public health
        aspects of tobacco control: setting the agenda for action by oral health professions
        across Europe. *Oral Health Prev. Dent.* 2006;4:19-26.

[7]   World Health Organization (WHO). WHO report on global tobacco epidemic. The
        MPOWER   package.   Geneva: WHO,   2005.   Available   at:
        http://www.who.int/tobacco/mpower/en/. Accessed May 26, 2008.

[8]   Centers for Disease Control and Prevention (CDC). 2004 Surgeon General's Report—
        The health consequences of smoking. Rockville: CDC, 2004. Available at:
        http://www.cdc.gov/tobacco/data_statistics/sgr/sgr_2004/index.htm. Accessed May 26,
        2008.

[9]   American   Lung   Association.   Tobacco   use.   Available   at:
        http://www.lungusa.org/site/c.dvLUK9O0E/b.4061173/apps/s/content.asp?ct=5328919.
        Accessed May 26, 2008.

[10]   Centers for Disease Control and Prevention (CDC). 2006 Surgeon General's Report—
        The health consequences of involuntary exposure to tobacco smoke. Rockville: CDC,
        2006. Available at: http://www.cdc.gov/tobacco/data_statistics/sgr/sgr_2006/index.htm.
        Accessed May 26, 2008.

[11]   Fried J. Tobacco cessation. In: Darby ML, Walsh MM, Eds. Theory and practice. 2nd
        ed. St. Louis: Saunders, 2003:589-603.

[12]   Green CR, Rodgman A. The Tobacco Chemists' Research Conference; a half-century
        of advances in analytical methodology of tobacco and its products. *Recent. Adv. Tob.
        Sci.* 1996; 22:131-304.

[13]   Hoffmann D, Hoffmann I. The changing cigarette, 1950-1995. *J. Toxicol. Environ.
        Health*. 1997; 50:307-364.

[14]   Davis JM. Tobacco cessation for the dental team: a practical guide. Part I: Background
        and overview. *J. Dent. Contemp. Dent. Pract.* 2005;6:1-6.

[15]   Tomar S, Asma S. Smoking-attributable periodontitis is the United States: findings
        from NHANES III. *J. Periodontol.* 2000;71:743-51.

[16]   Johnson GK, Hil M. Cigarette smoking and periodontal patient. *J. Periodontol.*
        2004;75:196-209.

[17]   Tomar SL. Smoking increases the incidence of tooth loss and smoking cessation
        reduces it. *J. Evid Base Dent. Pract.* 2008;8:105-107.

[18]   Hilgers KK, Kinane DF. Smoking, periodontal disease and the role of the dental
        profession. *Int. J. Dent. Hygiene.* 2004;2:56-63.

[19]   Neville BW, Day TA. Oral cancer and precancerous lesions. *CA Cancer J. Clin.*
        2002;52:195-215.

[20]   Fiore MC, Bailey WC, Cohen SJ, et al. Treating tobacco use and dependence. Clinical
        Practice Guideline. Rockville, MD: U.S. Department of Health and Human Services.
        Public   Health   Service.   June   2000.   Available   at: http://surgeongeneral.gov/
        tobacco/treating_tobacco_use.pdf. Accessed May 26, 2008.

[21]   Anczak J, Nogler RA. Tobacco cessation in primary care: maximizing intervention
        strategies. *Clin. Med. Res.* 2003;1:201-216.

[22]   Centers for Disease Control and Prevention (CDC). Tobacco use and cessation
        counseling--global health professionals survey pilot study, 10 countries, 2005. *MMWR
        Morb. Mortal. Wkly. Rep.* 2005;54:505-509.

[23] Gorin SS, Heck JJ. Meta-analysis of the efficacy of tobacco counselling by health care providers. *Cancer Epidemiol. Biomarkers Prev.* 2004;13:2012-2022.

[24] Gordon JS, Andrews JA, Crews KM, Payne TJ, Severson HH. The 5A's vs 3A's plus proactive quitline referral in private practice dental offices: preliminary results. Tob. Control. 2007;16:285-288.

[25] Warnakulasuriya S. Effectiveness of tobacco counseling in the dental office. *J. Dent. Educ.* 2002; 66:1079-1087.

[26] Brothwell DJ. Should the use of smoking cessation products be promoted by dental offices? An evidence-based report. *J. Can. Dent. Assoc.* 2001;67:149-154.

[27] Gansky SA, Eleison JA, Kavanagh C, Hilton JF, Walsh MM. Oral screening and brief spit tobacco cessation counseling: a review and findings. *J. Dent. Educ.* 2002; 66: 1088-1098.

[28] Gelskey SC. Impact of a dental/dental hygiene tobacco-use cessation curriculum on practice. *J. Dent. Educ.* 2002; 66: 1074-1078.

[29] Johnson NW. The role of the dental team in tobacco cessation. *Eur. J. Dent. Educ.* 2004;8:18-24.

[30] Carr AB, Ebbert JO. Interventions for tobacco cessation in the dental setting. *Cochrane Database Syst. Rev.* 2006;1:CD005084.

[31] Carr AB, Ebbert JO. Interventions for tobacco cessation in the dental setting. A systematic review. *Community Dent. Health* 2007;24:70-74.

[32] Gordon JS, Lichtenstein E, Severson HH, Andrews JA. Tobacco cessation in dental settings: research findings and future directions. *Drug Alcohol Rev.* 2006;25:27-37.

[33] Needleman I, Warnakulasuriya S, Sutherland G, Bornstein MM, Casals E, Dietrich T, Suvan J. Evaluation of tobacco use cessation (TUC) counselling in the dental office. *Oral Health Prev. Dent.* 2006;4:27-47.

[34] Ranney L, Melvin C, Lux L, McClain E, Morgan L, Lohr KN. Tobacco use: prevention, cessation, and control. *Evid. Rep. Technol. Assess.* 2006;140:1-120.

[35] Davis JM. Tobacco cessation for the Dental Team: A Practical Guide. Part II: Evidence-based Interventions. *J. Contemp. Dent. Pract.* 2005;6:1-11.

[36] Walsh MM, Ellison JA. Treatment of tobacco use and dependence: the role of the dental professional. *J. Dent. Educ.* 2005;69:521-537.

[37] Prochaska JO, DiClemente CC. Stages of change in the modification of problem behaviours. In: Hersen M, Eisler PM, Miller PM, editors. Progress on behaviour modification. Sycamore, IL: Sycamore Publishing; 1992: 27-76.

[38] Fagerström KO, Schneider NG. Measuring nicotine dependence; a review of the Fagerström Tolerance questionaire. *J. Behav. Med.* 1989;12:159-182.

[39] Pizzo G, Licata ME, Piscopo MR, Davis JM. *Pharmacotherapies for smoking cessation.* In: Jeffries TC. Progress in Smoking and Health Research. Happauge, NY: Nova Science Publishers, 2007:5-40.

[40] Lancaster T, Stead LF. Individual behavioural counselling for smoking cessation. *Cochrane Database Syst. Rev.* 2005;2:CD001292.

[41] Shaohua H, Pallonen U, McAlister AL, Howard B, Kaminski R, Stevenson G, Servos T. Knowing how to help tobacco users. Dentists' familiarity and compliance with the clinical practice guideline. *J. Am. Dent. Assoc.* 2006;137:170-179.

[42] Monson AL, Engeswick LM. Promotion of tobacco cessation through dental hygiene education: a pilot study. *J. Dent. Educ.* 2005; 69, 8:901-911.

[43] Rollnick S, Mason P, Butler C. Health behavior change - a guide for practitioners. Edinburgh: Churchill Livingstone, 1999

[44] Pizzo G, Piscopo MR, Pizzo I, Giuliana G. Smoking cessation counselling and dental team. *Ann. Ig.* 2006;18:155-170.

[45] John J. Tobacco cessation counselling interventions delivered by dental professionals may be effective in helping tobacco users to quit. Evid. Based Dent. 2006;7:40-1

[46] Hanioka T, Ojima M, Hamajima N, Naito M. Patient feedback as a motivating force to quit smoking. *Community Dent. Oral Epidemiol.* 2007;35:310-317.

[47] Parker DR. A dental hygienist's role in tobacco cessation. *Int. J. Dent. Hyg.* 2003;1:105-9.

[48] Albert D, Ward A, Ahluwalia K, Sadowsky D. Addressing tobacco in managed care: a survey of dentists' knowledge, attitudes, and behaviors. *Am. J. Public Health.* 2002;92:997-1001.

[49] Wyne AH, Chohan AN, Al Moneef MM. Attitudes of general dentists about smoking cessation and prevention in child and adolescent patients in Riyadh, Saudi Arabia. *J. Contemp. Dent. Pract.* 2006;7:1-8.

[50] John JH, Thomas D, Richards D. Smoking cessation interventions in the Oxford region: changes in dentists' attitudes and reported practices 1996-2001. *Br. Dent. J.* 2003;195:270-275.

[51] Albert DA, Severson H, Gordon J, Ward A, Andrews J, Sadowsky D. Tobacco attitudes, practices, and behaviors: a survey of dentists participating in managed care. *Nicotine Tob. Res.* 2005;7:S9-18.

[52] Cruz GD, Ostroff JS, Kumar JV, Gajendra S. Preventing and detecting oral cancer. Oral health care providers' readiness to provide health behavior counseling and oral cancer examinations. *J. Am. Dent. Assoc.* 2005;136:594-601.

[53] Dalia D, Palmer RM, Wilson RF. Management of smoking patients by specialist periodontists and hygienists in the United Kingdom. *J. Clin. Periodontol.* 2007;34:416-422.

[54] Albert DA, Ahluwalia KP, Ward A, Sadowsky D. The use of 'academic detailing! To promote tobacco-use cessation counseling in dental offices. *J. Am. Dent. Assoc.* 2004;135:1700-1706.

[55] Watt RG, McGlove P, Dykes J, Smith M. Barriers limiting dentists' active involvement in smoking cessation. *Oral Health Prev. Dent.* 2004;2:95-102.

[56] Ramseier CA, Mattheos N, Needleman I, Watt R, Wickholm S. Consensus Report: First European Workshop on tobacco use prevention and cessation for oral health professionals. *Oral Health Prev. Dent.* 2006;4:7-9.

[57] Wickholm S, McEwen A, Fried J, Janda M, Knevel R, Lädrach E, Persson L. Continuing education of tobacco use cessation (TUC) for dentists and dental hygienists. *Oral. Health. Prev. Dent.* 2006;4:61-70.

[58] Ramseier CA, Christen A, McGowan J, McCartan B, Minenna L, Öhrn K, Walter C. Tobacco use prevention and cessation in dental and dental hygiene undergraduate education. *Oral Health Prev. Dent.* 2006;4:49-60.

[59] Grinstead CL, Dolan TA. Trends in U.S. dental schools' curriculum content in tobacco use cessation 1989-93. *J. Dent. Educ.* 1994;58:663-667.

[60] Barker GJ, Williams KB. Tobacco use cessation activities in U.S. dental and dental hygiene student clinics. *J. Dent. Educ.* 1999;63:828-833.

[61]   Centers for Disease Control and Prevention. Use of smokeless tobacco among adults, United States, 1991. *MMWR Morb. Mortal. Wkly. Rep.* 1993;42:382.

[62]   Centers for Disease Control and Prevention (CDC). Tobacco use, access, and exposure to tobacco in media among middle and high school students - United States, 2004. *MMWR Morb. Mortal. Wkly. Rep.* 2005;54:297-301.

[63]   Rodu B, Jansson C. Smokeless tobacco and oral cancer: a review of the risks and determinants. *Crit. Rev. Oral. Biol. Med.* 2004;15:1252-263.

[64]   Fisher MA, Taylor GW, Tilashalski KR. Smokeless tobacco and severe active periodontal disease, NHANES III. *J. Dent. Res.* 2005;84:704-710.

[65]   Ebbert JO, Montori V, Vickers KS, Erwin PC, Dale LC, Stead LF. Interventions for smokeless tobacco use cessation. *Cochrane Database Syst. Rev.* 2007;4:CD004306.

[66]   West R, McNeill A, Raw M; Health Development Agency for England. Smokeless tobacco cessation guidelines for health professionals in England. *Br. Dent. J.* 2004;196:611-618.

[67]   Pizzo G, Licata ME, Davis J. Tobacco use by adolescents and young adults: oral health effects and cessation strategies. In: Lapointe MM, Ed. Adolescent smoking and health research. Hauppauge, NY: Nova Science Publishers, 2008:149-169.

[68]   Centers for Disease Control and Prevention (CDC). Cigarette use among high school students - United States, 1991-2005. *MMWR Morb. Mortal. Wkly. Rep.* 2006;55:724-726.

[69]   Marshall L, Schooley M, Ryan H, Cox P, Easton A, Healton C, et al. Youth Tobacco Surveillance - United States, 2001-2002. *MMWR Morb. Mortal. Wkly. Rep.* 2006;55:1-56.

[70]   The Global Youth Tobacco Survey Collaborative Group. Tobacco use among youth: a cross country comparison. *Tob. Control.* 2002;11:252-270.

[71]   Centers for Disease Control and Prevention (CDC). Use of cigarettes and other tobacco products among students aged 13-15 years - worldwide, 1999-2005. *MMWR Morb. Mortal. Wkly. Rep.* 2006;55:553-556.

[72]   Garg RH, Tandon S. Smoking habits of adolescents and the role of dentists. *J. Contemp. Dent. Pract.* 2006;7:1-7.

[73]   Shelley D, Cantrell J, Faulkner D, Haviland L, Healton C, Messeri P. Physician and dentist tobacco use counseling and adolescent smoking behavior: results from the 2000 National Youth Tobacco Survey. *Pediatrics.* 2005;115:719-725.

[74]   Albert DA, Severson HH, Andrews JA. Tobacco use by adolescents: the role of oral health professional in evidence-based cessation programs. *Pediatr. Dent.* 2006;28:177-187.

[75]   Grimshaw GM, Stanton A. Tobacco cessation interventions for young people. *Cochrane Database Syst. Rev.* 2006;4:CD003289

[76]   U.S. Department of Health and Human Services. Women and smoking: a report of the Surgeon General. Atlanta, GA: U.S. Department of Health and Human Services, Public Health Service, CDC, National Center for Chronic Disease Prevention and Health Promotion, Office on Smoking and Health; 2001. Available at: http://www.cdc.gov/tobacco/data_statistics/sgr/sgr_2001/index.htm. Accessed May 26, 2008.

[77]   Parkins KA. Smoking cessation in women. Special considerations. *CNS Drugs.* 2001;15:391-411.

[78] Fried JL. Women and tobacco: oral health issues. *J. Dent. Hyg.* 2000;74:49-55.

[79] Kenfield SA, Stampfer MJ, Rosner BA, Colditz GA. Smoking and smoking cessation in relation to mortality in women. *J. Am. Med. Assoc.* 2008;299:2037-2047.

[80] Lawrence T, Aveyard P, Cheng KK, Griffin C, Johnson C, Croghan E. Does stage-based smoking cessation advice in pregnancy result in long term quitters? 18-month postpartum follow-up of a randomized controlled trial. *Addiction.* 2005;100:107-116.

[81] Ershoff D, Quinn V, Boyd N, Stern J, Gregory M, Wirtschafter D. The Kaiser Permanente prenatal smoking-cessation trial: when more isn't better, what enough? *Am. J. Prev. Med.* 1999;17:161-168.

INDEX

B

E

F

H

J

K

N

S

T